BREAST CANCER

DIAGNOSIS & TREATMENT

Irving M. Ariel, M.D., F.A.C.S., M.S.

Professor of Clinical Surgery
New York Medical College
State University of New York at Stony Brook

Attending Surgeon
Long Island Jewish Hospital, New Hyde Park
Cabrini Medical Center, New York

Consultant Surgeon
Hospital for Joint Diseases and Orthopedic Institute
New York, New York

Joseph B. Cleary, M.D., F.I.C.S

Clinical Instructor in Surgery
New York Medical College, Valhalla, New York

Attending Surgeon, Doctors Hospital, New York

Staff Surgeon, Cabrini Medical Center, New York
and Westchester County Medical Center
Valhalla, New York

McGraw-Hill Book Company

New York St. Louis San Francisco Auckland Bogotá Hamburg Johannesburg
Lisbon London Madrid Mexico Milan Montreal New Delhi Panama Paris
San Juan São Paulo Singapore Sydney Tokyo Toronto

To all women who have suffered from breast cancer as exemplified by MARILYN FIXMAN (1928–1980), who died in the prime of life 15 years after a radical mastectomy. She personified femininity and loveliness and courageously helped candidates for mastectomy as a volunteer in "Reach for Recovery." She demonstrated that the time from the first diagnosis of breast cancer until death (if inevitable) could be productive and meaningful.

NOTICE

Medicine is an ever-changing science. As new research and clinical experience broaden our knowledge, changes in treatment and drug therapy are required. The editors and the publisher of this work have checked with sources believed to be reliable in their efforts to provide drug dosage schedules that are complete and in accord with the standards accepted at the time of publication. However, readers are advised to check the product information sheet included in the package of each drug they plan to administer to be certain that the information contained in these schedules is accurate and that changes have not been made in the recommended dose or in the contraindications for administration. This recommendation is of particular importance in connection with new or infrequently used drugs.

BREAST CANCER

1234567890 HALHAL 89876

ISBN 0-07-002190-2

This book was set in Times Roman by McGraw-Hill Information Systems and Technology; the editors were Robert E. McGrath, Thomas H. Kothman, and Mariapaz Ramos-Englis; the production supervisor was Thomas J. LoPinto. The cover was designed by Joe Cupani.
Arcata Graphics/Halliday was printer and binder.

Library of Congress Cataloging-in-Publication Data

Breast cancer.

Includes bibliographies and index.
1. Breast—Cancer. I. Ariel, Irving, M.
II. Cleary, Joseph B. (Joseph Brian), date
[DNLM: 1. Breast Neoplasms—diagnosis. 2 Breast
Neoplasms—therapy. WP 870 B8235]
RC280.B8B683 1986 616.99'449 86-20164
ISBN 0-07-002190-2

Contents

IV Detection and Diagnosis of Breast Cancer

V Treatment of Potentially Curable Breast Cancer

VI Treatment of Advanced Breast Cancer

Contributors

Martin D. Abeloff, M.D.
Associate Professor of Oncology and Medicine, The Johns Hopkins Oncology Center, The Johns Hopkins Hospital and Medical School, Baltimore, Maryland

Irving M. Ariel, M.D., F.A.C.S., M.S.
Professor of Clinical Surgery, New York Medical College and State University of New York at Stony Brook; Attending Surgeon, Long Island Jewish Hospital, New Hyde Park, Cabrini Medical Center, and Doctors Hospital, New York; Consultant Surgeon, Hospital for Joint Diseases and Orthopedic Institute, New York, New York

Oliver Beahrs, M.D.
Professor of Surgery, Emeritus, Mayo Medical School, Rochester, Minnesota

Maurice Black, M.D.
Director, Institute of Breast Diseases; Clinical Professor of Pathology, New York Medical Center and Westchester County Medical Center, Valhalla, New York

Arthur S. Caron, M.D.
Adjunct Attending Surgeon, Breast Service, Department of Surgery, Memorial Sloan-Kettering Cancer Center; Attending Surgeon, Doctors Hospital, New York, New York

Stephen K. Carter, M.D.
Senior Vice President, Anti-Cancer Research, Pharmaceutical Research and Development Division, Bristol-Myers Co., New York, New York

Angelo Cammarata, M.D., F.A.C.S., F.I.C.S.
Assistant Clinical Professor of Surgery, New York Medical College; Attending Surgeon, Breast Service, Cabrini Medical Center; Associate Attending Surgeon, Doctors Hospital and Metropolitan Hospital Medical Center, New York, New York

Florence Chu, M.D.
Associate Chairman, Department of Radiology, New York Hospital; Chief, Division of Radiology Oncology, Department of Radiology, New York Hospital; Consultant, Memorial Hospital for Cancer and Allied Diseases; Professor of Radiology, Cornell University Medical College, New York, New York

Joseph B. Cleary, M.D., F.I.C.S.
Clinical Instructor in Surgery, New York Medical College, Valhalla; Attending Surgeon, Doctors Hospital, New York; Staff Surgeon, Cabrini Medical Center, New York and Westchester County Medical Center, Valhalla, New York

Hiram S. Cody III, M.D.
Assistant Attending Surgeon, St. Lukes–Roosevelt Hospital Center; Instructor in Clinical Surgery, Columbia University College of Physicians and Surgeons, New York, New York

Andrew James Coldman, M.D.
Senior Statistician, Division of Epidemiology, Biometry, and Occupational Oncology, Cancer Control Agency of British Columbia, Vancouver, British Columbia, Canada

Robert Crichlow, M.D.
William and Bessie Allyn Professor of Surgery; Chairman, Department of Surgery, Dartmouth–Hitchcock Medical Center, Hanover, New Hampshire

Joseph P. Crowe, M.D.
Department of Surgery, Case Western Reserve University Hospital, Cleveland, Ohio

Leonid Deemarsky, M.D.†
Petrov Research Institute of Oncology, Leningrad, USSR

John M. Edwards, M.S., F.R.C.S.
Attending Surgeon, St. Thomas Hospital, London, England

Douglas B. Evans, M.D.
Resident in General Surgery, Dartmouth–Hitchcock Medical Center, Hanover, New Hampshire

Zvi Fuks, M.D.
Chairman, Department of Radiation Oncology, Memorial Sloan-Kettering Hospital, New York, New York

Francis J. Gillen, M.D.
Attending Surgeon, Plastic and Reconstructive Surgery, Doctors Hospital, New York, New York

Rita Girolamo, M.D.
Vice-Chairman of Radiology, Department of Radiology, New York Medical College, Valhalla, New York

James H. Goldie, M.D.
Head, Division of Medical Oncology, Cancer Control Agency of British Columbia; Clinical Professor of Medicine, University of British Columbia, Vancouver, British Columbia, Canada

William Goodson III, M.D., F.A.C.S.
Associate Professor of Surgery and Chief, Breast Screening Center, University of California Medical Center, San Francisco, California

Erza M. Greenspan, M.D.
Clinical Professor of Medicine (Oncology), The Mount Sinai School of Medicine; Attending Physician, Mount Sinai Hospital, New York, New York

†Deceased

James N. Ingle, M.D.
Consultant in Medical Oncology, The Mayo Clinic; Associate Professor of Oncology, Mayo Medical School, Rochester, Minnesota

Merrill Kies, M.D.
Associate Professor of Clinical Medicine, Medical Oncology Section, Northwestern University, Chicago, Illinois

Raymond D. LaRaja, M.D., F.A.C.S.
Associate Professor of Clinical Surgery, New York Medical College; Director of Surgery, Cabrini Medical Center; Attending Surgeon, VA Medical Center; Associate Attending Surgeon, Bellevue Medical Center, New York, New York

Henry Patrick Leis, Jr., M.D., F.A.C.S., F.I.C.S.
Clinical Professor of Surgery, Chief of the Breast Service, and Co-Director of the Institute of Breast Diseases at New York Medical College; Chief of Breast Surgery, Cabrini Medical Center, New York, New York; Clinical Professor of Surgery in Breast Surgical Oncology, University of South Carolina School of Medicine, Columbia, South Carolina

Gerson Lesnick, M.D.
Clinical Professor of Surgery, Emeritus, Mount Sinai School of Medicine (CUNY); Consultant Surgeon, Mount Sinai Hospital, New York, New York

Katherine Yue Yuin Li, M.D.
Professor and Head of the Department of Surgery, Shanghai First Medical College, Shanghai, Peoples Republic of China

Jane F. Lynch, B.S.N.
Instructor, Department of Preventive Medicine/Public Health, Creighton University School of Medicine and the Hereditary Cancer Institute, Omaha, Nebraska

Henry T. Lynch, M.D.
Professor and Chairman, Department of Preventive Medicine/Public Health and Professor of Medicine, Creighton University School of Medicine, Omaha, Nebraska

Andrea Manni, M.D.
Associate Professor of Medicine, Division of Endocrinology, The Milton S. Hershey Medical Center, The Pennsylvania State University, Hershey, Pennsylvania

Mohamed F. Manji, M.D.
Radiation Oncologist and Clinical Assistant Professor, University of British Columbia, Cancer Control Agency of British Columbia, Vancouver, British Columbia, Canada

Robert J. McKenna, M.D., F.A.C.S.
Clinical Professor of Surgery, University of Southern California School of Medicine, Wilshire Oncology Medical Group, Los Angeles, California

Curtis Mettlin, Ph.D.
Chief, Epidemiologic Research, Roswell Park Memorial Institute, Department of Health–New York State, Buffalo, New York

Michael P. Osborne, M.D., M.S., F.R.C.S., F.A.C.S.
Assistant Attending Surgeon, Department of Surgery, Memorial Sloan-Kettering Cancer Center; Associate Professor of Surgery, Cornell University Medical Center; Visiting Associate Physician, The Rockefeller University Hospital, and Adjunct Faculty Member, The Rockefeller University, New York, New York

Vincent R. Pennisi, M.D., D.D.S., F.A.C.S.
Clinical Associate Professor of Surgery (Plastic Surgery), University of California School of Medicine, St. Francis Memorial Hospital, San Francisco, California

Romulo Prudente, M.D.
Attending Pathologist, Department of Pathology, Doctors Hospital, New York, New York

Joseph Ragaz, M.D.
Medical Oncologist and Assistant Professor, University of British Columbia, Cancer Control Agency of British Columbia, Vancouver, British Columbia, Canada

Guy Robbins, M.D.
Consultant–Breast Service, Department of Surgery, Memorial Sloan-Kettering Cancer Center, New York, New York

Robert E. Rothenberg, M.D., F.A.C.S.
Clinical Professor of Surgery, New York Medical College; Director, Surgical Research, Cabrini Medical Center, New York, New York

Fernando A. Salinas, D.V.M.
Senior Research Scientist and Professor of Pathology, Faculty of Medicine, University of British Columbia; Senior Oncologist, Cancer Control Agency of British Columbia, Vancouver, British Columbia, Canada

Daniele Sarrazin, M.D.
Chief of the Breast Division, Department of Radiation–Oncology, Institüt Gustave Roussy, Villejuif, France

John H. Seashore, M.D.
Professor of Surgery and Pediatrics, Yale University School of Medicine, New Haven, Connecticut

V. R. Semiglazov, M.D.
Chief, Breast Tumors Department, Petrov Research Institute of Oncology, Leningrad, USSR

Joel H. Shaper, M.D.
Associate Professor of Oncology and Associate Professor of Pharmacology and Experimental Therapeutics, The Johns Hopkins Oncology Center, The Johns Hopkins Hospital and Medical School, Baltimore, Maryland

Zhen-Zhou Shen, M.D.
Lecturer in the Department of Surgery, Shanghai First Medical College, Shanghai, Peoples Republic of China

Richard V. Smalley, M.D.
Chief of Biological Resources Branch, Frederick, Maryland

Adrienne Snyderman, M.S.W.
Adjunct Instructor, UMDNJ–The Robert Wood Johnson Medical School; Consultant, The Comprehensive Breast Center, New Brunswick, New Jersey

Reuven K. Snyderman, M.D.
Professor and Chief, Section of Plastic and Reconstructive Surgery; Co-Director, The Comprehensive Breast Center, UMDNJ–The Robert Wood Johnson Medical School, New Brunswick, New Jersey

Phillip Strax, M.D.
Clinical Professor of Oncology, University of Miami School of Medicine, Miami, Florida; Associate Clinical Professor, Community and Preventive Medicine, New York Medical College, Valhalla, New York; Medical Director, Guttman Breast Diagnostic Institute, New York, and Strax Breast Cancer Detection Institute, Fort Lauderdale, Florida

Pin Kie Teng, M.D.
Director, Department of Pathology, Doctors Hospital, New York, New York

Mary Ann Tinker, M.D.
Associate Director of Surgery, Queens Hospital Center Affiliation of Long Island Jewish Medical Center; Assistant Professor of Surgery, State University of New York at Stony Brook; Staff Surgeon, Long Island Jewish Medical Center, Long Island, New York

Zelig A. Tochner, M.D.
Radiation Oncology Branch, National Cancer Institute, Bethesda, Maryland

Nicholas J. Toghia, J.D.
Partner, Acret and Perrochet, Lawyers, Los Angeles, California

Maurice Tubiana, M.D.
Department of Radiation Therapy, Institüt Gustave Roussy, Villejuif, France

Jerome A. Urban, M.D.
Consultant, Breast Service, Department of Surgery, Memorial Sloan-Kettering Hospital, New York, New York; Clinical Professor of Surgery, Cornell University Medical School; Attending Surgeon, Roosevelt Hospital and Doctors Hospital, New York, New York

T. Phillip Waalkes, M.D.
Professor of Oncology, The Johns Hopkins Oncology Center, The Johns Hopkins Hospital and Medical School, Baltimore, Maryland

Robert S. Weiss, Ph.D.
Professor of Sociology, University of Massachusetts, Boston, Massachusetts

Margery Wiesenthal
National Director of the American Cancer Society and National Coordinator of the Reach-to-Recovery Program, White Plains, New York

Richard E. Wilson, M.D.
Chief, Surgical Oncology, Brigham and Women's Hospital and Dana-Farber Cancer Institute; Professor of Surgery, Harvard Medical School, Boston, Massachusetts

Leslie Wise, M.D.
Chairman, Department of Surgery, Long Island Jewish Medical Center; Professor of Surgery, State University of New York at Stony Brook; Professor and Chairman, Department of Surgery, City University of New York Medical School, Long Island Jewish Medical Center, Long Island, New York

Ann J. Worth, M.D., F.R.C.P.
Director of Clinical Laboratories and Clinical Professor of Pathology, University of British Columbia, Cancer Control Agency of British Columbia, Vancouver, British Columbia, Canada

Reinhard E. Zachrau, M.D.
Co-Director, Institute of Breast Diseases, Associate Professor of Pathology, New York Medical College, Westchester County Medical Center, Valhalla, New York

Herman Zuckerman, M.D.
Assistant Clinical Professor of Radiology, Mount Sinai Hospital Medical School; Associate Radiologist, Beth Israel Hospital; Consultant, Roosevelt Hospital, New York, New York

Preface

A medical revolution had taken place in the management of patients with breast cancer. There was a change in the radical surgical approach which had been used for centuries. The radical mastectomy operation is now being replaced with less traumatic procedures. After conservative surgery, radiation therapy is strongly advocated as a means of destroying any residual cancer within the breast. The multiple disciplinary approach of treating breast cancer invited questions and speculations. The discoveries in chemotherapy, immunotherapy, endocrine therapy, etc., each play a role in the total treatment of the patient. There resulted an avalanche of studies from specialists advocating their own therapies. My approach was to present a current and true update regarding the indications, complications, and results for treating the different types and stages of breast cancer. A unified method for reporting end-results is presented so that the reader could decide what was the best method or combination of methods for various subsets of patients with cancer. It is the hope of this editor that the indications, techniques, complications, and end-results of each modality are objectively presented.

A review of the efforts made to cope with breast cancer in the past is developed in Chapter 1. The attitude of a physician evaluating a patient suspect or proved of having breast cancer is summarized in Chapter 2.

Since practically nothing is known about the exact etiology of breast cancer, a quest is necessary to discover which patients are at risk and which factors contribute to that risk. This subject is discussed in Chapter 3. Chapter 4 is devoted to the role of heredity in the etiology of breast cancer and Chapter 5 presents the physiologic and pathologic aspects of fibrocystic disease. Chapter 6 lists the criteria for the identification of high risk patients and the establishment of a special surveillance clinic for their monitoring.

Accurate and precise classification is mandatory and is presented in Chapter 7. At present there are about thirty different types of breast cancers which are based on pathologic criteria. The pathology of breast cancer is discussed in Chapter 8. The employment of relatively new chemical identifiers, the "hormone receptors," is discussed in Chapter 9. The body's mechanism is a most important factor in the efforts to control cancer and this is presented in Chapter 10.

Section IV discusses our present methods of detecting and diagnosing breast cancer. Chapter 11 presents the results of mammographic screening of many women and gives the number of cancer so diagnosed and their prognosis. Chapter 12 presents the effects of mammography in detecting, describing, and diagnosing breast cancer. Imaging techniques other than mammography as well as biologic markers that may give clues for the detection of breast cancer are presented in Chapters 13 and 14. Chapter 15 is devoted to the different techniques for obtaining a biopsy.

Section V presents various options open to the physician for "curing" a patient with breast cancer and covers Chapters 16 to 25.

The management of clinically nonpalpable breast cancer (although not early cancer) is presented in

Chapter 16. If the decision is made for local excision and radiotherapy, the indications and techniques of surgery are presented in Chapter 17, and the radiation factors and results in Chapter 18. The choice of operative procedures are then discussed. Chapter 19 discusses the role of modified mastectomy. Chapter 20 deals with the radical mastectomy, presenting the indications and accomplishments of each type of operation, while Chapter 21 covers extended radical mastectomy. Radiation therapy is discussed in some detail in Chapter 23.

The incidence, methods of treatment, and prognostic significance or regional recurrence are detailed in Chapter 24.

A philosophy is developing in that cytotoxic chemotherapy would be beneficial as the first line of attack and this is discussed in Chapter 25.

Chapter 26 deals with adjuvant cancer therapy, its beneficial results, indications, and complications.

The role of surgery that includes the incidents, prognostic significance, and results of surgical treatment of regional recurrences is discussed in Chapter 27. The role of hormone manipulation and cancer chemotherapy are presented in Chapters 28 and 29. The indications and accomplishments of radiation therapy as a palliative procedure are detailed in Chapter 30. The roles of interferon and other biologics in the management of advanced breast cancer are discussed in Chapter 31.

Rarely will a breast cancer grow to huge crippling proportions after exhausting all other forms of treatment and remain localized. In such instance interscapulomammothoracic amputation offers palliation and may even prolong life (Chapter 32).

An overview of accomplishments by the reconstructive surgeon is presented in Chapter 33.

Section VIII includes treatment of nipple disease and cancer (Chapter 34), inflammatory cancer (Chapter 35), and what one does with the opposite breast in a patient with cancer on one breast (Chapter 36). Breast disease in children is presented in Chapter 37.

Chapter 38 deals with the treatment of the pregnant woman who develops breast cancer during her pregnancy. Chapter 39 discusses the many unusual breast cancers, such as melanoma arising in the skin of the breast, or those rare cancers arising from the supporting structures. The rare development of cancer in the male breast is covered in Chapter 40.

Section IX represents a relatively new but well-deserved dimension in a medical book. It deals with the patient's reactions and rights. Chapters 41 and 42 discuss the emotional aspects of the patient, and Chapter 43 discusses a most worthwhile practice whereby women who had previously been subjected to a mastectomy come to the hospital to give solace to candidates for breast surgery.

The book closes with Chapter 45 that deals with the laws of different states to protect the patient against unscrupulous practices.

IMA

Acknowledgments

It is a pleasure to acknowledge our indebtedness to the many authorities whose notable contributions made this book possible.

The superior medical illustrations contribute greatly to the value of the text. We express our gratitude to each of the medical illustrators and to our own medical photographer, Mr. Harry Weissfishch. We join the other authors in acknowledging the generous cooperation of the many journals and publishers who freely permitted the use of graphic and statistical material; specific acknowledgments are given throughout the text.

Our research assistants, Ms. Maryanne Wagner, Ms. Ingegard Angerer, and Mr. Habib Hassouna have been most assiduous and competent in the gathering of statistical and referential data. Mrs. Pamela Bartle, our editorial associate, patiently typed complicated and sometimes unintelligible tapes into rough manuscripts from which the final copy was derived.

The following individuals and foundations have made basic contributions for this venture:

The Pack Medical Foundation
The Foundation for Clinical Research
The Janet K. Hetherington Fund
The Arnold and Muriel Rosen Cancer Fund
The Hudson Chapter of the Pack Medical Foundation, with special thanks to the late Rudolph J. DeAngelo
Mr. Ben Fixman
Mr. Everett Kouvler
Mr. Barry Epstein
Mr. Buddy Monarch

Finally we are most indebted to McGraw-Hill and especially to Mr. B.J. Clark, Mr. Robert E. McGrath, and Ms. Mariapaz R. Englis for their patience and industry in the preparation and production of this book.

Part One

Introduction

1

Breast Cancer A Historic Review: Is the Past Prologue?

Irving M. Ariel, M.D.

Let us not cast aside things that belong to the past, for only with the past can we weave the fabric of the future.

Anatole France

INTRODUCTION

Cancer of the breast is as ancient as medical history. The two major forces that have dominated the development of treatment policies are (1) the attitudes of women who suffer from cancer toward their breasts; and (2) developments in medical science, spurred on by medical pioneers.[59] This chapter will attempt to trace the development of treatment policies through the ages and explore how some present-day techniques have developed from ancient concepts and methods of treating breast cancer.[40]

It is a pleasure to acknowledge my great indebtedness for this brief historic review to many sources, especially to the erudite and comprehensive presentations of William A. Cooper,[19] Edward Lewison, David Schechter,[73] and the late George Degenshein;[22] and Bernice Sachs,[71] for her history of women's attitudes toward their breasts.

WOMEN'S ATTITUDES TOWARD THEIR BREASTS

How women perceive their breasts has been a dominant force through the ages. It determines the willingness or reluctance of women to lose their breasts, and the reluctance of surgeons to do that which women accept unwillingly. The female breasts have been acclaimed universally through the centuries as symbols of beauty.[87] In art, literature, theater, movies, television, and advertising, the female breasts are glorified. These modified sweat glands are defined in a mundane manner in Gray's *Anatomy* as follows:

> The mammae secrete the milk and are the accessory glands of the generative system.... In the female they are two large hemispherical eminences lying within the superficial fascia and situated on the front and sides of the chest; each extends from the second rib above to the sixth rib below, and from the side of the sternum to the mid-axillary line. Their weight and dimensions differ at different periods of life and in different individuals.[27]

These two hemispheres filled with adipose, glandular, and fibrous tissue have been the objects of constant medical debate regarding the treatment of the physiologic and pathologic changes that occur in them. In view of the attitudes, albeit often exaggerated, toward the female breast, is it any wonder that a woman with normal breasts except for the presence of an asymptomatic lump (and in some instances no lump, but a diagnosis made by mammographic examination) is loathe to have her breast amputated?[8,29] (Fig. 1-1.)

Historically, this is a complete turnabout. König, in 1893, wrote:

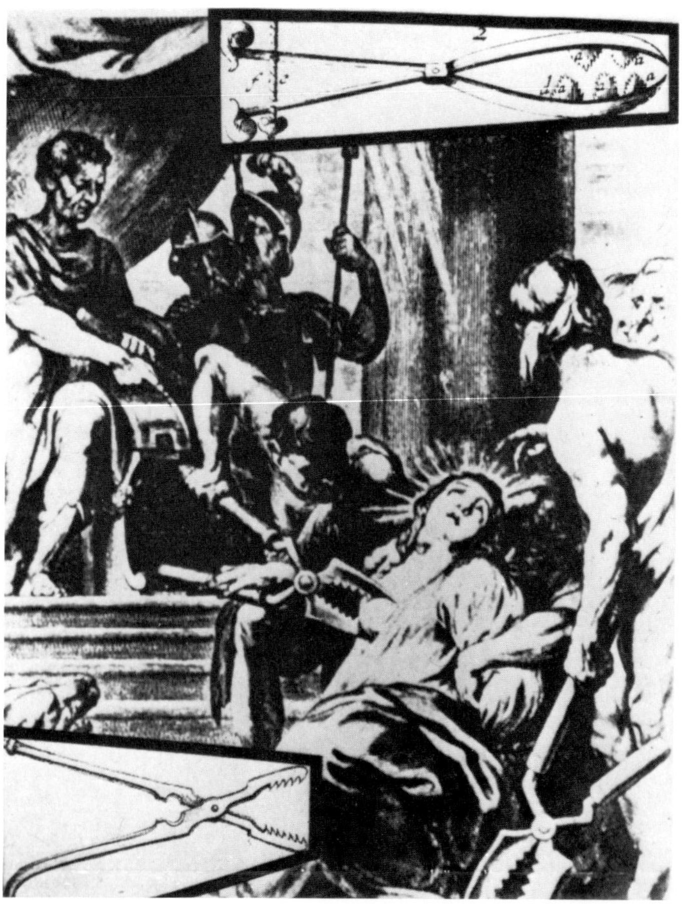

Figure 1-1 The martyrdom of St. Agatha by Anthony Van Dyck. The inserts: Top (from Scultetus) and bottom (from Milne) show the instruments used for removal of the breast as a means of torture, later developed to treat breast cancer.

> Before me I have fifteen preserved breasts of women from the past ten years. Most of them were taken from women who feared they had carcinoma. These women failed to calm down even after they had been told that their breasts were not cancerous but due to an infection (mastitis). . . .[43]

In these instances the women feared cancer more than they wanted to preserve their breasts, and underwent mastectomy at their own insistence. The situation has now changed in that many women believe that their breasts can be preserved in the presence of mammary cancer. This attitude, plus certain developments in medical circles, have influenced physicians to seek a means of curing the patient of her cancer and also preserve the afflicted breast. We must now consider if this approach is warranted.

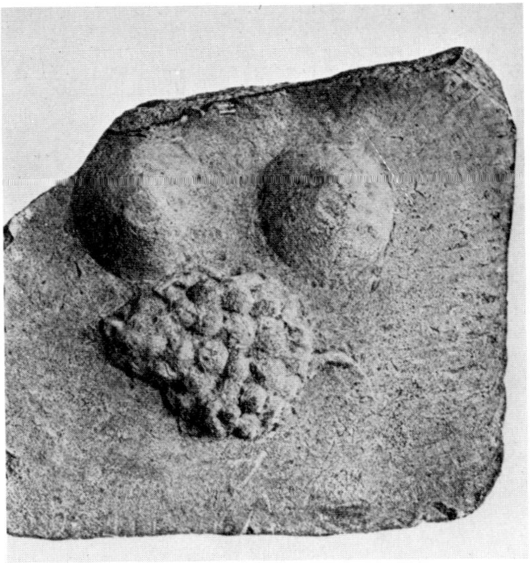

Figure 1-2 Votive offerings: Limestone slab found in the temple at Golgol, Cyprus (third to second century B.C.). A nodular tumor mass is beneath the two breasts. It is stated that this represents one of the earliest representation of "cancer" in art.

THE DEVELOPMENT OF MEDICAL SCIENCE IN THE TREATMENT OF BREAST CANCER

Breast cancer in the female is an ubiquitous disease which has been present from time immemorial and has killed many women all over the world. Generations of surgeons have boldly attempted every conceivable method of combating this disease. Through the ages there has been a gradual evolution in both the understanding of this form of cancer and in treatment methods.

Cancer has been with us from prehistoric times. Preserved relics, ancient bones, and paleopathologic remnants reveal that cancer is worldwide and afflicts all life, both plant and animal (Fig. 1-2). Dinosaurs of the Mesozoic period have shown signs of bone cancer. Cancer has been found in mummies from Egyptian pyramids, Etruscan tombs, and from Peru. A historic review of this disease and methods used to control it will help us understand better the enigma which confronts us today regarding the best treatment of breast cancer. As well, it will help prevent us from making the mistakes made in the past (Fig. 1-3).[12]

Ancient History

The Edwin Smith Surgical Papyrus

The very earliest medical record regarding medical history is the ancient Edwin Smith surgical papyrus (Fig. 1-4), covering a period of the Egyptian pyramid age (2nd millennium B.C.). Although we do not know the author, it is believed to represent teachings of the oldest known physician, Imhotep. J. H. Breasted, the late director of the Oriental Institute of the University of Chicago, who translated and made commentaries on this papyrus, states that the papyrus describes eight cases concerned with tumors of the breast:

> If you examine a man having bulging tumors on his breast, and you find that they have spread over his breast; and you place your hand upon his breast tumors and you find them to be cool, there being no

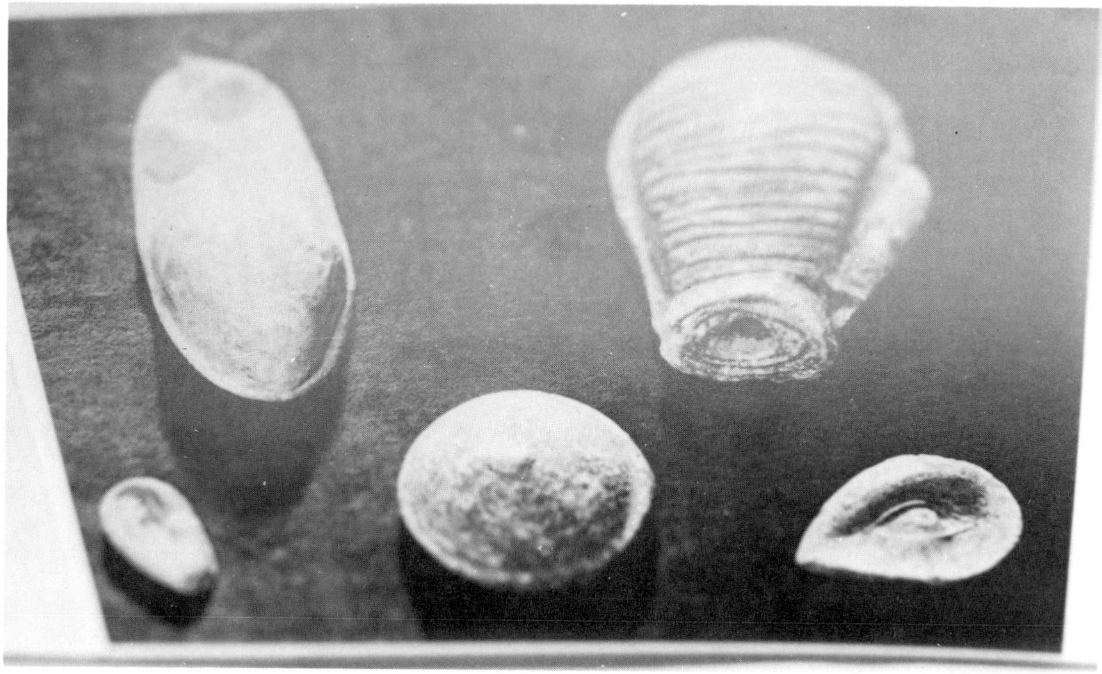

Figure 1-3 Votive offerings given during the Aesculapian period. The breast is seen in the middle part of the illustration.

> fever at all therein when your hand feels him; they have no granulations, contain no fluid, give rise to no liquid discharge, yet they feel protuberant to your touch, you should say concerning him: this is a case of bulging tumors I have to contend with.[11]

As for treatment of these bulging tumors, a simple statement is made: "There is no treatment."[11] This translation is followed by a brief commentary by a later physician, about 2500 B.C., as follows:

> Bulging tumors on his breast, it means the existence of swellings on the breast, large, spreading and hard; touching them is like touching a ball of wrapping; the comparison is to a green hemat fruit which is hard and cool under thy hand like touching those swellings which are on his breast.[11,23]

These hard, cool tumors are thus separated from inflammatory diseases or abscesses of the breast. Cauterization or "fire drill" was used for abscesses and no treatment whatsoever was advocated for cancers. Does this not sound like the teachings of some of today's physicians regarding the treatment of the primary tumor, which is a nihilistic approach?

The Ebers Papyrus and The Code of Hammurabi

The Ebers papyrus (2nd millennium B.C.) gives us a great deal of insight regarding the status of the surgeon at that time. A surgeon had to make one of three decisions on seeing a patient. He could say, "I can cure this patient," and thereby he made a contract to do so. He could say, "I cannot cure this ailment," and he then had to refuse to treat it at all because no allowances were made for therapeutic results short of cure. Or he could say, "I must observe longer before I know where I can cure." These notations gave rise to the code of Hammurabi (2250 B.C.).[17]

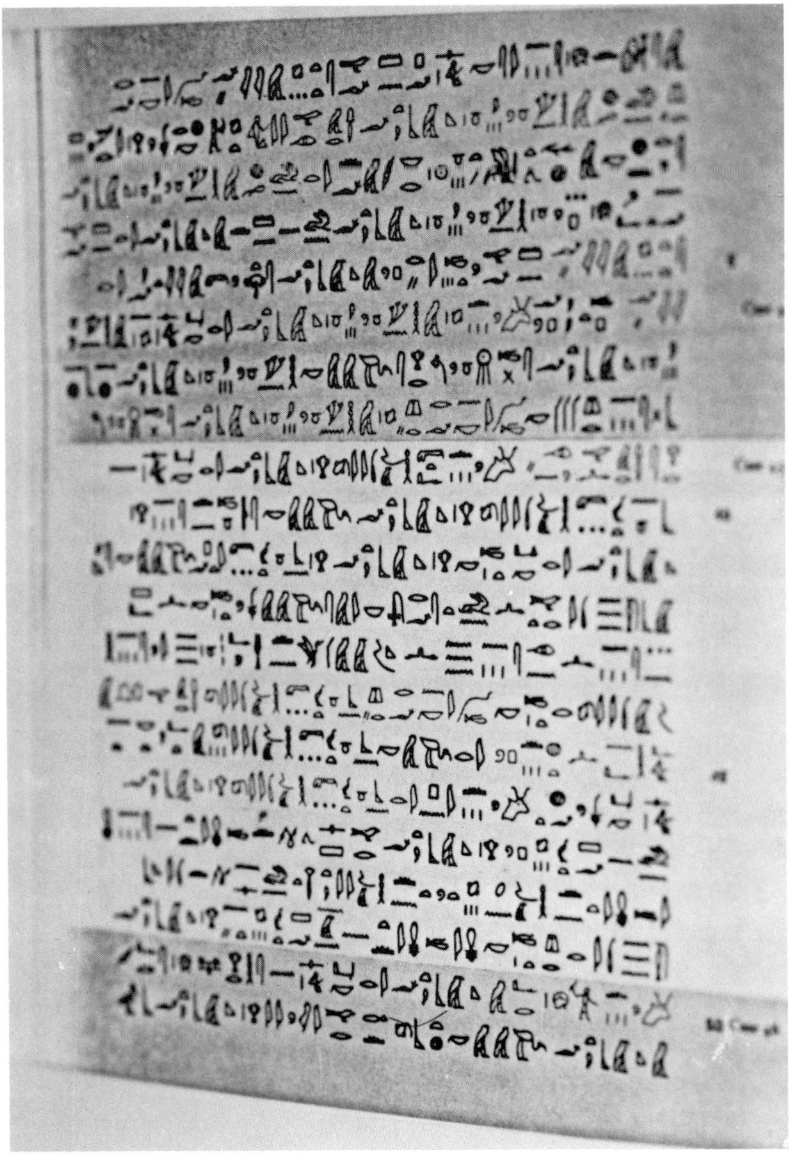

Figure 1-4 Hieroglyphic translation of case 45 from the Edwin Smith papyrus, the earliest medical record (3000-2500 B.C.). This applies to breast tumors. (*Translated by Henry Breasted, Chicago Press.*)

We learn from the code of Hammurabi that the medical profession in Babylon had advanced far enough in public esteem to be rewarded with adequate fees, carefully described and regulated by law. Thus, 10 shekels in silver was the statutory fee for treating a wound or a tumor or opening an abscess of the eye with a bronze lancet if the patient happened to be a gentleman. For a poor man or a servant the fee was 5 or 2 shekels, respectively. If the doctor caused the patient to lose his life or his eyes, he had his hands cut off, in the case of the gentleman, or had to render a value for a value in the case of a slave. (Modern malpractice fees seem mild in comparison to those days!) These fees were relatively high when one considers that yearly rent was 5 shekels for a middle-class dwelling, or one-fiftieth of a shekel for daily pay for an ordinary craftsman.[6]

Herodotus

The ancient Greek historian Herodotus,[39] who lived in the fifth century B.C. just prior to Hippocrates, relates a story of the Princess Atossa, who had a tumor of her breast. After a time, the tumor ulcerated and spread. False modesty prevented her from complaining about this tumor while it was small. But when it grew larger and gave her trouble, she sent for the famous physician, Democedes (525 B.C.), and he cured her of the disease from which she suffered. The type of treatment is not mentioned. The fact that she was cured is presumptive evidence that she did not have cancer. The case does demonstrate the attitude of women regarding their breasts, even during this very early period.

Hippocrates

The famous physician Hippocrates (400 B.C.)[41] makes little mention of breast cancer (Fig. 1-5). He does state that it was better to give no treatment for deep-seated cancers because treatment accelerated the dying process, but if one omitted treatment one might prolong life. The average life span at the time of Christ was about 18 years, so it is not surprising that breast cancer is mentioned so infrequently. Hippocrates established three precepts: that those diseases curable by medicine are best, those not curable by medicine are curable by the knife, and those not curable by the knife are curable by fire. Those that fire cannot cure are incurable. It is doubtful that he ever recommended surgery for breast cancer.

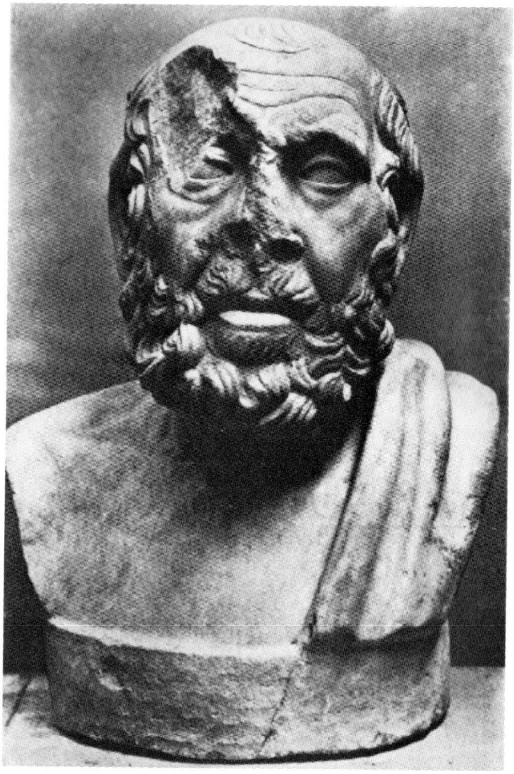

Figure 1-5 Hippocrates from a head recently discovered near Rome. (*Published by A. Lyon chez Jean Gregoire.*)

The Early Christian Era

A great scholar who lived between 30 B.C. and 38 A.D. was Aulus Cornealius Celsus,[14] who established the first classification of breast cancer. The early surgically curable precancers were classified as the *cacoethes*:

> First there is the cacoethes, then carcinoma without ulceration, then the fungating ulcer. None of these can be removed but the cacoethes; the rest are irritated by every method of cure. The more violent the operations the more angry they grow. Some use caustics, some burning irons, others remove the growth with the scalpel; after excision, even though a cicatrix be formed, it recurs, bringing with it the cause of death. Whereas at the same time most people, by using no violent methods to attempt the extirpation of the disease but only applying mild medications to soothe it, protract their lives, notwithstanding the disorder, to an extreme old age.[14]

Medical treatment consisted of venesection and purgatives. Local treatment consisted of applications of the juice of strichnos.

Galen

We next jump ahead about 200 years to Galen of Pergamon (131 to 203 A.D.), who was probably responsible for the first surgical treatment of breast cancer and who coined the term "crab" to describe cancer: "Just as a crab has legs on both sides of his body, so in this disease the veins extending out from the unnatural growth take the shape of crab's legs."[25] He further goes on to say:

> We have often cured this disease in the early stages, but after it has grown to a noticeable size no one has cured it without surgery. In all surgery we attempt to excise a pathologic tumor in a circle in the region where it borders on the healing tissue.[25]

Ligatures were frowned upon for it was believed that they caused extension of the disease. Galen also advised against removal of the pectoral muscle. As well, Galen introduced the concept of "humors" being responsible for cancer, a theory which dominated medicine for over a thousand years. Cancer was thought to be due to an excess of black bile.

Aetius of Ameda

Shortly after this time (372 A.D.) the Roman Empire had fallen, and the barbarians had invaded Europe. In 550 A.D. the Byzantine Empire was at its height. In the sixth century Aetius of Ameda was physician to the Byzantine Emperor Justinian.[2] Aetius described excision followed by cautery (see Fig. 1-6) and stated: "The first burns are for the sake of blooding and the last for the attention of eradicating the disease."[1,27] He described Leonides of Alexandria as a great physician, an astute clinician, and a careful surgeon. Although most of the doctors of the time had a nihilistic attitude toward cancer, Leonides actually performed courageous surgery, being careful not to operate on advanced cases. He was the first to describe nipple retraction as a clinical sign of breast cancer.

Aegineta

Paulus Aegineta,[1] a seventh-century Greek surgeon, agreed with the principles of Galen. He believed that cancers are formed from black bile:

> . . . if overheated it is attended with ulceration, and owing to the thickness of the humor, cancer of the breast is an incurable disease, for it can neither be repelled not dissolved: not yielding to purging of the whole body, resisting the milder applications and being exasperated by the stronger ones. The only chance for a radical cure consisted in making a complete excision of the part.[1]

Rhazes (841–926 A.D.), a great Arabic physician, warned that those who incise a breast cancer would merely produce an ulceration, and that only if the breast could be completely removed and the parts burned should an excision be done. If ulceration had taken place, he approved of using cooling applications.[4,22]

Haly Ben-Abbas, a Persian who died in 994, recommended excision of the breast, allowing bleeding to rid the body of melancholic humors. He disapproved of tying arteries. It is assumed he used pressure for hemostasis.[5,22]

Albucasis, during the first half of the eleventh century, stated: "As for me, I have never been able to cure a case nor have I known one who

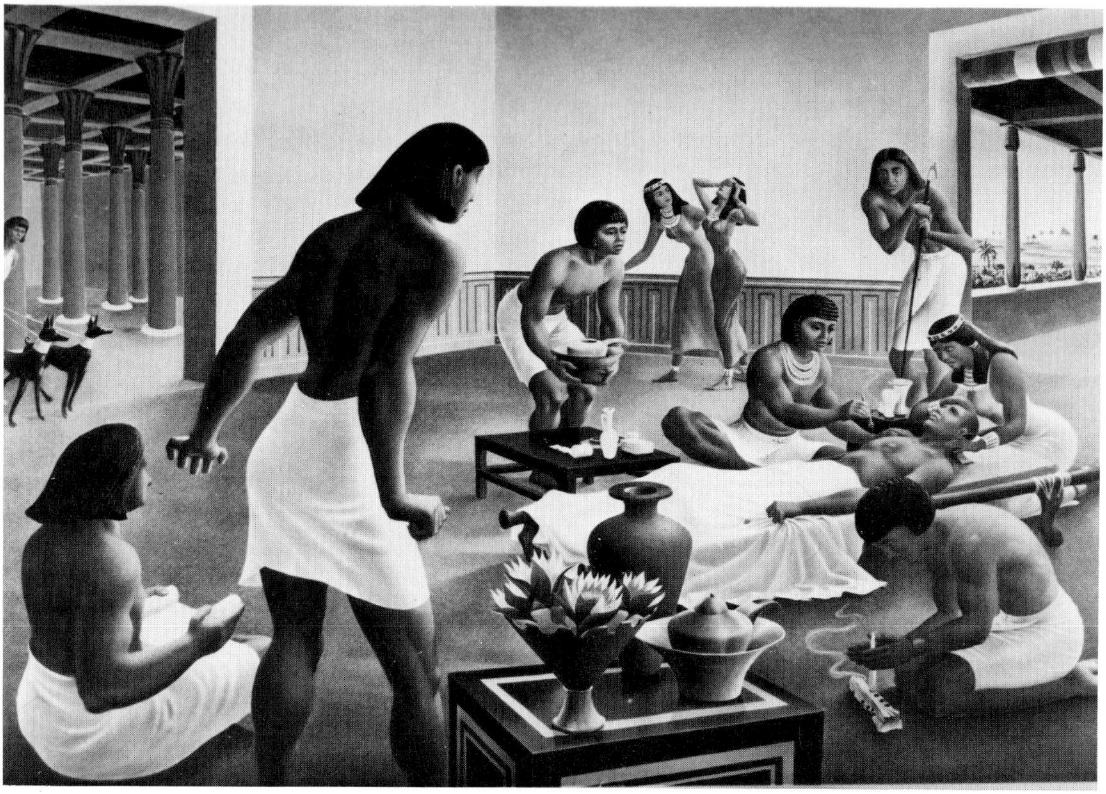

Figure 1-6 Artist's conception of treatment of breast disease by cauterization with the "fire drill." (*Courtesy of Lederle Laboratories.*)

has." Lanfrank[44] (1300) is considered the father of French surgery and was still using the method of Leonides despite the lapse of more than a thousand years.[22]

Guy de Chauliac, a fourteenth-century surgeon and the patron saint of the American College of Surgeons, recommended conservative treatment primarily, but if one could excise the entire mass, surgery might be done. He devised various unique instruments designed after instruments used for mutilation[15,73] for the rapid amputation of the breast.

A unique practice was performed by the Spanish surgeon Francisco Arceo (1493-1571). He divided the cancerous breast lengthwise and dissolved the tumor by means of a ligature. Fuchs (1501-1566), a German surgeon, compressed cancers of the breast by means of a lead plate.[70]

The Role of Religion

Religion played a role[28] and after the Council of Tours in 1162, religious fervor frowned on surgery and put a ban on the barbarous practice of surgery for breast cancer, a situation which lasted well into the fifteenth century.

The practice of exorcism dates back to time immemorial, as does the laying on of hands and other mystic practices. William Clowes,[16] physician to Queen Elizabeth, practiced exorcism for breast cancer. The simple ritual of the laying on of royal hands was the queen's counterpart of curing the "king's evil" (scrofula). The "royal touch" was said to have originated with Edward the Confessor, but served several of his successors who were somewhat skeptical of their own divine power of faith healing. William III possessed no self-delusion when he told his ailing subjects, "May God give you better health and better sense." When he discontinued the practice, he was accused of cruelty. Queen Elizabeth had a blessed ring which she wore suspended between her breasts. The ring had the presumed virtue of expelling infected air and preventing disease. Similar amulets of asafetida were worn until recently as protection against occult or evil influences, including breast cancer.

The Middle Ages

An important contributor to the development of the treatment of breast cancer was Ambroise Paré[64] (1510-1590; Fig. 1-7) who stated: "If the cancer was small, non-ulcerated, and situated in a region where it could be easily removed, the tumor should be excised, but one should go well beyond its boundaries." Large and ulcerated lesions were treated with sweet milk, vinegar, and ointments. Paré called attention to the fact that the primary breast cancer and the axillary extension to the breast were related.

Vesalius[85] (1514-1564) was one of the first who vigorously opposed Galen's doctrines and discarded the old anatomy. His anatomy book, published in 1543, marks the beginning of modern anatomy. Vesalius treated cancer by wide surgical excision and controlled bleeding by means of ligatures. Fabricius Ab Aquapendente[89] (1537-1619), teacher of William Harvey, performed radical surgery for cancer only at the patient's request and decried partial excision as worthless. This is an early example of the patient's role in the decision making involved in her treatment.

Nicholaes Tulp (1594-1674),[82] a Dutch anatomist who commissioned Rembrandt to

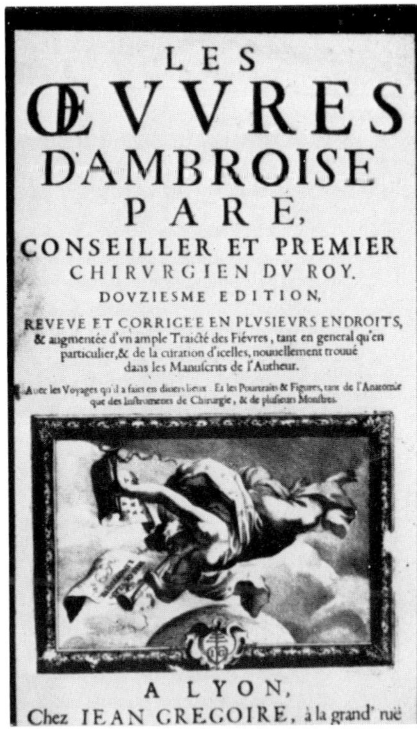

LES ŒVVRES D'AMBROISE PARE, CONSEILLER ET PREMIER CHIRVRGIEN DV ROY. DOVZIESME EDITION, REVEVE ET CORRIGEE EN PLVSIEVRS ENDROITS, & augmentée d'vn ample Traicté des Fiévres, tant en general qu'en particulier, & de la curation d'icelles, nouuellement trouué dans les Manuscrits de l'Autheur.

A LYON, Chez JEAN GREGOIRE, à la grand' ruë

Figure 1-7 Front page of the writings of Ambroise Paré, who favored excision of small nonulcerated tumors (1510–1590).

paint the now-famous *Anatomy Lesson*, showing Dr. Tulp doing an anatomy demonstration, believed that breast cancer was contagious and described a case in which the disease was passed presumably from mistress to her servant girl.

Scultetus[74] (1595-1645) described an operation in which heavy ligatures were passed through the breast. Traction was then applied as the breast was amputated, and bleeding from the operative area was quickly scarred with a hot iron (Fig. 1-8).

The Renaissance

LeDran (1685-1770)[45] once and for all put to sleep Galen's humoral theory and stressed the fact that cancer was a local lesion in its earlier stages and was spread by way of the

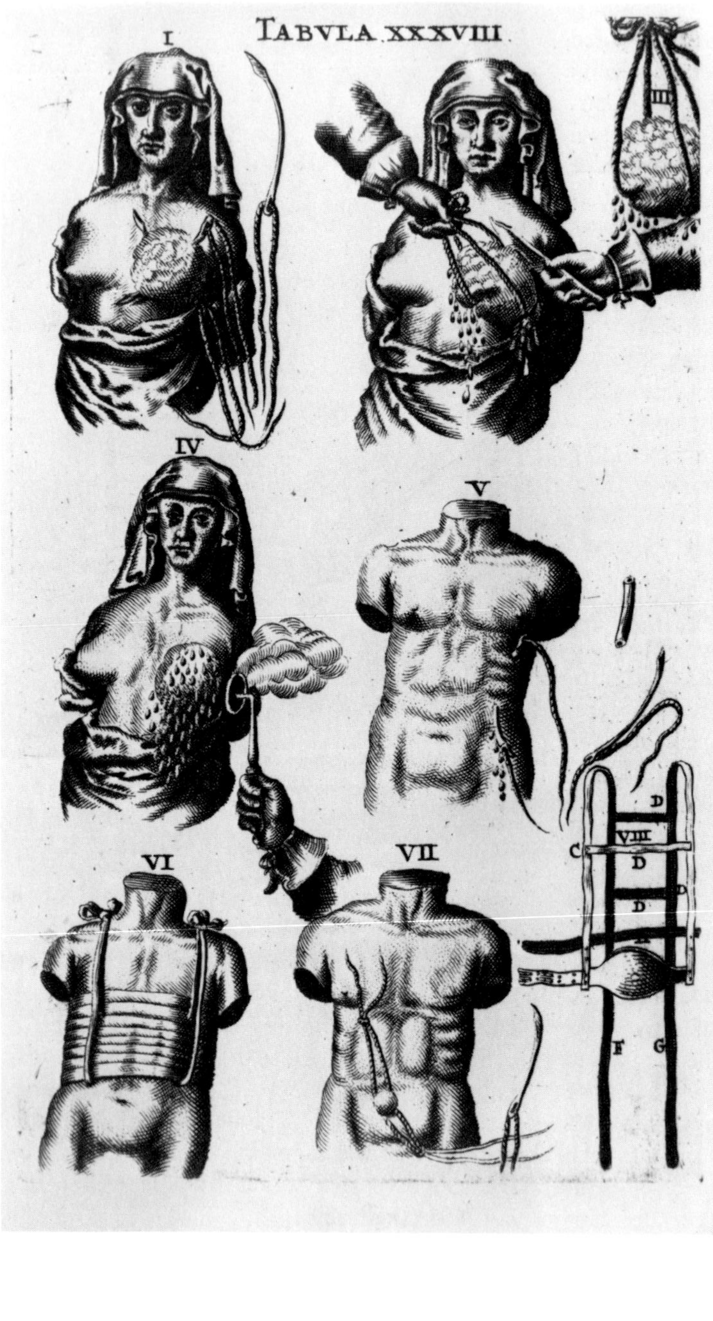

Figure 1-8 The operation for breast cancer as vividly illustrated by Scultetus (1595–1645). Leather thongs are sutured through the breast and used for traction as the breast is severed, after which the region is cauterized by the actual cautery. The Scultetus binder is still used.

lymphatics. He stressed early treatment, which consisted of a local excision with a lymph node dissection. He called attention to the fact that hope for cure was decidedly less when the axillary nodes were involved, which was the usual situation.[75]

Jean Louis Petit (1674-1750)[65] believed in wide surgical excision and stated that, although the breast tumor was carefully avoided during the operation, as little skin as possible was to be removed, with preservation of the nipple (Fig. 1-9). He is noted for his wide excision, careful removal of the axillary nodes, and appreciation of dissection in-continuity, at a time when major surgical procedures so often resulted in widespread infection and death. He further called attention to evaluating the pectoralis major muscle at a time before microscopic examination became available.

Period of Hopelessness

The latter part of the eighteenth century and the first half of the nineteenth century are characterized by pessimism and gloom regarding breast cancer. Alexander Monro (1773-1859)[57] stated that of 60 cases treated, only four were free of disease at the end of 2 years. The unscientific approach is emphasized by Velpeau in a lecture he presented before the Sydenham Society in 1856.[84] Among the various methods used for treating breast cancer by internal measures (largely influenced by Galen's teachings of the humors) were repeated bleedings, leeches, purgatives, and emetics. Various drugs were used to destroy the humors. As outlined by Velpeau, these included hemlock; iron; arsenic; mercury solutions; alkaline substances, including Vichy water; gold, which had been used for syphilis; preparations of iodine; etc. Regarding surgery, he stated:

> ... to destroy a cancerous tumor by surgical means is usually an easy matter and but little dangerous in itself; but the question arises, whether such a procedure affords a chance of radically curing the patient. This proposition remains undecided.[84]

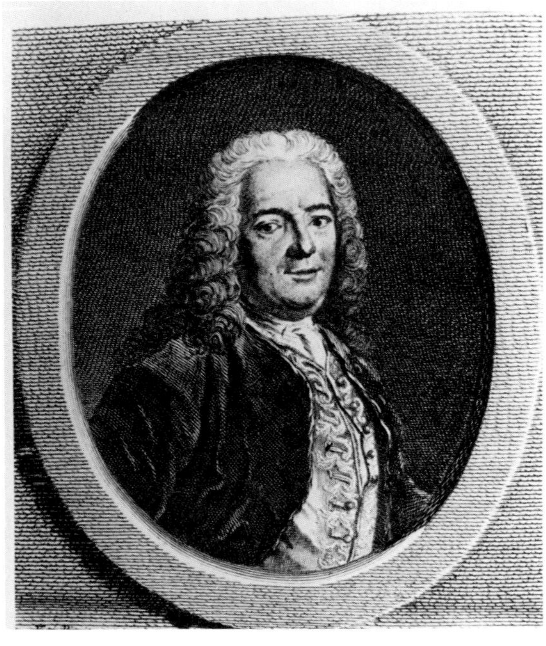

Figure 1-9 Jean Louis Petit (1674–1750), the first surgeon to form a unified concept of surgery for breast cancer: wide excision, en bloc resection with axillary dissection, and evaluation of the pectoral fascia.

He continued: "The disease always returns after removal, and operation only accelerates its growth and fatal termination." This pessimism is reflected by others of that time, as quoted by Velpeau. James Syme (1799-1870), a Scotsman, condemned the practice of palliative procedures in the treatment of cancer. He stated: "The only proceeding that deserves at all to be considered a remedy for cancer is removal of the morbid structure."[81]

It is to be recalled that all of this was done without the availability of microscopic anatomy (Fig. 1-10).[33] Schleiden (1838)[86] was among the first to appreciate the significance of the cell as a unit in plant structure, and Virchow[86] epitomized the matter by saying: "Omnis cellula e cellula." He advanced the concept that any normal cell can become a cancer cell as a result of irritation. Sir James Paget (1814-1899; Fig. 1-11),[62] without the availability of anesthesia or asepsis, stated: "We have to ask ourselves

Figure 1-10 Figure demonstrating the lymphatic drainage of the breast which influenced LeDran (1685-1770), who championed lymph node dissection. (*Courtesy of Ciba Pharmaceutical Co.*)

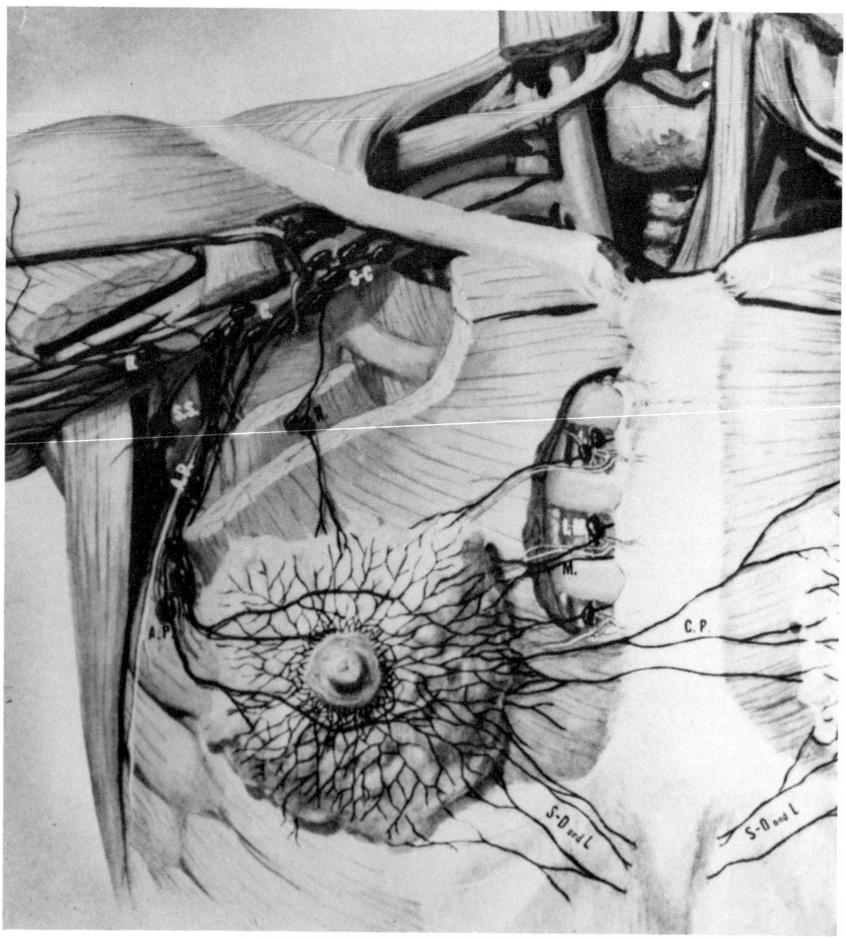

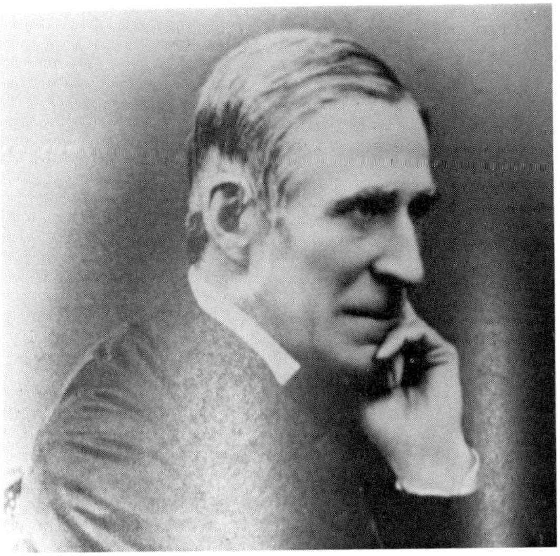

Figure 1-11 Sir James Paget (1814–1899), who first described Paget's disease of the nipple. Paget remained pessimistic regarding breast cancer.

whether it is probable that the operation will add to the length or comfort of life enough to justify incurring the risk of its own consequences." He had an operative mortality of 10 percent in 235 cases of breast cancer. Paget believed the disease to be hopeless, and stated:

> In deciding for or against removal of the cancerous breast, in any single case, we may, I think, dismiss all hope that the operation will be a final remedy for the disease. I would not say that such a thing is impossible; but it is so highly improbable that a hope of its occurring in any single case cannot be reasonably entertained.[62]

This pessimistic attitude was also voiced by Robert Liston (1794-1847): "No one can now be found so rash or so cruel as to attempt the removal of the glands thus affected whether primary or secondary."[51] In this pessimistic atmosphere, Velpeau favored thorough excision in preference to complete amputation, stating:

> If the disease requires, the pectoralis muscle should not arrest us. The smallest shade of the disease must be taken away, if we are determined not to lose any chance of success. However, should there appear to be any necessity of interfering with the bones or resecting the ribs we must not deceive ourselves. The return of the disease is then inevitable and it would have been better not to have undertaken the operation at all.[84]

His basic operation consisted of complete excision of the tumor with its overlying skin, with preservation of the nipple when possible, and only in certain cases amputation of the breast.

D. Hayes Agnew (1818-1892)[3] resorted to surgery solely for its moral effect. He believed that operation actually shortened rather than prolonged survival time. J. Pancoast (1805-1882)[63] emphasized the importance of excising axillary nodes with the breast in-continuity (Fig. 1-12). He made no mention of dividing the pectoralis muscles to gain access to the axilla. He was one of the first to practice approximation of the skin with adhesive tape (Fig. 1-13).

Beginning of the Modern Era

Resurgence of Surgery

In 1869, Richard Sweeting[80] reported something slightly different in that he advocated complete removal of the pectoralis major muscle. He espoused it as a routine part of the mastectomy.

Extension of surgical procedures to include amputation of the entire breast was advocated by Samuel D. Gross. He insisted that under the most favorable circumstances, that is, when the tumor was small and well circumscribed, and when the axillary nodes were not involved, the appropriate procedure was removal of the entire breast with overlying skin, but not an axillary dissection.[30] Samuel W. Gross (1880), son of Samuel D. Gross, advocated removal of the pectoral fascia while doing an in-continuity

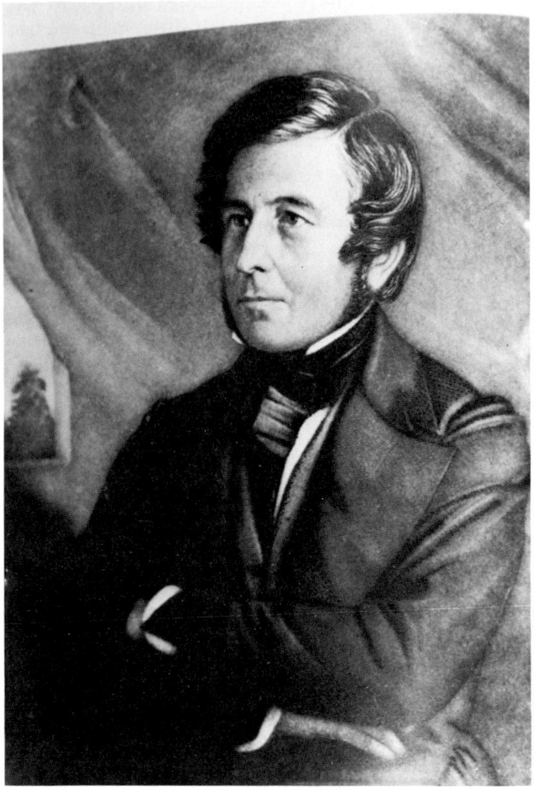

Figure 1-12 Joseph Pancoast (1805–1882) advocated resecting the breast and axillary lymph nodes in continuity. He did not favor excising the pectoralis muscles and made no mention of how he gained access to the axilla.

removal of the breast and the axillary lymph nodes.[31]

The intellectual basis for the radical mastectomy depends upon an understanding of the lymphatic spread of cancer.[83] Aselius (1627) was the first to demonstrate lacteals which he found in a recently fed dog. Mascagni (1787) and Sappey (1885), using mercury injections, clearly outlined the lymphatics of the breast, as quoted by Leeds.[47] Heidenhain (1889)[38] demonstrated microscopically that delicate extensions of breast parenchyma follow the pectoral fascia down into the muscle and that foci of carcinoma are often found in the same deep plane within the lymphatics. It was an anatomic concept based on the belief that the mastectomy operation must be extensive enough to prevent recurrence. Heidenhain suspected that such an operation would have to include excision of part of the pectoralis major muscle. He stated that the pectoralis was involved in most cancers and should be excised. No one had ever approached the problem in this sophisticated manner.

Charles H. Moore in 1867,[58] although he acknowledged that surgery was being performed earlier than before, asserted that it was not nearly so radical as required (Fig. 1-14). A century before, wide excision was the rule, but now the skin was undermined by dissection and after removal of the tumor, was reapplied. At times even the nipple and areola were preserved. Moore (Fig. 1-14) espoused the following major points: (1) During the operation the tumor should not be cut into, nor even seen. (2) Recurrence was determined by centrifugal dispersion from the primary site and not by any independent organic origin. (3) The entire mammary gland must be removed. (4) The removal of the breast is most likely to be incomplete at the sternal margin. (5) Unsound tissue adjacent to the lesion, such as skin, ought to be removed in-continuity with the whole; the skin and the nipple should be removed or the results may be disastrous. Moore did not remove the pectoral muscles. Three years later, Lister[50] described his technique of dividing but not removing the pectoral muscles. In 1877, Banks[9] wrote regarding the axillary lymph nodes: "As you cannot tell whether the glands are affected or not till you see them in your hand, let them be always removed and so increase the patient's chances of future immunity."

Through the ages one can trace a constant ongoing extension of the surgical treatment of breast cancer as new techniques were developed. These included (1) safer surgery with understanding of the anatomy and control of infection and transfusions; (2) development of anesthesia; and (3) better understanding of the

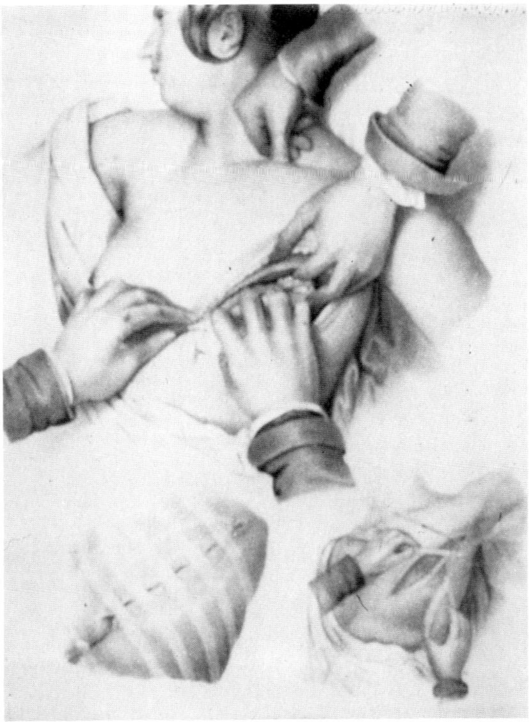

Figure 1-13 Mastectomy as practiced by Pancoast (1844). Note touch of modernism where adhesive strips rather than sutures were used.

biology of cancer, especially that cancer starts as a single entity and spreads by direct extension, lymphatic spread, and vascular dissemination. The various surgical approaches can be listed as follows: (1) Should an operation be done at all? (2) How much skin should be removed? (3) Should the underlying pectoralis major muscle be removed? (4) Should the axillary nodes be removed? (5) Should the nipple be removed? And (6) a combination of all the above, culminating in the radical mastectomy.

No Treatment At All

No treatment at all was the approach documented in the first records of breast cancer in world history. Early physicians advised no treatment. They must have tried some form of treatment and found it unsuccessful because it is unlikely that they would not have attempted some type of treatment. In the 1500s, Ambroise Paré[64] advised wide excision, but if the cancers were large, advanced, and ulcerated, he advised no surgery but only treatment with sweet milk, vinegar, and ointment. In England, Robert Liston (1794–1847)[51,52] advised against surgery if the axillary nodes were involved. Extension to the nodes was considered a contraindication for operation.

Much confusion existed regarding the origin of cancer. Was it related to the humors of Galen? Was it a manifestation of a constitutional disease, an infection, or a parasite? Could it be transmitted? In 1894, Keen made the following statement:

> There is no question at all in the present day that cancer is of local origin. In my earlier professional life, it was one of the disputed points constantly coming up in medical society as to whether it was local or from the first a constitutional dis-

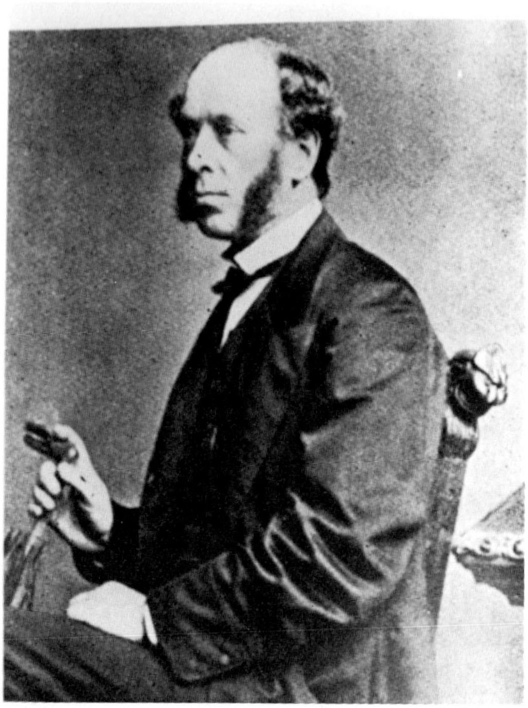

Figure 1-14 Charles Hewlett Moore (1867)—first conceived but did not implement the concept of radical mastectomy.

> ease, and if the latter it was said that no good could come from operating upon the breast. But this question of local origin is no longer confronting us. It is a thing settled. A point one. And women must be taught that this brings help to them. Don't wait, I beg of you, gentlemen and ladies, don't wait for that old classic symptom, retraction of the nipple, for in nearly one half of the cases it will not exist. I take no account of it. I make an incision into the tumor, and if it is malignant or suspicious, I amputate the entire breast.[42]

The same problem exists today regarding treatment of local-regional cancer, but for an entirely different reason. Instead of believing that cancer is a local manifestation of a systemic disease, some claim that when the patient is seen by the physician, although the cancer started locally it is disseminated and local control is meaningless.

The Axillary Nodes

The axillary nodes have always posed a problem regarding their treatment. Cervinius (1580) was one of the first to call attention to them and to remove them. It is unlikely that any previous surgeons tackled the nodes. Aetius[2] first mentioned axillary swelling which may have represented metastases. Henry LeDran (1685-1770),[45] a Frenchman, stressed the need for early surgery, and was the first to remove the axillary lymph nodes routinely. It took this length of time to repudiate Galen's humors. LeDran stressed the fact that cancer was a local lesion when early and spread by way of the lymphatics. He was the one who stressed a poor prognosis if the axillary nodes were involved. Benjamin Bell (1749-1886),[10] a Scotsman, stated that small cancers should be treated by total mastectomy and axillary dissection.

Bryant (1887) stated:

> When a cancer or carcinomatous growth ceases to be a local disease, it spreads in 3 methods, by continuous or local infection, by lymphatic infection, or by secondary vascular infection. One form may be more marked than another or all forms may coexist together.[12a]

Charles Moore,[58] an Englishman, was the one who advised amputation of the breast with axillary dissection in-continuity. Samuel D. Gross advocated amputation of the breast but sacrificed thoroughness by preserving the skin and the axilla. His son, Samuel W. Gross, corrected the omissions of his father and brought to America the Moore operation. The great German surgeons, Volkman, Billroth, and Heidenhain, advised routine removal of the lymph nodes in the late 1800s.

The Skin

Until the mid-1700s, a large mass of skin was usually removed. However, Benjamin Bell[10] was one of the first to state that unless the cancer had invaded the skin, thin skin flaps could be developed and thus facilitate closure, which is the technique followed today. The question of skin flaps has been debated for many years. Some, such as Haagensen,[32] advise very, very thin skin flaps; others say it doesn't matter. But at present, the development of skin flaps is mandatory in order to facilitate closure and as a precursor for adequate cosmetic reconstructive surgery at a later date.

Wide Excision or Amputation

The question of whether a wide excision or an amputation of the breast should be performed has dominated surgical thought throughout the ages. Aetius, Guy de Chauliac, Ambroise Paré, Vesalius, and Velpeau all advocated a wide excision, whereas Leonides, Aquapendente, Scultetus, Bell, and, of course, the surgeons of the later nineteenth century, all advised amputation, even for the smallest cancer.[51] It is, however, doubtful that they ever saw a small cancer, inasmuch as the combination of modesty of the woman and ignorance of the profession usually meant that the cancer had become rather large and widespread before attempts at eradication were made.[66]

The Pectoralis Muscle

The pectoralis muscle is now receiving a great deal of attention with the frequent performance of the modified mastectomy to preserve the form and function of the patient. There have been arguments both for and against its removal throughout the ages. Even when an amputation was done in those early days, the pectoral muscle was not removed. Jean Louis Petit[65] (1674–1750) removed the pectoral fascia and some of the fibers if they were involved. He believed that the roots of the cancer were the enlarged lymph nodes and removed them. He preserved the skin and sutured it to prevent hemorrhage. Earlier surgeons left the wound open. Petit also preserved the nipple.

At first, only the fascia was removed, but gradually more and more of the muscles were resected. Samuel D. Gross[30] removed only the fascia; Volkmann[88] in 1875 carried the incision down to the pectoral muscle: "Carrying the knife parallel with the fibers of the muscle and penetrating into their intricacies, the pectoral fascia is thus entirely removed." He stated that he adopted this procedure because on microscopic examination he found the fascia "carcinomatous" where he least expected it. He describes the resection of the pectoralis major muscle and, at times, the pectoralis minor in 38 patients with far-advanced cases, with a 3-year survival of 14 percent.

Heidenhain[38] (1889) stated that "a tumor, however freely moveable on the underlying parts has almost certainly advanced as far as the surface of the muscle." He believed cancer cells were propagated through the lymphatics by muscular action. He described 18 cases examined microscopically in which the superficial layer of the pectoralis major was involved.

Bryant (1887) stated: "When the pectoral muscle is infiltrated, it must be freely excised.[12a]

The Radical Mastectomy

Degenshein and Ceccarelli[22] give credit to the Frenchman Bartoleny Cabrol, who in 1590 performed the first radical mastectomy, much as it is done today (with the excision of the pectoral muscle). Moore[58] in 1867 presented a paper, "The Influence of Inadequate Operations on the Theory of Cancer," in which he actually described the radical mastectomy. He thus championed a new cause in the relatively futile era of surgery of the breast. Three years later, Joseph Lister (1837–1912)[50] supported and extended Moore's teachings. He cut the pectoralis muscle to expose the axilla and performed a meticulous axillary dissection. His aseptic technique, using carbolic spray, probably played a major role in the outcome of his patients. The microscope's availability led Speese, who studied the involvement of the muscle in 100 consecutive operative cases and found involvement in 25 of those cases, and involvement of the fascia in 18 cases, to advocate its routine removal (quoted by Wolff[91]).

The stage was thus set for William Halsted (1852-1923)[34-36] at Johns Hopkins Hospital to construct out of this sizable background of details a practical solution to the problem (Figs. 1-15 and 1-16). In 1894 he published a paper on the classical radical mastectomy as we know it today.[36] Ten days after Halsted's paper was published, on November 12, 1894, Willy Meyer presented before the New York Academy of Medicine a similar operation in which he also transsected the pectoralis minor muscle, thus making the radical mastectomy anatomically complete .[55]

The development of the radical mastectomy was a laborious and tedious process which actually started with Petit in 1739 [although occasionally performed earlier (1590)] and ended with Halsted in 1894.

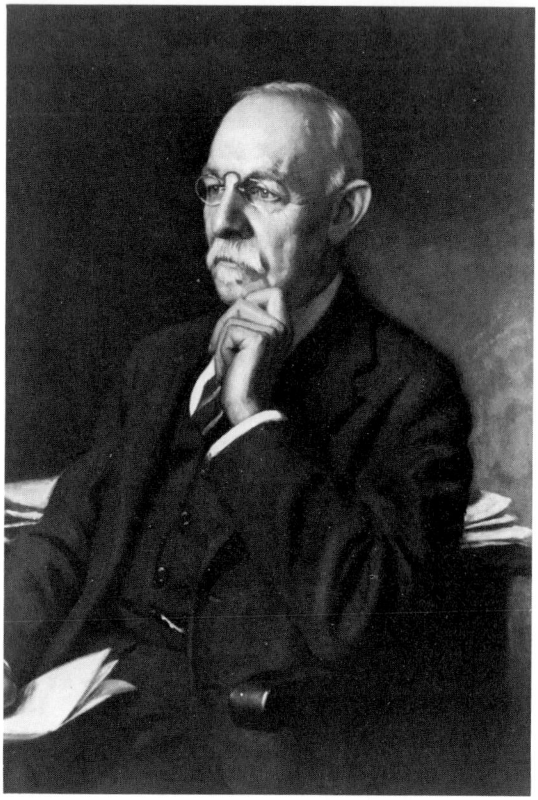

Figure 1-15 Dr. William Stewart Halsted.

> The story is not one of ordinary progression, but was frought with retrogressions that are prominent even today. The horror of sepsis, the need for anesthesia, and the wide acceptance of the incurability of cancer were prominent in delaying the development of surgery of the breast.[49]

The Englishman Charles H. Moore conceived the operation, the Germans began practicing the operation as conceived by Moore (Volkman, Billroth, Heidenhain), and two Americans, Halsted and Meyer, independently implemented the completed procedure.

Since the advent of the radical mastectomy, the operation has been extended in every direction. It has been extended proximally to include the neck dissection, associated with the radical mastectomy by Dahl Iverson,[21] with no improved survival rate. It has been extended to include the internal mammary nodes.[37] It has been extended by Wangensteen[89] to remove the entire chest plastron with a dissection of the mediastinal lymph nodes, and by Prudente to combine an interscapulomammothoracic amputation in selected situations.[69]

Now, almost 100 years after the development of the radical mastectomy, the tendency is for less and less surgery, in a 180-degree turnaround to surgical procedures practiced many years ago.[24] Is the change warranted?

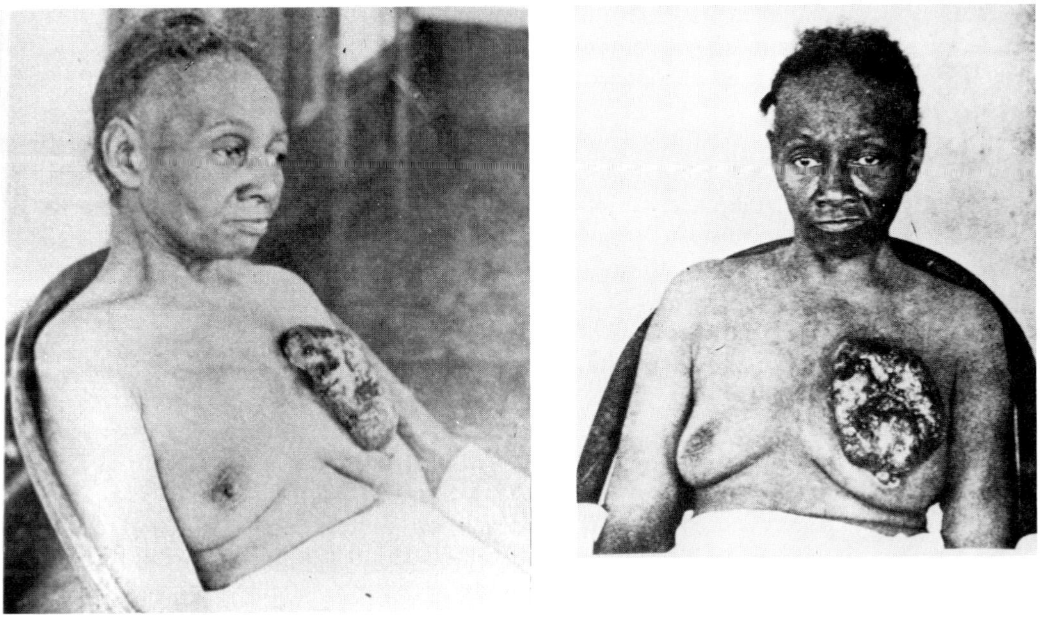

Figure 1-16 Two of Halsted's patients demonstrating the advanced stage of the cancer, usually seen at that time.

The Development of Radiation Therapy for Cancer of the Breast

Irradiation using orthovoltage generators as the sole means of treating breast cancer had been tried, but the results in the past had been poor.[7] Microscopic studies of the irradiated tissues did not reveal any changes from orthovoltage radiation therapy in four-fifths of the cases, and lymph nodes bearing cancer seemed unaffected from the irradiation. Preoperative irradiation[46] had been largely abandoned, but it is now receiving a resurgence. Simple mastectomy, or lumpectomy, with postoperative irradiation is being strongly advocated, using supervoltage irradiation and/or interstitial irradiation. Grace of Brooklyn, New York treated 40 patients by simply mastectomy with postoperative orthovoltage irradiation and reported a 44% 5-year "cure."[26] McWhirter after simple mastectomy and postoperative orthovoltage radiation therapy reported a 42% 5-year survival and a 25% 10-year survival for 1,345 patients treated between 1941 and 1962.[54] Modern radiation equipment and more reliable methods of radiation techniques are largely responsible for the increased use of radiation therapy and the improved results.

The advent of supervoltage x-ray therapy was first inaugurated in 1932. In 1935, Stone, Livingston, Sloan, and Chaffee built a million-volt generator, and reports regarding its initial use were encouraging.[79] In 1941, Kerst built the first betatron, which generated 20 million electron volts and was utilized by Roger Harvey in the treatment of cancer. The discovery by Ernest Orlando Lawrence of the cyclotron in 1932 contributed greatly to the development of radioactive isotopes. Two of these isotopes, cobalt-60 and radioactive cesium -137 are used for supervoltage therapy. Now, over 50 years since the supervoltage treatment units were described, are the observations that better results for breast cancer are being obtained by their use.

Most of the results are those of relatively short-term follow-up with only a few 10-year follow-up studies.[56] If continued good results are obtained for prolonged periods, mastectomy (both simple and radical) may be abandoned. It is too early to state.

Chemotherapy and Hormone Manipulation

Every form of chemical measure for treating cancer has been attempted from the earliest times until the present. Some of these include purgatives, blood-letting, weird diets, reptile venom, heavy metals, and thousands of others. It is lamentable that certain charlatans, both in and out of the medical profession, still practice some of these approaches, thereby depriving patients of methods which can be curative.

Some of the earliest chemicals used were arsenic, as administered in Fowler's solution; stilbamidine; and urethane. During World War II, when one of our liberty ships carrying nitrogen mustard hit a bomb in the Italian harbor of Barato, leukopenia occurred in the survivors,[90] and Gilman and colleagues started using nitrogen mustard for treating cancer of the lymphopoietic system. Since then many new drugs have been tested and clinically applied. The development of various drugs for cancer is an ongoing challenge.[60]

Hormone manipulation has been used for treating breast cancer, receiving its impetus from the studies of Huggins,[41a] which opened the road for hormone therapy. Before Huggins' observations, cancer cells were considered "wild" cells which did not adhere to body controls. His work demonstrated a varied response of the cancer cell to a given hormonal environment.

Inasmuch as orthovoltage radiation is considered inadequate for evaluation of radiation effects (beneficial and adverse) in today's setting, and because supervoltage irradiation, chemotherapy, and modern hormone treatment are relatively new, these disciplines do not lend themselves for historic evaluation as pertains to their exact role in the cure of cancer.

SUMMARY

The attitude of women toward their breasts, a factor that often prevented them from coming for early diagnosis and treatment, and the extreme importance of the breast to the modern woman are reasons for seeking means of curing breast cancers and at the same time of preserving the breasts.

Through the ages, there have been cults which practice magic, mysticism, and the administration of unorthodox medications, and they still flourish today. Pseudo-religion has played a role. The humors of Galen, as the etiology for cancer, dominated medical thought for over a thousand years. Treatment was aimed at ridding the body of humors. Today, some charlatans advocate purging and other mysterious medicants for treatment.

The code of Hammurabi in 2250 B.C. was a forerunner of modern malpractice.

Classification of breast cancer inaugurated by Celsus (around 30 A.D.) has been modified innumerable times until our present TNM system of classification was developed.

Vesalius instituted the anatomic approach, which prevailed for about 300 years before the histologic approach was introduced by Virchow with his classical doctrine, "omnis cellulla a cellula." Breast cancer was believed to be infectious but this was disproved.

Radical surgery was practiced by Aquapendente in 1550—but only at the patient's request, the first example of informed consent.

Early disagreements were between those who believed that breast cancer was beyond cure, and those surgeons who believed surgery could be beneficial. The surgeons were often severely criticized for their efforts until the latter part of the nineteenth century.

Breast cancer was believed to be a local manifestation of a systemic disorder until Keen demonstrated that it began locally and spread. Today it is claimed by some that it is already disseminated when the diagnosis is made and local treatment is useless.

Surgery for breast cancer first consisted of local excision plus cautery followed by amputation speedily done with instruments originally designed for breast mutilation. Then followed a period of local excision. In time, amputation was again advocated. Surgery gradually developed, as the lymphatic spread of cancer became known, to include amputation of the breast and an in-continuity dissection of the axillary lymph nodes and pectoral muscles—the Halsted radical mastectomy. This was later extended to include the internal mammary lymph nodes.

It must be recalled that most cancers at that time were huge, which necessitated the radical approach. In 1894, Keen stated that he was beginning to see patients with earlier cancers and claimed that 3 years after operation, if the patient had no evidence of cancer, she was cured. In 1985, Fisher,[24] after a median follow-up of patients for 3 years and 3 months with the aid of actuarial methods, claimed 5-year results for breast-preserving operations. We now know of the chronicity of this disease, which may take its toll 15 to 20 years after "curative" treatment.

Radiation therapy in the past was unsuccessful using radium implants and othovoltage irradiation. Recent use of supervoltage equipment, computer-assisted dosimetry, and well-trained radiologists have led many to advocate breast-sparing excision of the cancer plus radiation treatment. The results seem good, and although there are a few 10-year absolute follow-ups, a larger experience and longer follow-up are needed, especially for younger women. The development of mammography and xerography have been pivotal in the earlier diagnosis of breast cancer.

Advances in hormonal therapy and chemotherapy are monumental. The greatest advance, however, has been in professional and public education. Women are coming for treatment with smaller and smaller lesions (some nonpalpable), which has permitted a more conservative approach than was necessary at the turn of the century. The death rate continues at 27.1 per 100,000 women, and with all developments it becomes important to individualize patients for the treatment best suited to a given woman.

Surgery is based on lymphatic spread of the tumor. Today some claim vascular spread is dominant. Cancer can spread by one or more methods, as claimed by Bryant in 1887. Those who believe that local-regional treatment is of little value must recall that 80 to 95 percent of stage I cancers and 60 to 75 percent of stage II cancers are surviving 10 years and longer.

As more is learned about immunity and cancer, better results will be obtained. In the meantime, we must resort to the methods of the ancients—albeit with much more sophistication; namely, cutting out the cancer (surgery), burning it out (radiation treatment), or poisoning it (chemotherapy).

Time will be the final referee.

REFERENCES

1. Adams F: *Seven Books of Paulus Aegineta* (translated from the Greek). London, The Sydenham Society, 1846, p. 79.
2. Aetius: *Graeci Contractae ex Veteribus Medicinae Tetrabiblos*. Basileae, impensis Hier., Frobenii and Nic. Episcopii, 1542, sermo IV, cap. XLV, p. 884.
3. Agnew DH: *The Principles and Practice of Surgery*, vol. III. Philadelphia, J. B. Lippincott Co., 1883.
4. Albucasis A: *De Chirurgica, Arabice et Latine Cura Johannis Channing*, 3 vols. Oxonii, e typ. Clarendoniano, 1778.
5. Arrian, the Greek historian: *Anabasis of Alexander*, book 7, vol. 2. New York, Random House, 1942.
6. Aselli G: *Delactibus sine Lacteis*. Milan, Italy, J. B. Bidellum, 1627.
7. Baclesse F: La roentgentherapie seule dans le traitement des cancers du sein. *Int Union against Cancer* 8:129, 1952.
8. Banks WM: A plea for the more free removal

of cancerous growths. *Liverpool and Manchester Surgical Reports*, p. 192, 1878.

9. Banks WM: *Some Results of the Operative Treatment of Cancer of the Breast.* Edinburgh, Neill & Co., 1882.
10. Bell B: *A System of Surgery*, 6 vol. Edinburgh, C. Elliot, 1782–87.
11. Breasted JH: *The Edwin Smith Surgical Papyrus*, vol. 1. Chicago, University of Chicago Press, 1930, case 39, p. 363; case 45, p. 463.
12. Brothwell D, Sandtov AT: *Diseases in Antiquity.* Springfield, Illinois, Charles C Thomas, 1967.

12a. Bryant T: *The Diseases of the Breast.* London, Cassess and Co., Ltd. 1887.

13. Butter J: Practical observations on the compression of cancerous breasts. *Edinburgh Med J* 14:498, 1818.
14. Celsus AC: Translation by Greive J, Brook V, chap. 28, pp. 27 and 303.
15. Chauliac G: *De Chirurgica.* Vincentius de Portonuriis de Tridino de Monteferrato, 1510.
16. Clowes, W. Cited by Wolff, J., in ref. 91, vol. I, p. 49.
17. Code of Hammurabi. *The Cadillac Modern Encyclopedia.* New York, Cadillac Publishing Co., 1973, p. 1679.
18. Cooper A: *The Anatomy and Diseases of the Breast.* Philadelphia, Lea & Blanchard, 1845, p. 355.
19. Cooper W: The history of the radical mastectomy. *Ann Med History* 3:36, 1941.
20. Dahl-Iversen E: Examen ulterieur de 109 malades ayant subi l'operation radicale du cancer du sein, concernant essentiellement le rapport entre la decouverte microscopique et la frequence de la recidive. *Lyon Chir* 24:648, 1927.
21. Dahl-Iversen E: Carcinoma of the breast. *Official Tran Northern SA* p. 150, 1951.
22. Degenshein G, Ceccarelli F: The history of breast cancer. Part I, Early beginnings to Halsted. *Breast, Diseases of the Breast* 3:28, 1977.
23. Ebell B, translator: *Ebers Papyrus.* Copenhagen, Levin and Munksgaard, 1937.
24. Fisher B, et al: Five-year results of a randomized clinical trial comparing total mastectomy and segmental mastectomy with or without radiation in the treatment of breast cancer. *N Eng J Med* 312:665, 1985.
25. Galen C: *Opera Omnia.* C. G. Kuhn (ed). Leipzig, 1824.

25a. Gilman A: The initial clinical trials of nitrogen mustard. *Am J Surg* 105:574, 1963.

26. Grace EJ: Simple mastectomy in cancer of the breast. *Am J Surg* 35:512, 1937.
27. Gray H, Lewis WH: *Anatomy of the Human Body.* New York, Lea & Febiger, 1924, p. 1277.
28. Greenblatt RB: *Search the Scriptures.* Philadelphia, J. B. Lippincott Co., 1977, p. 98.
29. Greenblatt RB, Chadda S, Teresa AZ, Lewis A: Fibrocystic breast disease; pathophysiology, hormonology, treatment. *Contemp Surg* 24:49, 1984.
30. Gross SD: *A System of Surgery*, 2 vols. Philadelphia, Blanchard & Lea, 1859.
31. Gross SW: *A Practical Treatise on Tumors of the Mammary Gland.* New York, D. Appleton & Co., 1880.
32. Haagensen CD, et al: *The Lymphatics in Cancer.* Philadelphia, London and Toronto, W. B. Saunders, 1972.
33. Haddow A: Historical notes on cancer from the MSS of Louis Westerna Sambon. *Proc R Soc Med* 29:1015, Feb. 5, 1936.
34. Halsted WS: A clinical and histological study of certain adenocarcinomata of the breast. *Tr Am SA* 16:144, 1898 (reprinted); also *Ann Surg* 28:557, 1898.
35. Halsted WS: The results of radical operations for the cure of cancer of the breast. *Tr Am SA* 25:61 (reprinted); also *Ann Surg* 46:1, 1907.
36. Halsted WS: The original conception of the complete operation for cancer of the breast. *Surgical Papers by William Stewart Halsted*, vol 2. Baltimore, The Johns Hopkins Press, 1924, p. 101.
37. Handley RS, Patey DH, Hand BH: Excision of the internal mammary chain in radical mastectomy. *Lancet* 1:457, 1956.
38. Heidenhain L: *Centralbl f Chir* 16:53, 1889.
39. Herodotus: *Thalia*, lib. III, cap. 133. (Also quoted in Wolff J: *Die Lehre von der Krebskrankheit*, vol. 1, p. 4.)
40. Herodotus: *The Histories.* New York, Penguin Classic, 1967.
41. Hippocrates: Works edited by Jones WH and Withington ET (4 vols.). New York, Putnam, 1923–1931.

41a. Huggins CB, Stevens RE, Hodges CV: Studies on prostatic cancer. The effect of castration on advanced carcinoma on the prostate glands. *Ach Surg* 43:209, 1941.

42. Keen WW: Amputation of the female breast. *Cleve Med Gazette* 10(2):39, 1894.
43. König C: Mastitis chronica cystica. *Centralbl f Chir* 20:49, 1983.
43a. Krumbhaar EB, Krumbhaar HD: The blood and bone marrow in yellow cross gas (mustard gas); poisoning; changes produced in the bone marrow of fatal cases. *J Med Res* 40:497, 1919.
44. Lanfrank: *Chirurgia Magna*. London, T. Marshe, 1565.
45. LeDran HF: Mémoire avec un précis de plusieurs observations sur le cancer. *Mem de l'Acad roy de Chir* 3:1, 1757.
46. Lee BJ: End results in the treatment of cancer of the breast combined with preoperative and postoperative irradiation. *Am J Surg* 60:405, 1933.
47. Leeds SE: Three centuries of history of the lymphatic system. *Surg Gynecol Obstet* 144:927, 1977.
48. Lewison E: *Breast Cancer, Its Diagnosis and Treatment*. Baltimore, Williams and Wilkins, 1955.
49. Lewison EF: The surgical treatment of breast cancer, an historical and collective review. *Surgery* 34:904, 1953.
50. Lister J: *Collected Papers*, vol. 2. Oxford, Clarendon Press, 1902, p. 158; also *Lancet* 2:267, 1870.
51. Liston R: *Elements of Surgery with Notes by Samuel D. Gross*. Barrington J, Haswell D (eds). Louisville, Ky., 1846, p. 412.
52. Liston R: *Practical Surgery*. London, J. Churchill, 1873.
53. Margottini M, Bucalossi P: Le metastasi linfoghiandolari. Mammarie interne nel cancro della mammellae. *Oncologia* 23:70, 1949.
54. McWhirter R: The value of simple mastectomy and radiotherapy in the treatment of cancer of the breast. *Br J Radiol* 21:599, 1948.
55. Meyer W: An improved method of the radical operation for carcinoma of the breast. *N Y Med Rec* 46:716, 1984.
56. Mitchiner PH, Bailey GN, Price AK: Comparison of results of conservative and radical surgical treatment in carcinoma of the breast for decade 1924–33. *St Thomas Hosp Rept* 2:192, 1937.
57. Monro A: *Medical Essays*, quoted by Lewison E, in ref. 48, p.7.
58. Moore CH: On the influence of inadequate operations on the theory of cancer. *R Med Chir Soc* 1: 244, 1867.
59. Osler W: *The Leaven of Science, Aequanimitas and Other Addresses*. Philadelphia, Blakiston, 1932.
60. Pack GT, Ariel IM: A half century of effort to control cancer. *Surg Gynecol Obstet* 100:4, 309, 1955
61. Pack GT, Ariel IM: *Treatment of Cancer and Allied Disease*, vol. 4, 1960, p. 3.
62. Paget J: *Lectures, Surgical Pathology, Tumours*, vol. II. Longman, Brown, Green and Longman's, 1853.
63. Pancoast J: *A Treatise of Operative Surgery*. Philadelphia, Carey & Hart, 1844.
64. Paré A: *Les Oevres de M. Ambroise Paré*. Paris, G. Buoni, 1575.
65. Petit JL: *Traité des Maladies Chirurgicales*. Paris, T. F. Didot, jeune, 1774.
66. Poulsen K: Die Greschwulste der Mamma. *Arch Klin Chir* 42:593, 1891.
67. Power DA: The history of the amputation of the breast to 1904. *Liverpool Med Chir J* 42:29, 1934.
68. Preus J: *Biblical and Talmudic Medicine*. Translated by Rosner F. New York and London, Sanhedrin Press, 1978, p. 404.
69. Prudente A: Interscapulomammothoracic amputation, in Pact GT, Ariel IM (eds): *Treatment of Cancer and Allied Disease*, vol. 4. New York, Paul B. Hoeber, 1960, p. 133.
70. Riesman D: *The Story of Medicine in the Middle Ages*. New York, Paul Hoeber, 1935.
71. Sachs BC: Breasts: Sex symbols and releasers. *Breast, Diseases of the Breast* 4:26, 1979.
72. Schechter D: Breast mutilation in the Amazons. *Surgery* 51:554, 1962.
73. Schechter D, Swan H: Of saints, surgical instruments and breast amputation. *Surgery* 52:693, 1962.
74. Scultetus J: *Armamentarium chirurgicum Ulmae Suevorum*. B. Kühnen, 1655.
75. Severinus MA: *DeRecondita Absessuum Natura*, Neopoli, 1632.
76. Siegerist HE: *A History of Medicine*, vols. I and II. New York, Oxford University Press, 1951–1961.
77. Robbins GF (ed): *Silvergirl's Surgery—The Breast*. 1984.
78. Sappey MP: *Traité d'anatomie Déscriptive*, 4th ed. Paris, A. Delahage et E. Lucosnier, 1888.
79. Stone RS, Livingston MS, Sloan DH, Chaffee MA: A radio frequency high voltage apparatus for

x-ray therapy. *Radiology* 24:153, 159, 298–302, 1935.

80. Sweeting R: On a new operation for cancer of the breast. *Lancet* 1:323, 1869.
81. Syme J: *Principles of Surgery*. London, Syndenham Society, 1842.
82. Tulp N: *Observationes Medicae*. Amstelredami, 1652.
83. Turner-Warwick RT: The lymphatics of the breast. *Br J Surg* 46:574, 1958–1959.
84. Velpeau A: *A Treatise on the Diseases of the Breast and Mammary Region*, translated by Mitchell Henry. London, Sydenham Society, 1856.
85. Vesalius A: *De Humani Corporis Fabrica*, Basileae, 1543.
86. Virchow RL: *Aintersuchungen über die Entwichelung des Schädelgreindes im Geseinden und Krankhaften Zustände; Die Krankhaften Gerchwulste*, Berlin, G. Reidmer, 1857.
87. Virgil: *Aeneid.* New York, Bantam Books 1:695, 1972.
88. Volkmann R: *Beiträge zur Chirurgie*, Leipzig,. 1875, p. 329.
89. Wangensteen OH: Lewis FJ: Radical mastectomy with dissection of supraclavicular, mediastinal and internal mammary lymph nodes, in Pack GT, Ariel IM (eds): *Treatment of Cancer and Allied Disease*, vol. 4. New York, Hoeber, 1960, p. 122.
90. Wiltse W: The Medical Department. Medical Services in the Mediterranean and Minor Theaters. U.S. Army in World War II. The Technical Services, Office of the Chief of Military History, Dept. of the Army, 1965, pp 350-351.
91. Wolff, J. Die Lehre von der Krebskrankheit von den ältesten zeiten bis zur Gegenwart. Jena, Fischer, 1907–28.

2

Current Controversies Concerning Breast Cancer

Guy Robbins, M.D.

INTRODUCTION

Controversies concerning the utilization of "better methods" of diagnosing and treating women with breast carcinoma concern all of us, not just health professionals. Considerable confusion exists because of the plethora of radio and television talk shows and lay and professional publications which present innovative (often unproven) methods of coping with breast carcinoma. Physicians, potential patients, and their families must become knowledgeable regarding the current status of acceptable options that exist. There is dual patient and physician responsibility in acquiring this information.

EARLIER DIAGNOSIS AND TREATMENT

Local control of the disease is the goal of surgery and/or radiation therapy. Long-term survivals were limited until recently, usually because of delay in diagnosis and treatment. In the 1940s only 20 percent of patients treated for potentially curable breast carcinoma at Memorial Hospital had cancers less than 2 cm in diameter. One-third of the patients had lesions greater than 4 cm. In 1980 to 1981 35.6 percent of potentially curable patients with breast carcinoma had lesions less than 2 cm in diameter and only 12.4 percent had lesions greater than 4 cm in diameter. Those patients with lesions less than 2 cm had a 22 percent incidence of positive axillary nodes compared to a 53 percent nodal involvement if the cancer was greater than 4 cm in diameter.[1] Patients are seeking medical attention when the cancer is more localized and thus are more apt to have a better chance of having long-term survival than in the past, provided efforts to attain maximum local control of the carcinoma are instituted.

In 1933, Dr. James Ewing, then chief medical officer at Memorial Hospital in New York City, had become a proponent of radiation therapy as the primary treatment for breast carcinoma. For several years Dr. Frank Adair and his staff acquiesced to his recommendations of excising the dominant mass and then subjecting the patient to orthovoltage radiation therapy to the involved breast, the ipsilateral axilla, and supraclavicular areas. According to Dr. Adair,[1] the 5-year survival for patients subjected to tumor excision plus x-ray therapy was 26 percent. Those patients subjected to radical mastectomy had a 54 percent 5-year survival. Selection of patients, the utilization of various types of statistics, varied time intervals for survival figures, and questionable quality control of the reporting by pathologists, medical oncologists, surgeons, and radiation therapists have made it impossible to ascertain the true value of many of their reports. In addition, interested but not always knowledgeable consumers disseminate these data by appearing on talk shows and writing articles for lay publications. It is no wonder that potential patients, their families, and many health professionals are confused.

DIAGNOSIS

A patient's failure to seek medical advice after recognizing that her breasts have changed really cannot be considered as a controversial point, but it may well make the difference to the patient between being cured and being palliated. Through the educational programs of the American Cancer Society, the National Cancer Institute, health professionals, and others, patients are more conscious of the need for medical consultation when breast changes are noted.

In the 1940s, only 43 percent of the patients treated for potentially curable breast carcinoma at Memorial Hospital stated that they had noted a breast change in less than 2 months before seeking advice. In 1980 to 1981, 63 percent of our patients came to us in less than 2 months. In the 1940s 31 percent stated that they had waited over 6 months, while in 1980 to 1981 only 12 percent admitted to a greater than 6 months delay.[2]

There is controversy as to what types of abnormalities should be biopsied. Palpation of the mass or thickening and results of mammographic and sonographic studies are helpful but not definitive. Microscopic studies of biopsied breast tissue are essential. We have no faith in thermographic studies.

Specimens from aspiration biopsy of thickenings and solid masses should be utilized for histological diagnosis only if the involved pathologist has a broad and continuing experience in this particular area. A negative aspiration biopsy report requires additional biopsy (incisional or excisional).

When dealing with preclinical breast carcinoma (less than 1 cm), most pathologists prefer paraffin section studies. The increasing popularity of a two-stage procedure which separates breast biopsy from mastectomy is reasonable if the biopsy is done on an outpatient basis or in a surgical center with 1-day hospitalization. However, we have observed that many patients spend considerable time and money getting second, third, and fourth opinions, thus delaying definitive therapy for as long as 3 to 4 weeks. The psychological impact on the patient and her family during these weeks can be disastrous. We still prefer to carry out biopsy and therapy as a single procedure, provided our pathologist gives us positive diagnosis of carcinoma. If an outpatient positive biopsy is obtained, it is essential that receptor studies are performed.

PRETHERAPY EVALUATION

Prior to definitive therapy a general medical evaluation including the documentation of all medications (including aspirin) is recorded.

In addition to the clinical signs indicating that primary breast cancer is operable, such preoperative tests as roentgenography of the chest and screening profile, including serum liver function tests and calcium, potassium, and phosphorus determinations, should show no contraindication to surgery. Bone scans, a more sensitive indicator of unsuspected metastases than skeletal surveys, have been abnormal in 1.5 percent of patients with stages I and II disease, whereas 24 percent of patients with stage III disease had abnormal scans. Robbins et al. showed that within 10 years of treatment of primary breast cancer, only 19 percent (61/321) of patients had osseous metastases.[3]

Our practice is to obtain bone scans in patients with musculoskeletal symptoms, advanced borderline operable lesions, or abnormal screening blood test results, particularly alkaline phosphatase level. In addition, perioperative bone scans are obtained as a baseline determinant on all patients with pathologic involvement of axillary lymph nodes and all candidates for adjuvant chemotherapy or radiation therapy.

TREATMENT CONTROVERSIES

The prime objective of a treatment regimen for women with potentially curable breast cancer has been to provide the greatest chance for cure or long-term survival. If this could be done by preserving the major portion of the breast and still result in preservation of a reasonably acceptable breast and equal or better long-term survival of the affected patient, there would be no controversies. However, it has not been proven to the satisfaction of many that solid data supporting this concept are available.[4–6]

Physicians recommending treatment regimens for women with potentially curable breast carcinoma should be aware of some basic problems involved in the data regarding conventional and innovative approaches to the problem. Foremost is the presentation of *statistics* supporting a particular method of treatment. Response to a treatment regimen should not include only a relatively few number of patients followed for less than 10 years. The statistical method utilized should be clearly defined, and must be the *same* method used by the alternative method of treatment. Comparing experience during a 10-year period is quite different from giving data on patients all of whom were followed up for a minimum of 10-years. Unless there is documentation of quality control of surgery, radiation therapy, and pathology, the reporting of statistical data is less than valid. Multi-institutional studies are especially suspect in regard to quality control.

Local control is all that can be expected when surgery and/or radiation therapy are applied to the breast, chest wall, supraclavicular, internal mammary, and axillary areas. The controversies relate to which approach will produce the most effective results. Studies must break down data according to the size of the lesions and extent of nodal involvement. Loading a cadre of patients with lesions less than 2 cm in diameter, then comparing their survivals to a group of patients whose lesions are of greater diameter and therefore have more nodal involvement, does not provide for accurate evaluation.

Most reports on innovative approaches do not include large numbers of patients, statistics regarding complications, quality of survival of the involved patients, and 10- and 15-year survival figures broken down by the size of the lesions and nodal extent of disease. There is no way available to determine the extent of multicentric invasive and noninvasive carcinoma except by careful histologic study of the total breast. Mammograms often fail and manual palpation of the axilla is usually inaccurate at the 33 percent level. An additional fuzzy area exists in determining which breast carcinomas will be sensitive to the effects of radiation therapy. Most radiotherapists admit to this but do not seem to be concerned. Several therapists believe that treatment of noninvasive breast carcinomas is not warranted in spite of many studies that document the frequent presence of invasive carcinoma in breasts which have noninvasive carcinoma. Carefully acquired data from patients followed from 5 to 25 years have shown that as many as one-third of patients who have had biopsy demonstrating noninvasive carcinoma eventually are shown to have invasive carcinoma in their breasts.[7,8]

The carcinogenic effects of radiation therapy and chemotherapy are recognized, but are far from being quantitated when dealing with breast carcinoma, especially in the young. Perhaps this controversy will be settled, but until then it must be considered when recommending its utilization in the treatment plan.

Adjuvant therapy, be it chemotherapy and/or radiation therapy, is another controversial issue. Radiation therapy is aimed at control or destruction of microscopic foci of disease which may remain after a mastectomy or primary radiation to the breast and axilla. Chemotherapy may be of value in controlling occult systemic disease. Studies are under way to evaluate the combination of adjuvant radiation and chemotherapy. Although early reports regarding adjuvant chemotherapy were quite positive, long-term survival figures do not seem to have been affected by protocols using available drugs. Studies of results obtained following the use of antiestrogen drugs for patients whose cancers had positive estrogen and progesterone receptors seem to show considerable promise. There certainly is no controversy concerning the need for drugs that will destroy local and systemic deposits of breast cancer. Are they available for clinical use currently?

RECONSTRUCTION

Breast reconstruction following mastectomy has improved technically since the early 1970s. Many procedures have been suggested and discarded for more effective ones. We have observed that pushing for an immediate reconstruction (strictly a clinical experiment) is unfair to patient and surgeon. The patient is under tremendous stress at the loss of a breast and the surgeon requires serious documentation of the complications before considering the procedure as a practical, safe method of reconstruction.

PATIENT SUPPORT

Assistance in the readaptation of patients to society by nurses, social workers, physical therapists, the American Cancer Society's Reach for Recovery Program, and the YWCA Encore Program initially caused considerable controversy among surgeons. Many believed they were being usurped by these efforts. Currently there is a realization that most, if not all of these patients need structured physical and emotional support postoperatively and after hospital discharge. The efforts of these knowledgeable groups of health professionals and educators are supplying previously unmet needs and they are slowly being accepted by surgeons and patients alike.

GUIDELINES FOR SOLVING CONTROVERSIAL ISSUES

1 Patients and physicians must accept the fact that palpation, mammograms, sonograms, and thermograms cannot produce a definitive diagnosis of breast carcinoma.

2 Physicians must be more communicative with patients and their families by taking the time to explain the options facing patients with persistent breast thickenings, breast masses, firm axillary nodes, and serous or bloody nipple discharges.

3 Physicians must acquire and utilize expertise in interpreting statistical analyses presented in the defense of conventional and innovative diagnostic and therapeutic regimens.

4 Physicians must use language understandable to patients and their families when presenting options to them.

5 Physicians must explain the value of long-term survival data versus short-term figures.

6 They must explain the importance of multicentricity, carcinogenesis, and the need for evaluation of the opposite breast (contralateral biopsy).

7 Physicians must explain the potential values and shortcomings of adjuvant chemotherapy and radiation therapy.

8 In order to protect themselves from malpractice suits, physicians must keep detailed, legible office records, including recommendations and patients' responses to them, as well as written notations concerning telephone conversations with patients and their families.

Controversies have never been as strident even though they have existed for many years. Consumer involvement, the plethora of protocols, the deceitful use of statistical methods by investigators, the electronic and written media, the apparent emphasis of femininity over longevity by some women, and the ever-present threat of malpractice suits have spawned and nurtured many of the controversies concerning the management of women with breast cancer.

Perhaps a rational approach to these serious controversies will eventually evolve, and hopefully without increasing the loss in this generation of women because of breast carcinoma.

REFERENCES

1. Adair FE: Cancer of the breast. *The Practitioner* 115:473, November 1950.
2. Pilipshen SJ, Gerardi J, Bretsky S, Robbins GF: The significance of delay in treating patients with potentially curable breast cancer. *Breast* (10): 16, July–September 1984.
3. Robbins GF, Knapper WH, Barrie J: Metastatic bone disease developing in patients with potentially curable breast cancer. *Cancer* 29:1702, 1972.
4. Kinne DW. De Cosse J: New developments in the management of breast disease. *Surg Annu* (13): 163, 1981.
5. Osborne MP: Controversies in the management of primary breast cancer—A surgical analysis. *Cancer Investigation* 1(3):259, 1983.
6. De Cosse J, Kinne DW, Robbins GF: Controversies Concerning Breast Cancer—A Focus on Properly Managing the Patient. Brochure published by Breast Service, Department of Surgery, Memorial Sloan-Kettering Cancer Center, 1275 York Avenue, New York, NY 10021, 1982.
7. Hutter RVP, Foote FW Jr, Farrow JH: In situ lobular carcinoma of the female breast. Cancer Year Book Medical Publishers, 1968.
8. Betsill WL, Rosen PP, Lieberman PH, Robbins GF: Intraductal carcinoma, *JAMA* 239:1863, 1970.

Part Two

The Patient at Risk

3

Breast Cancer Risk Factors

Curtis Mettlin, Ph.D.

INTRODUCTION

The study of risk factors for breast cancer includes some of the important historical landmarks in cancer epidemiology.[1] Early in the eighteenth century, Ramazzini observed that breast cancer occurred more frequently among nuns, a risk which he incorrectly attributed to celibacy. In 1844, Rigoni-Stern quantified the relative risk of breast cancer in nuns as being five times that of the other female population. Most of the known risk factors for breast cancer, however, were not identified until recently. In this chapter, the major known risk factors for breast cancer will be described. Because the role of heredity is discussed elsewhere it will not be considered further here. (See Chap. 4.)

APPLICATIONS OF THE CONCEPT OF RISK

Epidemiologists usually focus on risk factors in identifying means of disease prevention. Perhaps the best-known example is the identification of cigarette smoking as a risk factor for lung cancer. However, it is not always the case that an identified risk factor lends itself to a preventive intervention. For example, having a family history of cancer is known to be a risk for an individual, but there is nothing one can do to prevent having a family history of cancer.

Seidman et al.[2] suggested that as much as 80 percent of breast cancer risk is not explained by known risk factors when considered either singly or in combination. They further demonstrated that most breast cancer patients do not have any of the known risk factors for the disease. The implication they drew was that "all women should be treated as at appreciable risk for breast cancer."

Even if the risk factors do not allow one to predict with precision who might develop breast cancer, risk factors may have other important uses with respect to female breast cancer. For example, awareness of risk factors may motivate women to seek appropriate screening and detection services.

Risk should be distinguished from cause. A risk factor may not be a sufficient or necessary antecedent to the onset of disease. However, implicit in the concept of risk is the notion that the presence of the risk factor has a known probability of association with disease occurrence. That probability can be so high as to nearly exclude other possible explanations of cause, such as with cigarette smoking and lung cancer. On the other hand, the association of a single risk factor with the disease occurrence may be so small as to require consideration of a number of different variables as having potentially equal or greater contributions to disease etiology. The latter situation tends to reflect our understanding of breast cancer etiology where the range of possible risk factors includes demographic characteristics such as social class and ethnicity, family history of disease, reproductive history, diet and obesity, previous breast disease, and exposure to a range of potential carcinogens including estrogens and ionizing radiation.

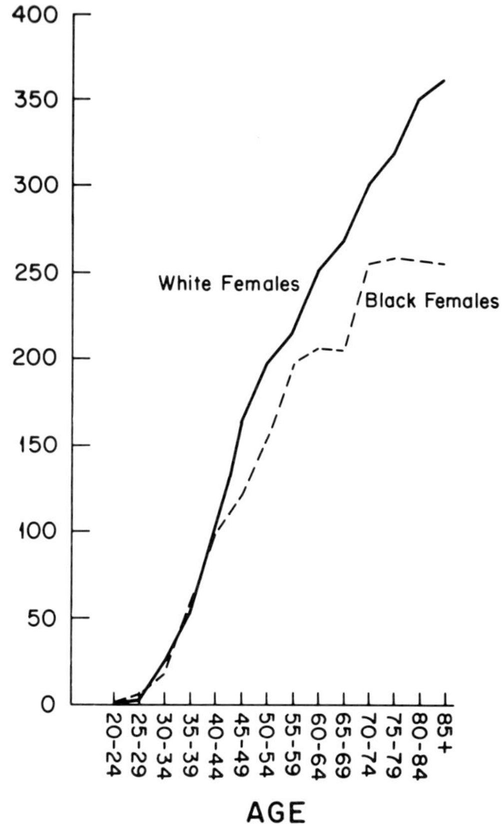

Figure 3-1 Age-specific incidence rates for female breast cancer in the United States, 1973–1977, by race. (*From Young, Percy, Asire.*[6])

PATTERNS OF OCCURRENCE

One of the reasons we have been able to identify so many risk factors for breast cancer is that large numbers of cases are available for study. Breast cancer is the most common cancer occurring among women. In the United States, 26 percent of incident cancers are breast cancers.[3] Analyses of cancer incidence trends by Devesa and Silverman have shown that the incidence rate for breast cancer has changed very little during the last four decades.[4]

Although common in both black and white women, the patterns of incidence and mortality do differ between these two groups. Figure 3-1 shows the age-specific incidence rates for female breast cancer in the United States during the 1973 to 1977 period for blacks and whites. These data suggest that the incidence rates are the same among younger women, but among older women, white female rates are greater than those of black females. Austin et al. have shown that the incidence rates for black and white women do not differ for women born after 1925.[5] This suggests that the incidence differential observed among older women may disappear in future years. The cumulative lifetime risk (from age 0 to 74) of incidence of breast cancer for white women in the United States is estimated to be 8.2 percent, and for black women, 7.0 percent.[6]

Figure 3-2 shows the age-specific death rates for white females and black females in the United States. Although the risk of death at

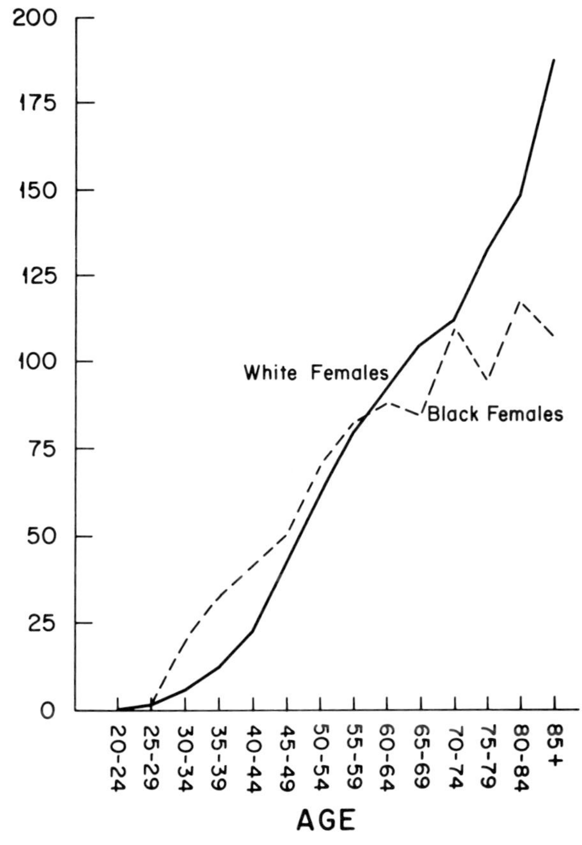

Figure 3-2 Age-specific mortality rates for female breast cancer in the United States, 1973–1977, by race. (*From Young, Percy, Asire.*[6])

older ages is less among black females, reflecting their lower incidence rate, the risk of death is greater among young black women. Overall, the cumulative lifetime risk of breast cancer death in the United States is the same for black and white women, 2.7 percent. The reasons for the greater mortality rate among younger black women has been the subject of considerable speculation. Possible factors involved in this include a later stage of diagnosis of breast cancer among young black women, a lower rate of estrogen receptor assay among black patients, differences in medical care, or differences in histologic types of cancers diagnosed in blacks compared to whites.[7–9]

The pattern of breast cancer mortality varies markedly when examined on an international scale. Figure 3-3 shows the age-adjusted death rates from breast cancer in 1976 from 40 countries.[10] Several developed nations have rates that exceed those of the United States. In contrast, there are some nations where breast cancer is relatively rare. Japan, for example, has a highly developed medical record system that reports little breast cancer mortality. Other Asian populations have similarly low rates. These international variations have prompted researchers to investigate aspects of culture and environment that may affect breast cancer risk, most particularly diet. Studies of breast cancer in Japanese women and their descendants who migrate to Hawaii and the continental United States indicate the the risk of breast cancer increases as the population migrates, giving

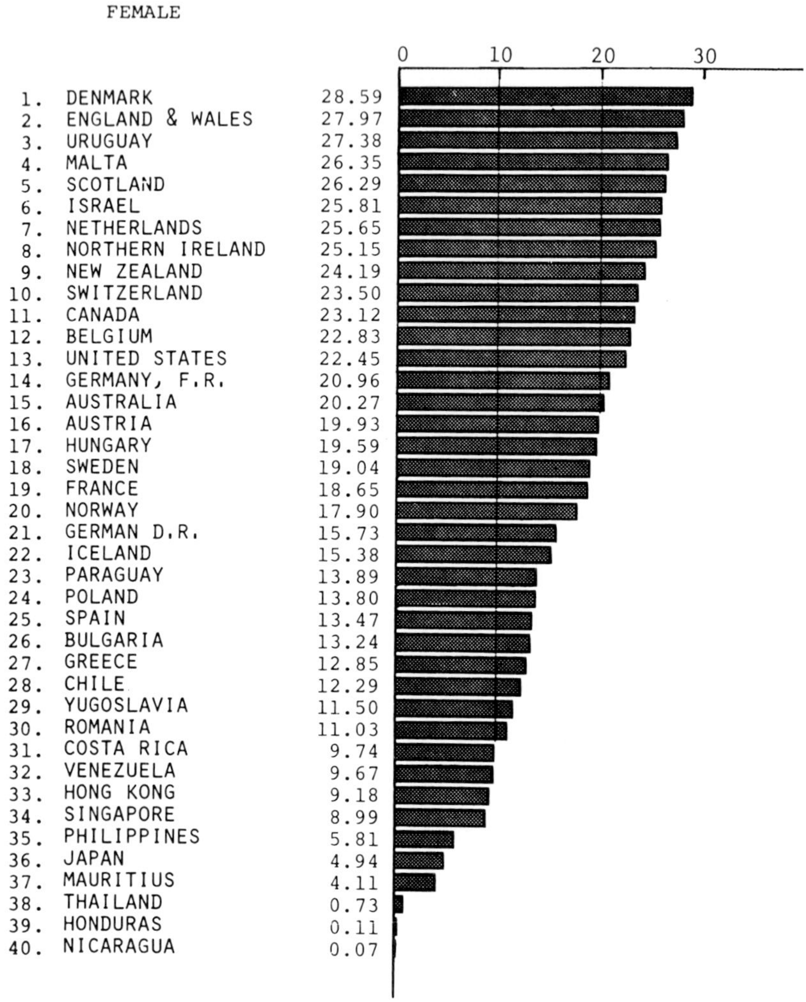

Figure 3-3 Age-adjusted death rates for breast cancer in 1976 from 40 countries. (*From Segi Institute.*[10])

further credence to the concept that environmental and cultural factors may contribute to the international variations observed.[11]

REPRODUCTIVE FACTORS

Although celibacy was first suspected, parity has been determined to be the relevant indicator of risk. Nulliparous women have significantly greater risk than parous women, but little additional protective benefit appears to result from additional pregnancies beyond the first.[12]

Age at the time of the first live birth is also significant. MacMahon has shown that breast cancer risk increases with increases in age at which the woman bears her first full-term child.[12] Women whose first delivery occurs after the age of 35 have a threefold greater risk than those first parous before the age of 18. Janerich has suggested that the protective effect of early first pregnancy may relate only to cancers occurring after the age of 40.[13] He suggests that early age at first pregnancy actually may promote the occurrence of breast cancer in younger women. Given that breast cancer in younger women is relatively rare, even accepting Janerich's hypothesis, the net effect of early age of first pregnancy on breast cancer incidence has to be regarded as protective.

Additional factors related to reproduction which are associated with breast cancer risk include early menarche, late menopause, and surgical menopause. The protective effect appears to be greater when the operation occurs at a younger age. Overall, the protective effect of surgical menopause has been estimated as involving a 40 percent reduction of risk.[12]

BENIGN BREAST DISEASE

A history of benign breast disease has been shown to confer a two- to threefold increase in risk for the subsequent occurrence of breast cancer.* Coombs and Lilienfeld conducted a prospective study of 747 women diagnosed at Roswell Park Memorial as having benign breast diseases during the 1957 to 1965 period.[14] Follow-up of this group and of a matched control population through mailed questionnaires, tumor registry reports, and death certificates, showed that the age-adjusted incidence of breast cancer was three times higher in the benign breast disease group than in the control group. Hutchinson et al. determined rates of breast cancer in a group of 1489 women treated for biopsy proven benign breast disease in a single surgery practice from 1940 to 1975.[15] Follow-up of the population showed that 66 of the women subsequently developed breast cancer. This number was two times greater than expected on the basis of the risk of the general population. However, as MacMahon points out, it is not common for a breast cancer patient to report a history of benign breast disease.[12] Only 5 percent of breast cancer patients report earlier benign breast conditions. This observation further confirms the observation that most breast cancers occur among women who have no established risk factor.

*The histologic subtype of benign breast disease is a significant factor when considering the malignant potential. (See Chap. 5.)

EXOGENOUS ESTROGENS

Does the use of oral contraceptives affect the risk of breast cancer? Given the very large number of women in the United States who have been exposed for some portion of their reproductive lives to oral contraceptives, it is an exposure that would be of public health significance if it has effects on breast tumorigenesis. Fortunately, most published reports suggest little impact on breast cancer risk from use of oral contraceptives. The Centers for Disease Control (CDC) has reported on the analysis of 689 breast cancer patients compared to 1077 control subjects.[16] The study is significant not only for the number of patients involved but also for the fact that the pattern of use in a number of women dates back 15 years and there was opportunity to examine longer-term exposure to oral contraceptives. The overall result was that oral contraceptive use had a relative risk of 0.9 compared to never having used oral contraceptives. The level of risk is not significantly less than 1.0 and it is not possible to assert a protective effect for oral contraceptive use, but the data clearly contradict the suggestion that oral contraceptive use may be associated with increased risk. Neither duration of oral contraceptive use nor the length of time since the first use appeared to influence breast cancer risk. It had been hypothesized that certain subcategories of women such as those with benign breast disease or a family history of cancer may be at increased risk of breast cancer when these risk factors are combined with oral contraceptive use. This hypothesis was not supported in the CDC data.

In England, Vessey et al. have reported on a 12-year study of oral contraceptive use and breast cancer risk.[17] The findings were regarded as reassuring because few statistically significant differences in oral contraceptive use were found between breast cancer and control groups. Kelsey et al. reported a case control study of patients seen in several large hospitals in Connecticut and found no significant association between the use of oral contraceptives and the risk of breast cancer.[18]

Several studies have examined the possible relationship between breast cancer and the use of estrogens following menopause. The findings have been negative, with no consistent pattern of elevated risk of breast cancer being associated with use of menopausal estrogens. The Drug Epidemiology Unit in Boston compared patterns of conjugated estrogen and other forms of noncontraceptive estrogen use among 1610 women with breast cancer and 1606 control subjects[19] This study did not support the hypothesis that noncontraceptive estrogen use represents a source of risk for breast cancer. No effects were evident among premenopausal or postmenopausal women, among persons with benign breast disease, or among persons with a family history of breast cancer. No combination of noncontraceptive estrogen use and any other known risk factor for breast cancer suggested an interaction that resulted in increased risk.

Thus, the general thrust of epidemiologic evidence on the relationship of exogenous estrogen use to breast cancer risk has been to suggest no significant breast cancer risk. However, Greenwald has pointed out a number of issues which justify continuing research on this question.[20] These issues include the fact that oral contraceptive use is a relatively recent phenomenon and few long-term data are available. Furthermore, there are subcategories of risk status and combinations of risk factors that may increase the potential risk from oral contraceptive use beyond that which has been observed in studies to date.

RADIATION EFFECTS

Exposure to ionizing radiation increases the risk of breast cancer in women. This has been shown in a number of epidemiologic studies. McGregor et al. followed 63,275 female Nagasaki and Hiroshima atomic bomb survivors.[21] They observed a dose-response relationship to neutron and gamma radiation that yielded an overall absolute risk per rad of 1.9 excess cases per 1 million women years at risk. Women 10 to 19 years old at the time of exposure experienced much greater excess risk of breast cancer than did women older than 35 at the time of exposure.

Shore et al. followed 571 women who had been treated with x-rays for acute postpartum mastitis.[22] Compared to a control population, the relative risk of exposure to a mean dose of 347 rads to both breasts rose to 3.6 20 years following exposure. In this study, the excess risk was estimated to be eight to ten excess cases per rad per million women years. Boice and Monson followed 1047 women who received an average of 102 fluoroscopic examinations over a period of several years as part of their course of tuberculosis therapy.[23] Their estimate of the excess risk of this exposure was 6.2 excess "cases" per rad per million women years. They observed higher risk for women whose exposure to repeated fluoroscopic examinations initially occurred before the age of 30. Female radium dial workers have been studied by Adams and Brues, who located 1180 dial workers first employed before 1930.[24] These women exhibited a 50 percent greater risk of death from breast cancer compared to the comparably aged general female population.

Exposure to relatively high doses of ionizing radiation significantly elevates breast cancer risks. Furthermore, there is some consistency in the data suggesting that exposure during adolescence poses greater risk than exposure at later ages. The evidence concerning the effects of radiation on breast carcinogenesis has been important in evaluating the risk and benefits of mammography. Because of the very low doses involved in mammographic examinations relative to other studies of radiation carcinogenesis, there are no direct estimates of risk based on the observation of women exposed to routine mammographic examinations. However, extrapolations of risk based on the high dose data when combined with the benefits estimated to be derived from early detection of breast cancer from mammographic examinations, suggest that the far greater effect of mammography is to increase life expectancy.[25]

DIET

Dietary factors have recently become objects of intensive research with respect to their role in the etiology of breast cancer. Part of the basis for this interest is the fact that international variations in breast cancer rates suggest substantial differences which may be attributable to dietary differences. Because diet is a factor to which everyone is exposed, the public health importance can be very significant. Of greatest interest has been the possible role of dietary fat in elevating breast cancer risk. Other nutritional factors are also under investigation.

The interest in the role of dietary fat and breast cancer has been stimulated by experimental data involving the study of mammary tumors in mice or rats. Carroll and Khor showed that animals exposed to the carcinogen 7,12-dimethylbenz(a)anthracene (DMBA) and fed diets containing 10 and 20 percent by weight of corn oil developed more mammary adenocarcinomas than animals fed 0.5 percent and 5 percent corn oil diets.[26] The high-fat-diet rats bore more tumors per rat, more rats bore tumors, and the tumors began to appear more rapidly among the high-fat-diet group. Carroll and Hopkins and others further showed that fewer tumors are produced in animals fed saturated fats than in those fed unsaturated fats.[27]

The high unsaturated fat diet known to be associated with promotion of rat mammary tumors has been suggested as reflecting the average American diet in which 40 percent of the calorie intake is from dietary fat. Indeed, age-adjusted mortality rates of breast cancer exhibit a high correlation with international patterns of per capita fat consumption.[28] Mettlin has suggested that within the United States, the lower risk of breast cancer among black women may be attributable to their less frequent intake of fats and oils.[29] Similarly, Seventh-Day Adventists, who have a lower than average fat intake because of vegetarian dietary practices, have been shown to have lower cancer death rates than the general population.[30]

Under the hypothesis that diet might affect cancer risk by influencing circulating lipid levels, the association of breast cancer with serum cholesterol has been investigated. Hiatt et al. studied a cohort of 95,179 women for whom serum cholesterol, lipoproteins, and total lipid measures had been obtained.[31] Follow-up of the cohort revealed 1035 cases of breast cancer. They observed that the level of blood lipids has no value in predicting subsequent breast cancer risk. Under the hypothesis that breast cancer and gallstone disease share intake of dietary fat as a common etiologic factor, Adami et al. studied breast cancer incidence in a cohort of 11,678 women who had undergone cholecystectomy.[32] Follow-up after 11 to 14 years of observation revealed an incidence of breast cancer not significantly greater than that among comparably aged women in the general population. Thus, these data suggest that breast cancer does not share etiologic factors with gallstone disease, and that if dietary fat is related to one of the diseases, it possibly is not related to the other.

Some retrospective studies comparing the reported dietary habits of breast cancer patients with a comparable control population have suggested that more frequent consumption of high-fat-containing foods characterizes these patients relative to controls. For example, elevated risks have been associated with use of butter as opposed to margarine, and the more frequent consumption of beef and pork, which are common sources of animal fats in the western diet.[33,34] Not all studies are consistent in this regard, however. Patients entering Roswell Park from 1957 to 1965 were interviewed regarding their dietary habits and food consumption habits.[35] Analysis of 2024 breast cancer patients compared to 1463 control patients showed no differences in reported fat intake.

Dietary fat intake in the United States on a per capita basis has been increasing throughout this century. Between 1913 and 1976 total fat consumption in the United States increased 27 percent, from 125 g per person per day to 159 g per person per day. The greatest proportion of this increase is attributable to increased use of separated fats and oils such as margarine, vegetable oil, and shortening.[36] Thus, the overall effect is not only an increase in dietary fat content, but also a high proportion of polyunsaturated fat. In light of these trends in dietary fat intake and the predictions of the laboratory data, one might expect to observe increased rates of breast cancer associated with this changing dietary pattern. However, breast cancer incidence among white women in the United States has been virtually unchanged for the last four decades. Although there may be many interacting factors that would obscure a relationship between changes in dietary fat intake and breast cancer incidence, the overall association does not suggest that significant reduction in breast cancer risk would be associated with a reversal of the historical trend of increasing dietary fat intake.

In addition to dietary fat, there are a number of nutritional aspects of the western diet that are under investigation with respect to their possible inhibitory effects in breast carcinogenesis. For example, the antioxidants butylated hydroxyanisole (BHA) and butylated hydroxytoluene (BHT) are widely used as food preservatives. Experimental data on rat mammary gland carcinogenesis show that both BHA and BHT inhibit DMBA-induced neoplasia.[37] Studies of Ip and others at Roswell Park have shown that selenium is capable of reducing the tumor yield and extending the latency period preceding tumor appearance in animals challenged with DMBA.[38] Additionally, it has shown that a combination of sodium selenite and retinyl acetate supplementing the diet have additive effects in reducing the incidence of DMBA-induced tumors.[39] Studies in humans are lacking. In one study at Roswell Park, we did observe a reduction in risk associated with a higher intake of vitamin A.[35] This was only apparent among the older women and the reduction in risk was relatively modest. Wald et al. recently reported on a prospective study of 5004 women in Guernsey for whom plasma samples had been collected and stored.[40] Retinol, beta carotene, and vitamin E levels later were measured in samples from 39 women who subsequently developed breast cancer and from 78 controls who did not. Their findings indicated that although the retinol and beta carotene levels did not differ between the cases and controls, low plasma vitamin E levels showed a clear association with higher risk of cancer. Over the range of levels studied, there was a fivefold increase in risk associated with low plasma levels of vitamin E.

It is possible that important modification of risks may result from some combination of dietary factors such as the reduction in fat as well as the improvement of nutritional status with respect to some vitamins or trace elements in the diet. *Although the potential for dietary manipulation of breast cancer risk is substantial, its true nature and significance is not yet established.*

CONCLUSION

Breast cancer is among the most epidemiologically studied cancers. A large number of environmental and individual traits have been associated with risk for this disease. In this selective review of risk factors, we have focused on those categories of risk for which there have been substantial consistency in research results. However, in all these areas there is a need for refinement and further focus to identify and understand the biological mechanisms involved.

REFERENCES

1. Shimkin MD: Some historical landmarks in cancer epidemiology, in Schottenfeld D (ed.): *Cancer Epidemiology and Prevention*. Charles C Thomas, Springfield, Illinois, 1975.
2. Seidman H, Stellman SD, Mushihski MH: A different perspective on breast cancer risk factors; some implications of the nonattributable risk. *CA* 32:301, 1982.
3. American Cancer Society: *Cancer Facts and Figures, 1984*, American Cancer Society Inc, New York, 1984.
4. Devesa SS, Silverman DT: Cancer incidence and mortality trends in the United States: 1935–1974. *J Natl Cancer Inst* 60:545, 1978.
5. Austin H, Cole P, Wynder E: Breast cancer in black American women. *Int J Cancer* 24:541, 1979.
6. Young JL, Percy CL, Asire AJ: Surveillance, Epidemiology and End Results: Incidence and Mortality data, 1973–1977. *Natl Cancer Inst Monograph 57*, DHEW Publication (NIH) 81-2330, Washington, D.C. U.S. Government Printing Office, 1981.
7. Mohla S, Sampson CC, Khan T, Enterline JP, Lefall L, White JR, Gabriel BW, Hunter JB: Estrogen and progesterone receptors in breast cancer in black Americans. *Cancer* 50:552, 1982.
8. Nemoto T, Vana J, Natarajan N, Bedwani R, Mettlin C: Observations on short-term and long-term surveys of breast cancer by the American College of Surgeons. I. Significance of the number of axillary nodes, and II. Estrogen receptor assay in the U.S. in 1977, in Murphy GP (ed.): *International Advances in Surgical Oncology* 4:209, 1981.
9. Vana J, Bedwani R, Mettlin C, Murphy GP: Trends in diagnosis and management of breast cancer in the U.S. from the surveys of the American College of Surgeons. *Cancer* 48:1043, 1981.
10. Segi Institute of Cancer Epidemiology: *Age-adjusted Death Rates for Cancer for Selected Sites in 43 Countries in 1977*. Segi Institute Publication, Nagoya, Japan, 1982.
11. Buell P: Changing incidence of breast cancer in Japanese-American women. *J Natl Cancer Inst* 51:1479, 1973.
12. MacMahon B, Cole P, Brown J: Etiology of human breast cancer: A review. *J Natl Cancer Inst* 50:21, 1973.
13. Janerich DT: Pregnancy, breast cancer risk and maternal-fetal genetics. *Lancet* 1:327 (June 2), 1979.
14. Coombs J, Lilienfeld AM, Bross IDJ, Burnett WS: A prospective study of the relationship between benign breast diseases and breast carcinoma. *Prev Med* 8:40, 1979.
15. Hutchinson WP, Thomas DB, Hamlin WB, Roth GJ, Peterson AV, Williams B: Risk of breast cancer in women with benign breast disease. *J Natl Cancer Inst* 65(1), 1980.
16. The Centers for Disease Control Cancer and Steroid Hormone Study: Long-term oral contraceptive use and the risk of breast cancer. *JAMA* 249:1591, 1983.
17. Vessey M, Baron J, Doll R, McPherson K, Yeates D: Oral contraceptives and breast cancer: Final report of an epidemiological study. *Br J Cancer* 47:455, 1983.
18. Kelsey JL, Holford TR, White C, Mayer ES, Kilty SE, Acheson RM: Oral contraceptives and breast disease. *Am J Epidemiol* 107:236, 1978.
19. Kaufman DW, Miller DR, Rosenberg L, Helmrich SP, Stolley P, Schohenfeld D, Shapiro S: Noncontraceptive estrogen use and the risk of breast cancer. *JAMA* 252:63, 1984.
20. Greenwald P, Nasca PC, Burnett WS, Howe HL, Houton J: Breast cancer: Epidemiology and screening. *NY State J Med* 84:47, 1984.
21. McGregor DH, Land CE, Choi K, et al: Breast cancer incidence among atomic bomb survivors, Hiroshima and Nagasaki, 1950–1969. *J Natl Cancer Inst* 59:799, 1977.
22. Shore RE, Hempelmann LH, Kowaluk E, et al: Breast neoplasms in women treated with x-rays for acute postpartum mastitis. *J Natl Cancer Inst* 59:813, 1977.

23. Boice JD Jr, Monson RR: Breast cancer in women after repeated fluoroscopic examinations of the chest. *J Natl Cancer Inst* 59:823, 1977.
24. Adams EE, Brues, AM: Breast cancer in female radium dial workers first employed before 1930. *J Occ Med* 22:583, 1980.
25. American Cancer Society: *Guidelines for the Cancer-related Check-up: Recommendations and Rationale. CA* 30:194, 1980.
26. Carroll KK, Knor HT: Effects of level and type of dietary fat on incidence of mammary tumors induced in female Sprague-Dawley rats by 7,12-dimethylbenz(a)anthracene. *Lipids* 6:415, 1971.
27. Carroll KK, Hopkins GJ: Dietary polyunsaturated fat versus saturated fat in relation to mammary carcinogenesis. *Lipids* 14:155, 1978.
28. Wynder EL, Hyams L, Shigematsu T: Correlations of international cancer death rate: An epidemiological exercise. *Cancer* 20:113, 1967.
29. Mettlin C: Diet and the epidemiology of human breast cancer. *Cancer* 53:605, 1984.
30. Phillips RL: Role of lifestyle and dietary habits in risk of cancer among Seventh-Day Adventists. *Cancer Res* 35:3513, 1975.
31. Hiatt RA, Friedman GD, Bawol RD, Ury HK: Breast cancer and serum cholesterol. *J Natl Cancer Inst* 68:885, 1982.
32. Adami HO, et al: Cholecystectomy and the incidence of breast cancer: A cohort study. *Br J Cancer* 49:235, 1984.
33. Miller AB, Kelly A, Choi NW, et al: A study of diet and breast cancer. *Am J Epidemiol* 107: 499, 1978.
34. Lubin JH, Burns PE, Blot WJ, Ziegler RG, Lees AW, Fraumeni JF: Dietary factors and breast cancer risk. *Int J Cancer* 28:685, 1981.
35. Graham S, Marshall J, Mettlin C, Rzepka T, Nemoto T, Byers T: Diet in the epidemiology of breast cancer. *Am J Epidemiol* 116:68, 1982
36. Brewster L, Jacobson MF: The changing American diet. Center for Science in the Public Interest, 1978.
37. Wattenberg LW: Inhibition of carcinogenic and toxic effects of polycyclic hydrocarbons by phenolic antioxidants and ethyoxyquin. *J Natl Cancer Inst* 48:1425, 1972.
38. Ip C: Factors influencing the anticarcinogenic efficacy of selenium in dimethylbenz(a)anthracene-induced mammary tumorgenesis in rats. *Cancer Res* 41:2683, 1981.
39. Ip C, Ip MM: Chemoprevention of mammary tumorgenesis by a combined regimen of selenium and vitamin A. *Carcinogenesis* 2:915, 1981.
40. Wald NJ, et al: Plasma retinol, B-carotene and vitamin E levels in relation to the future risk of breast cancer. *Br J Cancer* 49:321, 1984.

4

Heredity in Breast Cancer

Henry T. Lynch, M.D.
Vincent R. Pennisi, M.D., D.D.S.
Jane F. Lynch, B.S.N.

INTRODUCTION

Familial breast cancer was recognized in the Roman medical literature of 100 A.D.[1] There is now substantial evidence that a subset (at least 5 percent) of all patients with breast cancer has a hereditary etiology.[2,3]

It is important to distinguish between "familial" and "hereditary" breast cancer. We define *familial* breast cancer as an aggregation of breast cancer within a family which could be due to chance alone, to common environmental exposures, or which could even be a result of primary genetic factors. The data are usually insufficient to ascribe a clear-cut hereditary etiology.[1] On the other hand, when we discuss *hereditary* breast cancer, we infer that there is sufficient information within the pedigree to signify that primary genetic factors are of major etiologic importance.[4,5]

Certain clinical features aid immeasurably in assessing the significance of genetic factors. We refer to them as cardinal clinical features of hereditary breast cancer,[1,6] and they include the following:

1 Significant *early* age of onset of breast cancer, with the average age being 44, as opposed to the general population estimates of about age 60.[7]

2 An excess of *bilateral* breast cancer. Our results indicate that the cumulative risk to the contralateral breast over a 20-year period among patients with hereditary breast cancer is 46 percent.[8]

3 Hereditary breast cancer is *heterogeneous* and may show differing tumor combinations in kindreds which are integral to specific hereditary breast cancer syndromes (Fig. 4-1).[9] For example, breast cancer may appear in association with carcinoma of the ovary in the so-called breast/ovarian carcinoma syndrome (Fig. 4-2),[10] or it may appear in an exceedingly complex setting characterized by *S*arcoma; *B*reast cancer and brain tumors; *L*ung cancer, laryngeal carcinoma, and leukemia; and *A*drenal cortical carcinoma (SBLA syndrome) (Fig. 4-3).[11] Breast cancer may also appear as an integral component of

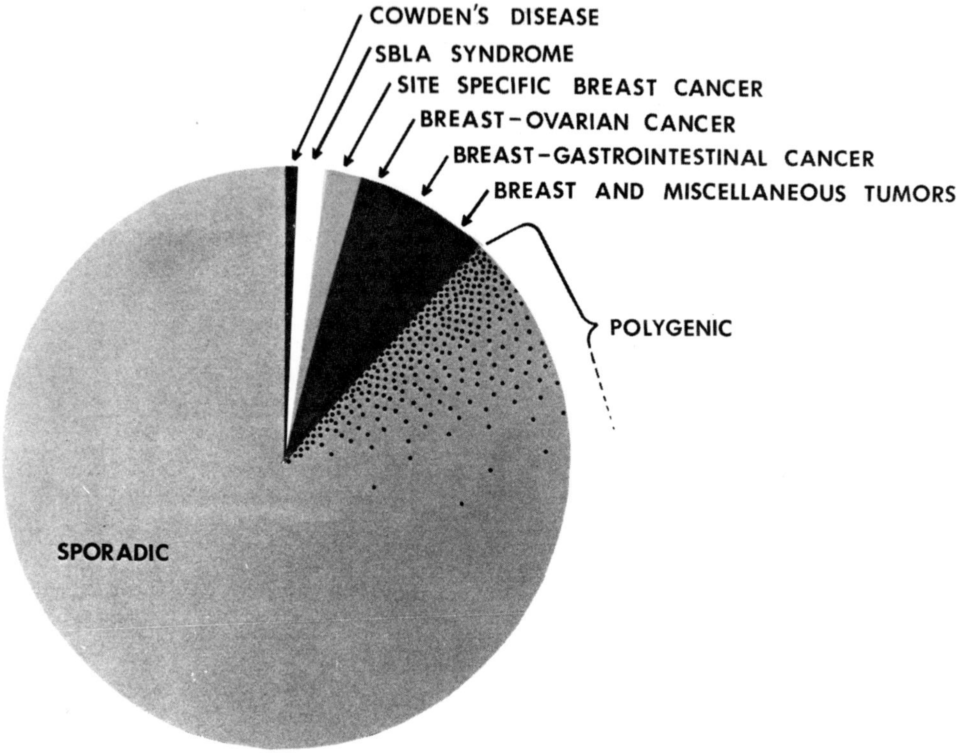

Figure 4-1 Schematic illustrating hereditary breast cancer syndromes. (*From Lynch et al.*[6])

certain cancer-associated genodermatoses.[12] This is clearly seen in Cowden's disease, an autosomal dominantly inherited disorder which has features of multiple trichilemmomas (a cutaneous sign which is virtually pathognomonic for this syndrome) (Fig. 4-4), virginal hypertrophy of the breasts, an increased frequency of carcinoma of the thyroid, and possibly colon cancer secondary to multiple adenomatous polyps. These patients are at an inordinately high risk for bilateral breast cancer. We have recently learned of the occurrence of breast cancer in a 21-year-old woman with Bloom's syndrome, an autosomal recessively inherited genodermatosis (courtesy of Stephen Lichter, M.D.).

4 Hereditary breast cancer segregates within kindreds in accord with an autosomal dominant mode of inheritance, as evidenced by studies of segregation analysis.[13] These analyses have shown heterogeneity of the disease, as evidenced by the monitored tumor associations. In addition, the breast cancer susceptibility gene shows putative linkage with glutamic-pyruvic transaminase (GPT).[14]

MAGNITUDE OF HEREDITARY BREAST CANCER

In order to derive a crude estimate of the frequency of hereditary breast cancer, we evaluated family histories on 225 consecutive patients with verified breast cancer in Creighton's oncology clinic.[3] We excluded all patients who were referred for genetic evaluation in order to avoid biasing our sample. We found that 13 percent of the patients fulfilled criteria for familial breast cancer, while 5 percent fit our hereditary criteria. The remaining 82 percent were considered to be sporadic (Fig. 4-5). We consider our estimate of 5 percent as being hereditary to be highly conservative.

A certain percentage of so called sporadic occurrences will have been the result of a fresh mutation in the germinal lines of one of their parents. Short of a biomarker which can *unequivocally* define the cancer-prone genotype, we will have to await the test of time to determine their etiology through prospective studies of the families. On the other hand, over the course of time the family histories of some of the sporadics may prove to be hereditary once clearer patterns of tumor expression emerge within their kindreds.

OBTAINING AN INFORMATIVE FAMILY HISTORY

We have developed the concept of the "modified nuclear pedigree" as a practical measure for the assessment of family history. This covers all *first-degree* relatives (parents, siblings, children) and *second-degree* relatives (both maternal and paternal sets of grandparents, aunts, and uncles) (Fig. 4-6). We focus on these latter individuals since they are more likely to be informative given their older ages, and cancer correlates with advancing age. Hereditary breast cancer is most probably autosomal dominantly inherited. This means that the deleterious gene is present on one of the autosomal chromosomes, as opposed to the X or Y chromosomes. Hence, *males* may be harbingers of the deleterious genotype and transmit this to their daughters, who may then express the phenotype (cancer), while their sons (dependent upon cancer-prone genotype) may or may not express cancer. This is why it is essential to study both maternal *and* paternal lineages of the kindred. Heretofore, attention has been focused by many physicians only upon the *maternal* lineage. The pedigree in Fig. 4-2 illustrates maternal *and* paternal transmission of hereditary breast cancer, in addition to the heterogeneity of this problem.

Once an informative portion of the pedigree is discerned, it may then become necessary to extend the pedigree to more remote relatives to assess fully the significance of the transmission of breast cancer and/or its association with other forms of cancer. Figure 4-2 shows an example of this problem in a family which has been classified as having the hereditary breast and ovarian carcinoma syndrome.

BIOMARKERS ASSOCIATED WITH BREAST CANCER-PRONE GENOTYPE

There is thus a dire need for the recognition of biomarkers which will aid in the definition of breast cancer susceptibility genes. Because of the problems of heterogeneity in hereditary breast cancer, any single biomarker may not be linked to *all* forms of hereditary breast cancer. At the present time, great effort is being expended toward identifying biomarkers in this disease.[1–3] (See Chap. 14.)

One promising example has been described by Fishman et al., who studied blood and 12-h daily urine samples which were collected throughout a single menstrual cycle in 30 women at high risk for familial breast cancer.[15] These data were then compared with an equal number of meticulously matched controls. Abnormal estrogen conjugation was observed at the periovulatory stage of the menstrual cycle in the women who were at high risk for familial breast cancer. Plasma androsterone sulfate was significantly lower in these high-risk subjects, while the plasma estrone and estradiol glucuronides showed a decreased trend. There was a trend for increased urinary estrone and estradiol glucuronides among these high-risk subjects.

Another potentially informative biomarker in hereditary breast cancer is increased in vitro hyperdiploidy, in the presence of normal tetraploidy, in cultured skin fibroblasts

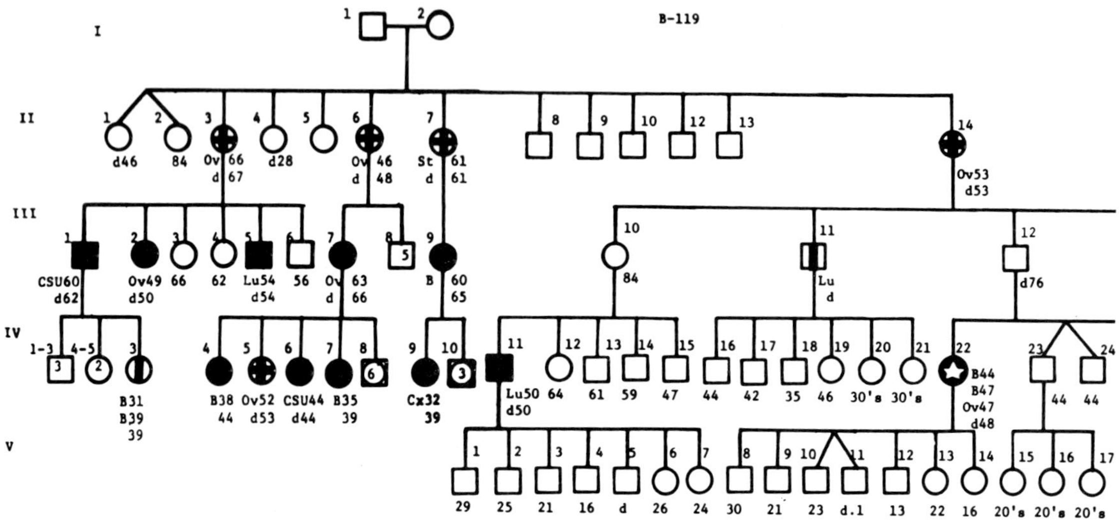

Figure 4-2 Updated pedigree of a family showing breast cancer in association with ovarian and other cancers. Note that males III-1 and III-12 were apparently harbingers of the deleterious gene and transmitted breast cancer to their daughters. (*Previously reported in Lynch et al.*[10])

from affected and high-risk members of breast cancer-prone kindreds.[2,3] These findings, while preliminary, merit testing on additional families (See Fig. 4-7).

SEGREGATION ANALYSIS AND GENE LINKAGE

Eighteen large kindreds from Creighton's Breast Cancer Family Resource were investigated to test the hypothesis that a single gene increased breast cancer susceptibility, and that such a gene may segregate according to Mendelian laws in some families.[13] Sixteen of the pedigrees showed findings consistent with an autosomal dominant mode of inheritance, while the two remaining families fit an environmental hypothesis. Heterogeneity by tumor association was observed.

In a companion paper, in seven families with primarily premenopausal breast cancer and five families showing the combination of breast and ovarian cancer, a dominant susceptibility allele was shown to be putatively linked to the genetic marker glutamic-pyruvic transaminase (GPT), with a lod score of 1.95 at zero recombination.[14]

The data require cautious interpretation. In any family with possible GPT linkage, women who carry the hypothetical susceptibility allele would be at high risk for breast cancer, whereas relatives who do not carry that allele would not be at an increased breast cancer risk. The GPT genotype, however, is not associated with breast

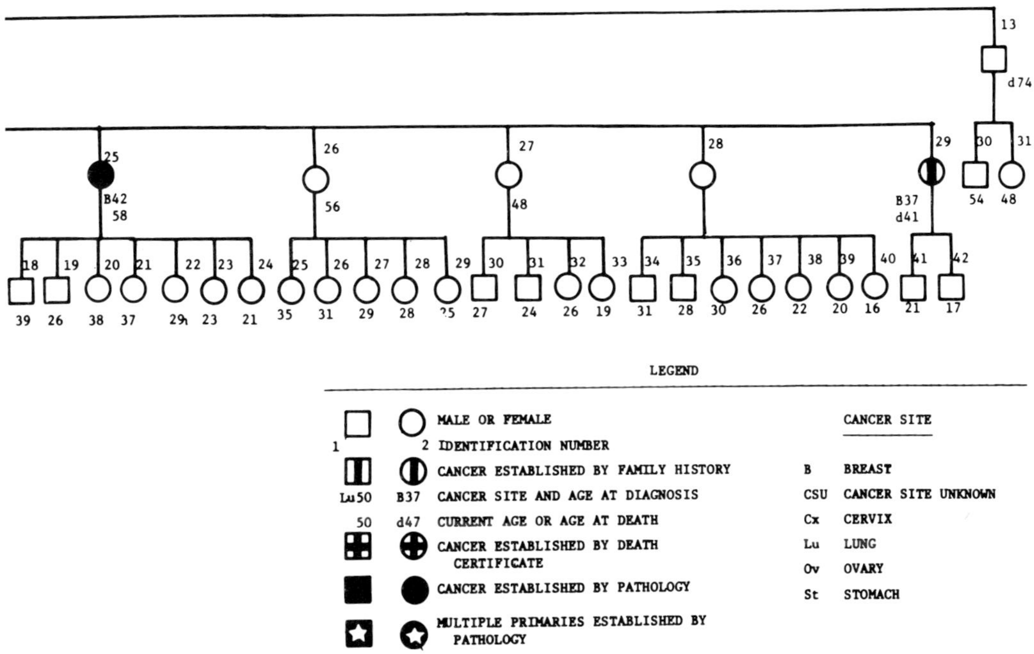

cancer in the general population, and therefore this cannot be used as a screening test. GPT has been assigned to the short arm of chromosome 16. Genes for a regulator of interferon production and a regulator of antiviral state are believed to be located on this same chromosome. Hence, it would be interesting to investigate linkage between these loci and hereditary breast cancer.

We stress the potential value of linkage studies for research as well as for clinical utility because it would be possible to (1) detect genetically susceptible young women from high-risk families *prior* to clinical symptoms; (2) counsel highly selected cases who would become candidates for surgical prophylaxis; (3) determine if more than one genetically influenced form of breast cancer exists, an assumption that we have confidence in on a clinical basis, but which we would like to confirm through further linkage studies; (4) investigate why some genetically susceptible women do *not* develop breast cancer; (5) scrutinize the role of environment in genetically susceptible women more critically; and (6) study biochemical and physiologic mechanisms by which a gene increases breast cancer susceptibility, by comparing young women who have not yet developed breast cancer with other young women in the same family who are at low risk (by linkage analysis). This would enable comparison of appropriate immunologic, biochemical, and endocrinological parameters

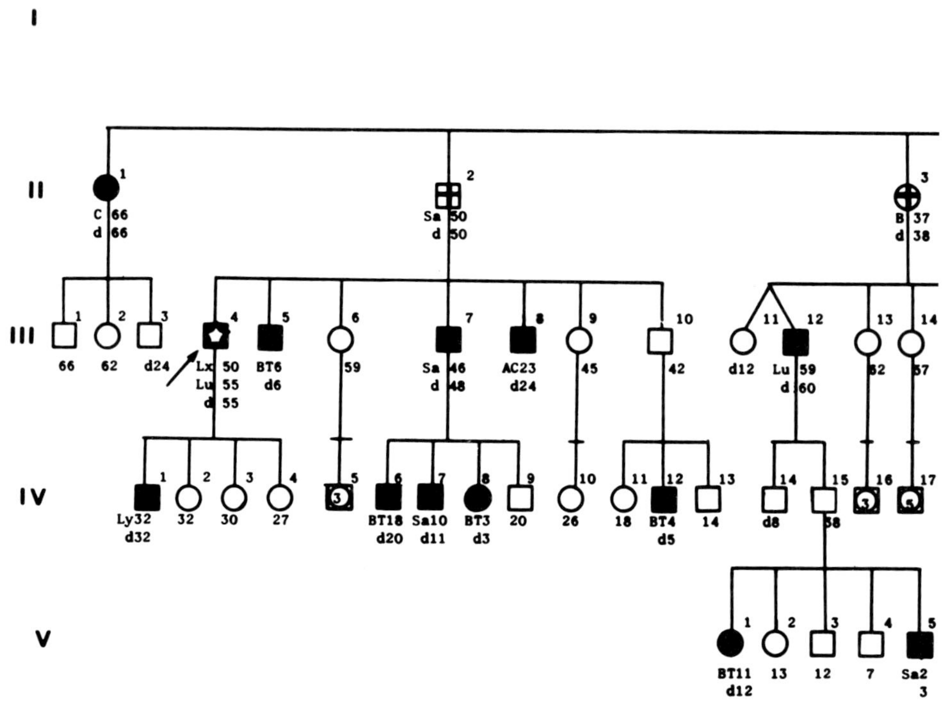

Figure 4-3 Updated pedigree of a family with the SBLA syndrome. (*From Lynch et al.*[3])

among these high- and low-risk young women and would be potentially informative in understanding how breast cancer susceptibility genes are expressed. The implications for prevention of familial breast cancer would then become legion.

EDUCATION, PREVENTION, AND CONTROL: THE HEREDITARY CANCER INSTITUTE

Major obstacles to the achievement of effective preventive care may be that listeners (patients as well as physicians) do not perceive provided information as being relevant. Screening of the general population is not cost-effective.

Preventive health care and patient education are relevant, cost-effective, and crucial, especially to the highest cancer risk population known, namely, those first-degree relatives of *hereditary* breast cancer patients. Within a clearly defined hereditary breast cancer pedigree, women who are at 50 percent risk will be the parents, siblings, or progeny of a breast cancer-affected patient. Because of variable age

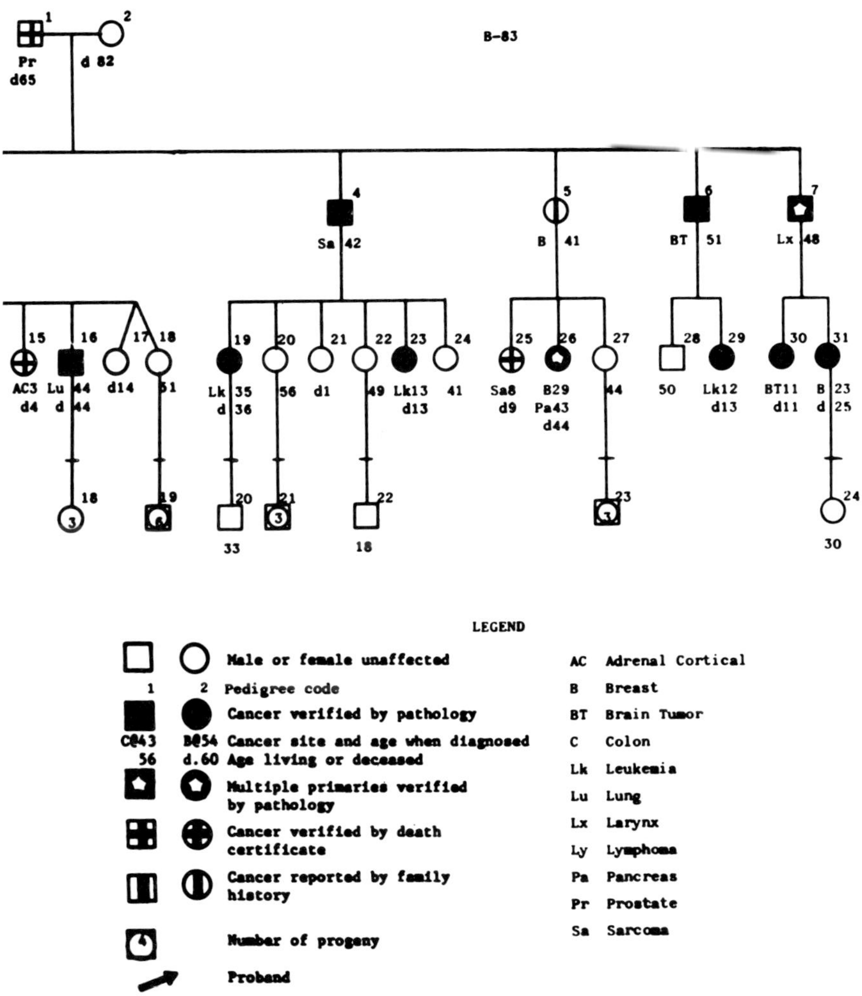

of onset, the parent or sibling may not yet have expressed the cancer phenotype. It may be more difficult to define the risk to progeny in the case of paternal transmission since the father may not express breast cancer due to sex-influenced or sex-limited factors. The most difficult area in managing high-risk patients centers around the need for an accurate delineation of genetic risk status. In certain settings this may be accomplished with relative ease, as when the cardinal features of hereditary breast cancer are striking. Such an example would be a patient whose mother and maternal aunt had early-onset, bilateral breast cancer. The occurrence of the disease in the patient's sister would crystallize the issue. The patient would then clearly be at 50 percent risk for development of breast cancer. However, of greater difficulty would be a situation where there is a negative history on the patient's maternal side, but the patient's paternal grandmother may have had early-onset breast cancer. A paternal great-aunt also may have been affected at an early age. Bilaterality may or may not have been present. If her father

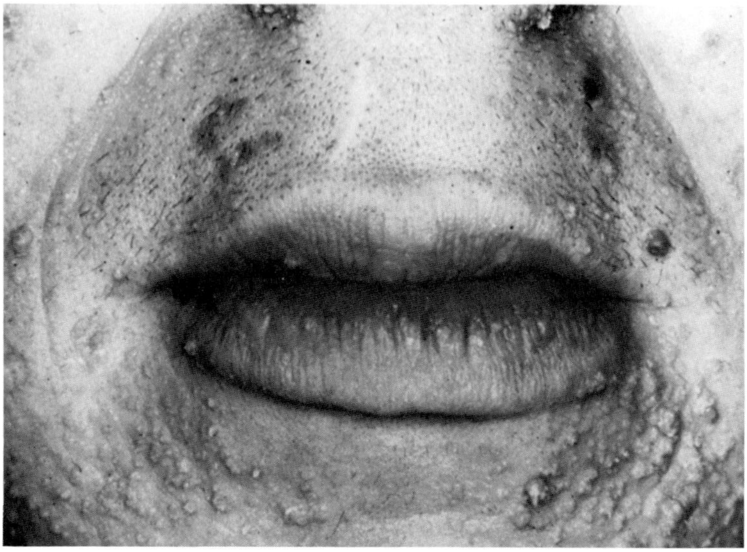

Figure 4-4 Facial trichilemmomas from a 35-year-old woman with oral fibromas, hypothyroidism, xanthomas, vitiligo, and severe fibrocystic disease of the breasts. Prophylactic bilateral simple mastectomies were performed. [*By permission of Brownstein MH, in Lynch HT (ed): Genetics and Breast Cancer. Van Nostrand Reinhold, New York, 1981.*]

had affected sisters, this would then increase the likelihood that he might be a carrier of the deleterious gene. The issue would then become clearer if the patient's sister manifested early-onset breast cancer. In certain of these types of complex circumstances, it will be prudent for the physician to consult with a medical geneticist who is knowledgeable in the area of cancer genetics.

In many circumstances, environmental risk factors such as dietary factors, alcohol consumption, excess estrogen intake, smoking, and the proliferative form of fibrocystic breast disease may interact with the deleterious cancer-prone genotype and could represent additive risk factors incorporated into the overall risk assessment and preventive program.

One such example of how perplexing this issue is concerns the absence of a protective effect of early age at first pregnancy in hereditary breast cancer. Specifically, Lynch et al. have shown that the generally accepted dictum of an early term first pregnancy providing a protective effect against the development of breast cancer may not be applicable to the hereditary breast cancer population (Fig. 4-8).[16]

Preventive implications are legion, once breast cancer-prone families are identified. Our Hereditary Cancer Institute (HCI) is a reference center which furnishes information concerning all aspects of hereditary cancer. There are over 100 well-established hereditary cancer syndromes, over 70 of which are autosomal dominantly inherited. Information about highly targeted, pragmatic cancer preventive care programs are available for patients and physicians.*

*The Hereditary Cancer Institute, California and 24th Streets, Omaha, Nebraska 68178.

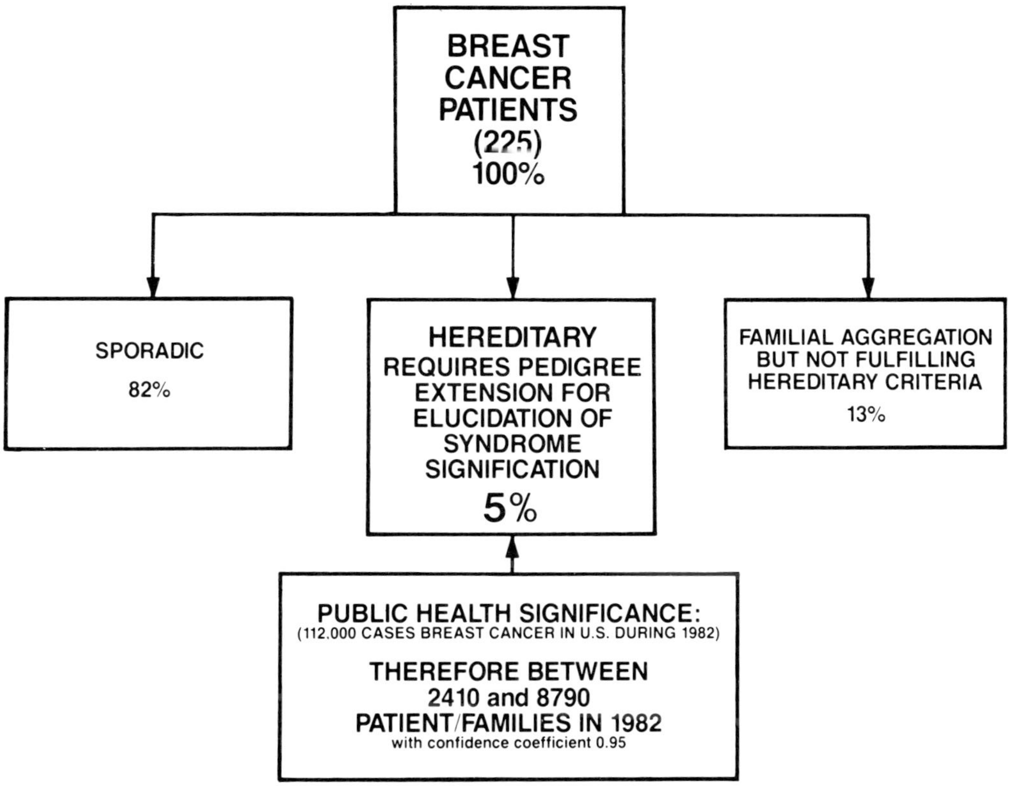

Figure 4-5 A schematic breakdown of 225 consecutively ascertained patients with breast cancer with respect to the percentage of those showing familial, hereditary, or sporadic breast cancer. (*From Lynch et al.*[3])

We recommend the following guidelines for high-risk women who are members of hereditary breast cancer families:

1 Instruct all patients about self-breast examination and have them perform this procedure periodically to assure that they are doing this examination correctly.

2 Provide a rationale as well as the statistical figures showing the benefit relevant to improved survival through earlier detection. Stress the need to have their breasts evaluated by their physician at least twice per year. We also discuss in detail the importance of biopsy when indicated.

3 We recommend that a baseline mammogram be performed on women at 50 percent risk for breast cancer by age 25. These are to be repeated every 2 to 3 years or more frequently if clinical and mammographic findings warrant.

GENETIC COUNSELING

When a patient is clearly at risk for hereditary breast cancer, genetic counseling should be initiated. This is integrated with all facets of the medical management of the patient. This entire process should be both patient- and physician-centered. Thus, genetic counseling involves a meticulous delineation of the family history, interpretation of its significance to the patient and her close relatives, diagnosis, treatment, and prognosis. For genetic counseling to be effective, it must sensitively embrace all the psychodynamic issues relevant to the subject

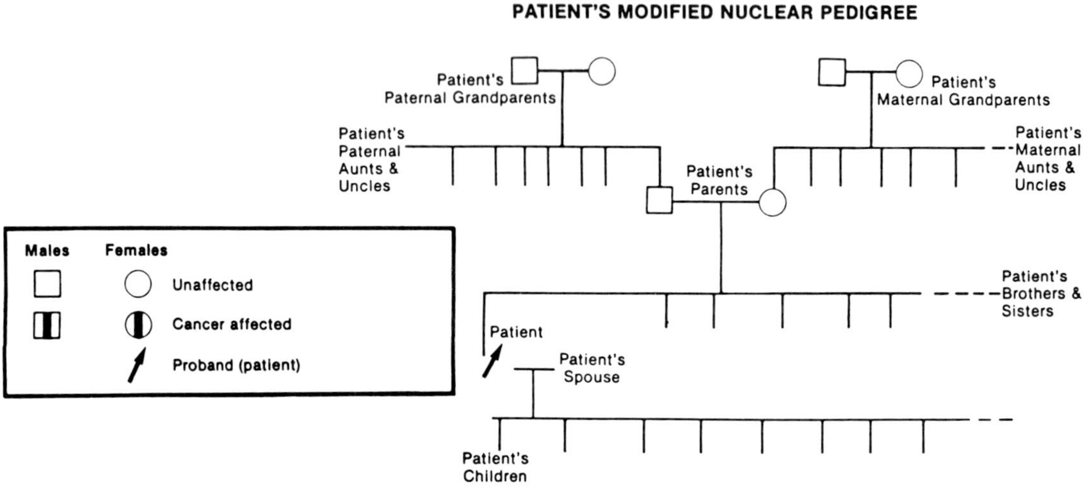

Figure 4-6 Diagram representing a modified nuclear pedigree.

disorder, a matter which may be particularly emotionally burdensome when dealing with the breast.[17,18]

PROPHYLACTIC SUBCUTANEOUS MASTECTOMY (PSM)

We prefer this operation because it is most acceptable to patients. Although this operation has many shortcomings and is not universally accepted, it fulfills a specific need for this subset of patients.[19–23]

Because of the dearth of knowledge about genetic indications for PSM, we provided initial guidelines which are intended specifically for the management of consultands* from breast cancer-prone families who may be considered as candidates for intensive surveillance and/or selective-elective prophylactic surgery.[4,5] The guidelines are as follows:

1 Ascertain histologic verification of cancer occurrences among the consultand's parents, siblings, offspring, grandparents, aunts, and uncles. If the consultand has a strong *maternal* history of breast cancer, as evidenced by histologically confirmed mammary carcinoma in her mother, plus any combination involving her sisters, maternal grandmother, and maternal aunts, then the consultand is herself at high risk for the disease and should be considered for PSM. If the consultand has a strong *paternal* history of breast cancer, as evidenced by histologically confirmed mammary carcinoma in the paternal grandmother or one or more paternal aunts, then the issue becomes more complicated. In this situation, the consultand should be a candidate for PSM if one or more of her sisters has already developed breast cancer. Clinical judgment for PSM is strengthened further in those more rarely occurring circumstances when *both* the maternal and paternal histories are positive for breast cancer and when close relatives have manifested premenopausal breast cancer and/or bilateral disease. Histological verification is essential in decision making because of the confounding errors from hearsay evidence supplied by family relatives and/or death certificates.

2 Extend the consultand's pedigree to other second-degree relatives and, when possible, even further, since such investigation could reveal significant tumor associations consonant with one of several familial breast cancer-prone syndromes.

*Consultand is the index case, i.e., the family member who first brings a family to the attention of the doctor.

3 Evaluate the consultand for additional risk factors believed to contribute to breast cancer, including age at menarche, menopause, obesity, presence of chronic cystic mastitis with histologic verification of proliferative changes, past radiation exposure to the chest and breast area, and socioeconomic/ethnic background. In addition, the age of the consultand relative to the age at cancer onset among her relatives may generally provide indications for the timeliness of initiating intensive surveillance and/or PSM. While there may be exceptions to the clustering of age of cancer onset in a given family, consultands who have passed through high-risk age intervals should remain under surveillance, but their need for PSM will lessen.

4 When considering prophylactic surgery, carefully assess and evaluate the consultand's attitudes and feelings, not only about her cancer risk, but also her psychological status and her emotional response to cancer per se, including the presence or absence of cancer phobia. She should be advised that her body image may be changed and that erogenous zones of the breast may be altered. Explanation of all these issues should be given to the consultand's husband and he should play an important role in decision making.

5 A detailed description of the surgical procedure (PSM), including the extent of possible morbidity, as well as the cosmetic results available through advanced technology in the hands of skilled surgeons, should be provided. She should also be made fully cognizant of the fact that all breast tissue is not removed, and therefore breast cancer risk still exists. The decision to undergo PSM carries an approximate 50 percent false-positive rate when based on the best possible familial breast cancer risk estimate.

6 A consultand with histologically verified unilateral breast cancer who meets the criteria of hereditary breast cancer, and who is psychologically and medically suitable (i.e., no evidence of widespread metastases or serious chronic debilitating disorders), should be advised to undergo PSM of the opposite breast.

7 Consultands from families prone to hereditary breast and ovarian carcinoma require special consideration for both target organs. Those consultands from breast and ovarian cancer-prone families who have breast cancer initially should undergo PSM of the contralateral breast (as stated in paragraph 6).

8 Ideally, the decision-making process for PSM should embrace consultation from an informed medical geneticist, a second surgical opinion, and most importantly, close interaction of the medical team with the consultand and her husband.*

ALTERNATIVE SURGICAL METHODS

There are alternative surgical methods to prophylactic subcutaneous mastectomy. The indications are the same and the usual criteria must be met.

The most radical approach to this problem is the complete amputation of both breasts. This certainly removes at least 95 percent of breast tissue. However, this form of total mastectomy will leave the female patient with an unsightly chest which may be acceptable to a few, but is unacceptable to most women.

Total mastectomy with immediate or delayed reconstruction is to be considered for certain patients.[25]

SUMMARY

Breast cancer etiology and control remain important challenges of this century. Perhaps for the first time in dealing with human breast cancer, we can talk about *hereditary* breast cancer with credibility, based upon laborious investigations of countless extended families.[1–11] Further credence from these clinical studies has been provided by segregation analysis,[13] and gene linkage studies with putative linkage of the breast cancer susceptibility gene to the GPT locus on the small arm of chromosome 16.[14] Endocrine patterns in hereditary subsets have also been informative. These have shown abnormal

**Editorial note*: Although subcutaneous mastectomy removes the bulk of breast tissue, there are no adequate data to demonstrate that it reduces the incidence of breast cancer.

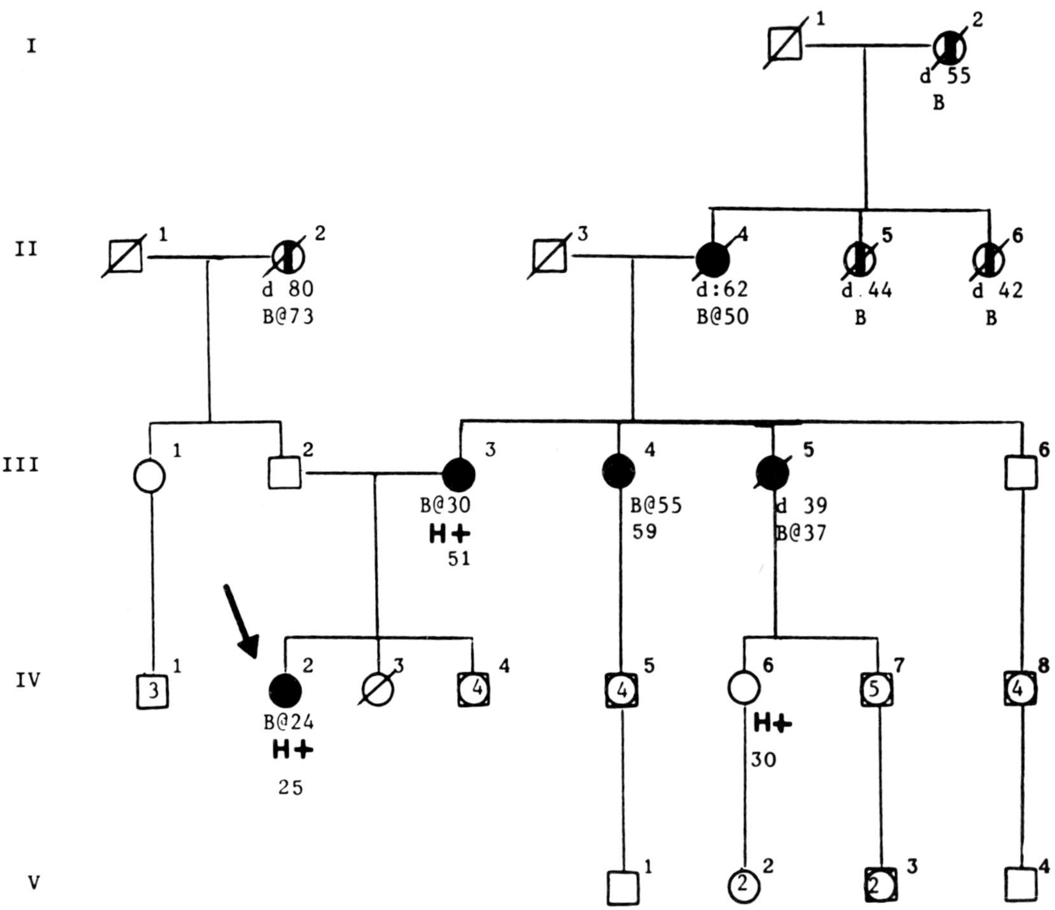

estrogen conjugation at the periovulatory stage of the menstrual cycle in those women who are at high risk for this disease. These patients demonstrated plasma andosterone sulfate which was significantly lower, while the plasma estrone and estradiol glucuronides showed a decreased trend, with a trend for an increase in urinary estrone and estradiol sulfates in concert with a significant decrease of urinary estrone and estradiol glucuronides.[15]

We now estimate that the hereditary subset constitutes about 5 percent of all breast cancer occurrences while an additional 13 percent of all breast cancer occurrences show familial aggregation (Fig. 4-5).

Descriptively, we see certain cardinal clinical features which characterize hereditary breast cancer. Foremost are early age of onset, excess of bilaterality, and heterogeneity as evidenced by certain patterns of tumor combinations within specific breast cancer genotypes (the most heralded of which are the hereditary site-specific and hereditary breast and ovarian cancer variants), and a consistent pattern of autosomal dominant transmission as evidenced clinically for many years[1] and now supported by segregation analysis.[13] There is also the possibility of an increased occurrence of medullary breast cancer in the hereditary variety.[1-3] Recently, we have

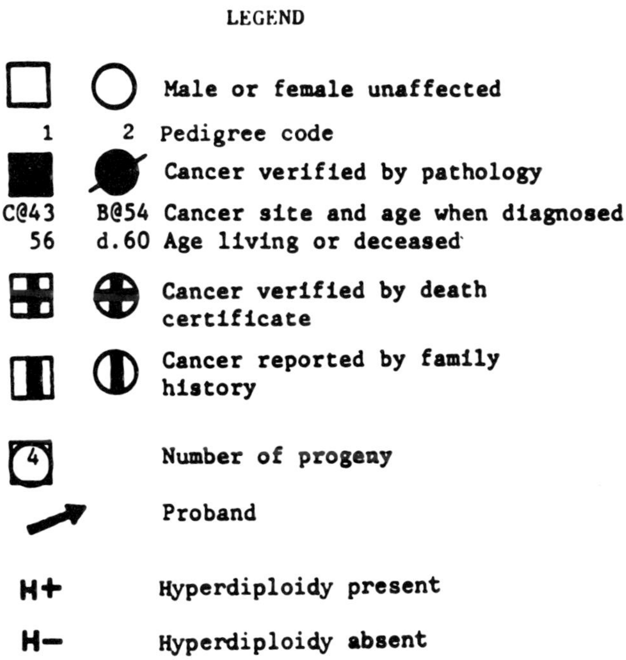

Figure 4-7 Pedigree of a hereditary breast cancer family showing the occurrence of in vitro hyperdiploidy. (*From Lynch et al.*[2])

observed improved survival in the hereditary variety of breast cancer when compared, stage for stage, with the large American College of Surgeons' Audit Series.[1,26,27] These latter observations may possibly be influenced by the putative excess of medullary breast cancer in the hereditary variant.[1] However, these provocative survival findings remain enigmatic and warrant further intensive investigation.

These improved survival findings raise many questions: Are there inborn immunological factors in the hereditary variant, which are less effective in control of this disease than in the sporadic variant? May less radical surgical approaches to the hereditary variant be utilized? Is the hereditary variety of breast cancer more or less likely to respond favorably to radiation therapy than its sporadic counterpart? Are there pharmacogenetic factors which afford advantage to certain forms of chemotherapy in the hereditary variety of breast cancer when compared to sporadic occurrences of this disease? Are patients with hereditary breast cancer more apt to benefit from specific forms of hormonal therapy when compared to sporadic breast cancer? Surprisingly, we have no systematic data on these important questions. However, we should begin addressing these issues.

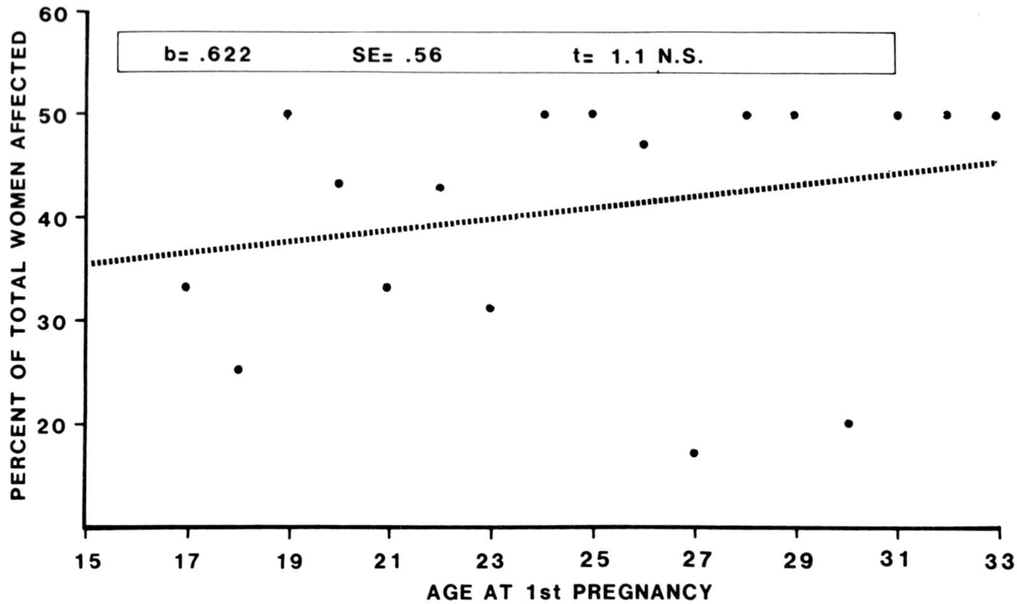

Figure 4-8 Percentage of females affected as a function of age at first pregnancy in the Creighton Hereditary Breast Cancer Family Resource. (*From Lynch et al.*[16])

The most important concern at this time is education of the patient and physician so that both parties can participate prudently and efficiently in identifying and managing hereditary breast cancer.

Many of the high-risk patients exhibit a paradoxical delay emanating from the conflict engendered by knowledge of the disease occurring excessively in their family coupled with evidence of its morbidity and mortality, all acting in concert with the stereotype given the breast in our society.[1,28] The physician should encourage patients at high risk to begin exercising some of the strict surveillance measures which are advocated.

We are hopeful that through Creighton's Hereditary Cancer Institute, we will be able to mount national and international programs directed toward hereditary cancer, with particular attention to breast cancer.

REFERENCES

1. Lynch HT: *Breast Cancer Genetics*. New York, Van Nostrand Reinhold Co., 1981.
2. Lynch HT, Albano WA, Layton MA, Lynch JF, Costello KA, Tindall SL, Wagner CA, Cheng SC: Genetic predisposition to breast cancer. *Cancer* 53:612, 1984.
3. Lynch HT, Albano WA, Heieck JJ, Mulcahy GM, Lynch JF, Layton MA, Danes BS: Genetics, biomarkers, and control of breast cancer: A review. *Ca Genet Cytogenet* 13:43, 1984.
4. Lynch HT, Harris RE, Organ CH, Lynch JF: Management of familial breast cancer, Part I. *Arch Surg* 113:1053, 1978.
5. Lynch HT, Harris RE, Organ CH, Lynch JF: Management of familial breast cancer, Part II. *Arch Surg* 113:1061, 1978.
6. Lynch HT, Albano WA, Organ CH, Schmitz GD, Lynch JF: Surveillance and management of hereditary breast cancer. *Breast* 7:2, 1982.
7. Lynch HT, Guirgis H, Brodkey F, Maloney K, Lynch PM, Rankin L, Lynch JF:

Early age of onset in familial breast cancer: Genetic and cancer control implications. *Arch Surg* 111:126, 1976.

8. Harris RE, Lynch HT, Guirgis HA: Familial breast cancer: Risk to the contralateral breast. *J Natl Cancer Inst* 60:955, 1978.
9. Lynch HT, Krush AJ, et al: Tumor variation in families with breast cancer. *JAMA* 222:163, 1972.
10. Lynch HT, Harris RE, Guirgis HA, Maloney K, Carmody L, Lynch JF: Familial association of breast/ovarian cancer. *Cancer* 41:1543, 1978.
11. Lynch HT, Mulcahy GM, Harris RE, Guirgis HA, Lynch JF: Genetic and pathologic findings in a kindred with hereditary sarcoma, breast cancer, brain tumors, leukemia, lung, laryngeal, and adrenal cortical carcinoma. *Cancer* 41:2055, 1978.
12. Lynch HT, Fusaro RM: *Cancer-Associated Genodermatoses*. New York, Van Nostrand Reinhold Co., 1982.
13. Go RCP, King M-C, Bailey-Wilson J, Elston RC, Lynch HT: Genetic epidemiology of breast cancer and associated cancers in high risk families, Part I. *J Natl Cancer Inst* 71:455, 1983.
14. King M-C, Go RCP, Lynch HT, Elston RC, Terasaki PI, Petrakis NL, Rodgers GC, Lattanzio D, Bailey-Wilson J: Genetic epidemiology of breast cancer and associated cancers in high risk families, Part II. *J Natl Cancer Inst* 71:463, 1983.
15. Fishman J, Bradlow HL, Fukushima DK, O'Connor J, Rosenfeld RS, Graepel GJ, Elston R, Lynch H: Abnormal estrogen conjugation in women at risk for familial breast cancer at the periovulatory stage of the mentrual cycle. *Cancer Res* 43:1884, 1983.
16. Lynch HT, Albano WA, Layton MA, Kimberling WJ, Lynch JF: Breast cancer, genetics, and age at first pregnancy. *J Med Genet* 21:96, 1984.
17. Lynch HT: *Dynamic Genetic Counseling for Clinicians*. Springfield, Charles C Thomas, 1969, p. 354.
18. Lynch HT, Lynch PM, Lynch JF: Genetic counseling and cancer, Kessler S (ed): *Genetic Counseling: Psychological Dimensions*. Academic Press, 1979, p. 221.
19. Woods JE, Masson JK, Irons GB: Experience with subcutaneous mastectomy. *Surgery* 80:422, 1976.
20. Freeman BS: Subcutaneous mastectomy for benign breast lesions with immediate or delayed prosthetic replacement. *Plast Reconstr Surg* 30:676, 1962.
21. Pennisi VR, Capozzi A, Perez FM: Subcutaneous mastectomy data: A preliminary report. *Plast Reconstr Surg* 59:53, 1977.
22. Pennisi VR, Capozzi A, Perez FM: Subcutaneous mastectomy data: An interim report. *Breast* 5:18, 1979.
23. Pennisi VR, Capozzi A: Subcutaneous mastectomy: An interim report on 1244 patients. *Ann Plast Surg* 12:340, 1984.
24. Personal communication of current data by Pennisi.
25. Dowden RV, Horton CE: Total mastectomy for premalignant disease with immediate reconstruction, in Gant TE, Vasconez LO (eds): *Post-Mastectomy Reconstruction*. Baltimore/London, Williams and Wilkins, 1981, p. 113.
26. Albano WA, Recabaren JA, Lynch HT, Campbell AS, Mailliard JA, Organ CH, Kimberling WJ: Natural history of hereditary cancer of the breast and colon. *Cancer* 50:360, 1982.
27. Lynch HT, Albano WA, Recabaren J, Lynch PM, Lynch JF, Elston RC: Prolonged survival as a component of hereditary breast and nonpolyposis colon cancer. *Med Hypoth* 7:1201, 1981.
28. Lynch HT, Krush AJ: Delay: a deterrent to cancer detection. *Arch Environ Health* 17:204, 1968.

5

Fibrocystic Breasts: Diagnosis, Treatment, and Association with Cancer

Irving M. Ariel, M.D.
Pin Kie Teng, M.D.
Romulo Prudente, M.D.

INTRODUCTION

One of the greatest rewards in the practice of medicine is the treatment of a patient with a benign breast cyst. The patient may have recently discovered a large mass in her breast and is most fearful that it represents a cancer. On examination, it is easy to discern the smooth outline signifying a benign cyst. After aspiration of the fluid, the mass disappears. It gives the physician great satisfaction to explain to the patient what it was and see the patient's expression of relief. The authors do not examine the cyst fluid, since several thousand such aspirations and examinations of the fluid for cellular content invariably have shown no indication of malignancy. A few authors have claimed to find signs of malignancy by analyzing cyst fluid, but the yield is very low. However, if a residual mass is palpated after aspiration of the fluid or if the aspirated fluid is bloody, a biopsy is indicated.

What of the patient who presents with multiple nodules, either painful or painless, each varying in size and blending into the surrounding breast tissue without being sharply demarcated? These patients may be said to suffer from fibrocystic disease, a catchall phrase for approximately 50 subsets of disease entities. These include Cooper's disease, Reclus' disease, Schimmelbusch's disease, mazoplasia, mammary dysplasia or dystrophy, adenofibroma, intracanalicular fibroadenoma, ductal papilloma, papillomatosis, gross cystic disease, mammary duct ectasia, cystophorous desquamative epithelial hyperplasia, fibroadenomatosis, mastodynia, florid and sclerosing adenoses, and a host of other names.[5] New entities are constantly being added to this catchall diagnosis, such as microglandular adenosis,[6] granulomatous mastitis,[7] fibromatosis,[8] and others.

If, on aspiration or biopsy of a suspicious mass, the pathologist records one or at times a number of diagnoses, the physician must be able to determine which of these pathologic subsets are potentially dangerous from the standpoint of forming cancer, which are physiologic, and which are a temporary result of hormonal changes. The breast responds to hormonal changes from the time the child is in utero until death. It is very sensitive and undergoes constant changes, answering the ebb and flow of numerous metabolic changes associated with procreation.

Chronic cystic mastitis was first described by Velpeau[9] in 1838 as *induration en masse.* This condition has probably existed from time immemorial, but was not designated a disease entity until Velpeau's classic description. Later, he used the term "chronic induration" and, after giving a concise and complete description, added, "celibacy and the disturbance of menstruation and of uterine functions has seemed to me its regular associates." In 1893 König[10] believed it to be of inflammatory origin and called it "chronic cystic mastitis." This is essentially a misnomer as there is very little if any inflammatory component, but rather an overgrowth of the normal constituents of the breast parenchyma with modest deposition of lymphocytes in certain instances.

Brodie[10a] (1840) described the nature of the disease and suggested it be called "sero-cystic tumor of the breast." Reclus[10b] (1883) was the first to use the microscope and concurred with Brodie's description. In France the disease is sometimes referred to as *maladie Reclus.* Reclus discussed a young patient referred to a famous breast specialist, Dr. Broca, who incorrectly diagnosed the disorder as being cancer because of a family history of cancer, albeit outside the breast. The importance of a family history is thus shown. Schimmelbusch (1892) suggested the term "cystic adenoma" but König felt the name cystic adenoma should be dropped as it was anatomically incorrect. Bloodgood, working with Halsted, divided the cysts into three types: adenomatous, ectasic, and adenocystic. The latter was associated with carcinoma.

PHYSIOLOGY OF THE BREAST

The breast is derived partially from the mesoderm and partially from the ectoderm, which gives rise to the acinar and ductual cellular elements. It first becomes apparent after the third month of gestation. The ducts are lined by columnar epithelium resting on a basement membrane. The alveolae are small and solid, being filled with a mass of granular polyhedral cells. Beginning with the first menses, the acini are well developed, with a patent lumen containing secretions. The stroma is somewhat vascular with lymphocytic infiltration. Involutionary changes appear about the fourth day of the cycle and progress to the twelfth day. These changes are characterized by closure of the acinal lumina so that many become extinct. Secretions and lymphocytes disappear. Beginning about the fifteenth day of the cycle, signs of reactivation appear and multiply, and the lumina become distinct and again contain secretions.

With pregnancy, there is hypertrophy of all aspects of the breast, and with lactation, milk is produced. The breast suffers a loss of elasticity and tends to become prolapsed with lactational involutions. The glandular portion and major ducts are more distinctly palpable because of the decrease in surrounding fat.

Menopausal and Senile Involution

With the onset of menopause, involutionary changes begin to appear in the glandular portion of the breast. These are characterized mainly by atrophy of the lobular structures which are replaced with fat and connective tissue. Fibrosis of surrounding remnants of the suspensory ligament may partly isolate segments of fatty tissue and thus form soft pseudolobulations. As a result of incomplete involution, remnants of lobular structures may persist and appear as multiple, relatively soft, and indistinct thickenings.

HORMONE PHYSIOLOGY

The above changes noted on microscopic examination are the result of hormonal changes associated with the menarche, menses, pregnancy, lactation, and senility.

The development of the ductal elements depends on estrogen stimulation, whereas acinar and alveolar growth depends on estrogen-progesterone. Growth hormone, ACTH, corticoids, insulin, thyroxine, and androgens all play facultative roles. During the follicular phase of the menstrual cycle, estrogens induce minimal mitoses, but estrogen and progesterone provoke considerable mitotic activity. This is opposite to the activity which occurs in the endometrium with regressive changes and which occurs with deciduation of the endometrium. Greenblatt[11] calls attention to an important biologic property of estradiol, which is the induction of progesterone receptors.

The changes which occur during menstruation are excellent examples of the exact synchronization of the response of the breast to hormonal changes. Under the influence of sex steroids, breast size becomes greater because of lobular edema, infiltration of perilobular stroma with fluid, and the appearance of some intra-alveolar secretory activity. During menses, moderate intra-alveolar secretion occurs as a consequence of estrogen-progesterone withdrawal, permitting a limited milk secretory action of prolactin. Mammary blood flow is increased. Under the influence of estrogen, a histamine effect occurs which contributes to breast edema. A diminution of thyroid hormones may contribute to the proliferative hyperplasia. During pregnancy and lactation, all elements increase under the combined influences of estrogens, progesterone, and prolactin. After delivery, with diminution of sex steroids, the presecretory alveolar epithelium is converted into active milk synthesizing and releasing cells, resulting in lactation. If milk is regularly withdrawn, the mammary epithelium continues to secrete milk; estrogens can antagonize the effects of prolactin on milk synthesis. The symptoms of fibrocystic disease improve during pregnancy and lactation.

Under cyclic hormonal influences, inappropriate glandular-alveolar responses may occur, particularly after 30 years of age. With the onset of menopause, considerable regression begins to take place, although residual lesions may remain well into old age. The hormonal and histological complexity of this target gland seems to invite these chordant responses of stimulation and regression, depending upon the endocrine milieu. Many other factors, including environment, stress, diet, menarche, and parity, play a role.

Incidence of Fibrocystic Disease

Chronic cystic mastitis has been described by Love, Gelman, and Silen[12] as a nondisease. With newer knowledge about the earliest forms of breast cancer and the various subsets included under this generic heading, we would term it "the nondisease disease entity."

The breast has been called by some investigators a premalignant lesion. Hutter[13,14] defines premalignancy as "the state preceding the development of malignant characteristics"; in this broad context he considers the female breast to be a premalignant organ. Fibrocystic disease is the most common lesion of the female breast. Stout[15] states that "almost all women over 30 years of age, regardless of the marital or lactational history, have affected mammary glands to a greater or lesser degree." On a clinical basis, evidence of some fibrocystic disease will be found in about 40 percent of women between 20 and 45 years of age, and on autopsy, histologic evidence of fibrocystic disease was found in 53 percent of patients as evidenced by Frantz and associates.[16] Love et al.[12] state that fibrocystic change occurs clinically in 50 percent and histologically in 90 percent of women. The essential change of fibrocystic disease consists of hyperplasia of all mammary cells (lobular and ductal cells, and fibroblasts). The final diagnosis depends upon which histologic changes dominate. It is impossible to evaluate the true incidence of this disorder, since given its broad general definition it is ubiquitous. The pathologist must cease using the generic term and employ a more precise classification.

Histologic Variants

Hyperplasia is the most frequent finding and might be considered the common denominator of most breast pathology. All the tissues of the breast, including the lobular epithelium, the ductal epithelium, and the connective tissue are involved (Figs. 5-1, 5-2, and 5-3). However, usually one tissue predominates thus leading to different nomenclatures.

Adenosis is a synonym for hyperplasia of the lobular epithelium. It is identified by an increase in the size and/or number of lobules. In simple adenosis, the duct cells are normal single layers but they maintain their orientation to the basement membrane. Multilayering, loss of polarity, and reduction in the diameter of the duct lumina are signs of atypia. When the lesion is extensive or when the degree of atypia is marked, the term "florid adenosis" is used (Fig. 5-4).

Increased connective tissue is often seen in the hyperplasia. The ingrowth of the young fibroblastic cells will often separate the ducts of the enlarged lobules, producing a variant called "sclerosing adenosis" (Fig. 5-5) If localized, it is referred to as stromal fibrosis, fibrous dysplasia, fibrous mastopathy, fibrous tumor, or fibromatosis.

Blunt-duct adenosis represents a stage of physiologic lobular atrophy rather than an intrinsic lesion of fibrocystic disease. Blunt-duct adenosis often results from an unfolding of the lobule of the associated terminal duct.

Figure 5-1 Interlobular and intracellular ductal hyperplasia beside an intraductal papilloma. The hyperplasia involves the whole mammary unit.

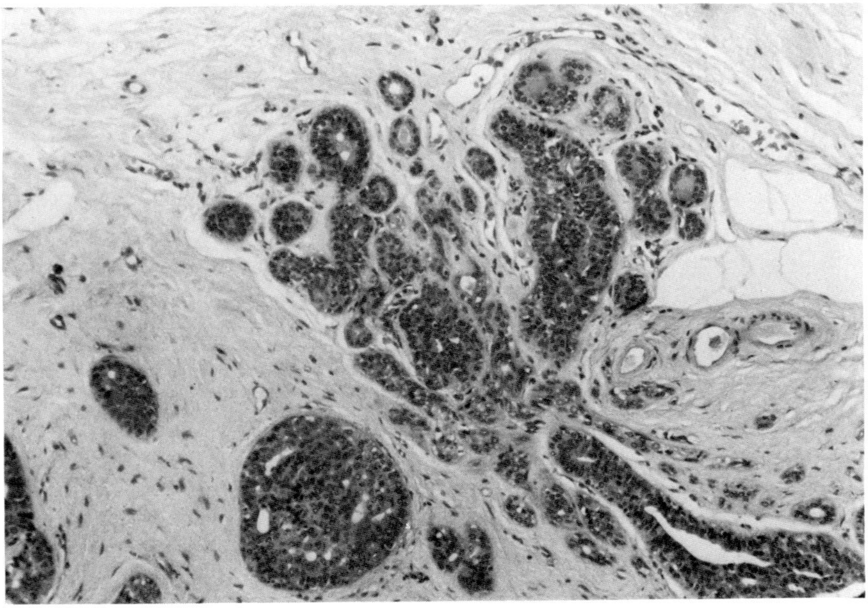

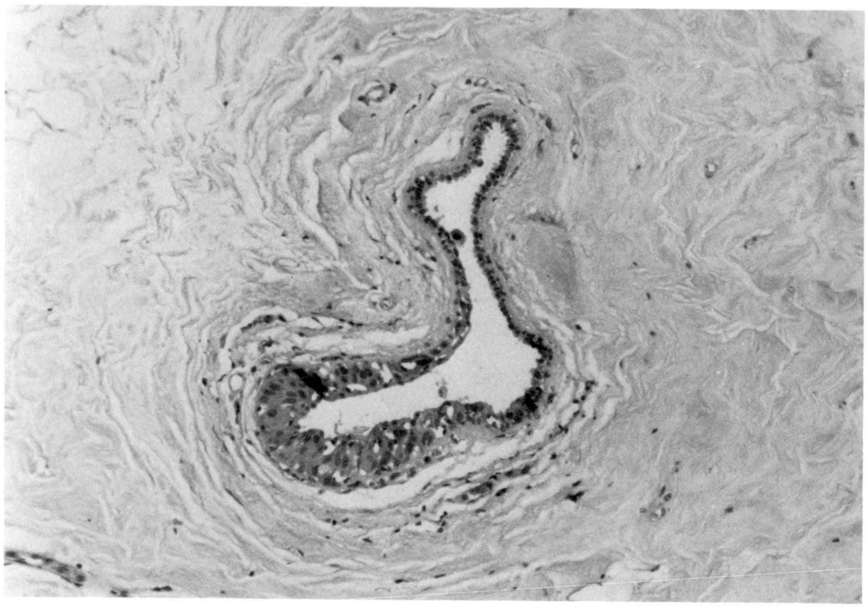

Figure 5-2 Atypical interlobular duct hyperplasia. Gradual neoplastic changes of the lining cells which become several layers thick. The nuclei are pleomorphic and hyperchromatic without papillary formation.

Hyperplasia of the duct epithelium results in an increase in duct diameter and length, and the consequent folding of the duct itself. The simplest form of papillary duct hyperplasia, also called "duct papilloma or papillomatosis," consists of infolded ridges of connective tissue (Figs. 5-6 and 5-7). Atypia is present when secondary papillomas, composed of epithelium and fibroblasts, deviate from the normal. In advanced stages, cells may bridge the lumen of the ducts, producing in cross section an irregular cartwheel appearance. The atypia can progress to in situ carcinoma. Different degrees of atypism, location in the duct system, and extent of the atypia have been classified by Black and Chabon[17] for their malignant potential. (See Chap. 10.)

Apocrine metaplasia is a conversion of the epithelium to bulky columnar cells with prominent eosinophilic cytoplasm (Fig. 5-8). In themselves they are not particularly dangerous, but when marked hyperplasia and atypia occur, there is the possibility that they may develop into cancer.

Cysts, the result of duct hyperplasia, at first contain normal-appearing cells, but with continuation of hyperplastic changes, intracystic papillomas are formed. With increasing pressure from the cyst fluid, the cells become flattened and may disappear completely. The unprotected surrounding connective tissue may undergo thickening or inflammatory changes.

Clinical Picture

Symptoms are monotonously similar, consisting of pain, nodularity, and tenderness. Both breasts are usually involved and the symptoms are either sporadic (usually premenstrual) or continuous. No specific types give rise to special symptoms. From a symptom standpoint they can all be grouped together. A deviant space-occupying mass on physical examination will

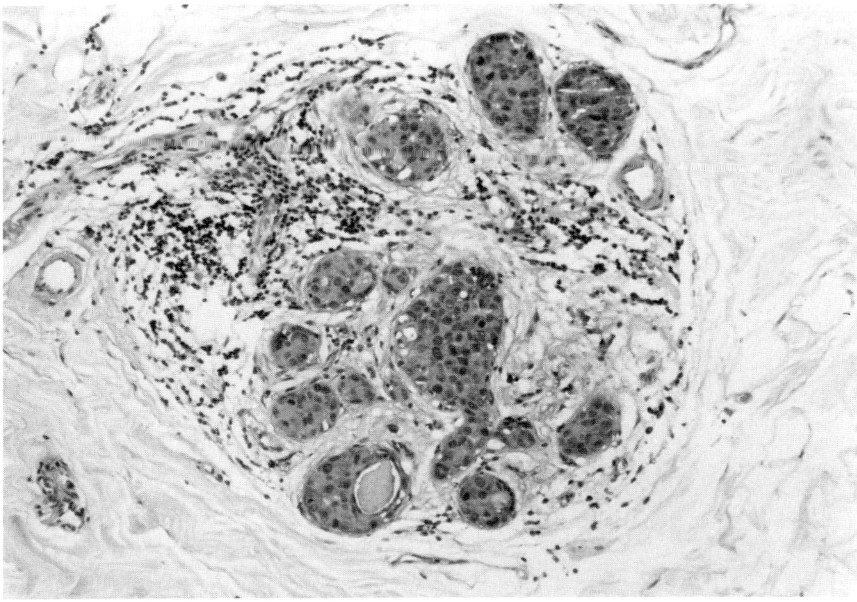

Figure 5-3 Lobular hyperplasia with atypia. Atypical hyperplasia of the epithelial structure is limited to the lobules which still maintain a lobular appearance.

dictate the need for a biopsy; the results will dictate if further treatment is indicated.

Virginal hypertrophy is seen in young girls. It is often asymptomatic and no treatment is indicated. It is usually due to an overgrowth of fibrous tissue and is self-limiting.

Mazoplasia occurs in girls in their late teens and presents as a painful, tender swelling, usually in the tail of the breast. Encouragement with explanation is the treatment of choice.

Chronic cystic mastitis. Most cases of fibrocystic disease occur in women in their mid-30s and 40s. Patients usually describe the symptoms as a persistence with increased severity of premenstrual symptoms. When cysts develop, there is an associated dull, heavy feeling which the patient can usually palpate herself. Pain referred to the breast must be distinguished from true breast pain. Such causes as cervical or dorsal radiculitis, Tietze's syndrome (costochondritis), shingles (herpes zoster), etc., must be excluded. Cancer rarely causes pain, and if pain exists in a patient with cancer it is usually from some other cause.

During pregnancy and lactation symptoms usually disappear, as they usually do also after menopause. Physical examination is usually unproductive unless there is dominant mass. Leis at al.[5] describe the sensation of the nodularity as "running your hands over a plate of peas." They further state that "areas of thickening develop that are two-dimensional (height and width) rather than the three-dimensional findings characteristic of a true mass or lump."

Changes that may occur involving the nipple are described in Chap. 34.

The Possible Relation of Fibrocystic Disease to Cancer

Fibrocystic disease is so ubiquitous that saying it is related to cancer is akin to the statement of Hutter that the female breast is premalignant.

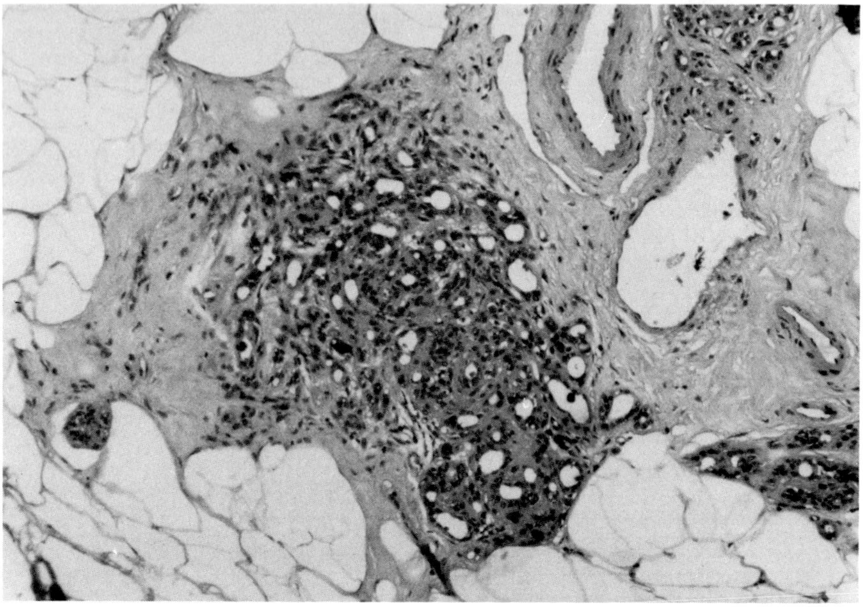

Figure 5-4 Florid adenosis. There is an increase in number of the terminal mammary ductules and the size of the lobules. The ductules are so crowded that intralobular connective tissue is hardly discernible. This condition should be distinguished from myoepithelial proliferation, in which the cells have clear cytoplasm and sharp cytoplasmic outlines.

With increased knowledge, it becomes necessary for pathologists to be more precise in their histologic diagnoses. Histologic studies of breasts removed for cancer show the same incidence of fibrocystic disease as those not removed for cancer.[12] Black et al.[18] reported that a woman with duct hyperplasia with atypia has a five times greater chance of developing breast cancer. Thus, hyperplasia with atypia is considered precancerous. These changes in the larger terminal ducts are more dangerous than similar changes in the smaller ducts. This conclusion remains dubious according to Gallager and Martin,[19] who state that hyperplasia and atypia are stages that epithelium must traverse en route to becoming cancer; this stage may never progress, but rather remain stationary, or it may even revert to normal.

The relationship of cysts to the incidence of cancer has been reported to be, respectively, 4 times the expected incidence of the population,[4] 3.5 times,[3] and 2.4 times.[5] However, no such increased incidence of cystic disease with cancer has been claimed by some.[20] We have not observed any increased association of cancer in patients with simple cysts, and treat them with simple aspiration in practically all instances. We follow such patients every 6 months by simple physical examination, and if any question arises, a mammogram is performed.

Foot and Stewart[20] planned a study to determine whether or not there is any characteristic "soil" in the breast which would predispose toward the formation of cancer. They reviewed 300 cancerous breasts and 200 breast specimens removed for benign conditions. The two lesions associated with cancer were atypical ductular papillomatosis and atypical lobular hyperplasia.[20]

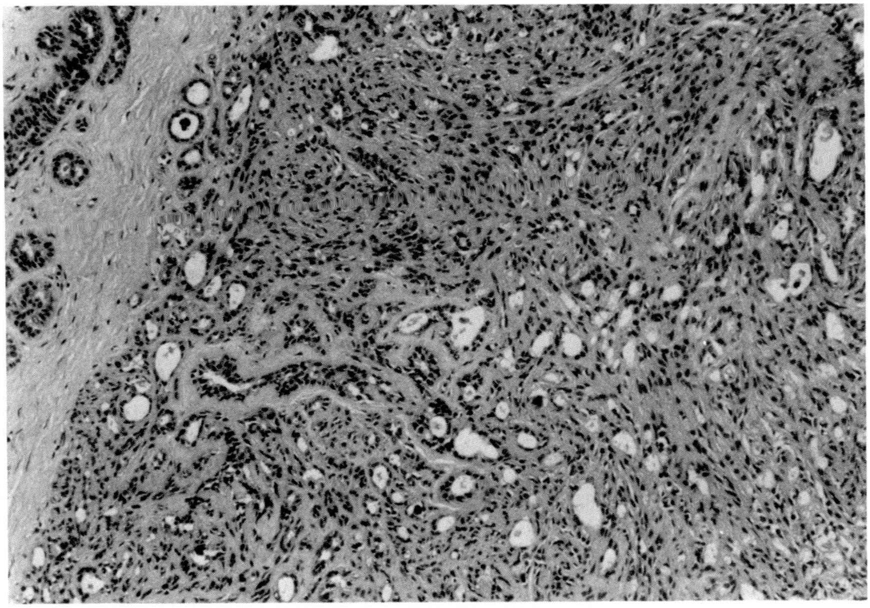

Figure 5-5 Sclerosing adenosis. Ductules are compressed between the bands of dense fibrocollagenous tissue which replace the normal loose intralobular stroma. Sometimes, the atrophic ductules distorted by the fibrosing process can simulate a scirrhous carcinoma.

McDivitt, Stewart, and Berg[21] state:

> It is useless, however, to talk about the importance of the cystic proliferative complex unless one can translate discussion into appropriate treatment for the patient. This requires segregation of various significant and insignificant patterns. As yet, such segregation does not exist in any practical form, and it would require a very long, extensive and preplanned study to accomplish this.

They go on to say: "There is no epidemiologic evidence to support an association between benign breast disease and carcinoma. . . ."[11]

Spratt et al., in a study of 10,000 women with chronic cystic mastitis performed by the Breast Cancer Detection and Demonstration project, found no relation between the incidence of mastitis and breast cancer.[22]

In a prospective study to understand better the premalignant changes in as unrelated a group of women as is possible to obtain, Moskowitz et al.,[23] after taking biopsies from 10,500 self-selected women, concluded that in intraductal and in situ lobular carcinomas the determining insult occurs at a relatively early age. Atypical hyperplasia is quite likely premalignant, but "nonobligate." The role of hyperplasia without atypia remains enigmatic. Patients with gross fibrocystic disease are at greater risk than the general population; this conclusion is heralded by some but denied by others. Dupont and Page[23a] reevaluated 10,366 women who had biopsies of their breasts and followed them for a median period of 17 years. Women having proliferative disease without atypical hyperplasia had a risk of cancer that was 1.9 times the risk in women with nonproliferative lesions (95 percent confidence interval, 1.2 to 2.9). The risk in women with atypical hyperplasia (atypia) was 5.3 times that in women with nonproliferative lesions (95 percent confidence interval, 3.1 to 8.8). A family history

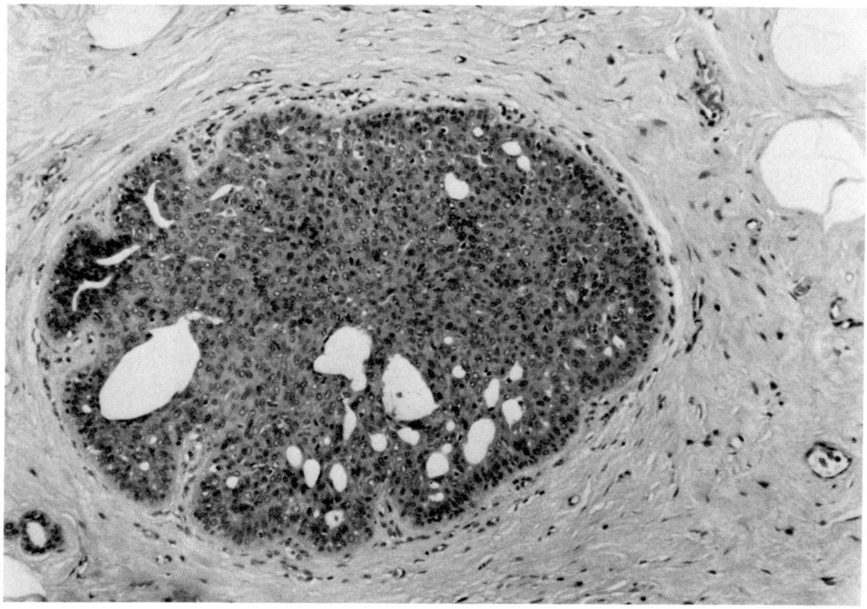

Figure 5-6 Intraductal papilloma. Proliferative epithelial lining of the ducts projects into the lumina and crosses it in forming bridges.

of breast cancer had little effect on the risk in women with nonproliferative lesions. However, the risk in women with atypia and a family history of breast cancer was eleven times that in women who had nonproliferative lesions without a family history (95 percent confidence interval, 5.5 to 24).[23a]

Etiology

An evaluation of proposed tentative etiologic factors may give some insight to a possible relationship of fibrocystic disease to cancer. Inasmuch as fibrocystic disease is related to hormone imbalance, various studies have been performed to identify a possible hormonal abnormality. None has been identified. Women with Stein-Leventhal syndrome (who are anovulatory) do not suffer from mammary dysplasia. No correlation can be discerned in women who received exogenic estrogens.

As the breasts participate in cyclic changes, they are often part of the premenstrual syndrome. A reversible "medical oophorectomy" was obtained in 50 women, accomplished through daily administration of the gonadotropin-releasing hormone (GnRH). Agonist has been claimed by Muse et al.[24] to have the most favorable results, including relief of breast pain.

The association between oral contraceptives and breast pathology has been extensively investigated. LeVolse et al.,[25] who studied 205 premenopausal women, discovered that those with fibrocystic disease in which epithelial atypia was minimal or absent, were takers of birth control pills. In women with marked atypia, there was no significant difference in frequency of long-term users compared to women who had never used oral contraceptives. These authors believe that a spectrum of cystic disease exists and that long-term use of oral contraceptives protects against forms of fibrocystic disease not firmly associated with an increased risk of breast cancer, but does not protect against premalignant forms.

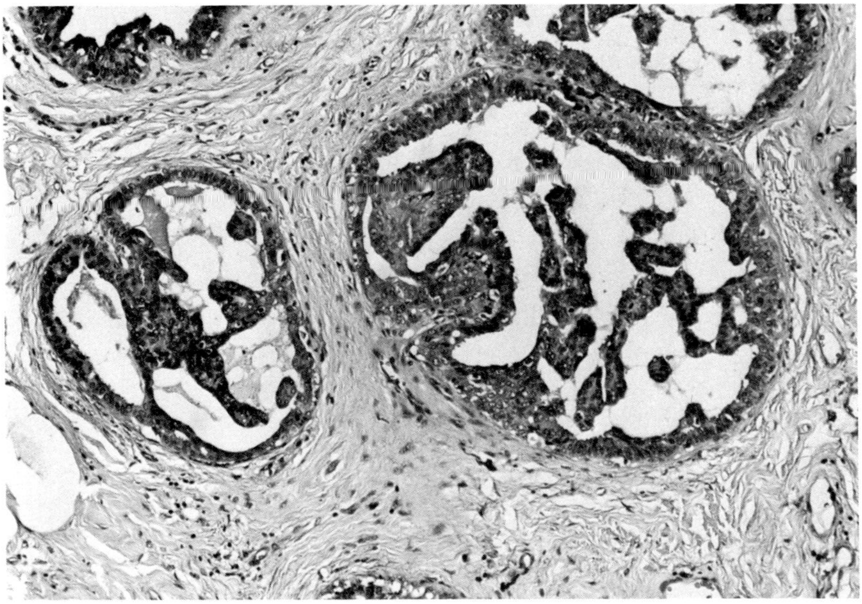

Figure 5-7 Atypical intraductal papillomas. The ductal epithelial cells are more pleomorphic and hyperchromatic, obliterating the lumen.

Other studies have demonstrated little if any association between oral contraceptives and fibrocystic disease.[25,27,28] In fact, oral contraceptives will often relieve the symptoms. Ariel[26] demonstrated marked relief of symptoms in 54 of 110 women with fibrocystic disease after administration of Enovid (norethynodrel with mestranol). There was no relationship between the incidence of fibrocystic disease and the future development of cancer in his series.

Biochemical examination of cyst fluid that could lead to a better knowledge of this disease entity has been unrewarding. These studies include estrogen and progesterone receptors (Jacquemier et al.),[29] cyclic adenosine 3',5'-monophosphate receptor proteins (Handschin et al.),[30] isozyme patterns (Balinsky),[31] electrolyte and androgen conjugate composition (Miller et al.),[32] circulating autoantibodies (Tsakraklides et al.),[33] alpha-lactalbumen (Bahu et al.),[34] various steroid hormones (Bradlow et al.),[35] and polypeptide hormones, especially GhCG and prolactin (Greenblatt et al.).[11] This demonstrates the intense activity being devoted to understanding the mechanism of this diverse disease entity. Clinical application of these studies awaits their better understanding.

Breast cancer has been related to ionizing radiation[37] and to diethylstilbestrol (DES) intake, in which the cancer occurs many, many years after exposure, but no mention is made regarding fibrocystic disease preceding development of the cancer and the effects of the radiation or DES in the etiology of fibrocystic disease. A recent attempt to follow women who received DES in utero has been unsuccessful.[36]

Greenberg et al.[38] studied the incidence of breast cancer in 3033 women who had taken DES in pregnancy and concluded cautiously that the incidence of breast cancer is slightly increased in women given DES, but other factors may play a role. No mention was made in their study regarding fibrocystic disease.

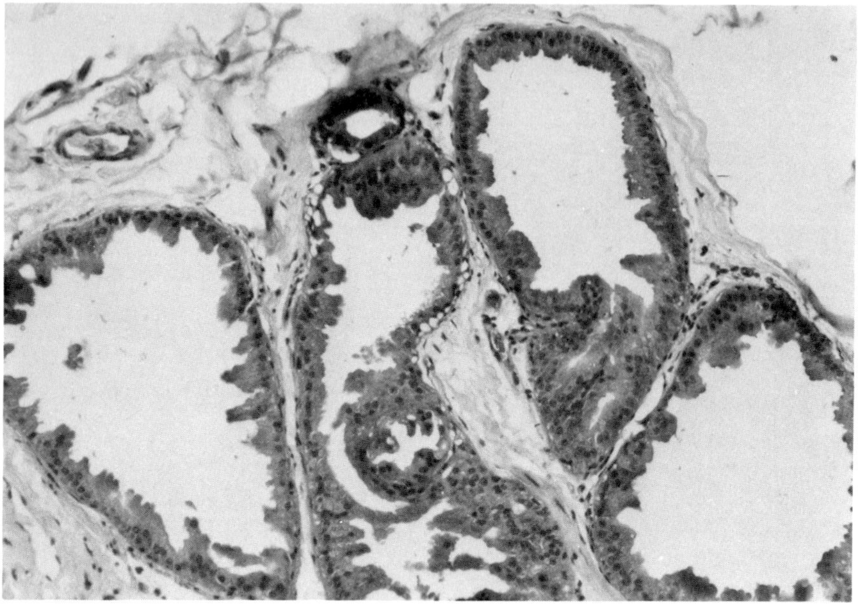

Figure 5-8 Apocrine metaplasia. The lining cells are like those of apocrine sweat glands. They are large and tall, with eosinophilic opaque cytoplasm, projecting sometimes into the dilated ducts.

Thus, the overriding questions of any patient with fibrocystic disease are as follows:

1 Are any of the nodules cancer?
2 What subgroup of chronic cystic disease does the patient have?
3 What can be done to give relief and reduce the risk of cancer?

History, physical examination, mammography, and, where indicated, an aspiration, or formal biopsy, are the ways the actual diagnosis can be made. There are no convincing data to support or refute that treatment will diminish the risk of cancer.

TREATMENT

Treatment will tax any physician who sees many cases of fibrocystic disease. The main concern is whether or not there is an underlying cancer and which of the masses are potentially malignant. In women with one large gross cyst, aspiration is all that is necessary, and cytologic examination does not as a rule reveal any information. However, if the aspirate is hemorrhagic, if there is a residual mass after aspiration, or if the mammogram after aspiration reveals abnormalities, then a local excision is indicated. In any patient with severe fibrocystic disease, we have repeat mammograms performed, preferably every 6 months. If any change is observed in the mammogram, then an aspiration or formal biopsy of the region of change is performed.

Treatment fluctuates between medical or surgical, and depends on the severity of the symptoms plus the concern of the doctor regarding the possibility of cancer. As cancers are most commonly asymptomatic, if a cancer is discovered in a patient who has pain, the pain is usually the result of some other cause. Symptoms will vary from sporadic discomfort, which is often self-limiting, to extremely painful and tender breasts, from which the woman suffers day and night. For sporadic self-limiting mastodynia no treatment is necessary. Aspirin or any analgesic is prescribed, and the patient is advised to wear an uplift bra and to sleep with the bra if symptoms so dictate. For the more persistent form, a variety of medical treatments have been recommended:

Dietary Measures

1 Methylxanthine caffeine: This substance, present in coffee, colas, etc., was found by Minton et al.[39] to exacerbate the symptoms. Severely reducing intake may give dramatic relief and reduce the need for biopsy. This has been confirmed by some and denied by others.[40]

2 Vitamin E: 400 to 600 units taken daily, helps to diminish symptoms and nodularity, as claimed by London et al.[41]

3 Dietary fat: Wynder et al.,[42] after intensive epidemiologic and environmental data, concluded that a significant factor in the development of breast cancer is dietary fat. Whether excessive fat plays a role in chronic mastitis has not been investigated, but it is a good idea to place the patient on a low-fat diet.

4 Vitamin B complex: When it was believed that excess circulating estrogen was the cause for mastitis, and following the observations of Biskind, Biskind, and Biskind[43] that estrogen is more readily metabolized by the liver in the presence of vitamin B, its administration became popular in the past.

We have found that some patients enjoy mild relief when under the above regimen while others do not respond.

Controlling Associated Gynecologic Problems

Since the early studies of Taylor[44] and Pierce and Slaughter[45] demonstrated an association between gynecologic disorders and mastitis, each patient should have a careful gynecologic examination and corrective measures instituted.

Hormone Manipulation

Since the precise nature of an imbalance has not been determined, treatment is empirical. The following are some of the hormonal agents that have been advocated:

1 Oral contraceptives for 3 or 4 months, according to the usual schedule. To this may be added additional progesterone, 5 to 10 mg each day during the last 5 days, if indicated.

2 Tamoxifen: Years ago, androgen administration was the treatment of choice. With the advent of antiestrogenic agents without associated complications of androgen administration, administration of antiestrogenic hormones is often beneficial.[46] We have used tamoxifen citrate, 10 mg orally two or three times a day, as a second-line modality if dietary measures fail, with success in some and no benefit in others.

3 Danazol: An antigonadotropin, when used in the treatment of endometriosis, was found to give relief of pain and decrease in nodularity by Greenblatt and associates.[11,47] They originally treated 130 patients with severe mastitis and obtained satisfactory results in 70 percent. Minor side effects, of which the most common are muscle cramps, acne, oily hair, weight gain, and amenorrhea, were usually self-limiting and occurred in less than 20 percent of treated patients. A dose of 100 to 400 mg per day is given, depending on the severity of the disease. A limiting factor of this treatment is that it takes at least 3 to 6 months for the complete response to be obtained. It is the treatment of choice for refractory severe mastitis. Usually all the nodularity will disappear, but if a residual nodule persists after the others have disappeared, it should be biopsied.

4 Thyroid hormone: Some claim hypothyroidism to be a contributing cause of mastitis and advise administration of thyroid hormones. The dose used by Estes[48] is 0.1 mg levothyroxine per day, with rapid relief of pain in 47 percent of 19 patients treated. We have had limited success with administration of thyroid to patients.

Miscellaneous

1 Diuretics: As some edema is associated with breast symptoms, administration of any diuretic for a short period will often give some relief.

2 Ibuprofen: Although there are many antiinflammatory drugs, and inflammation plays a most minor role in this disease, administration of 400 mg of ibuprofen three times a day has been found helpful for some patients. This may be due to a prostaglandin effect.

3 Analgesics: Given for a short period of time for severe pain, analgesics can provide some relief if other measures have not been successful.

If the above measures fail and if the patient does not want to become pregnant (nearly all symptoms and signs of mastitis disappear during pregnancy and lactation), then surgical measures should be considered.

Reassurance is a most important function which the physician can perform. Every woman with moderate to severe symptoms due to fibrocystic disease is fearful that she is suffering from cancer.

Surgical Treatment

A carefully placed incision for biopsy is indicated for the presence of any dominant mass and if a mammogram is suspicious. Other indications for a patient with fibrocystic disease include:

Sudden increase in breast size
Appearance of unexplained erythema or edema
Any retraction signs
Any unexplained nipple discharge (exclusive of a milky discharge)
Any nipple changes

We do not advise nor practice subcutaneous mastectomy for fibrocystic disease. In rare instances we recommend reduction mammoplasty for relief of severe symptoms, not for protection from cancer.

CONCLUSION

Fibrocystic disease (chronic cystic mastitis) is present to some degree in most women. It increases with age and tends to disappear after menopause. The underlying changes are largely due to alterations in the hormonal milieu. Cystic changes are associated with menstruation (which aggravates symptoms) and with pregnancy and lactation, when symptoms subside. Coincidently, the maturating changes which occur with menarche and the involutionary changes during menopause contribute to the overall changes. Fibrocystic disease becomes a clinical problem for two major reasons:

1 Controlling extreme and persistent pain and nodularity
2 Determining whether the observed nodules are cancerous or precancerous

Patients with fibrocystic disease are said by some to manifest a higher incidence for developing cancer, varying from two to four times the normal population. This is the result of two practices:

a. Patients in whom symptoms and signs cause the physician to biopsy the lesions; thus the data are skewed to a subset of patients more prone to develop cancer.
b. Examination of breasts amputated for cancer may show other changes considered preneoplastic.

Fibrocystic disease as a general term is so all-inclusive that it includes many subentities, physiologic and pathologic. As such, the term is meaningless and the pathologist must classify the entities into specific subsets. At the very least, the disease should be classified into:

1 Proliferative fibrocystic disease (10 to 15 percent of all patients)
  a. With atypism
  b. Without atypism
2 Nonproliferative disease (85 to 90 percent of all patients)

A family history can help identify patients with proliferative disease and atypia. These patients can then be placed in a high-risk category, as the risk is eleven times that of women without a family history and nonproliferative mastitis. (See Chap. 6.)

Inasmuch as there are no noninvasive techniques for determining the types of fibrocystic disease from which a woman may suffer, biopsies should be liberally performed where suspicion exists and careful surveillance maintained for extended periods.

Treatment is for symptomatic relief. There are no data that medical treatment will prevent formation of cancer. Indications for surgery are very few, although at present 85 percent of all surgery upon the breast (exclusive of cosmetic surgery) is performed for benign entities.

REFERENCES

1. Leis HP Jr: Risk factors for breast cancer: An update. *Breast* 6:21, 1980.
2. Hinton CP, Hughes RG: Repeated aspiration of breast cysts. A safe procedure. *Br J Surg* 7:145, 1968.
3. Harrington E, Lesnick G: The association between gross cysts of the breast and breast cancer. *Breast* 7:13, 1981.
4. Haagensen CP: *Diseases of the Breast*, 2d ed. Philadelphia, W. B. Saunders, p. 155, 1971.
5. Leis HP Jr, Cammarata A, LaRaja R, Cruz E: Fibrocystic disease. *The Female Patient* 8:56, 1983.
6. Tavassoli FA, Norris HG: Microglandular adenosis of the breast. A clinical pathologic study of eleven cases with ultrastructural observation. *Am J Surg Path* 7:731, December 1983.
7. DeHertogh DA, Rossof AH, Harris AA, Economou SG: Prednisone management of granulomatous mastitis. *N Engl J Med* 303:799, 1980.
8. Chen KTY: Fibromatoses of the breast. *Breast* 10:25, 1984.
9. Velpeau J: Quoted by Farrow JH, in Pack GT, Ariel IM (eds): *Treatment of Cancer and Allied Diseases*, vol. 4, p. 55, 1060.
10. König P: Mastitis chronica, cystica. *Central Bl Chin* 20:49, 1893.

10a. Brodie R: Lectures on sero-cystic tumors of the breast. *London Med Gazette* 25:808, 1840.

10b. Reclus P: Cystic disease of the breast. *Rev Chir* 3:761, 1883.

11. Greenblatt RB, Chaddha S, Teran AZ, Lewis A: Fibrocystic breast disease: Pathophysiology, hormonology, treatment. *Contemp Surg* 24:49, 1984.
12. Love SN, Gelman RS, Silen W: Sounding board. Fibrocystic disease of the breast—a non-disease? *N Engl J Med* 307(16):1010, October 14, 1982.
13. Hutter RVP: What is a premalignant lesion? in Gallager HS (ed): *Early Breast Cancer—Detection and Treatment*. New York, Wiley, 1975.
14. Hutter RVP: Definition of precancerous mastopathy and minimal breast cancer. 2d Annual Breast Cancer Symposium, New York Met. Breast Cancer Group. New York, 1975.
15. Stout AP: *Human Cancer*. Philadelphia, Lea & Febiger, 1932.
16. Frantz VK, Pickren JW, Melcher GW, Auchincloss H Jr: Incidence of chronic cystic disease in so-called "normal breasts"; study based on 225 post-mortem examinations. *Cancer* 4:762, 1951.
17. Black MM, Chabon A: In situ carcinoma of the breast, in Sommers SC (ed): *Pathology Annual*, New York, 1969.
18. Black MM, Barclay TH, Cutler SJ, et al: Association of atypical characteristics of benign breast lesions with subsequent risk of breast cancer. *Cancer* 29:338, 1972.
19. Gallager HS, Martin JE: Early phases in the development of breast cancer. *Cancer* 24:1170, 1969.
20. Foote FW Jr, Stewart FW: Comparative studies of cancerous versus noncancerous breasts: Role of so-called chronic cystic mastitis in mammary carcinogenesis. *Ann Surg* 121:197, 1945.
21. McDivitt RW, Stewart FW, Berg JW: *Tumors of the Breast: Atlas of Tumor Pathology*, 2d series. Fascile 2, 1968, p. 16.
22. Spratt JS, Kuhns JG, Buchanan JB, et al: Association of types of chronic cystic mastopathy, xeromammographic patterns and cancer. *Cancer* 55:1372, 1985.
23. Moskowitz M, Seshagirarao P, Rulles P: Lists of observations on the natural history of carcinoma of the breast. *Breast—The Diseases of the Breast* 3:14, 1977.

23a. Dupont WD, Page DL: Risk factors for breast cancer in women with proliferative breast disease. *N Engl J Med* 312:146, 1985.

24. Muse KN, Cetel NS, Futtermann LA, Yen SC: Effects of "medical ovariectomy." *N Engl J Med* 311:1345, 1984.
25. LeVolse VA, Stradel BV, et al: Fibrocystic breast disease in oral contraceptive users. *N Engl J Med* 299:381, 1978.
26. Ariel IM: Enovid therapy (norethynodrel with mestranol) for fibrocystic disease. *Am J Obstet Gynecol* 117:453, 1973.

27. Balinsky D, Platz CE, Lewis JW: Enzyme activities in normal, dysplastic, and cancerous human breast tissues. *J Natl Cancer Inst* 72(2):217, February 1984.
28. Hsieh CC, Crosson AW, Walker AM, Trapido EJ, MacMahon B: Oral contraceptive use and fibrocystic breast disease of different histologic classifications. *J Natl Cancer Inst* 72(2):285, February 1972.
29. Jacquemier JD, Rolland PH, Vague D, Lieutaud R, Spitalier JM, Martin PM: Relationships between steroid receptor and epithelial cell proliferation in benign fibrocystic disease of the breast. *Cancer* 49(12):2534, June 15, 1982.
30. Handschin JC, Handloser K, Takahashi A, Eppenberger U: Cyclic adenosine 3':5'-monophosphate receptor proteins in dysplastic and neoplastic human breast tissue cytosol and their inverse relationship with estrogen receptors. *Cancer Res* 43(6):2947, June 1983.
31. Balinsky D, Platz CE, Lewis JW: Isozyme patterns of normal, benign, and malignant human breast tissues. *Cancer Res* 43(12, pt. 1):5895, December 1983.
32. Miller WR, Dixon JM, Scott WN, Forrest AP: Classification of human breast cysts according to electrolyte and androgen conjugate composition. *Clin Oncol* 9(3):227, September 1983.
33. Tsakraklides E, Anastassiades OT, Gogas J, Renieri N: Circulating autoantibodies in patients with fibrocystic disease of the breast. *J Cancer Res Clin Oncol* 106(3):219, 1983.
34. Bahu RM, Mangkornkanck-Mark M, Albertson D, Fors E, Molteni A, Battifora H: Detection of alpha-lactalbumin in breast lesions and relationship to estrogen receptors and serum prolactin. *Cancer* 46(8):1775, October 15, 1980.
35. Bradlow HL, Rosenfeld RS, Kream J, Fleisher M, O'Connor J, Schwartz MK: Steroid hormone accumulation in human breast cyst fluid. *Cancer Res* 41(1):105, January 1981.
36. Nash S, Tilley BC, Kurland LT, Gundersen J, Barnes AB, Labarthe D, Donohew PS, Kovacs L: Identifying and tracing a population at risk: The DESAD Project experience. *Am J Public Health* 73(3):253, March 1983.
37. Land CE, Boice JD Jr, Shore RB: Breast cancer risk from low dose exposure to ionizing radiation, results of parallel analyses of three exposed populations of women. *J Natl Cancer Inst* 65:353, 1979.
38. Greenberg ER, Barnes AM, Ressegene L, et al: Breast cancer in mothers given diethylstilbestrol in pregnancy. *N Engl J Med* 311:1393, 1984.
39. Minton JP, Abou-Issa H, Reiches N, Roseman JM: Clinical and biochemical studies on methylxanthine-related fibrocystic breast disease. *Surgery* 90(2):299, August 1981.
40. Marshall J, Graham S, Swanson M: Caffeine consumption and benign breast disease: A case-control comparison. *Am J Public Health* 72(6):610, June 1982.
41. London RS, Solomon DM, London ED, et al: Mammary dysplasia; clinical response and urinary excretion of 11-deoxy-17 ketosteroids and pregnandiol following alpha-tocopherol therapy. *Breast* 4:19, 1978.
42. Wynder EI, Cohen LA, Hill P, et al: Nutrition and the etiology and prevention of breast cancer, in Strax P(ed): Control of Breast Cancer Through Mass Screening. Littleton, MA, PFG Publishing Co., 1979, p. 89.
43. Biskind MS, Biskind GR, Biskind LH: Nutritional deficiency in the etiology of mastitis. *Surg Gynecol Obstet* 78:49, 1944.
44. Taylor HC Jr: The relation of chronic mastitis to certain hormones of the ovary and pituitary and to coincident gynecologic lesions. *Surg Gynecol Obstet* 62:129, 1936.
45. Pierce VV, Slaughter NN: The association of breast and pelvic disease. *Cancer* 1:468, 1948.
46. Ricciardi I, Ianniruberto A: Tamoxifen induced regression of benign breast lesions. *Obstet Gynecol* 54:80, 1979.
47. Greenblatt B, Ben-Nun I: Danazol in the treatment of mammary dysplasia. *Drugs* 19(5):349, May 1980.
48. Estes NC: Mastodynia due to fibrocystic disease of the breast controlled with thyroid hormone. *Am J Surg* 142(6):764, December 1981.

6

The Identification of Enhanced Risk Patients and Their Management in a Special Surveillance Breast Clinic

Michael P. Osborne, M.D.
Joseph P. Crowe, M.D.

INTRODUCTION

Recently, substantial data have accumulated delineating possible risk factors for breast cancer. Family history, parity, age at first pregnancy, total duration of active menses, and variations in hormonal milieu have been studied.[40,55] Certain benign breast conditions predispose to malignant disease. The risk associated with several of these factors has been postulated to be cumulative. Despite efforts to define women at high risk, the incidence of breast cancer is increasing. Current estimates indicate that 1 in 10 women in the United States will develop breast cancer in her lifetime.

Three promising areas deserving attention as possible markers of breast cancer risk are (1) genetic susceptibility, (2) histologic precursor lesions, and (3) endocrine biomarkers. A long-term prospective study is currently under way at Memorial Sloan-Kettering Cancer Center to evaluate these factors with the formation of a Special Surveillance Breast Clinic. Eligibility criteria include either a strong family history of breast cancer or a finding of epithelial atypia on a prior breast biopsy. Over 300 patients have registered in the Special Surveillance Breast Clinic as of December 1985. From this cohort of high-risk women who have not yet developed breast cancer, various factors in the spectrum of preneoplasia can be studied. A specific abnormality of endocrine metabolism has been recently observed in women with breast cancer[66] and in nonaffected women at increased risk.[60a] This abnormality may serve as a biomarker to study the effects of potential chemopreventive agents in this high-risk population. An in-depth assessment of genetic profiles, breast biopsy pathology, psychological motivation, and compliance with conventional measures of early breast cancer detection will provide a comprehensive evaluation of this population.

DEFINED RISK FACTORS

Genetic Factors

Patients entered into the Special Surveillance Breast Clinic provide a prospective comprehensive data base from which various genetic aspects of breast cancer may be studied.

Although a positive family history has long been recognized as a risk factor in breast cancer,[1,53] the underlying role of genetic factors remains elusive. There exist two avenues by which a genetic mechanism may contribute to development of cancer. One is in the form of a major gene. In such families, breast cancer segregates in a recognizable mendelian dominant pattern and first-degree female relatives of gene carriers are at high risk (50 percent) of developing breast cancer.[2,54] Another feature that has been observed in some of the hereditary families is the development of breast cancer in a male; however, such families are rare and in general males are unaffected and provide little information as to whether aggregation of breast cancer in a family is inherited, environmentally determined, or the result of a chance occurrence.

Furthermore, it is recognized that breast cancer, like other heritable diseases, must frequently lack the complete penetrance of the deleterious gene. The appearance of so-called skipped generations and apparent paternal transmission without involvement may be in part explained by this phenomenon.

In addition to families in which susceptibility to breast cancer appears to be inherited via a major gene, other disorders have been described in which breast cancer is only part of the total phenotypic expression. Cowden's disease is a clear example of genetic transmission of breast cancer as a dominant single gene trait. Primarily expressed as multiple cutaneous trichilemmomas and oral fibromas, Cowden's disease should be considered a reliable preclinical marker of genetic breast cancer and any woman with bilateral breast cancer and a strong family history should be investigated for the possibility of this autosomal dominant disease.[22] Other genetic syndromes that involve breast cancer include the SBLA (Sarcoma, Breast, Leukemia, and Adrenal) syndrome; the breast and ovarian syndrome, etc.[51]

The second avenue for genetic influence is through genes with small effect, or polygenes. These genes, for instance, might be exerting their influence on physiological variables related to the menstrual cycle, hormone levels, weight, or menarche—in other words, on traits that have a bearing on risk of developing breast cancer, and thus they indirectly exert an effect. Environmental factors in the form of nutrition, exercise, etc., also participate and interact with genes that control phenotypic expression of such physiological traits. Since the environmental and polygenic effects are intermingled, it is more common to speak of their joint contribution in the form of multifactorial inheritance. To the extent that such factors are shared by relatives, aggregation of breast cancer in relatives may reflect a multifactorial pattern of transmission as compared to a pattern defined by a major locus. As a final caveat, one must keep in mind the fact that breast cancer has a naturally high incidence, and therefore it is not unlikely that one might observe families with more than one affected individual solely on the basis of chance.

An important condition for diagnosis of genetic breast cancer is that the physician must have obtained a complete family history of the patient. In most instances, patients with a familial association or, more importantly, with a true genetic trait will be suspected at the initial interview. With construction of a full genealogy, identification of a genetic disorder can be made by the cancer geneticist.[52]

There are two ways in which familial risk of breast cancer is being determined in the Special Surveillance Breast Clinic. Each method has unique strengths. The first method is *an empirical definition of risk*, determined by the frequency of affection observed among families with a similar family history—for example, the frequency of affection in women with sisters who have breast cancer. Empiric risk estimates used in the Special Surveillance Breast Clinic are based upon figures published by Anderson,[3,4] Ottman et al.,[61] and Kelsey and Hildreth[42] (Table 6-1). These estimates raise problems in relation to bias in ascertainment by family history or hospital base. For these reasons, the use of relative risks is considered inappropriate by some investigators as the controls may not fully represent the general population.

A second method of determining risk, known as *analytic risk*, has been developed based upon prediction from a model of disease transmission. In this analysis the analytic risks are based on the mixed model parameters which were estimated from segregation analysis of 200 breast cancer pedigrees (Table 6-2).[75] The model postulates that breast cancer in some families is due to a major gene where penetrance increases as a function of age. Clustering in other families may be due to chance due to a high frequency of sporadic cases, also functionally related to age.[76]

The empiric and analytic risks shown in Tables 6-1 and 6-2 can be converted to percentages by multiplying the value by 100. The advantage of analytic risk estimation is that demographic features of the disease in a pedigree, such as age and sex, can be taken into consideration through use of a liability indicator, and consequently a more specific risk can be specified for each pedigree. Such information is lost in empiric figures which represent the mean risk as averaged across different pedigrees that have the same relatives affected.

Endocrine Factors

At present most of the epidemiologically recognized risk factors for breast cancer are considered to be endocrine-related. Thus, it is conceivable that the inherited genetic defect could be an endocrine-related enzymatic abnormality. Lemon[48,49] has postulated that the genetic defect results in an impaired estrone and estradiol hydroxylation to estriol by aryl hydroxylases. A further dimension to an endocrine hypothesis is offered by Sherman and Korenman,[68] who suggest that during critical times of life, termed *estrogen windows*, there is an excess of estrogen relative to progesterone.[45] They propose that this excessive unopposed estrogen stimulation may provide a setting favorable for the development of breast cancer.

Many studies have been unable to find consistent abnormalities in blood or urinary estrogen or estrogen-metabolite levels in breast cancer populations, which has cast some skepticism on these hypotheses. Fishman et al.[26,27,29] studied daily endocrine profiles of postpubertal premenopausal women judged to be at high risk for breast cancer and compared these with matched normal low-risk controls. An abnormality in estrogen conjugation, apparent only at a specific time of the menstrual cycle, was identified. Significant differences were found in lower urinary estrone and estradiol glucuronide levels in the genetically susceptible group. These differences were most pronounced in the luteal periovulatory phase, suggesting a decreased conversion of estradiol and its metabolite estrone to glucuronide conjugates. No differences were identified in the circulating estrogen levels.[26]

This work led Fishman and Martucci[28] and Schneider et al.[66] to an intriguing alternative hypothesis of endocrine dysfunction that may explain these shifts in estrogen conjugation in high-risk women. These investigators demonstrated a 50 percent increase in 16-alpha-hydroxylation of estradiol in women with breast cancer compared to matched controls. Preliminary studies in women at high risk for breast cancer development have suggested that this abnormality may be present prior to the development of detectable cancer.[60a] It will be of importance to investigate the mode of inheritance

Table 6-1 Empiric Risks for Frequently Observed Family Histories of Breast Cancer

Relatives with Breast Cancer						
Degree	**No.**	**Relative(s)**	**Menopause**	**Laterality**	**Empiric Risk**	**Reference**
First	1	Mother	—	—	0.14–0.21	Kelsey and Hildreth[42]
First	1	Sister	—	—	0.14–0.21	
First	1	Sister	—	Uni	0.17	
			Pre	Bil	0.56	
			Pre	Uni	0.08	Ottman et al.[61]
			Post	Bil	?	
			Post	Uni	0.18	
Second	1	Grandmother	—	—	?	
Second	1	Aunt	—	—	?	
First	2	Mother and sister	—	—	0.32	Anderson[4]
			Pre	Uni and		
			Pre	Bil	0.50	
			Pre	Uni and		
			Pre	Uni	0.33	
			Pre	Bil and		
			Post	Uni	0.23	Anderson and Williams[5]
			Pre	Uni and		
			Post	Bil	0.23	
			Pre	Uni and		
			Post	Uni	0.10	
			Post	Bil and		
			Post	Uni	0.28	
			Post	Uni and		
			Post	Uni	0.16	
First	2	Sister and sister	—	—	0.11	Anderson[4]
			Pre	Bil and		
			Pre	Uni	0.50	
			Pre	Uni and		
			Pre	Uni	0.18	
			Pre	Bil and		
			Post	Uni	0.11	Anderson and Williams[5]
			Pre	Uni and		
			Post	Bil	0.11	
			Pre	Uni and		
			Post	Uni	0.08	
			Post	Uni and		
			Post	Uni	0.05	
First and second	2	Mother and grandmother	—	—	0.27	Anderson[4]
	2	Sister and grandmother	—	—	0.19	Anderson[4]
	2	Mother and aunt	—	—	0.14	Anderson[4]
	2	Sister and aunt	—	—	0.19	Anderson[4]

Pre = premenopausal; Post = postmenopausal; Uni = unilateral; Bil = bilateral (after Williams, personal communication).

Table 6-2 Analytic Risks for Breast Cancer by Pedigree Types*

Relative(s)	Menopause	Analytic Risks: Major Gene Model	Analytic Risks: Multifactorial Model
Mother or sister			
	Pre	0.13	0.14
	Post	0.09	0.12
Grandmother or aunt			
	Pre	0.10	0.10
	Post	0.08	0.09
Mother and sister or sister and sister			
	Pre/pre	0.29	0.23
	Pre/post	0.24	0.20
	Post/post	0.17	0.17
Mother and grandmother or mother and aunt			
	Pre/pre	0.28	0.18
	Pre/post	0.23	0.16
	Post/post	0.16	0.14
Sister and grandmother or sister and aunt			
	Pre/pre	0.26	0.19
	Pre/post	0.20	0.16
	Post/post	0.14	0.15

*After Williams and Anderson.[75]

of 16-alpha-hydroxylation of estradiol in relation to the inheritance of breast cancer. This can be accomplished by examining the joint pattern of inheritance using a bivariate model for segregation analysis. The bivariate analysis will be used to determine whether breast cancer and 16-alpha-hydroxylase are inherited in a correlated manner and, if so, whether this association is the consequence of a major gene with pleiotropic effects on each trait, correlated multifactorial contributions, or shared environmental factors.

Studies suggesting the presence of abnormal levels of 16-alpha-hydroxyestrone would seem to fit a "window" hypothesis. Ordinarily, 16-alpha-hydroxyestrone, even though present in small quantities, does not bind to plasma carrier proteins and would in theory be "biologically" available. In its own right, 16-alpha-hydroxyestrone is a potent estrogen and has been shown to bind to estrogen receptor proteins.[28] During the susceptible "window" periods, 16-alpha-hydroxyestrone may gain access to the nucleus of the cell and with its demonstrated ability to form covalent adducts with nuclear histones,[12] 16-alpha-hydroxyestrone could potentially exert its estrogenic effects indefinitely.

A strong family history of breast cancer indicating genetic susceptibility may be the most reliable marker currently available for assessment of breast cancer risk. A family history is easily obtained information and should lead to an increased index of suspicion on the part of the physician. Management of patients at enhanced risk should be based on strict surveillance. The high-risk patient with an autosomal dominant family pattern has a lifetime chance of developing breast cancer of 50 percent and this does not account for other organ systems at risk. Strict surveillance of such high-risk patients can lead to early detection and cure of the disease. Focusing on this enhanced risk group may by extrapolation have substantial influence on the future control of breast cancer in the general population.

The Special Surveillance Breast Clinic provides a population of high-risk women in whom genetic and endocrine biomarkers may be quantitated. Possible means to alter the 16-alpha-hydroxyestrone biomarker could provide leads to effective strategies for chemoprevention. (See Chap. 4.)

Histopathologic Factors

Discovery of early or "minimal" breast cancer with its high cure rates has stimulated interest in the identification of a preneoplastic lesion. The literature relating a prior breast biopsy for benign breast disease to the subsequent risk of breast cancer is confusing (Table 6-3) but a pattern has emerged suggesting that certain defined histopathologic lesions are the true progenitors.[47] Any preneoplastic lesion should have a characteristic appearance of features considered to be precursors of malignancy. The definition of specific histologic features which predispose to malignant change is controversial and difficult to ascertain. Foote and Stewart postulated an association between breast carcinoma and proliferative breast disorders.[30]

Gallager and Martin[32] stated that hyperplasia and carcinoma are phases of a similar process and considered epithelial hyperplasia as a nonobligate premalignant condition, whereas atypical hyperplasia was a definite phase of epithelial alteration necessary for the development of frank carcinoma.

Atypical epithelial proliferation is a histologically identifiable finding which may be a true precursor lesion of in situ or invasive breast cancer.[6,9,13,18,24,34,62] Since atypical, proliferative mammary lesions are not identifiable pathologically as malignancy, a situation analogous to cervical dysplasia, they appear to lie in transition between benign epithelium and carcinoma. Recently, Black and Kwon published data suggesting an interaction among diverse risk factors and atypical hyperplastic breast epithelium.[11]

Table 6-3 Proposed Relative Risks of Prior Benign Breast Disease on the Subsequent Risk of Breast Cancer (Risk for "Normal" Population of Women = 1)

References	Increased Risk
Warren[72]	2.5–4.5
Claggett et al.[14]	5.0
Lewison and Lyons[50]	2.6–3.6
Kiaer[43]	4.0
Copeland[17]	3.0–7.0
Davis et al.[20]	1.2–2.5 (1.73)
Davis[19]	1.2–4.4 (2.5)
Veronesi and Pizzocoro[71]	1.5–4.5 (2.0)
Potter et al.[63]	4.8
Humphrey and Swerdlow[38]	1.3–6.4
Chardot et al.[15]	7.5
Steinhoff and Black[69]	3.0
Haagensen[36]	4.1
Black et al.[10]	5.0 (2.5–11.7)
Ashikari et al.[7]	up to 18.0
Donnelly et al.[23]	2.9–10.0
Monson et al.[56]	2.5
Kodlin et al.[44]	2.7 (2.5)
Page et al.[62]	2.0–6.0
Coombs et al.[16]	3.0
Hutchinson et al.[39]	2.1
Average	3.98

Detailed grading systems for pathologic risk have been devised. A numerical grading system was created by Black and Chabon based on both anatomic location within the breast and, more importantly, histologic degree of atypia.[9] The atypia is graded numerically from 1 to 5: (1) normotypic, normoplastic; (2) normotypic, hyperplastic; (3) minimal but distinct atypia; (4) well-defined atypia; and (5) in situ carcinoma. Grade 2 lesions would show an increase in cell number and/or size, without loss of normal polarity or the myoepithelial cell layer. Grade 3 lesions have a loss of the myoepithelial cell layer with monomorphic proliferation and some loss of cell polarity. Within a grade 3 the individual cell, although somewhat enlarged, can be normal in appearance. Grade 4 precancerous mastopathy demonstrates similar but more pronounced changes compared to grade 3, showing clear loss of cellular and nuclear polarity. An obvious cellular aberration and advanced degree of monomorphic atypical proliferation are present in grade 5 lesions.

Wellings et al. have suggested that certain atypical breast lobules (type A) may be precancerous.[73,74] In their subgross study of 196 human breast specimens, they identified a lesion similar to the murine hyperplastic alveolar nodule which is known to be a precancerous lesion. They proposed a grading system for epithelial atypia.[73] Lesions ranged from "grade I" (mild atypia) to "grade V" (in situ carcinoma). In grade I change, the cells retain polarity and have normal-appearing nuclei. Grade II lesions have some pleomorphism, slight loss of polarity, and occasional bridging of the lumina. Anaplasia is distinctly unusual in grade II lesions. Grade III lesions characteristically have partial or complete filling of the lumina, prominent cellular pleomorphism, moderate anaplasia, and a progressive loss of stromal support. Severe anaplasia without definite stromal support is present in grade IV change. There may be monomorphic epithelial cells filling ductules as well in grade IV change. Grade V is defined as in situ ductal carcinoma.

While strong evidence exists for the premalignant nature of epithelial hyperplasia and atypia, evidence is lacking to support the exact premalignant nature of fibrocystic breast disease.[16,20,31]

With these questions in mind, Rush and Kramer have hypothesized that the complex of chronic cystic mastitis is found to some extent in all aging women.[46,64] While this may be true, the demographic profile of women with hyperplastic atypical changes of the breast is not known.

Surveillance of a patient with preneoplastic atypia must include an evaluation of the epidemiologic traits previously recognized as risk factors for breast carcinoma.[55,60,67] (See also Chap. 5.)

MANAGEMENT OF PATIENTS AT ENHANCED RISK FOR BREAST CANCER

Controversies exist over what constitutes optimal management of patients with proliferative fibrocystic breast disease as well as those women with a genetic predisposition through a family history of breast cancer. The problem of accurate and early diagnosis and subsequent treatment grows more acute with the mounting evidence that atypical hyperplastic epithelium is the precursor lesion. Determination of the time interval required for transformation of the premalignant lesion to carcinoma is of prime importance. The spectrum of management of enhanced-risk patients ranges from careful observation to true prophylactic surgery. The question of prophylactic surgery in these women is difficult to resolve. Whether simple excision of an area containing the atypical lesions is sufficient, or whether complete ablation of the breast tissue would be preferable, is as yet undetermined. Any management decision must account for the tendency toward multicentricity of these hyperplastic atypical areas.

Through large prospective mass screening programs, both regular breast self-examination and annual mammography have been found to be effective complementary means toward early detection of breast cancer.[8,70] While physical examination and breast self-examination constitute an integral part of management, mammography can detect earlier cancers and is recommended annually for these high-risk patients. We do not regard mammography as capable of predicting risk. It has been estimated that an aggressive approach to breast cancer screening may reduce breast cancer mortality by 20 to 50 percent.[33,59] At present, an approach to the high-risk patient must include these two methods of early detection. For this high-risk group, the physician's examination may have the least impact on early detection. Until a reliable biomarker of both preclinical and premalignant disease is available, breast self-examination, annual mammography, and regular physician examinations will constitute the core approach to management of high-risk patients in a Special Surveillance Breast Clinic.

Clinical Protocol

Enrollment criteria in our Special Surveillance Breast Clinic requires either a strong family history of breast cancer and/or a prior breast biopsy showing atypical precursor lesions. In accord with hereditary risk factors as defined by Anderson and Williams,[5] an effort is being made to recruit women with family members who have developed breast cancer at an early age or who have bilateral breast cancer. A detailed history is obtained from each patient during an initial registration interview with a nurse, geneticist, and physician. This history is designed to provide a prospective data base for this unique population of high-risk patients. Included in the evaluation is an assessment of genetic risk through an in-depth family history, and details of the patient's gynecologic, obstetric, and medical history are obtained. Special attention is given to the patient's prior breast disease history. Any excessive exposure to radiation, particularly in the neck and chest regions, is noted. A thorough breast examination is carried out, which is the baseline evaluation. An introduction to breast self-examination is provided through the use of a slide/tape demonstration followed by instruction in breast self-examination by a trained nurse using both the patient and models. A baseline mammogram is obtained depending on individual indications. Finally, psychological evaluation of these women at enhanced risk for breast cancer development is included during the initial phase of entry into the clinic. At the outset it would seem most important to understand the motivational forces guiding women to seek management in such a breast clinic.

For those women who have had a breast biopsy demonstrating premalignant epithelial changes and for those women who might, during the course of their participation in the Special Surveillance Breast Clinic, require a breast biopsy, a uniform approach to the evaluation of their biopsy specimens has been developed. An effort is made to obtain all prior breast biopsy material on every patient entered into the clinic, which is evaluated by one pathologist. Ductal and lobular epithelium is assessed for its degree of hyperplasia and/or atypia. The presence of cysts, duct papillomatosis, sclerosing adenosis, apocrine metaplasia, mastitis, and fibroadenomas are specifically noted. The possible presence of lobular carcinoma in situ or intraductal carcinoma must be determined.

To conclude the initial clinic visit the physician discusses risk factors and the importance of the methods of early breast cancer detection with the patient. In the absence of a proven biomarker for breast cancer risk, early detection by breast self-examination, mammography, and regular examinations by a physician are together the only available means to achieve early diagnosis and improved survival for the breast cancer patient. Continued emphasis is placed on this combined approach at subsequent clinic visits.

Although patients are given an overall impression of the research activities at the initial evaluation, the opportunity to participate in them is presented at the second or third visit. Detailed studies of endocrine metabolism, with particular focus on the 16-alpha-hydroxylation of estradiol, are performed. If an abnormality of 16-alpha-hydroxylation can be correlated with a precise index of risk, then this endocrine abnormality would be used as a biomarker.

A second phase project for those women who elect to participate in these endocrine studies will be an assessment of various putative chemopreventive agents and their ability to alter favorably the endocrine biomarker. Through this prospective and detailed approach to the evaluation of chemopreventive agents, ultimately a true measure of their effective reduction of breast cancer risk may be possible through large randomized trials.

Clinic visits are scheduled every 4 to 6 months: All patients are encouraged to practice breast self-examination between clinic visits and this is reinforced at clinic visits by the nurse. Patients are told that if interim concerns emerge, they should not hesitate to return sooner. This diligent surveillance program allows for immediate evaluation, including biopsy if necessary, of all new masses or suspicious mammogram findings.

Initial evaluation of the clinic composition has shown that two-thirds were accrued on the basis of a positive family history, and one-third had significant breast biopsy changes. Approximately 40 percent of those with a family history as their risk factor had a sporadic pattern of family history, and the remaining 60 percent had a pedigree consistent with true familial breast cancer. Within this latter group one-third had a disease pattern suggesting an autosomal dominant transmission of breast cancer.[63a]

With an appreciation that genetic factors and atypical hyperplastic epithelium, together with a constellation of other attendant risk factors, may provide a triggering mechanism for malignant transformation, scrupulously careful observation of these women is mandatory.

REFERENCES

1. Anderson DE: A genetic study of human breast cancer. *J Natl Cancer Inst* 48:1029, 1972.
2. Anderson DE: Genetic study of breast cancer. Identification of a high risk group. *Cancer* 34:1090, 1974.
3. Anderson DE: Familial predisposition, in Schottenfeld D, Fraumeni JF, Jr (eds): *Cancer Epidemiology and Prevention*. Philadelphia, W. B. Saunders, 1982, p. 483.
4. Anderson DE: Breast cancer in families. *Cancer* 40:1855, 1977.
5. Anderson DE, Williams WR: Implications of a family history of breast or colon cancer, in Chaganti RSK, German JL (eds): *Genetics in Clinical Oncology*. Oxford University Press, 1985, pp. 241-256.
6. Ashikari H, Huvos AG, Snyder RE, Lucas JC, Hutter RVP, McDivitt RW, Schottenfeld D: A clinicopathologic study of atypical lesions of the breast. *Cancer* 33:310, 1974.
7. Ashikari H, Huvos AG, Snyder RE, Sharma R, Kirch R, Schottenfeld D: A clinicopathologic study of atypical lesions of the breast—further followup. *Path Res Pract* 166:48, 1980.
8. Baker LH: Breast cancer detection demonstration project: Five year summary report. *CA* 32:194, 1982.
9. Black MM, Chabon AB: In situ carcinoma of the breast. (Classification System), in Sommers AC (ed): *Pathlogy Annual*. New York, Appleton-Century-Crofts, 1969, p. 185.
10. Black MM, Barclay THC, Cutler SJ, Hankey BF, Asire AJ: Association of atypical characteristics of benign breast lesions with subsequent risk of breast cancer. *Cancer* 29:338, 1972.
11. Black MM, Kwon S: Precancerous mastopathy: Structural and biological considerations. *Path Res Pract* 166:491, 1980.
12. Bucala R, Fishman J, Cerami A: Formation of covalent adducts between cortisone and 16-alpha-hydroxyestrone and protein-possible role in the pathogenesis of cortisol toxicity and systemic lupus erythematosus. *Proc Natl Acad Sci USA* 79:3320, 1982.
13. Cardiff RD, Wellings SR, Faulker LJ: Biology of breast preneoplasia. *Cancer* 39:2734, 1977.
14. Claggett OT, Plimpton NC, Root GT: Lesions of the breast: The relationship of benign lesions to carcinoma. *Surgery* 15:413, 1944.
15. Chardot C, Arroy AV, Parache RM: *Bull Cancer (Paris)* 57:251, 1970.
16. Coombs LJ, Lilienfeld AM, Bross IDS, Burnett SW: A prospective study of the relationship

between benign breast disease and breast carcinoma. *Prev Med* 8:40, 1979.

17. Copeland MM: The treatment of mammary dysplasia with special reference to microcystic and macrocystic disease of the breast. *Am J Surg* 106:382, 1963.
18. Dao TL: The question of "preneoplastic" lesions. *J Surg Oncol* 4:397, 1972.
19. Davis JB: Cystic disease of the breast: Its relationship to mammary carcinoma. *Prog Clin Cancer* 3:221, 1967.
20. Davis HH, Simons M, Davis JB: Cystic disease of the breast—relationship to carcinoma. *Cancer* 17:957, 1964.
21. De Waard F: The epidemiology of breast cancer; review of prospects. *Int J Cancer* 4:577, 1969.
22. Donegan WL, Spratt JS (eds): *Cancer of the Breast.* Volume V in the series, *Major Problems in Clinical Surgery.* Philadelphia, W. B. Saunders Co., 1979, Epidemiology, p. 14.
23. Donnelly PK, Baker KW, Carney JA, O'Fallon WM: Benign breast lesions and subsequent breast carcinoma in Rochester, Minnesota. *Mayo Clin Proc* 50:650, 1975.
24. Dupont WD, Page DL: Risk factors for breast cancer in women with proliferative breast disease. *New Engl J Med* 312:146, 1985.
25. Fisher ER: The pathology of breast cancer as it relates to its evolution, prognosis and treatment, in Baum M (ed): *Clinics in Oncology*, vol. 1, no. 3. Philadelphia, W. B. Saunders, November 1982, p. 703.
26. Fishman J, Fukushima D, O'Connor J, Rosenfeld RS, Lynch HT, Lynch JF, Guirgis H, Maloney K: Plasma hormone profiles of young women at risk for familial breast cancer. *Cancer Res* 38:4006, 1978.
27. Fishman J, Fukushima DK, O'Connor J, Lynch HT: Low urinary estrogen glucuronides in women at risk for familial breast cancer. *Science* 204:1089, 1979.
28. Fishman J, Martucci C: Biological properties of 16-alpha-hydroxyestrone: Implications in estrogen physiology and pathophysiology. *J Clin Endocrinol Metab* 51:611, 1980.
29. Fishman J, Bradlow HL, Fukushima DK, O'Connor J, Rosenfeld RS, Graepel GJ, Elston R, Lynch H: Abnormal estrogen conjugation in women at risk for familial breast cancer at the periovulatory stage of the menstrual cycle. *Cancer Res* 43:1884, 1983.
30. Foote FW, Stewart FW: Comparative studies of cancerous versus noncancerous breasts. *Ann Surg* 121:6, 197, 1945.
31. Frantz VK, Pickren JW, Melcher GW, Auchincloss H, Jr: Incidence of chronic cystic disease in so-called normal breasts. A study based on 225 postmortem examinations. *Cancer* 4:762, 1951.
32. Gallager HS, Martin JE: Early phases in the development of breast cancer. *Cancer* 24:1170, 1969.
33. Greenwald P, Mascal PC, Lawrence CE, et al: Estimated effect of breast self-examination and routine physician examination on breast-cancer mortality. *N Engl J Med* 299:265, 1978.
34. Gullino PM: Natural history of breast cancer progression from hyperplasia to neoplasia as predicted by angiogenesis. *Cancer* 39:2697, 1977.
35. Haagensen CD: *Diseases of the Breast.* Philadelphia, W.B. Saunders, 1956, p. 162.
36. Haagensen CD: *Diseases of the Breast*, 2d ed. Philadelphia, W.B. Saunders, 1971, p. 170.
37. Humphrey LJ, Swerdlow M: Relationships of benign breast disease to carcinoma of the breast. *Surgery* 52:841, 1962.
38. Humphrey LJ, Swerdlow MA: Large duct epithelial hyperplasia and carcinoma of the breast. *Arch Surg* 97:592, 1968.
39. Hutchinson WB, Thomas DB, Hamlon WB, Roth GJ, Peterson AV, Williams B: Risk of breast cancer in women with benign breast disease. *J Natl Cancer Inst* 65:13, 1980.
40. Kalache A: Risk factors for breast cancer: A tabular summary of the epidemiological literature. *Br J Surg* 68:797, 1981.
41. Karpas OM, Leis HP, Oppenheimer A, Mersheimer WL: Relationship of fibrocystic disease to carcinoma of the breast. *Ann Surg* 162:1, 1965.
42. Kelsey JL, Hildreth NG: *Breast and Gynecologic Cancer Epidemiology.* Boca Raton, Florida, CRC Press, 1983, pp. 5-79.
43. Kiaer W: *Relation of Fibroadenomatosis ("Chronic Mastitis") to Cancer of the Breast.* Copenhagen, Munksgaard, 1954, p. 69.
44. Kodlin P, Winger EE, Morgenstern NL, Chen U: Chronic mastopathy and breast cancer—a follow-up study. *Cancer* 39:2603, 1977.

45. Korenman SG: Estrogen window hypothesis of the etiology of breast cancer. *Lancet* 1:700, 1980.
46. Kramer WM, Rush B Jr: Mammary duct proliferation in the elderly. A histopathologic study. *Cancer* 31:130, 1973.
47. Lagios MD: Human breast precancer: Current status, in DeCosse JJ (ed): *Cancer Surveys*, vol. 2, no. 3. Oxford University Press, 1983, p. 383.
48. Lemon HM, Wotiz HH, Parsons L, Mozden PJ: Reduced estriol excretion in patients with breast cancer prior to endocrine therapy. *JAMA* 196:1128, 1966.
49. Lemon HM: Review: Genetic predisposition to carcinoma of the breast. *J Surg Oncol* 4:255, 1972.
50. Lewison EF, Lyons JG: Relationship between benign breast disease and cancer. *Arch Surg* 66:94, 1953.
51. Lynch HT, Lynch PM, Albano WA, Edney J, Orgon CH, Lynch JF: Hereditary cancer: Ascertainment and management. *CA* 29:21, 1979.
52. Lynch HT, Follett RL, Lynch PM, Albano WA, Maillard JL, Pierson RL: Family history in an oncology clinic. *JAMA* 242:1268, 1979.
53. Lynch HT (ed): *Genetics and Breast Cancer*. New York, Van Nostrand Reinhold Co., 1981, p. 196.
54. Lynch HT, Fain PR, Golgor D, Albano WA, Maillard JA, McKenna P: Familial breast cancer and its recognition in an oncology clinic. *Cancer* 47:2730, 1981.
55. MacMahon B, Cole P, Brown J: Etiology of human breast cancer: A review. *J Natl Cancer Inst* 50:21, 1973.
56. Monson RR, Yen SS, MacMahon B, Warren S: Chronic mastitis and carcinoma of the breast. *Lancet* 2:224, 1976.
57. Moskowitz M, Russell P, Fidler J, Sutorius D, Law EJ, Holle J: Breast cancer screening—preliminary report of 207 biopsies performed in 4,128 volunteer screenees. *Cancer* 36:2245, 1975.
58. Moskowitz M, Pemmaraju S, Russell P, Gardella L, Gartside P, De Groot I: Observations on the natural history of carcinoma of the breast, its precursors and mammographic counterparts. *Dis Breast* 3:14, 1977.
59. Moskowitz M: The predictive value of certain mammographic signs in screening for cancer. *Cancer* 51:1007, 1983.
60. Nomura A, Comstock GN, Tonascia JA: Epidemiologic characteristics of benign breast disease. *Am J Epidemiol* 105:505, 1977.
60a. Osborne MP, Bradlow HL, Hershcopf, Fishman J: A potential marker for the risk of breast cancer: Abnormal estradiol 16 alpha hydroxylation. *Soc Surg Oncol 37th Ann Meeting* May 13-17, 1984. New York Abstract #36.
61. Ottman R, Pike MC, King MC, Henderson BE: Practical guide for estimating risk for familial breast cancer. *Lancet* 2:553, 1983.
62. Page DJ, Vanderzwagg R, Rogers LW, Williams LT, Walker WE, Hartmann WH: Relation between component parts of fibrocystic disease complex and breast cancer. *J Natl Cancer Inst* 61:1055, 1978.
63. Potter JF, Steinbaugh WP, Woodward SC: Can breast carcinoma be anticipated? A followup of benign breast biopsies. *Ann Surg* 167:829, 1968.
63a. Recabaren J, Osborne MP, Rosen PP, Chaganti R, Kinne DW, De Cosse JJ: A special surveillance breast clinic: Analysis of risk factors. *Proc Am Soc Clin Oncol* 3:6, 1984.
64. Rush BF, Kramer WM: Proliferative histological changes and occult carcinoma in the breast of the aging female. *Surg Gynecol Obstet* 117:425, 1963.
65. Sandison AT: An autopsy study of the adult human breast. *Natl Cancer Inst Monogr* 8:1, 1962.
66. Schneider J, Kinne DW, Fracchia A, Pierce V, Anderson KE, Bradlow HL, Fishman J: Abnormal oxidative metabolism of estradiol in women with breast cancer. *Proc Natl Acad Sci USA* 79:3047, 1982.
67. Shapiro S, Strax P, Venet L, Fink R: The search for risk factors in breast cancer. *Am J Public Health* 58:820, 1968.
68. Sherman BM, Korenman SG: Inadequate corpus luteum function: A pathophysiological interpretation of human breast cancer epidemiology. *Cancer* 33:1306, 1974.
69. Steinhoff NG, Black WC: Florid cystic disease preceding mammary cancer. *Ann Surg* 171:501, 1970.
70. Strax P: Results of mass screening for breast cancer in 50,000 examinations. *Cancer* 37:30, 1976.
71. Veronesi U, Pizzocoro G: Breast cancer in women subsequent to cystic disease of the breast. *Surg Gynecol Obstet* 126:529, 1968.

72. Warren S: The relation of "chronic mastitis" to carcinoma of the breast. *Surg Gynecol Obstet* 71:257, 1940.
73. Wellings SR, Jensen HM, Morcum RG: An atlas of subgross pathology of the human breast with special reference to possible precancerous lesions. *J Natl Cancer Inst* 55:231, 1975.
74. Wellings SR: Development of human breast cancer. *Adv Cancer Res* 31:287, 1980.
75. Williams WR, Anderson DE: Genetic epidemiology of breast cancer: Segregation analysis of 200 Danish pedigrees. *Genetic Epidemiol* 1:7, 1984.
76. Williams WR, Lalouel JM: Genetic risk, in Morton N, Rao DC, Lalouel JM (eds): *Methods in Genetic Epidemiology*. New York, S. Karger, 1983, p. 188.

Part Three

Basic Considerations: Classification, Pathology, Receptors, and Immunology

7

Classification and Staging of Breast Cancer

Oliver H. Beahrs, M.D.

INTRODUCTION

Staging of cancer of the breast or cancer at any anatomic site is a shorthand method of grouping like cases of cancers together to determine biologic behavior of the lesions, appropriate forms of treatment, and to permit critical evaluation of end results of management, prognosis, and survival of patients. It is generally accepted that a solid tumor begins as a single focus in the anatomic part of origin and over time increases in size, expanding at the primary site, and at some point spreading to regional tissues by direct extension and by lymphatic vessels to regional lymph nodes. In some instances, multicentric lesions might be present and, as a rule, the number of lesions are noted, but the more extensive lesion is the one that is staged. A cancer of the breast may also spread early or late to distant sites such as the pleura, bone, and other tissues away from the breast and its regional lymphatics, thus becoming a generalized disease.

Staging of a cancer is an expression of the anatomic extent of the disease. Even though there are other parameters that affect treatment and prognosis such as the cellular type of lesion, the degree of undifferentiation of the lesion, and possibly biologic markers, at present these parameters are not considered in describing the anatomic extent of the disease. These findings, however, should always be recorded since they also enter into decision making in the management of a breast cancer and also in evaluating the end results.

The American Joint Committee on Cancer, in making its recommendations regarding staging of breast cancer, has utilized TNM symbols—T representing the primary tumor, N the absence or involvement of regional lymph nodes, and M the presence or absence of distant metastasis. An attempt has been made to keep definitions relatively simple, but for research purposes the various TNM categories can be expanded depending on the information desired in the research study. With increased knowledge regarding the origin, function, and biologic behavior of some tumors of the breast, biologic markers and hormone receptors may be established as important or even more so than anatomic factors in staging. If this should prove to be true, then certainly this information will be incorporated in any recommendations regarding staging of cancer of the breast or cancer at other anatomic sites. In the meantime, the recommendations of the American Joint Committee on Cancer regarding staging of cancer of the breast follows.

The staging system for cancer of the breast applies to in situ carcinoma and to infiltrating cancer of the breast. Histologic verification is mandatory and the cell type must be recorded. Unconfirmed cases must be reported separately.

Although there have been minor differences in the recommendations for staging of cancer of the breast by the Union Internationale Contre le Cancer (UICC) and the AJCC in the past, the recommendations of the UICC are now consistent with those of the AJCC.

ANATOMY

Primary Site The mammary gland consists of glandular tissue within a dense fibroareolar stroma situated on the anterior chest wall. Deep to the breast is the fascia overlying the pectoralis major, which in turn covers the ribs and intercostal muscles of the first six intercostal spaces.

Nodal Stations The breast lymphatics drain by way of three major routes—axillary, transpectoral, and internal mammary trunks—into numerous surrounding first station nodes such as axillary (low, middle), axillary apex, and infraclavicular (referred to as levels I, II, and III, respectively), and internal mammary, interpectoral, and subclavicular. Supraclavicular nodes are juxtaregional on the homolateral side. Disease involvement in all other nodes—cervical, contralateral supraclavicular, and internal mammary—is equivalent to distant metastases.

Metastatic Sites All distant visceral sites are potential sites of metastatic disease. The four major sites are bone, lung, brain, and liver, but this widely metastasizing disease has been found in virtually all remote sites.

RULES FOR CLASSIFICATION

Clinical-Diagnostic Staging In the clinical-diagnostic stage, the following are required: physical examination, including careful inspection of skin and palpation of mammary glands and regional nodes; determination of the degree of fixation with and without flexing pectoral muscles; routine laboratory studies and hemograms; and chest films. Bilateral breast imaging by a validated technique such as x-ray mammography is recommended. Also, pathologic examination of the primary cancer or other tissues to establish the diagnosis of breast cancer is required. In other words, all data obtained prior to definitive treatment is used for clinical-diagnostic staging.

Postsurgical Resection–Pathologic Staging The postsurgical resection–pathologic stage includes the following:

1 All data used for clinical-diagnostic staging
2 Pathologic examination of the primary cancer, the entire breast, and all levels of axillary lymph nodes as with standard or modified radical mastectomy

TNM CLASSIFICATION

Primary Tumor (T)

Definitions for the primary tumor (T) for clinical-diagnostic classification are the same as those for postsurgical resection–pathologic classification.

TX Minimum requirements to assess primary tumor cannot be met.

T_0 No evidence of primary tumor.

T_{is} *In situ* cancer (in situ lobular, pure intraductal, and Paget's disease of the nipple without palpable tumor).

(*Note:* Paget's disease with a demonstrable tumor is classified according to size of the tumor. Inflammatory carcinoma should be reported separately.)

T_1† Tumor 2 cm or less in greatest dimension

T_{1a} No fixation to underlying pectoral fascia or muscle

T_{1b} Fixation to underlying pectoral fascia or muscle

i. tumor $\leq$ 0.5 cm

ii. tumor $>$ 0.5 $\leq$ 1.0 cm

iii. tumor $>$ 1.0 $\leq$ 2.0 cm

T_2† Tumor more than 2 cm but not more than 5 cm in its greatest dimension

T_{2a} No fixation to underlying pectoral fascia or muscle

T_{2b} Fixation to underlying pectoral fascia or muscle

T_3† Tumor more than 5 cm in its greatest dimension

T_{3a} No fixation to underlying pectoral fascia or muscle

T_{3b} Fixation to underlying pectoral fascia or muscle

T_4 Tumor of any size with direct extension to chest wall or skin

Chest wall includes ribs, intercostal muscles, and serratus anterior muscle, but not pectoral muscle.)

T_{4a} Fixation to chest wall

T_{4b} Edema (including *peau d'orange*), ulceration of the skin of the breast, or satellite skin nodules confined to the same breast

T_{4c} Both of the above

Nodal Involvement (N)

The definition of N categories varies somewhat as to time period of staging, as follows.

†Dimpling of the skin, nipple retraction, or any other skin changes except those in T_{4b} may occur in T_1, T_2, or T_3 without changing the classification.

Definitions for Clinical-Diagnostic Stage

NX Regional lymph nodes cannot be assessed clinically.

N_0 Homolateral axillary lymph nodes not considered to contain growth.

N_1 Movable homolateral axillary nodes considered to contain growth.

N_2 Homolateral axillary nodes considered to contain growth and fixed to one another or to other structures.

N_3 Homolateral supraclavicular or infraclavicular nodes considered to contain growth or edema of the arm. (Edema of the arm may be caused by lymphatic obstruction and lymph nodes may not then be palpable.)

Definitions for Surgical-Evaluative and Postsurgical Resection–Pathologic Stage

NX Regional lymph nodes cannot be assessed (not removed for study or previously removed).

N_0 No evidence of homolateral axillary lymph node metastasis.

N_1 Metastasis to movable homolateral axillary nodes not fixed to one another or to other structure.

N_{1a} Micrometastasis $\leq$0.2 cm in lymph node(s).

N_{1b} Gross metastasis in lymph node(s).

I Metastasis more than 0.2 cm but less than 2.0 cm in one to three lymph nodes

II Metastasis more than 0.2 cm but less than 2.0 cm in four or more lymph nodes

III Extension of metastasis beyond the lymph node capsule (less than 2.0 cm in dimension)

IV Metastasis in lymph node 2.0 cm or more in dimension

N_2 Metastases to homolateral axillary lymph nodes that are fixed to one another or to other structures

N_3 Metastasis to homolateral supraclavicular or infraclavicular lymph node(s)

(*Note:* Edema of the arm may be caused by lymphatic obstruction, and lymph nodes may not then be palpable. Homolateral internal mammary nodes considered to contain growth are included in N_3 for surgical-evaluative classification and postsurgical resection-pathologic classification.)

Distant Metastasis (M)

All time periods

MX Minimum requirements to assess the presence of distant metastasis cannot be met.
M_0 No (known) distant metastasis.
M_1 Distant metastasis present.
Specify_____

Specify sites according to the following notations:

Pulmonary, PUL
Osseous, OSS
Hepatic, HEP
Brain, BRA
Lymph nodes, LYM
Bone marrow, MAR
Pleura, PLE
Skin, SKI
Eye, EYE
Other, OTH

POSTSURGICAL RESECTION RESIDUAL TUMOR (R)

This does not enter into staging tumor but may be a factor in deciding management.

R_0 No residual tumor
R_1 Microscopic residual tumor
R_2 Macroscopic residual tumor
Specify_____

HISTOLOGIC TYPE OF CANCER

Cancer, NOS*
Ductal
- Intraductal (in situ)
- Invasive with predominant intraductal component
- Invasive, NOS*
- Comedo
- Inflammatory†
- Medullary with lymphocytic infiltrate
- Mucinous (colloid)
- Papillary
- Scirrhous
- Tubular
- Other
- Specify_____

Lobular
- In situ
- Invasive with predominant in situ component
- Invasive

Nipple
- Paget's disease, NOS*
- Paget's disease with intraductal carcinoma
- Paget's disease with invasive ductal carcinoma

Other
- Specify_____

*Not otherwise specified.

HISTOLOGIC GRADE

G_1 Well differentiated
G_2 Moderately well differentiated
G_3-G_4 Poorly to very poorly differentiated

Use whichever indicator is most appropriate (term or G + number).

STAGE GROUPING

Always indicate time of classification.

Clinical-Diagnostic (cTNM), Surgical-Evaluative (sTNM), and Postsurgical Resection-Pathologic (pTNM) Staging

Stage T_{is} *In situ*
Stage X Cannot stage
Stage I T_{1ai}, N_0, M_0
T_{1aii}, N_0, M_0
T_{1aiii}, N_0, M_0

†Inflammatory carcinoma is a clinicopathologic entity characterized by diffuse brawny induration of the skin of the breast with an erysipeloid edge, usually without an underlying palpable mass. Histologically infiltrating mammary carcinoma diffusely permeates dermal lymphatics. (Inflamed cancers that are clinically similar to the above owing to inflammation, infection, or necrosis but that lack microscopic dermal lymphatic permeation are *not* classified as inflammatory carcinoma.)

Stage I T_{1bi}, N_0, M_0
T_{1bii}, N_0, M_0
T_{1biii}, N_0, M_0
Stage II T_0, N_{1a} or N_{1b}, M_0
T_{1a} or T_{1b}, N_{1a} or N_{1b}, M_0
T_{2a} or T_{2b}, N_0, M_0
T_{2a} or T_{2b}, N_{1a} or N_{1b}, M_0
Stage IIIA T_0, N_2, M_0
T_{1a} or T_{1b}, N_2, M_0
T_{2a} or T_{2b}, N_2, M_0
T_{3a} or T_{3b}, N_0, M_0
T_{3a} or T_{3b}, N_1, M_0
T_{3a} or T_{3b}, N_2, M_0
Stage IIIB Any T, N_3, M_0
Any T_4, any N, M_0
Stage IV Any T, any N, M_1

Measurements of 2 cm or less for T_{1a}, T_{1b}, and N_{1b} do not necessarily need to be recorded.

PERFORMANCE STATUS OF HOST (H)

Performance status of the host should be recorded because this information at times is pertinent to the treatment of the patient.

8

Pathology of Breast Cancer

Pin Kie Teng, M.D.

INTRODUCTION

In the daily practice of oncology and in medical conferences, clinicians ask why pathologists do not get together and decide on a simple pathologic classification on which clinicians may rely as an aid in determining treatment policies and prognosis, and to permit comparison of results on an international scale.[12,16,17,21,22] The profession has labored from the time of Hippocrates to classify breast lesions. Celsus, at the time of Christ, offered the first classification:

1 Cacoethes—early or precancerous lesions
2 Carcinoma without ulceration
3 Fungating tumors

This clinical classification has been modified many times and is essentially an anatomic diagnosis describing the extent of the cancer. It is discussed fully in Chap. 7 as the TNM classification. The other method of classifying breast lesions is the microscopic appearance of the lesions. The true picture of the neoplasm is often modified by the varied response of the breast to the presence of the cancer, often resulting in bizarre histologic alterations.

A suitable pathologic classification would describe the intrinsic appearance of the lesion and the vagaries of response by the breast, such as a marked lymphocytic or desmoplastic reaction, an apparent defense mechanism, or in others, the absolute absence of such a response.[8]

No matter how scientific the classification, it is no good if it does not help pathologists and clinicians communicate on therapeutic decision making and prognosis.

Classification is not a mere academic exercise. In the past when there was only one treatment for a cancer or noncancer of the breast, a diagnosis of malignant or benign lesion would suffice. But today, since there are alternative treatments, both primary and adjuvant, a precise classification is a major factor in the choice of therapy. The prevalence of treatment trials is

Table 8-1 Carcinoma of the Breast

Carcinoma in the nipple	
Paget's disease	
Carcinoma of mammary ducts	
Noninfiltrating	Intraductal carcinoma
	Intracystic carcinoma
	Solid duct carcinoma
Infiltrating	Scirrhous carcinoma
	Papillary carcinoma
	Comedo carcinoma
	Mucinous carcinoma
	Medullary carcinoma
Carcinoma of mammary lobules	
Noninfiltrating lobular carcinoma in situ	
Infiltrating lobular carcinoma	
Rare carcinomas	
Tubular carcinoma	
Adenoid cystic carcinoma	
Inflammatory carcinoma	
Apocrine carcinoma	
Lipid-rich carcinoma	
Carcinoma arising from fibroadenoma	
Carcinoma with metaplasia	
Osseocartilaginous formation	
Fibromyxomatous sarcoma-like formation	
Squamous cell formation	
Clear cell carcinoma	
Non-Paget's carcinoma in the nipple	
Signet-ring-cell carcinoma	
Small-cell carcinoma	

another important factor for an accurate classification, since the latter is essential in the stratification that assures comparability.

A classification should be practical, related to reality, and specific; one and only one place for each entity. It should have common features in grouping and subgrouping entities. Classification of breast cancer is complicated because of the protean nature of the disease itself. In the International Histological Classification of Breast Tumors by the World Health Organization, breast cancer is divided as follows:

1 Noninfiltrating intraductal and intralobular
2 Infiltrating intraductal and intralobular
3 Special histological variants
   a Medullary
   b Papillary
   c Cribriform
   d Mucous
   e Lobular
   f Squamous cell
   g Paget's
   h Carcinoma arising in intracanalicular fibroadenoma

The pathology group of the National Cancer Institute (NCI) Breast Cancer Task Force presented a more exhaustive classification. A few rare carcinomas, such as signet-ring-cell[10] and lipid-rich carcinoma, were added by the National Cancer Institute (Pathology Group) in 1973.[11,19,23,27]

In this chapter, the pathology of carcinoma of the breast is presented by anatomic site and distribution: nipple, mammary ducts, mammary lobules, and rare carcinoma (see Table 8-1).[2,5,25]

IN SITU VERSUS INFILTRATING CANCER

It is the opinion of some pathologists that all cancers are fully malignant, capable of metastasizing and killing, whether infiltrating or not. In the study of a tumor, if the malignant cells are not seen to penetrate the duct wall or invade the breast stroma at some points, this does not justify the conclusion that infiltration has not taken place. It only means that the cells are not infiltrating at the sites studied. The small portion of the total carcinomatous epithelium in any individual carcinoma, even when a great many microscopic sections are studied, can only suggest in a general way whether or not infiltration has actually occurred. It cannot be regarded as decisive.[3,6,8]

HISTOLOGIC GRADING

Histologic grading of breast cancer for degree of malignancy and prognosis has not been accepted unanimously. The reason is that grading is subjective. It varies from pathologist to pathologist, from specimen tissue blocks to tissue blocks, from area to area on the same slide, and with the number of slides examined. Histologic grading is useful if used in light of the size of the primary lesion and the regional extent of the involvement. It can help to predict the behavior of the malignant tumor. There are, however, many other factors which affect prognosis. (See Chap. 10.)

BREAST CANCERS PRESENTING ON THE NIPPLE

Paget's Disease

Gross The lesion is sharply defined. The infiltrated area is dusky, erythematous, showing scaling, oozing, and crusting, at times extending to the surrounding skin.

Microscopic There are typical large Paget's cells in the epidermis of the nipple devoid of prickles with round pale-staining nucleus and a much lighter abundant cytoplasm, scattered

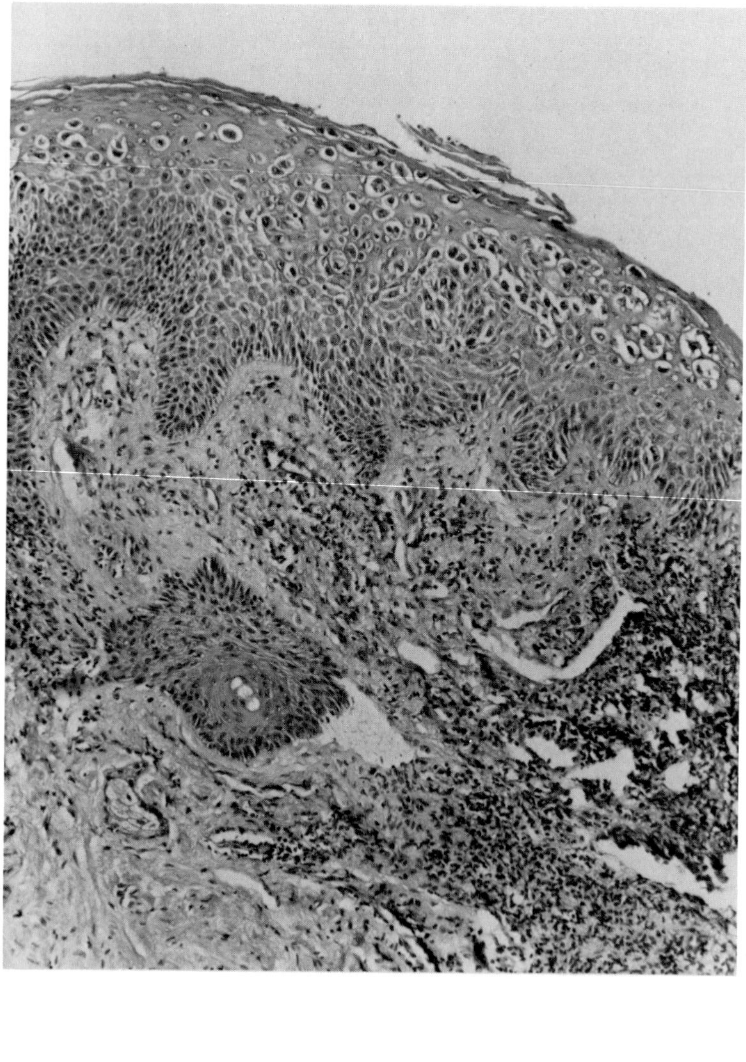

Figure 8-1 Paget's disease of nipple: Large opaque or slightly granular Paget's cells grow upward to the superficial layer of the epidermis of the nipple. The upper dermis is infiltrated by chronic inflammatory cells. ×85

in groups or singly. The dermis shows moderately chronic inflammation. Paget's cells do not invade the dermis, but may extend along the lactiferous ducts of the breast. Recent study suggests strongly the underlying ducts are the tissue of origin (Fig. 8-1).[4,15,18]

CARCINOMA ARISING FROM MAMMARY DUCTS

Noninfiltrating Ductal Carcinoma (Intraductal Carcinoma)

Noninfiltrating ductal carcinoma is considered as carcinoma in situ of the mammary duct. Consequently the prognosis is good if adequate excision is made, even if multicentric. Cure is highly possible. It is being diagnosed more frequently because of public and professional awareness.

Gross This tumor has a segmental distribution in the mammary ducts involving large, medium, or small segments. Multiple grayish, soft, small nodules are noted on a white, firm, fibrous stroma.

Microscopic The dilated lumens of the mammary ducts are partially filled by atypical ductal lining cells in single or multiple layers without well-vascularized stalks. The epithelial projections may bridge the opposite side of the dilated lumen or obliterate the lumen in cribriform pattern (Fig. 8-2). The obliterated lumens of the ducts do not have central necrosis, as do the comedo carcinomas (Fig. 8-3).

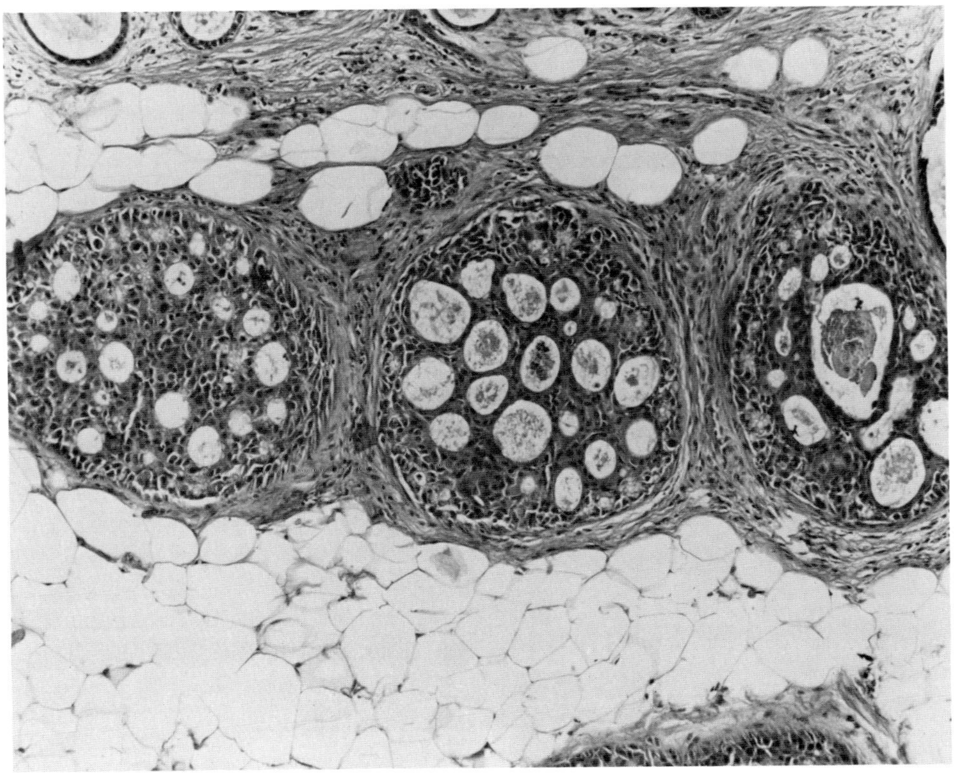

Figure 8-2 Noninfiltrating intraductal papillary carcinoma: Regularly arranged, small round spaces lined by relatively uniform epithelial cells give the tumor a characteristic cribriform pattern. ×85

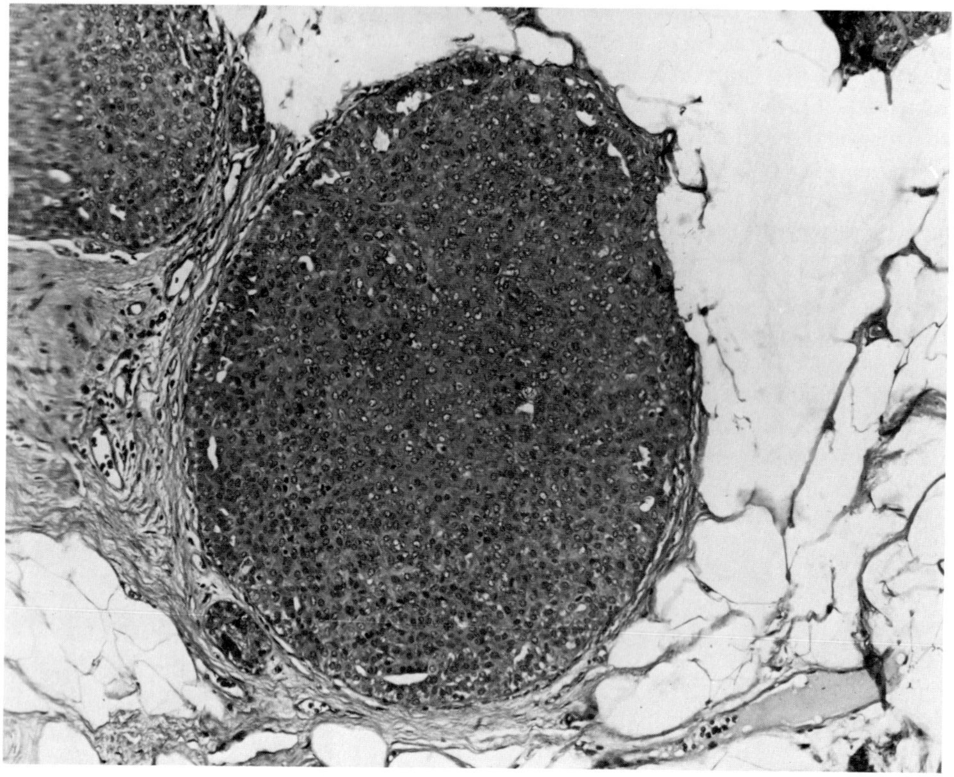

Figure 8-3 Noninfiltrating solid intraductal carcinoma: The dilated duct is completely filled with proliferating ductal lining cells with slightly hyperchromatic and pleomorphic nuclei. Rare atypical mitoses are seen. The basement membrane of the duct is not broken. ×85

The distinction between atypical intraductal papilloma and intraductal papillary carcinoma is extremely difficult in some cases. Cribriform pattern, single-layer epithelial cells, delicate or absence of connective stroma, especially disturbance in cell polarity, are most helpful in diagnosis of papillary carcinoma.

Infiltrating Ductal Carcinoma

Scirrhous Carcinoma

Gross This tumor is the most common and constitutes about three-fourths of all breast cancers. It is well outlined, and is stony hard, producing a grating sound when cut. When retracted from the surrounding tissue, the cut surface is grayish white, smooth, and cartilaginous-like, with chalky streaks or dots.

Microscopic Nests or strands of compressed round to polyhedral epithelial cells are in a mass of dense collagenous fibrous stroma. The tumor cells vary from uniform to slightly pleomorphic. The microscopic diagnosis is made more on disturbance of the normal mammary histologic pattern than on the characteristic malignant cytologic features which could be blurred by the fibrotic process of the stroma (Fig. 8-4).

Papillary Carcinoma

Gross The tumor is well outlined, but not

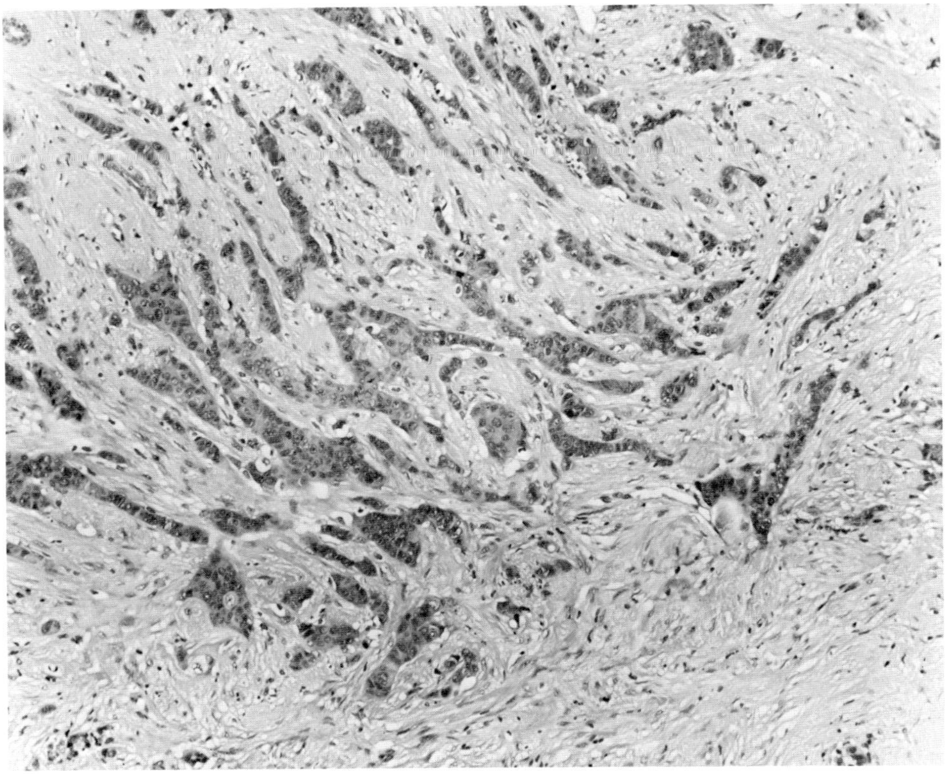

Figure 8-4 Scirrhous carcinoma, infiltrating duct carcinoma with fibrosis: Solid strands of malignant epithelial cells are spread in a disorderly fashion in a dense, productive fibrous stroma. ×85

encapsulated. It is soft, translucent, friable, and sometimes bulky. Necrosis is common.

Microscopic Histologically, this tumor is similar to noninfiltrating intraductal carcinoma. The papillae are present, but composed of ductal epithelial cells with pleomorphic and hyperchromatic nuclei in disorderly arrangement. The surrounding stroma is infiltrated by tumor cells (Fig. 8-5).

Comedo Carcinoma

Gross The name of this tumor comes from its resemblance to the comedo of skin with slightly elevated, yellowish, soft "plugs" on a smooth, grayish, firm surface of the breast tissue. The plugs are necrotic tissue in the centers of solid enlarged mammary ducts filled with malignant epithelial lining cells. Their presence on a hard surface is unmistakable.

Microscopic Enlarged, solid mammary ducts are completely filled by large anaplastic epithelial lining cells with hyperchromatic, pleomorphic nuclei, and loss of polarity. Their atypicality is more than that in an intraductal papillary carcinoma. Most of the comedo carcinomas are infiltrating, which feature can be determined by microscopic examination, although grossly it appears confined (Fig. 8-6).

Mucinous Carcinoma (Colloid)

Gross Well-outlined, bulky, translucent, soft gel-like lobules are in firm whitish fibrous tissue,

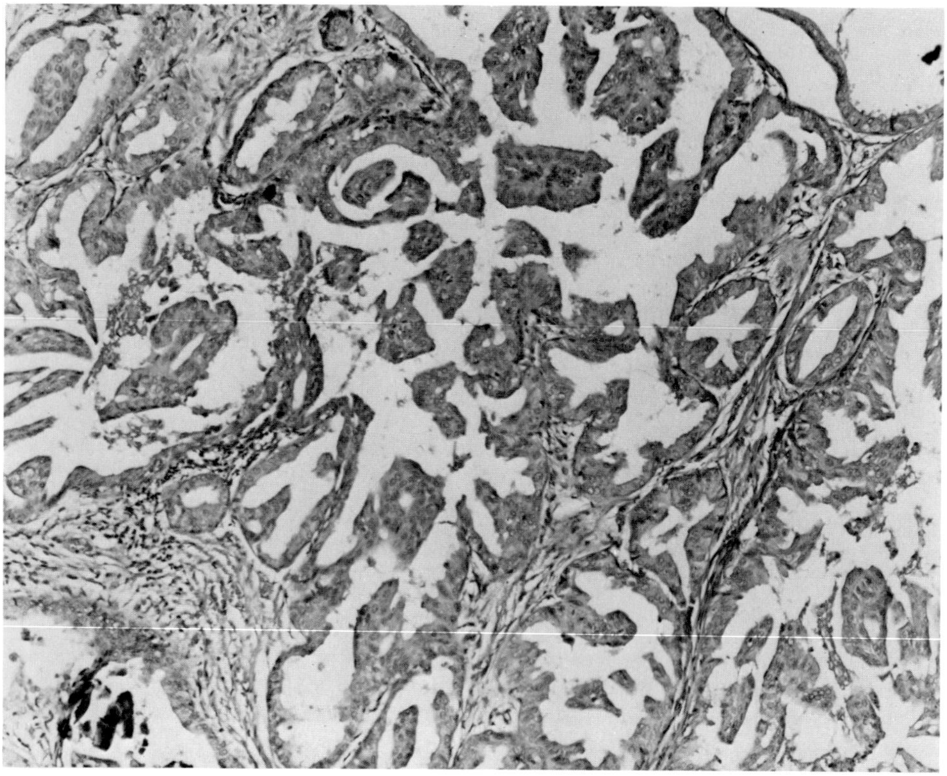

Figure 8-5 Infiltrating papillary carcinoma: Papillae project into the lumen of a duct, forming bridges. The nuclei are hyperchromatic and pleomorphic. Infiltration is in the lower right edge of the photo. ×85

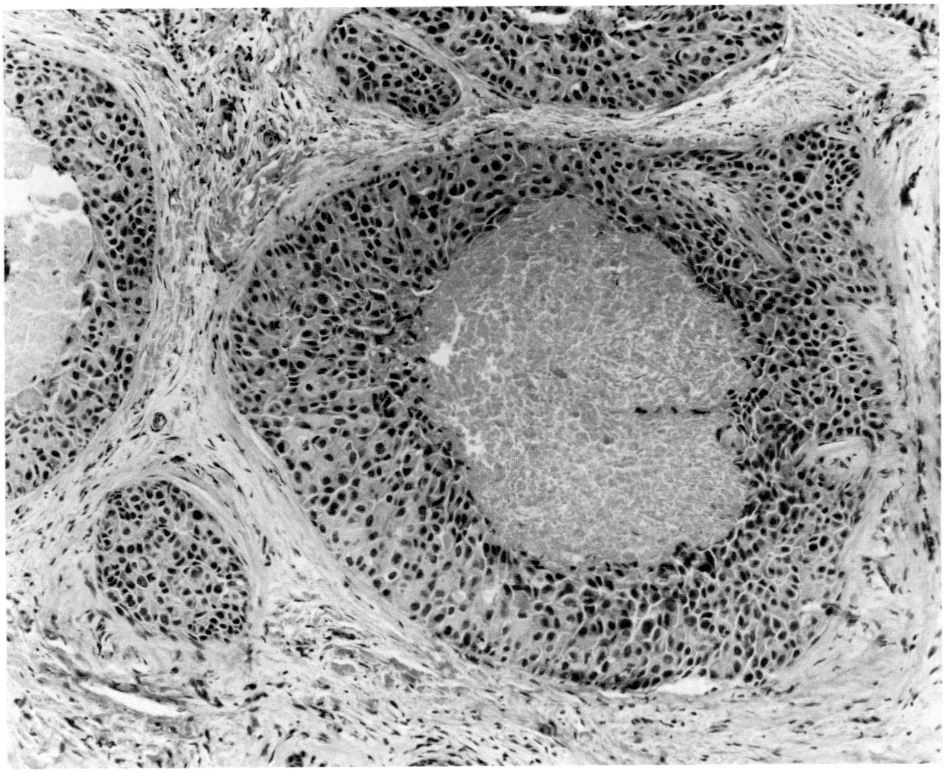

Figure 8-6 Comedo carcinoma: Two distended ducts are lined by several layers of malignant cells. The necrotic centers resemble comedones of skin. ×85

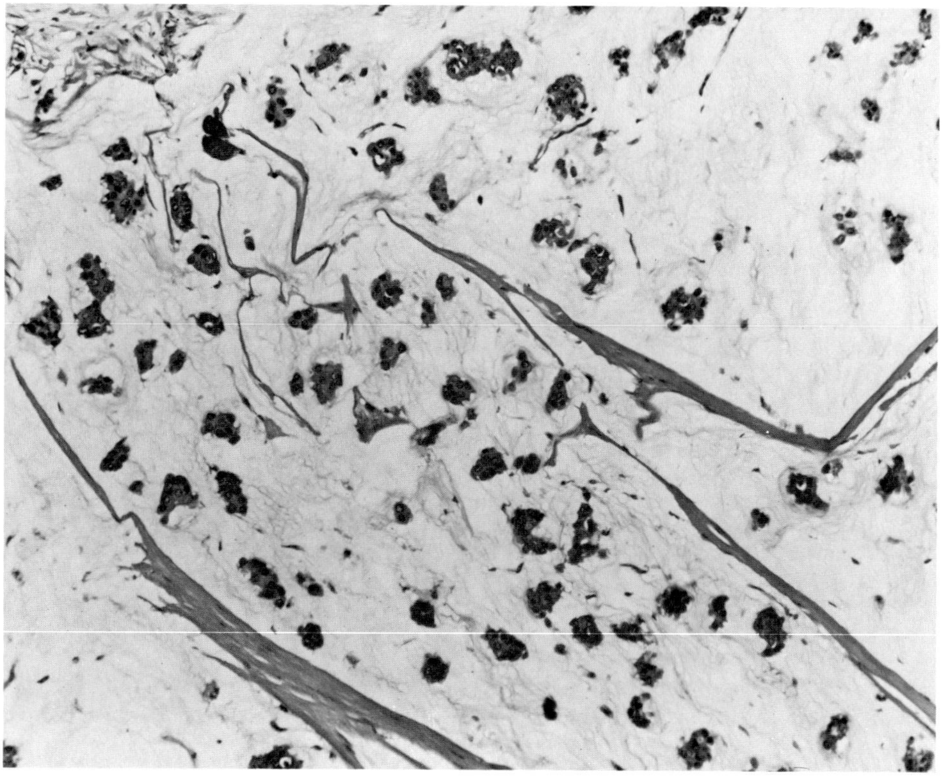

Figure 8-7 Mucinous carcinoma: Clusters of cells and small glands of relatively uniform epithelial calls are embedded in a mucinous pool. ×85

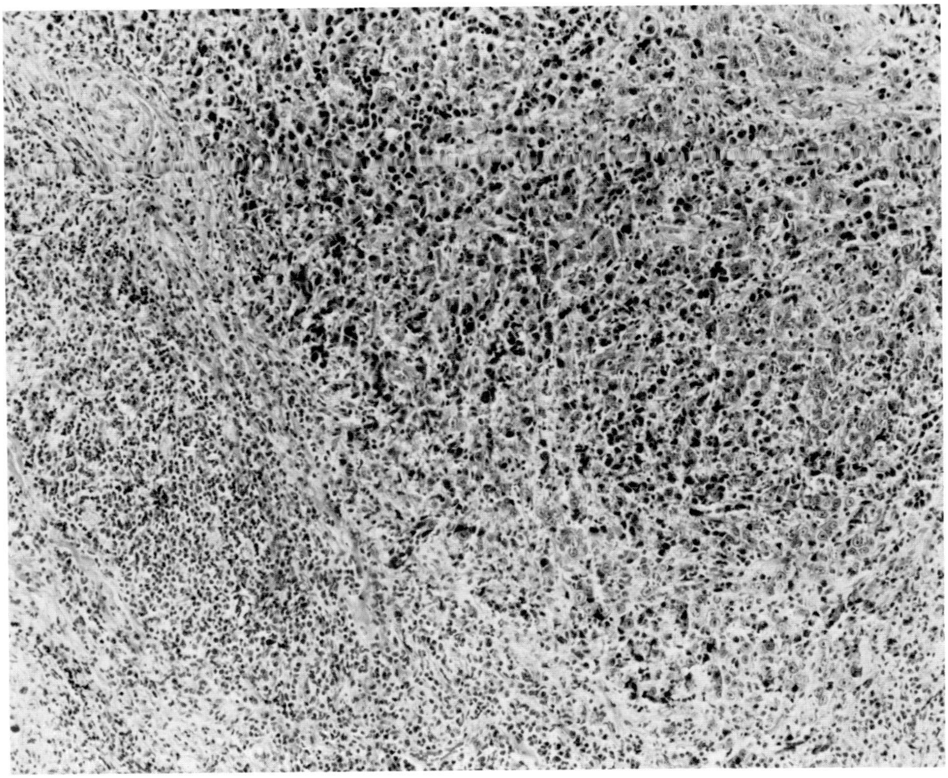

Figure 8-8 Medullary carcinoma: Large polyhedral, malignant epithelial cells with vesicular nucleus diffusely intermingle with lymphocytes, rendering frozen section examination difficult. × 85

measuring an average 1 cm in diameter. Gross appearance is typical, conveying a feeling of limited growth. Rarely, it may be mistaken for myxoid degenerated fibroadenoma.

Microscopic Well-differentiated glands lined by columnar epithelial cells with some secretion in the lumens are seen in a large pool of mucin. Sometimes the tumor cells are not well-differentiated and appear in clusters. Inflammatory reaction is seldom present (Fig. 8-7).

Medullary Carcinoma

Gross These circumscribed tumors are large, bulging, fleshy, soft, and grayish, measuring up to 10 cm in diameter. It does not have the loose, fibrous formation of scirrhous carcinoma.

Microscopic Medullary carcinoma is composed of an irregular mass of poorly differentiated epithelial cells arranged in sheets, without any fibrotic stroma. Sometimes it is heavily infiltrated by lymphocytes. This renders microscopic examination difficult, especially on frozen section of the small tumor cell type (Fig. 8-8).[13,26]

CARCINOMA ARISING FROM MAMMARY LOBULES

Lobular Carcinoma in Situ

Gross There is no palpable or visible mass. The tumor is indistinguishable from ordinary breast tissue.

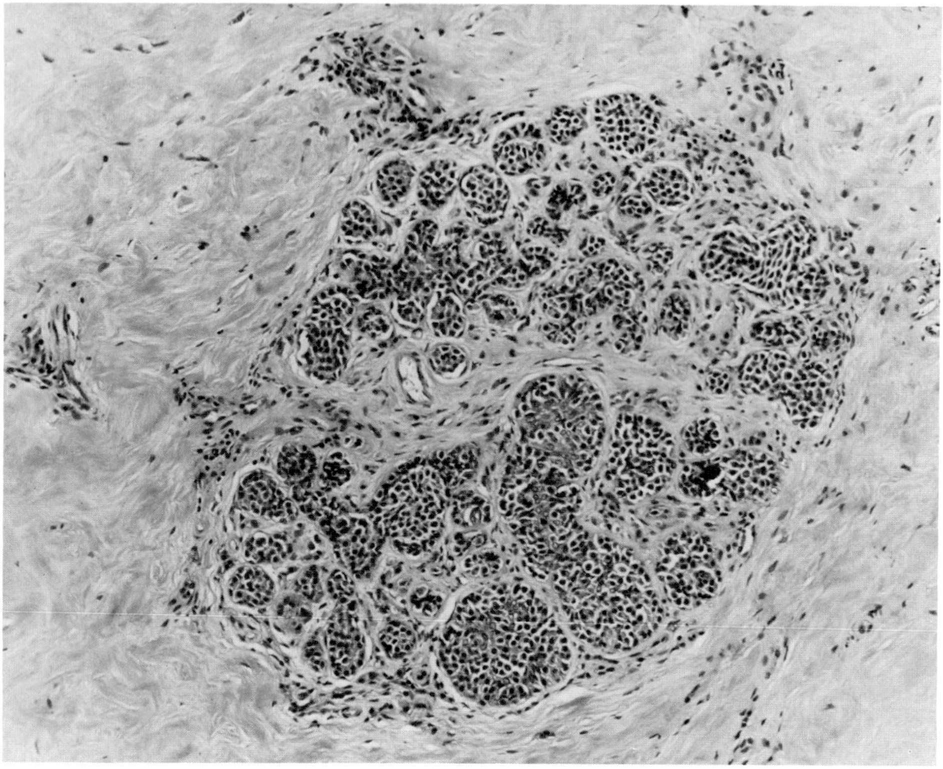

Figure 8-9 Lobular carcinoma in situ: Shown as mammary lobule of solid terminal ductules filled with cohesive tumor cells with indistinct cytoplasmic margin. The uniform nuclei are equally spaced. ×85

Microscopic Well-circumscribed lobule or lobules are packed with solid, enlarged, terminal mammary ductules filled with evenly spaced, enlarged epithelial lining cells. The nuclei are uniformly round. The cytoplasmic membrane is vague. The shape of the mammary lobules is preserved, and the basement membrane of the ductules is intact (Fig. 8-9). This lesion is not infrequently bilateral.

Infiltrating Lobular Carcinoma

Gross The gross appearance of this tumor is like that of scirrhous carcinoma. It is gray-white, poorly outlined, and irregular. The cut surface is smooth and very firm, without chalky streaks.

Microscopic The tumor cells of the terminal ductules of the mammary lobules break through the basement membrane of the ductules, distort the lobular structure, and invade the surrounding stroma in the form of strands, clusters, or small sheets of poorly differentiated cells with hyperchromatic and pleomorphic nuclei. Malignant features definitely are more impressive than those of a noninfiltrating lobular carcinoma (Fig. 8-10). Some pathologists emphasize the presence of "Indian file" or rows of single cells in width in a fibrotic stroma as an indication of lobular origin instead of ductal origin (Fig. 8-11). But these "Indian files" are also found in scirrhous carcinoma. Special stains for myoepithelial cells and electron microscopy are

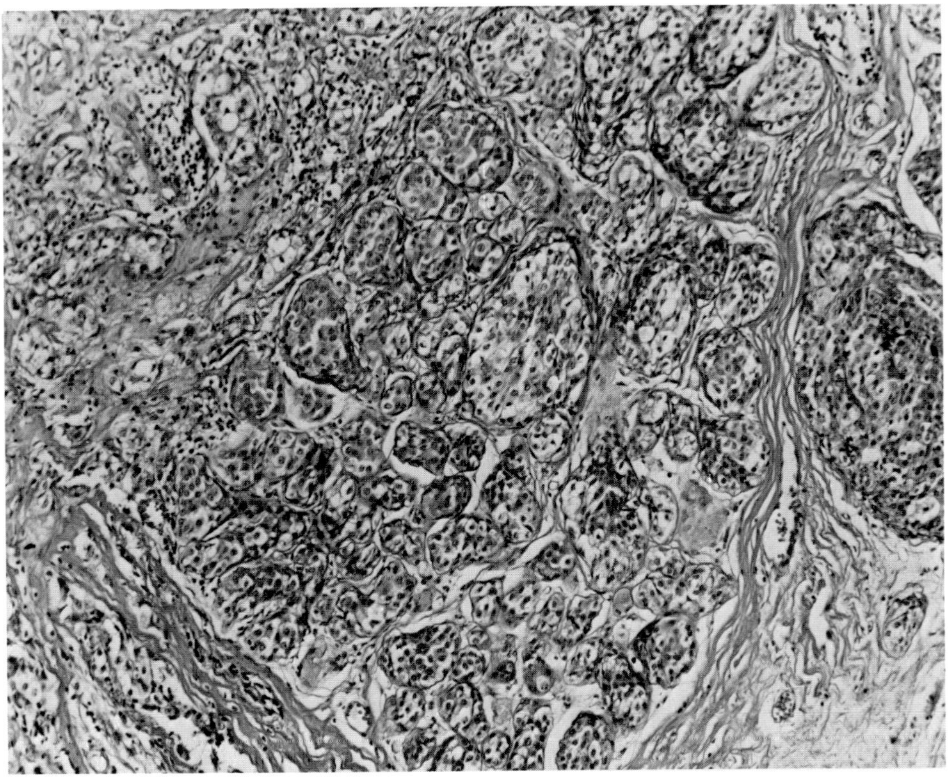

Figure 8-10 Infiltrating lobular carcinoma: On the right side of the photograph there is a lobular carcinoma in situ. Next to it is a lobular carcinoma infiltrating the stroma of the rest of the tumor. ×85

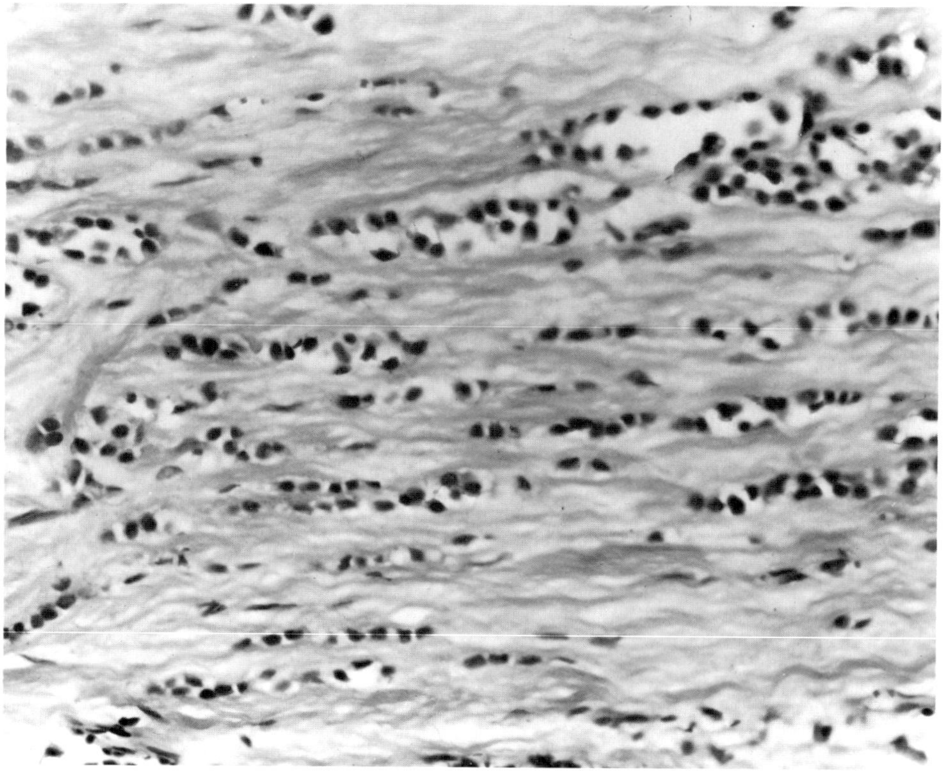

Figure 8-11 Infiltrating lobular carcinoma: So-called "Indian file" linear stromal infiltration of lobular carcinoma is thought to be from the terminal ductules and not from major ducts. ×340

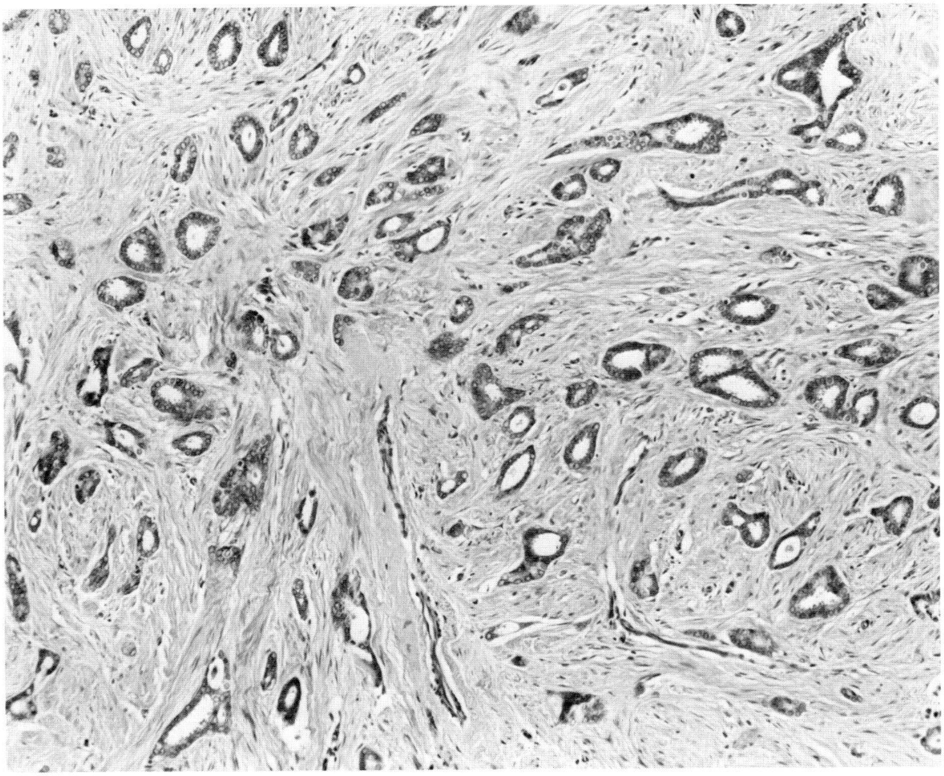

Figure 8-12 Tubular carcinoma: Tubules of uniform diameters are evenly embedded in a dense, fibrous stroma. The epithelial cells are not atypical. ×85

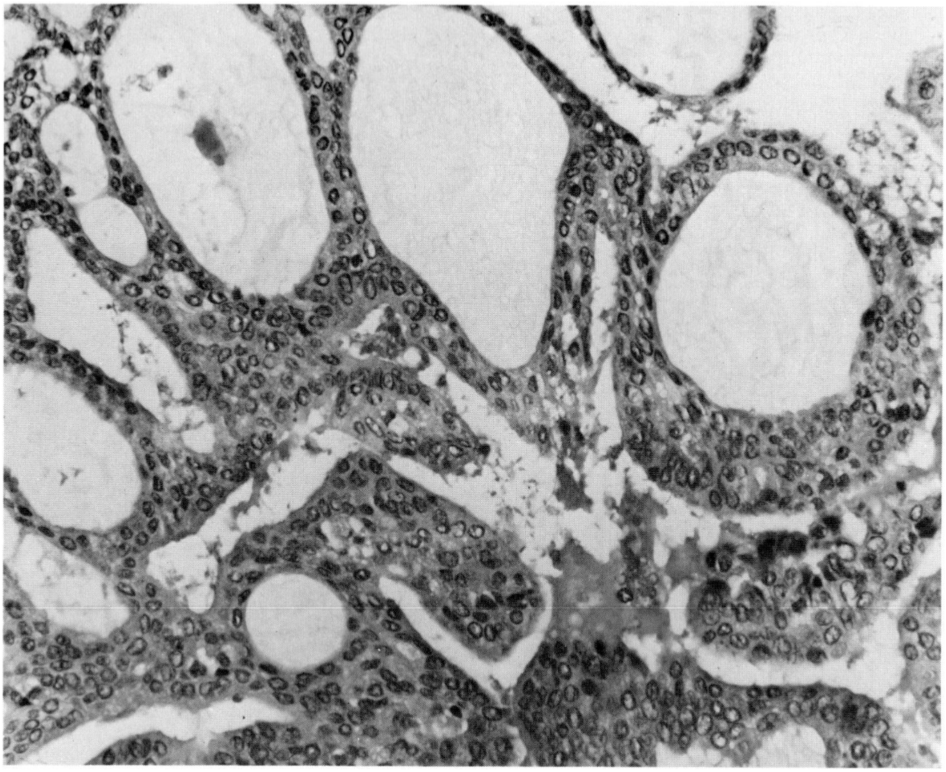

Figure 8-13 Adenoid cystic carcinoma: Large cystic glandular structures are compact. Some of them contain secretion but no papillae. This tumor should be distinguished from cribriform intraductal carcinoma. ×213

essential to determine the invasiveness in borderline cases. Many sections should be examined microscopically, because this lesion is often multicentric.

RARE BREAST CARCINOMAS

The following breast carcinomas are rare. Because of their very small number, their prognosis, clinical evaluation, and treatment have not been studied statistically. Their gross appearances do not have constant features.

Tubular Carcinoma

Gross It is indistinguishable from scirrhous carcinoma of the breast, and is of slow growth. Prognosis is good.

Microscopic An orderly formation of tubules of one or two layers of epithelial cells is embedded in a dense, sometimes hyaline fibrous tissue. The tubules are relatively uniform in size and evenly distributed. The lining cells of the tubules are uniformly cuboidal. There is no secretion in the lumens (Fig. 8-12).

Adenoid Cystic Carcinoma

This is a rare form of duct carcinoma, composed of groups of small cysts with some secretion mimicking the adenoid cystic carcinoma of the salivary gland (Fig. 8-13). Prognosis is favorable.

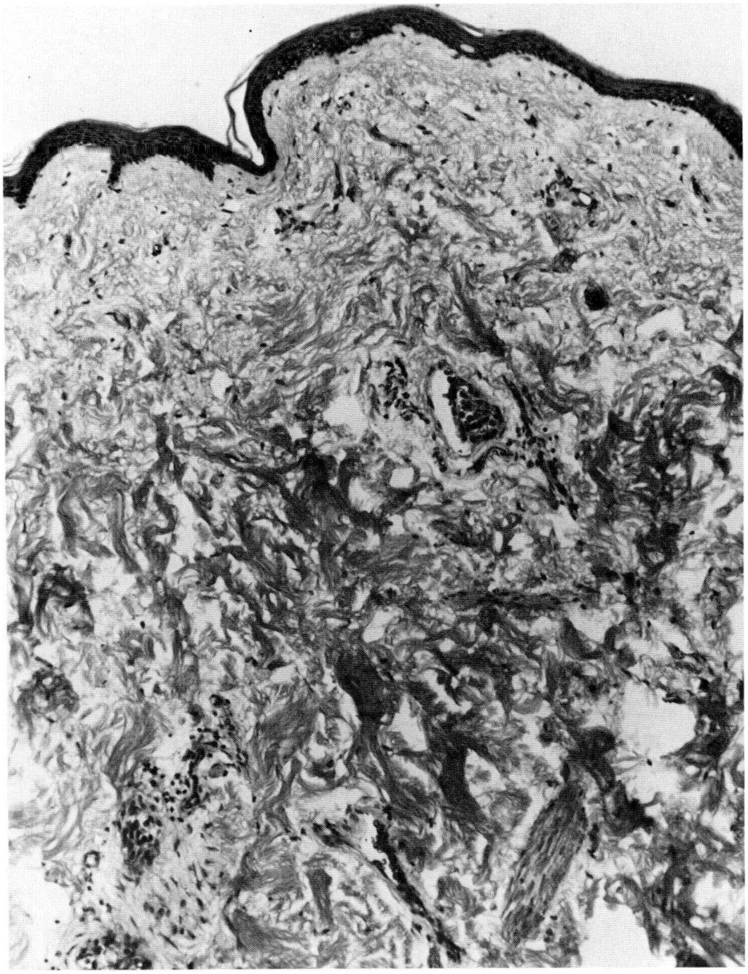

Figure 8-14 Inflammatory carcinoma: The lymphatic vessels in the dermis are plugged by loose cancer cells with little perivascular leukocytes. ×85

Inflammatory Carcinoma (See Chap. 35)

Inflammatory carcinoma has clinical features as well as histological findings (Fig. 8-14). It is not common and prognosis is poor.

Microscopic There are plugs of tumor cells in or around the capillaries and lymphatic vessels among collagen fibers in an edematous dermis. The inflammatory cells around the vessels and the dermis are composed of neutrophils, lymphocytes, and some eosinophils. The permeated vessels could be below the epidermis or erode into it.[7]

Apocrine Carcinoma

Apocrine metaplasia of the breast is common. When these metaplastic cells with abundant eosinophilic cytoplasm become hyperchromatic and pleomorphic, they extrude their cytoplasm into the lumen of the glands as intraluminal projection. The myoepithelial lining is usually discernible. This carcinoma constitutes about 0.3 percent of all breast cancers, and its prognosis is no worse than the others (Fig. 8-15).[10]

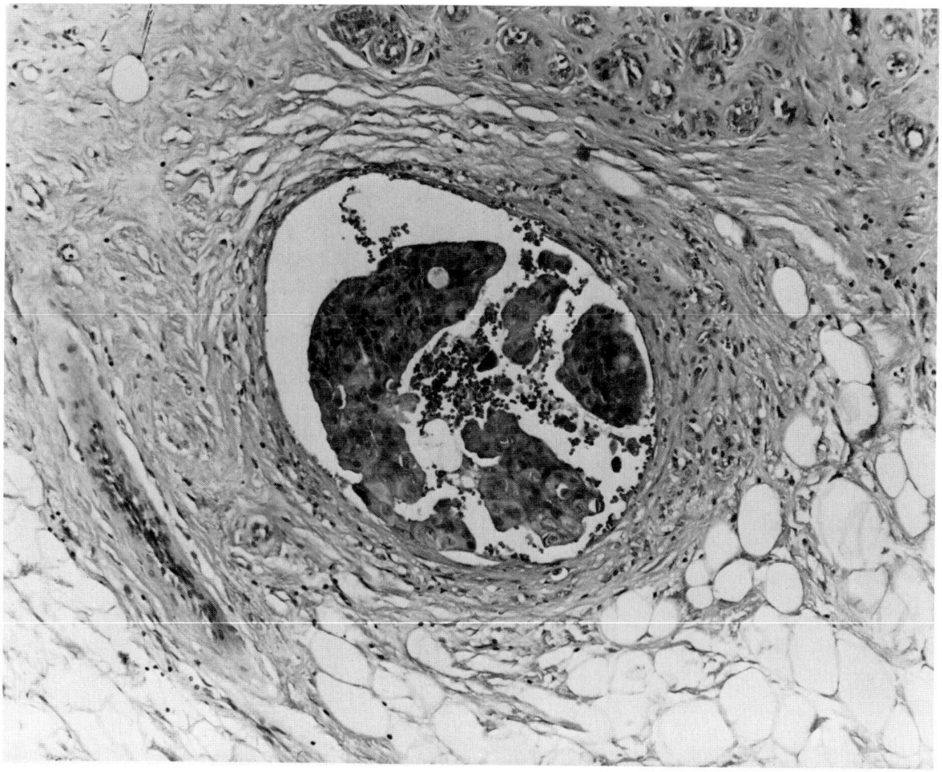

Figure 8-15 Apocrine carcinoma: Papillae of large cells with abundant eosinophilic cytoplasm project into the lumen. The nuclei are frankly malignant. ×85

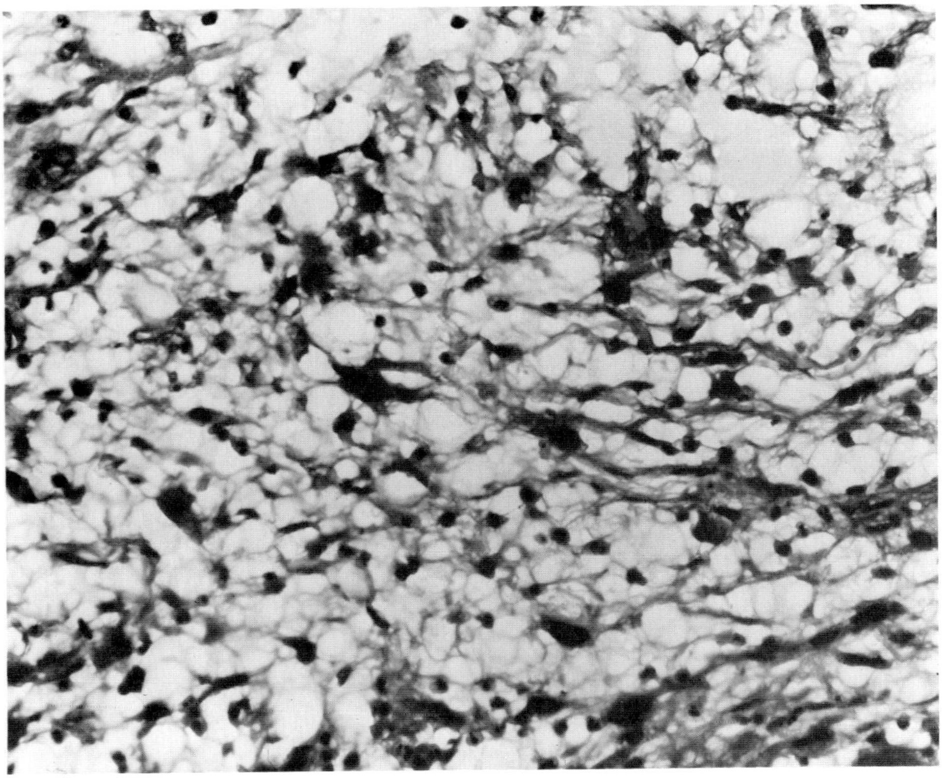

Figure 8-16 Carcinoma arising from fibroadenoma: Typical fibroadenoma pattern remains. The epithelial cells are atypical or frankly malignant. The stroma is hyperplastic, but benign. ×85

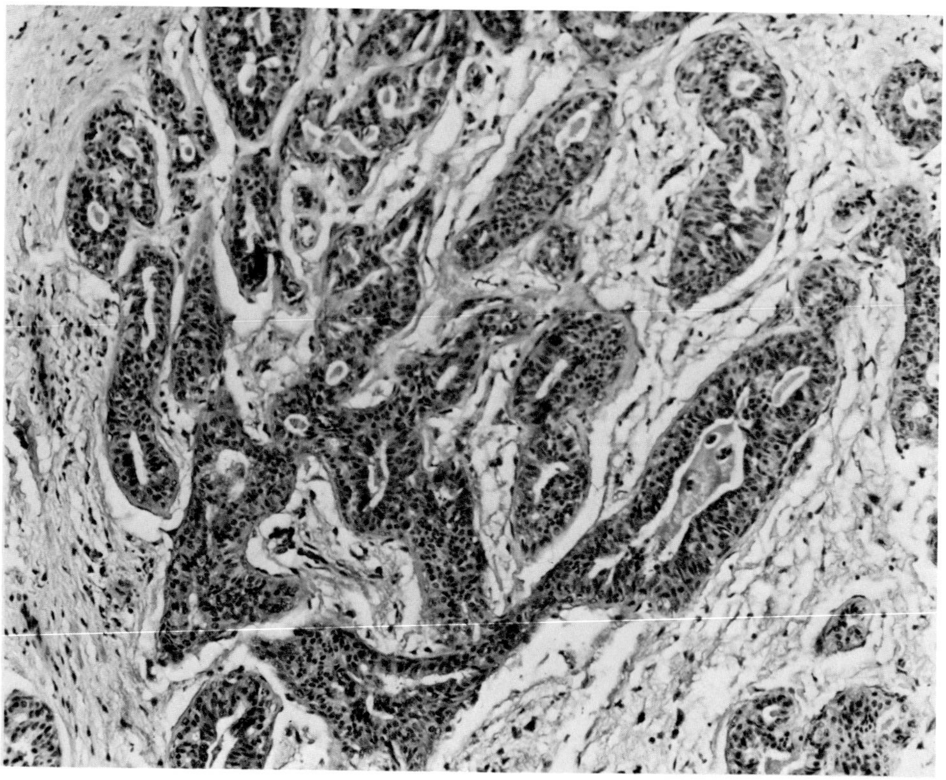

Figure 8-17 Lipid-rich carcinoma: Seen are sheets of large cells with clear vacuolated cytoplasm and small nuclei pushed to one side of the cells. ×213

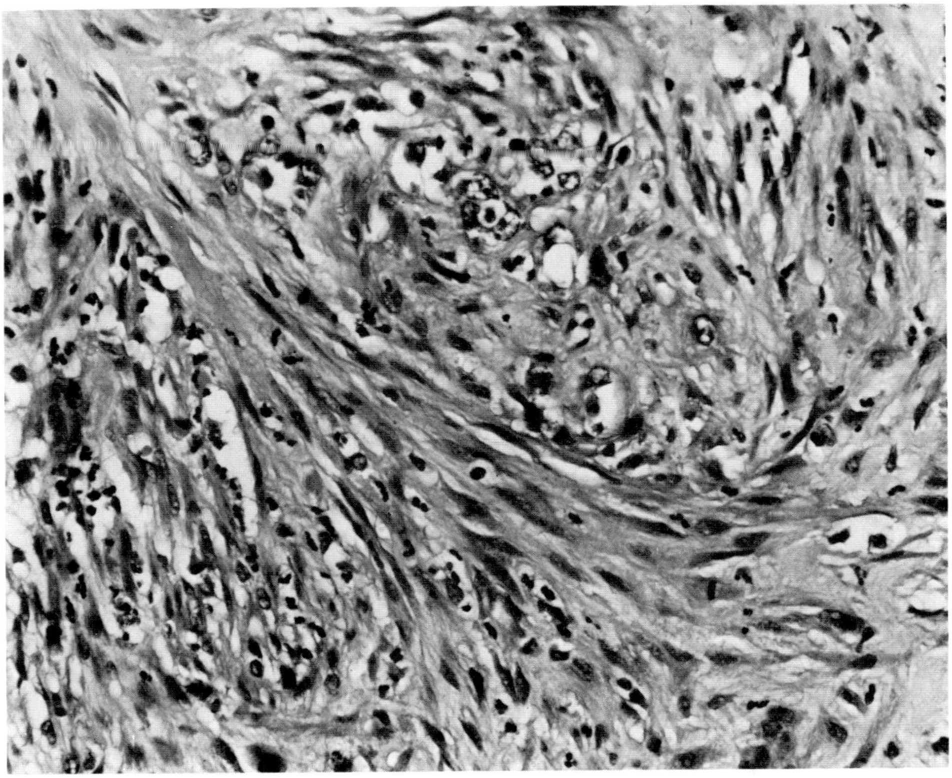

Figure 8-18 Carcinoma with pseudofibrosarcomatous changes: Interwoven bundles of fusiform cells with hyperchromatic pleomorphic nuclei are mixed with some ugly-looking mononuclear giant cells. ×213

Carcinoma Arising from Fibroadenoma

This tumor occurs 20 years later than the peak incidence of fibroadenoma. The preoperative diagnosis is that of fibroadenoma. The pathologic diagnosis is made only microscopically. The typical fibroadenomatous pattern remains, containing atypical to frankly malignant epithelial cells of the ducts. The stromal cells are hyperplastic, but not malignant (Fig. 8-16).[1,14]

Lipid-rich Carcinoma

This tumor is associated with ductal or lobular carcinoma. Its incidence is 1.5 percent of all breast cancer, if lipid change of a part of a cancer is accepted as a criterion. The tumor cells are large and less uniform in size. The cytoplasm is clear and abundantly rich in neutral lipid. Normally, the mammary epithelial cells contain some lipid. The lipid-rich carcinoma may be an extreme expression of lipid content. This tumor tends to be aggressive (Fig. 8-17).[9,24]

Carcinoma of Breast with Pseudosarcomatous Metaplasia of the Epithelial Cells

Beside the poorly differentiated malignant cells in clusters or glands, the epithelial cells change to spindle shape with hyperchromatic and pleomorphic nuclei, arranged in interwoven bundles. Occasional giant cells are present. Special

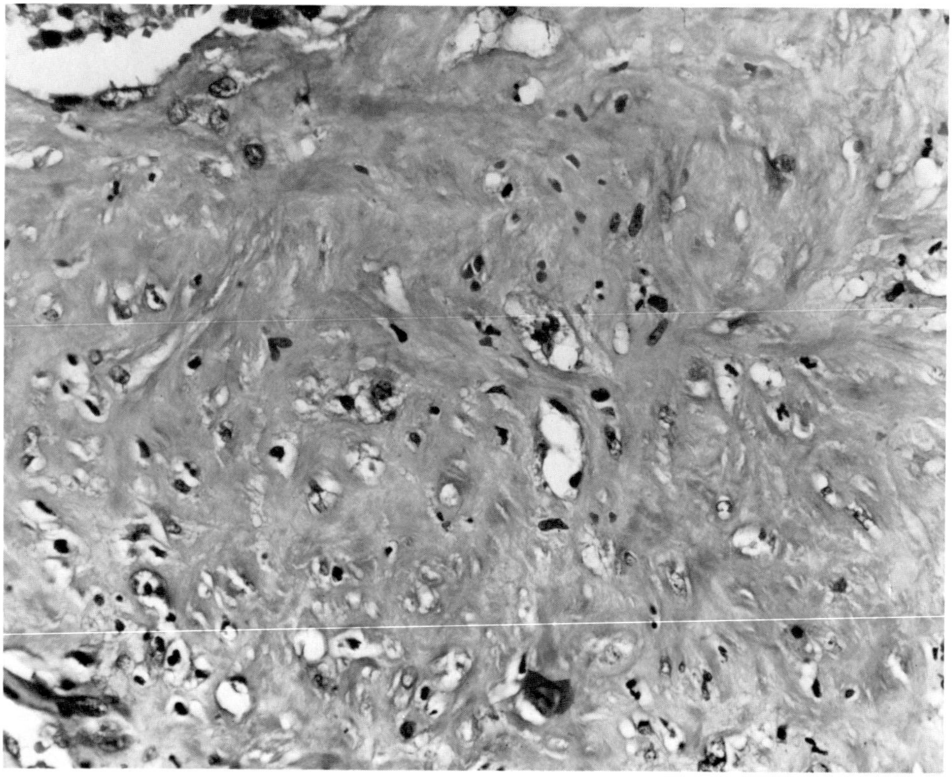

Figure 8-19 Carcinoma with cartilage metaplasia: Some cartilage cells are embedded in a hyaline cartilage matrix in an infiltrating duct cell carcinoma. ×213

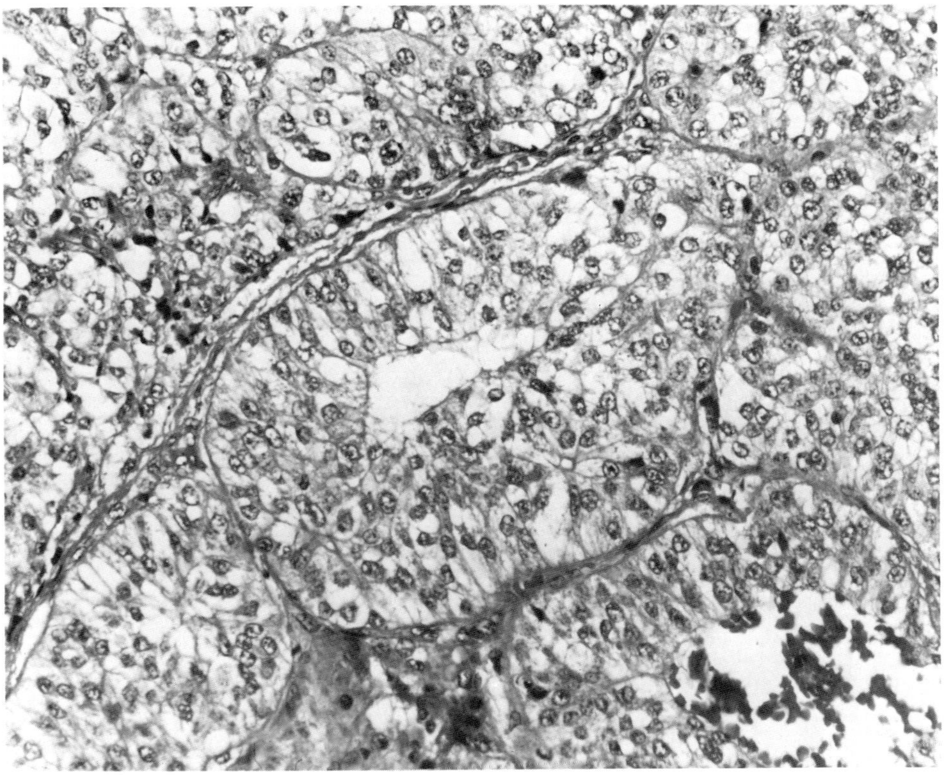

Figure 8-20 Clear cell carcinoma: Large, cylindrical, uniform epithelial cells with clear cytoplasm are palisading on a fibrous septa or radiating around a small vessel like a rosette. Clinical investigation for other primary site was negative. ×213

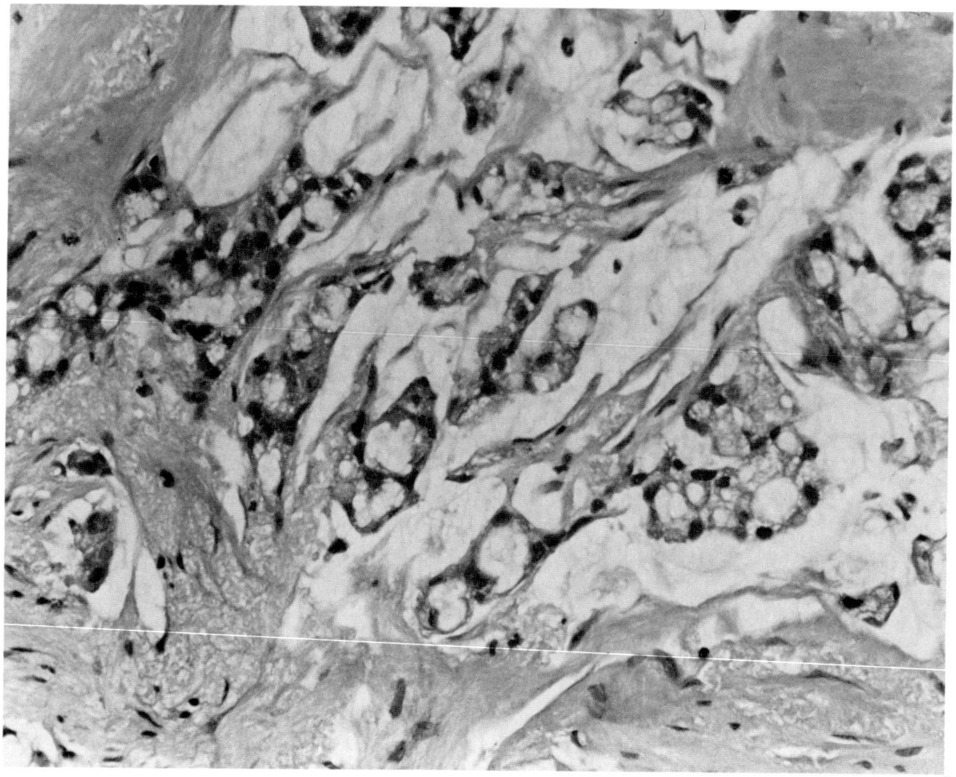

Figure 8-21 Signet-ring-cell carcinoma: Abundant cytoplasm expands the cells, pushing the small nuclei to one side, resembling signet rings. ×213

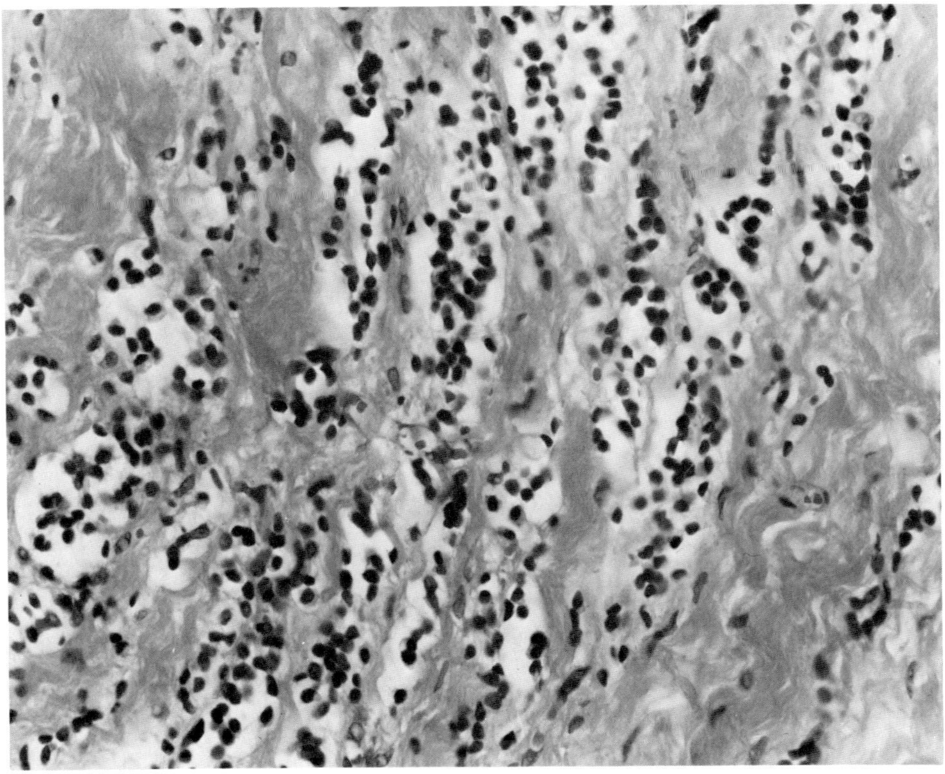

Figure 8-22 Small-cell carcinoma: Clusters of uniform, small, round cells with scanty cytoplasm are embedded in fibrotic stroma. These cells look like lymphocytes. Their arrangement distinguishes them from haphazardly scattered lymphocytes. ×213

stains and electron microscopic examination show that these cells are of epithelial origin. Bony cartilaginous and squamous metaplasia are infrequently seen (Figs. 8-18 and 8-19).[28]

Clear Cell Carcinoma of the Breast

Only a few cases are reported. Its incidence and prognosis are unknown. It is composed of sheets of large clear cells like those in renal cell carcinoma. In some areas, these cells grow around vessels in a pseudo-rosette or palisade over thin, fibrous septi (Fig. 8-20). Investigation for other primary sites of clear cell carcinoma is negative.

Small Cell Carcinoma and Signet-Ring-Cell Carcinoma

Pure small cell carcinomas are extremely rare. So-called small cell carcinomas in needle biopsy or aspiration cytologic smears are actually infiltrating lobular carcinomas when examined on histologic slides in most cases. Like small cell carcinomas of the other sites of the body, such as the lung, kidney, and thyroid, it is very difficult to distinguish from lymphoma or leukemic infiltrate; special staining is necessary (Fig. 8-22). In poorly differentiated medullary carcinoma, heavily infiltrated by lymphocytes, it is almost impossible to diagnose on frozen section examination.[13,26]

Signet-ring-cell carcinoma of the breast, as its appellation indicates, refers to malignant epithelial cells that resemble a signet ring (Fig. 8-21). Malignant signet ring cells were originally described in the metastatic carcinoma of gastrointestine and in the ovary. Signet-ring-cell carcinoma of the breast is very rare. Statistics and prognosis have not been sufficiently established to be of clinical value.[20]

REFERENCES

1. Austin W, Fidler H: Carcinoma developing in fibroadenoma of the breast. *Am J Clin Pathol* 23:688, 1953.
2. Azzopardi J, Ahmed A, et al: *Problems in Breast Pathology*. Philadelphia, W. B. Saunders, 1979.
3. Bettelheim R, et al: Prognostic significance of peritumoral vascular invasion in breast cancer. *Br J Cancer* 50(6):771, December 1984.
4. Bussolati G, Pich A: Mammary and extramammary Paget's disease, an immunocytochemical study. *Am J Pathol* 80:117, 1975.
5. Cooperman A, et al: Breast cancer: An overview. *Surg Clin North Am* 64(6):1031, December 1984.
6. Durand M: Evaluation of prognostic facts in breast cancer. *Bull Cancer* 71(4):331, 1984.
7. Ellis D, Teitelbaum S: Inflammatory carcinoma of the breast. A pathologic definition. *Cancer* 33:1045, 1974.
8. Fisher E: The impact of pathology on the biologic, diagnostic and therapeutic consideration in breast cancer. *Surg Clin North Am* 64(6):1073, December 1973.
9. Fisher E, Gregorio B, et al: Lipid in invasive cancer of the breast. *Am J Clin Pathol* 68:558, 1977.
10. Forsman L, et al: Antiserum against formalin fixed human milk fat globule glycoprotein for immunohistochemistry of normal and malignant apocrine epithelium. *Acta Path Microbiol Immunol Scand (A)* 92(5):331-7, 1984.
11. Gallager H, et al: Problems in the classification of breast cancer. *Radiol Clin North Am* vol. 21, no. 1, March 1983.
12. Gallager H, et al: *Newer Understanding of Breast Cancer. Current Concept in Breast Cancer and Tumor Immunology*. Medical Examination Publishing Co., 1974.
13. Giffler R, Kay S: Small cell carcinoma of the male mammary gland. A tumor resembling infiltrating lobular carcinoma. *Am J Clin Pathol* 66:715, 1976.
14. Goldman R, Friedman N: Carcinoma of the breast arising in fibroadenoma with emphasis on lobular carcinoma. A clinicopathologic study. *Cancer* 23:544, 1969.
15. Gudjonsdottir A, Hagerstrand I, et al: Adenoma of the nipple with carcinomatous development. *Acta Pathol Microbiol Scand (A)* 79:676, 1971.
16. Haagesen C: *Diseases of the Breast*, 2d ed., Philadelphia, W. B. Saunders, 1971.
17. Henderson C, Canellos G: Cancer of the breast. The past decade. *N Engl J Med* Jan 3-10, 1980.
18. Inglis K: The essential difference between the epidermal changes in Paget's disease of the nipple and those in Bowen's precancer dermatosis. *J Pathol Bacteriol* 64:637, 1952.
19. International histological classification of tumors. No. 2, Histological typing of breast tumors. World Health Organization, 1977.
20. Kondo Y, et al: Signet-ring-cell carcinoma of the breast. *Acta Pathol Jn* 34:875, July 1984.
21. McDivitt R, Stewart F, et al: *Tumors of the Breast. Atlas of Tumor Pathology*. Armed Forces Institute of Pathology, 1968.
22. McDivitt R, et al: *The Breast*. International Academy of Pathology Monograph, 1984.
23. Pathology Working Group, Breast Cancer Task Force: Standardized management of breast specimens. *Am J Clin Pathol* 60:789, 1973.
24. Ramos C, Taylor H: Lipid rich carcinoma of the breast. A clinicopathologic analysis of 13 examples. *Cancer* 33:812, 1974.
25. Symposium on Breast Cancer: *Surg Clin North Am* 64(6):1029, December 1984.
26. Toker G, Goldberg J: The small cell lesion of mammary ducts and lobules, in *Pathology Annual* (ed), 12:217. New York, Appleton-Century-Crofts, 1977.
27. Trojani M, et al: Classification of breast cancer. Comparative review apropos of a series of 876 cancers classified according to WHO in 1981. Discussion of problems of terminology and criteria for definition of histological types. *Arch Anat Cytol Pathol* 32(3):133, 1984.
28. Willis R: Squamous cell mammary carcinoma of predominantly fibrosarcoma-like structure. *J Pathol Bacteriol* 76:511, 1958.

9

Hormone Receptors

Andrea Manni, M.D.

INTRODUCTION

The hormone dependency of human breast cancer has been known since 1896, when Beatson first observed tumor regression in premenopausal patients following oophorectomy.[1] These observations have been amply confirmed.

Traditionally, endocrine treatment of breast cancer consists of hormone ablative and hormone additive therapy.[2] The former involves the removal of endocrine glands such as the ovaries in premenopausal patients, and adrenals and pituitary, which secrete hormones potentially involved in supporting tumor growth, in postmenopausal patients. Hormone additive therapy consists of the administration of pharmacologic doses of hormones such as estrogens, androgens, progestins, and glucocorticoid.

Significant improvement in our ability to treat breast cancer has been achieved with the introduction of newer forms of endocrine therapy such as the antiestrogen, *tamoxifen*,[3] and the estrogen biosynthesis inhibitor, *aminoglutethimide*.[4] These two forms of treatment are highly effective and safe, and have virtually replaced the need for major surgical procedures such as adrenalectomy and hypophysectomy.

There are two features which make endocrine therapy particularly attractive. One is the long duration of remission which is observed in responding patients, usually averaging about $1\frac{1}{2}$ years. The other is the relative lack of significant side effects, particularly with the newer forms of endocrine therapy using tamoxifen and aminoglutethimide. Since endocrine therapy will benefit only approximately one-third of *unselected* patients with metastatic breast carcinoma,[5] it is desirable to identify those patients who are likely to benefit from this therapy. This was reported in 1971, when Jensen et al. observed for the first time that the presence of cytosolic estrogen receptors in a tumor biopsy specimen predicted response to endocrine therapy.[6]

The rationale for receptor measurement is that the binding of a hormone to its own receptor is the initial and essential step for hormonal action to occur. Thus, it is logical to expect that if a breast cancer has maintained hormone receptors, its growth, like that of normal breast tissue, can still be influenced by alterations in the hormonal milieu of the host. If, on the other hand, in the process of dedifferentiation, the tumor has lost its ability to bind hormones with high affinity, its growth can no longer be expected to be affected by hormonal manipulations.

Approximately 500 mg of tumor tissue is required for assay by standard techniques. The specimen must not be placed in a fixative, and should be frozen at −20°C or lower without delay. Current investigations with immunochemical assay are demonstrating the ability to determine receptor protein in specimens as small as needle aspiration biopsy samples.

ESTROGEN RECEPTORS

Factors Affecting Estrogen Receptor Status

Overall, approximately 60 percent of human breast carcinomas contain a measurable amount of cytoplasmic estrogen receptors.[7] Tumors from premenopausal patients tend to be less frequently estrogen receptor-positive, and even when positive, tend to have a lower receptor concentration.[8] One possible explanation is that the higher plasma estrogen level in premenopausal patients may occupy the receptors and translocate them to the nucleus, thus making them unavailable for measurement in most assay systems, which only detect unoccupied cytoplasmic receptors. This hypothesis, however, has not been fully supported. It appears, in fact, that perhaps increasing age rather than menopausal status may correlate with estrogen receptor positivity.[9]

Estrogen receptor status also seems to correlate with tumor histology. Several reports,[10,11] but not all,[12] have demonstrated that tumors that are well differentiated are estrogen receptor-positive more frequently than poorly differentiated tumors. Significant correlation has been found between estrogen receptor status and cell kinetics.[13] It has been observed that estrogen receptor-negative breast cancers have a significantly larger fraction of cells in the S phase than do their estrogen receptor-positive counterparts. This finding points to the more aggressive biologic behavior of estrogen receptor-negative tumors.

Primary tumors tend to be estrogen receptor-positive more frequently than metastatic tumors.[14] This suggests that in some cases breast cancer may change its biologic behavior at the time of recurrence. In an individual patient, however, the concordance in receptor status between primary and metastatic tumors is approximately 80 percent.[15] Thus, the receptor measurement performed at the time of mastectomy can be reliably utilized to determine endocrine therapy at the time of relapse. If, however, metastatic tissue is available for biopsy, a second receptor measurement should be performed to optimize the selection of therapy.

Intervening Endocrine Therapy

Intervening systemic therapy, particularly in the form of endocrine therapy, has also been found to affect estrogen receptor status. Several investigators have observed that following endocrine therapy, estrogen receptor-positive tumors manifested a decrease in their receptor content.[16–18] This finding can probably be best explained by a heterogeneous population of receptor-positive and negative cells coexisting in the same neoplasm. Endocrine therapy is expected to affect only the receptor-positive subpopulation, thus leaving predominantly hormone-independent cells. Among the various forms of endocrine therapy, the antiestrogen tamoxifen deserves special mention in regard to its effect on the estrogen receptor status of the tumor. Because tamoxifen binds to the estrogen receptor, a tumor can potentially be misclassified as estrogen receptor-negative if the biopsy is performed while the patient is on antiestrogen therapy. Furthermore, in view of the long life of tamoxifen, receptor measurement is not reliable for probably 2 months after antiestrogen therapy has been discontinued.[19]

Predicting Response of Metastatic Breast Cancer to Endocrine Therapy

Unselected patients with metastatic breast cancer have approximately a 30 percent chance of responding to endocrine therapy. Several clinical trials have now firmly established that the likelihood of response to endocrine therapy is between 50 and 65 percent when estrogen receptors are present, whereas it is at best 10 percent when they are absent.[3,20,21] Thus, estrogen receptor measurement is particularly accurate in identifying patients with hormone-independent, estrogen receptor-negative tumors, who should be spared unnecessary endocrine manipulations and treated instead with combination chemotherapy. It is not clear why some (although very few) estrogen receptor-negative tumors regress after hormonal therapy. One plausible explanation is that there may have been receptor loss due to technical problems in the transport and storage of the sample or in the assay conditions. Considering the unstable and thermolabile nature of these proteins, it is remarkable that there are only so few false-negative results.

Positive estrogen receptor status is somewhat less accurate in predicting response to endocrine therapy, since at least 35 percent of tumors harboring estrogen receptors will fail to benefit from hormonal therapy. One likely explanation for this is tumor cell heterogeneity. Immunohistochemical methods have consistently shown that breast tumors are heterogeneous in nature, being composed of both estrogen receptor-positive and estrogen receptor-negative cells.[22,23] It is possible that a tumor composed primarily of estrogen receptor-negative cells, and thus hormone-independent, may possess enough estrogen receptor-rich cells to produce a positive biochemical assay. This hypothesis is supported by the fact that a direct correlation has been observed between the total concentration of estrogen receptor and the likelihood of response to endocrine treatment. When the concentration of cytosolic estrogen receptor has been found to exceed 100 fmol/mg cytosol protein, the likelihood of objective response to endocrine therapy has neared 80 percent.[24]

An alternative and perhaps additional explanation exists for the fact that some estrogen receptor-positive tumors do not benefit from endocrine therapy. It is possible that in the process of dedifferentiating, some tumors may retain the ability to bind estradiol and thus be estrogen receptor-positive, but they may have lost the ability to carry on subsequent steps of estrogen action such as migration of the estrogen receptor complex to the nucleus, stimulation of messenger RNA, and initiation of mitogenesis. Thus, assessment of the integrity of the estrogen action pathway beyond the initial binding of the hormone to its cytosolic receptor may better identify those tumors whose growth is still under hormonal influence. In agreement with this hypothesis, some investigators have observed that tumors which contained both nuclear and cytoplasmic receptors had a higher response to endocrine therapy than did those tumors containing only cytoplasmic receptors.[25,26] In the author's opinion, however, the role of nuclear estrogen receptors in clinical management of breast cancer remains to be established.

At present, the integrity of the estrogen action pathway can be assessed by measurement of progesterone receptors, the synthesis of which depends upon an intact estrogen action.[27]

Predicting Response of Metastatic Cancer to Cytotoxic Chemotherapy

Cytotoxic chemotherapy is, in general, more effective against rapidly dividing cells. Since estrogen receptor-negative tumors have a higher growth fraction than their estrogen receptor-positive counterparts, as shown by the higher labeling index,[13] it was logical to test whether absence of estrogen receptor would predict response to cytotoxic chemotherapy. In an initial retrospective analysis, Lippman et al. did indeed observe that patients with receptor-negative tumors had a much higher response to cytotoxic chemotherapy than patients with receptor-positive tumors.[28] In contrast, Kiang et al. observed a higher response to chemotherapy in patients with estrogen receptor-positive breast cancer.[29] Following these two initial conflicting reports, numerous clinical trials have been published.[30,31] When all data are combined, 53 percent of 231 patients with positive estrogen receptor responded to chemotherapy. A virtually identical response to chemotherapy was observed in 303 patients with receptor-negative tumors (50 percent). Thus, at present it is fair to summarize that estrogen receptor status has no predictive value in terms of response to cytotoxic chemotherapy.

Predicting Response of Early Breast Cancer to Endocrine Treatment

Human breast cancer is regarded by many as a systemic disease from the time of initial clinical presentation. Thus, considerable emphasis has recently been placed on early systemic treatment of breast cancer soon after removal of the primary tumor in the attempt to eradicate micrometastasis. Although the results of these adjuvant trials are still preliminary, it appears that the estrogen receptor status of the primary tumor may predict which patients are likely to benefit from endocrine therapy. In two separate prospective studies, women with positive axillary nodes were randomly assigned to receive chemotherapy or chemotherapy plus the antiestrogen tamoxifen for either 1 or 2 years.[32,33] Both studies showed that only in the subgroup of patients with positive estrogen receptors could a statistically significant beneficial effect be obtained from the addition of tamoxifen to chemotherapy. In contrast, in patients with estrogen receptor-negative tumors, no difference in disease-free survival was observed between the group treated with chemotherapy plus antiestrogen versus that treated with chemotherapy alone. In addition, as in the case of metastatic disease, the absolute level of estrogen receptors seems to influence the outcome of treatment.[32] In one study, it has been clearly shown that the higher the level of estrogen receptors, the greater was the benefit on disease-free survival from addition of tamoxifen to chemotherapy. On the other hand, in a clinical trial where tamoxifen alone was compared to no treatment in early breast cancer, the beneficial effect of tamoxifen in terms of prolongation of disease-free survival was not affected by the estrogen receptor status.[34] Thus, the role of estrogen receptor measurement in the selection of adjuvant therapy of breast cancer remains to be fully established. In the author's opinion, however, most preliminary evidence suggests an important role of the estrogen receptor status in predicting at least prolongation of disease-free survival by adjuvant endocrine therapy.

Estrogen Receptor Status as a Prognostic Variable

Several clinical trials have shown that patients with estrogen receptor-positive primary tumors have a significantly increased disease-free survival.[35,36] The prognostic value of the estrogen receptor status appears to be independent of other variables such as menopausal status, tumor size, axillary node status, and adjuvant treatment used. *These findings emphasize that hormone-dependent tumors as identified by positive estrogen receptors have a better prognosis than their hormone-independent counterparts.* This concept is further supported by the observation that estrogen receptor-positive breast cancer tends to be histologically more differentiated[10,11] and has a slower growth rate as evidenced by usually low labeling index.[13] The prognostic value of the estrogen receptor status in the primary tumor has potentially important therapeutic implications. It is conceivable, in fact, that among women with negative nodes breast cancer, traditionally considered to have a good prognosis, the subgroup of patients with receptor-negative tumors, and thus at higher risk of relapse, may benefit from early aggressive adjuvant therapy.

PROGESTERONE RECEPTORS

Predicting Response to Hormonal Therapy

The observation that progesterone receptor synthesis depends upon estrogen action[27] has made progesterone receptor measurements very attractive to test the integrity of the estrogen action pathway. Thus, it was logical to expect that the presence of progesterone receptors in addition to the estrogen receptors could more accurately identify hormone-responsive tumors.[37,38]

It is now well established that tumors lacking both estrogen and progesterone receptors have virtually no chance of regression following hormonal therapy. In contrast, the likelihood of response to endocrine treatment is between 75 and 80 percent in patients with both estrogen and progesterone receptor-positive tumors. It should be noted, however, that at least 20 percent of tumors positive both for estrogen and progesterone receptors still fail to benefit from endocrine therapy. The reason for this lack of response is presently not understood. One possible explanation is that the effect of estrogen on mitogenesis may be independent from the effect on progesterone receptor synthesis.[39,40] Thus, it is possible that in some tumors estrogens may still be able to stimulate progesterone receptor biosynthesis but may have lost the ability to influence tumor growth. These tumors would then be hormone-independent, despite the presence of both estrogen and progesterone receptors.

Approximately 20 percent of patients have tumors that are positive for estrogen receptors but negative for progesterone receptors. This finding would suggest that these tumors are hormone-independent, since estradiol is still able to bind to the cytosolic receptor but is unable to express its full action as shown by the absence of progesterone receptors. In reality, however, approximately 30 percent of patients belonging to this category benefit from endocrine therapy.[7] There are at least three possible explanations for this finding. If the biopsy is done during the luteal phase of the menstrual cycle in premenopausal women, the high plasma progesterone concentration may make detection of progesterone receptors impossible by standard techniques.[41] An additional circumstance where progesterone receptors may be falsely negative is in the case of older postmenopausal patients whose endogenous estrogens may be too low to induce progesterone receptor synthesis. This hypothesis is supported by the observation that at least in some patients the progesterone receptor status could be changed from negative to positive following short-term administration of estrogens.[42] Finally, an additional possibility is that in some tumors, estrogens may have lost the ability to stimulate progesterone receptor synthesis but may still be able to stimulate mitogenesis since the two mechanisms may be totally independent.[39,40]

As expected, the fraction of patients with negative estrogen receptors and positive progesterone receptors is very small, approximately 5 percent, since progesterone receptor synthesis depends on estrogen action. It is conceivable, then, that in these patients the estrogen receptor may be falsely negative due to technical problems. It is also possible that at least in premenopausal women, the estrogen receptors may be primarily located in the nucleus rather than the cytoplasm due to high circulating levels of estrogens. In either case, these tumors would be expected to be hormone-responsive. In agreement with this hypothesis, it has been observed that up to 50 percent of patients with negative estrogen receptors but positive progesterone receptors respond to hormonal therapy.[43]

Progesterone Receptor as a Prognostic Variable

It has been observed that patients whose primary tumors are positive for progesterone receptors have an overall increased disease-free survival, irrespective of any treatment.[44–46] The role of progesterone receptor as an independent prognostic factor has been recently well illustrated by Clark et al.[47] These investigators noted that in a group of patients with stage II (positive axillary nodes) breast cancer who were receiving adjuvant therapy, both estrogen and progesterone receptors were positively correlated with time to recurrence. When, however, the data were analyzed in a multivariate model which included several additional prognostic variables, it was observed that only the number of positive nodes and the presence of progesterone receptors significantly predicted longer disease-free survival. These data indicated that the progesterone receptor may actually be more important than the estrogen receptor as a prognostic factor. Although the data are still preliminary and a longer period of follow-up will be necessary, they nevertheless suggest that the presence of progesterone receptors successfully identifies a group of breast cancer patients with a favorable prognosis. Furthermore, these investigators observed that the duration of disease-free survival was correlated with the absolute concentration of progesterone receptors. These findings support the concept that the hormone dependency of human breast cancer is not an "all or nothing" phenomenon but rather a spectrum.

In the author's opinion, both estrogen and progesterone receptors should be measured in every patient with primary breast cancer because of their important therapeutic and prognostic implications.

OTHER RECEPTORS

Because of the possible influence of multiple hormones on the growth of human breast cancer, it is logical to test whether receptors for hormones other than estrogen and progesterone are present in breast cancer specimens and whether they are helpful in predicting response to hormonal therapy.

Prolactin receptors have been detected in up to 50 percent of human mammary cancers.[48,49] In our experience, there is no correlation between the presence of estrogen and prolactin receptors.[49] We observed that prolactin receptors could be found in either estrogen receptor-negative or positive tumors. We also found that the presence of prolactin receptors was of no value in predicting response to antiestrogen therapy.[49] It may be, however, that the presence of prolactin receptors may be a specific predictor of response to either a prolactin-lowering agent such as bromocriptine or hypophysectomy. In this regard, we have attempted to correlate the presence of prolactin receptors with response to hypophysectomy in patients who had relapsed on antiestrogen therapy.[50] We found that the prolactin receptor status had no predictive value under these circumstances. The data, however, are preliminary, and further studies are needed.

Both androgen and glucocorticoid receptors have been measured in breast cancer specimens.[51–54] The androgen receptor is usually positive in about 30 percent of the tumors while the glucocorticoid receptor has been found to be positive in up to 50 percent of breast tumors in some studies. Allegra et al. measured estrogen, progesterone, glucocorticoid, and androgen receptors in the same tumors and observed a high correlation among all these receptors.[54] The role, however, of either glucocorticoid or androgen receptors in predicting response to endocrine therapy is far from being established. Allegra et al. suggest that glucocorticoid receptor positivity may increase the predictability of response to endocrine therapy in estrogen receptor-positive tumors.[55] The data, however, are again preliminary.

Thus, a significant proportion of human breast carcinomas contain receptors for other hormones besides estrogen and progesterone. At this time, the role of these other receptors in the clinical management of breast cancer has not been demonstrated.

REFERENCES

1. Beatson GT: On the treatment of inoperable cases of carcinoma of the mamma: Suggestions for a new method of treatment, with illustrative cases. *Lancet* ii:104, 1896.
2. Kennedy BJ: Hormone therapy in cancer. *Geriatrics* 25:106, 1970.
3. Manni A, Trujillo JE, Marshall JS, Brodkey J, Pearson OH: Antihormone treatment of stage IV breast cancer. *Cancer* 43:444, 1979.
4. Santen RJ, Wells SA: The use of aminoglutethimide in the treatment of patients with metastatic carcinoma of the breast. *Cancer* 46:1066, 1980.
5. Manni A, Pearson OH, Marshall JS, Arafah BM: Sequential endocrine therapy and chemotherapy in metastatic breast cancer: Effects of survival. *Breast Cancer Res Treat* 1:97, 1981.
6. Jensen EV, Block GE, Smith S, Kyser K, Desombre, ER: Estrogen receptors and breast cancer response to adrenalectomy. *Natl Cancer Inst Monogr* 34:55, 1971.
7. Cowan K, Lippman M: Steroid receptors in breast cancer. *Arch Intern Med* 142:363, 1982.
8. Seibert K, Lippman M: Hormone receptors in breast cancer. *Clin Oncol* 1:735, 1982.
9. Elwood JM, Godolphin W: Oestrogen receptors in breast tumours: Associations with age, menopausal status and epidemiological and clinical features in 735 patients. *Br J Cancer* 42:635, 1980.
10. Hahnel R, Vivian AB: Biochemical and clinical experience with the estimation of estrogen receptors in human breast carcinoma, in McGuire WL (ed): *Estrogen Receptors in Human Breast Cancer.* New York, Raven Press, 1975, p. 205.
11. Thoreson S, Tangen M, Stoa KF, Hartveit F: Oestrogen receptor values and histological grade in human breast cancer. *Histopathology* 5:527, 1981.
12. Rosen PP, Menendez-Botet J, Nisselbaum JS, Urban JA, Mike V, Fracchia A, Schwartz MK: Pathological review of breast lesions analyzed for estrogen receptor protein. *Cancer Res* 35:3187, 1975.
13. Kute TE, Muss HB, Anderson D, Crumb K, Miller B, Burns D, Dube LA: Relationship of steroid receptor and cell kinetics and clinical status in patients with breast cancer. *Cancer Res* 41:3524, 1981.
14. Knight WA, Osborne CK, Yochmowitz MG, McGuire WL: Steroid hormone receptors in the management of human breast cancer. *Ann Clin Res* 12:202, 1980.
15. Mobbs BG: Effect of time and therapy on the hormone receptor status of breast carcinomas. *Can Med Assoc J* 127:217, 1982.
16. Kiang DT, Kennedy BJ: Factors affecting estrogen receptors in breast cancer. *Cancer* 40:1571, 1977.
17. Allegra JC, Barlock A, Huff K, Lippman ME: Changes in multiple or sequential estrogen receptor determinations in breast cancer. *Cancer* 45:792, 1980.
18. Heuson JC, Leclercq G: Quantitative aspects of estrogen receptors in the strategy of breast cancer treatment, in Wittliff JL, Dapunt O (eds): *Steroid Receptors and Hormone-Dependent Neoplasia.* New York, Masson, 1980, p. 239.
19. Hull DF, Clark GM, Osborne CK, Chamness GC, Knight WA, McGuire WL: Multiple estrogen receptor assays in human breast cancer. *Cancer Res* 43:413, 1983.
20. McGuire WL: Steroid receptors and clinical breast cancer, in Bresciani F (ed): *Perspectives in Steroid Receptor Research.* New York, Raven Press, 1980, p. 239.
21. Lippman ME, Allegra JC: Quantitative estrogen receptor analyses: The response to endocrine and cytotoxic chemotherapy in human breast cancer and disease-free interval. *Cancer* 46:2829, 1980.
22. Nenci I: Receptor and centrile pathways of steroid action in normal and neoplastic cells. *Cancer Res* 38:4204, 1978.
23. Mercer WK, Carlson CA, Wahl TM: Identification of estrogen receptors in human breast cancer cells by immunofluorescence. *Am J Clin Pathol* 70:330, 1978.

24. McGuire WL, Chamness GC, Horwitz KB, Zava DL: Hormones and their receptors in breast cancer, in O'Malley B, Birnbaumer L (eds): *Receptors and Hormone Action*. New York, Academic Press, 1978, p. 401.
25. Maass H, Jonat W: The current state of clinical relevance of receptor determination in breast cancer, in Wittliff J, Dapunt O (eds): *Steroid Receptors and Hormone Dependent Neoplasia*. New York, Masson, 1980, p. 257.
26. Leake RE, Lang L, McArdle C, Smith DC: Soluble and nuclear oestrogen receptor status in human breast cancer in relation to prognosis. *Br J Cancer* 43:67, 1981.
27. Horwitz K, McGuire WL: Estrogen control of progesterone receptor and estrogen receptor in human breast cancer. *J Biol Chem* 253:2223, 1978.
28. Lippman ME, Allegra JC, Thompson EB: The relation between estrogen receptors and response rate to cytotoxic chemotherapy in metastatic breast cancer. *N Engl J Med* 298:1223, 1978.
29. Kiang DT, Frenning DH, Goldman AI: Estrogen receptor and responses to chemotherapy and hormonal therapy in advanced breast cancer. *N Engl J Med* 299:1330, 1978.
30. Jonat W, Maass H, Stolzenbach G, Trams G: Estrogen receptor status and response to polychemotherapy in advanced breast cancer. *Cancer* 46:2807, 1980.
31. Samal B, Singhakowinta A, Brooks SC: Estrogen receptors and response of breast cancer to chemotherapy. *N Engl J Med* 299:604, 1978.
32. Fisher B, Redmond C, Brown A, Wickerham DL, Wolmark N, Allegra J, Escher G, Lippman M, Savlov E, Wittliff J, Fisher ER, Plotkin D, Bowman D, Wolter J, Bornstein R, Desser R, Frelick R: Influence of tumor estrogen and progesterone receptor levels on the response to tamoxifen and chemotherapy in primary breast cancer. *J Clin Oncol* 1:227, 1983.
33. Pearson OH, Hubay CA, Marshall JS, Gordon NH, McGuire WL, Mansour EG, Herman RE, Jones JC, Flynn WJ, Eckert C: Adjuvant endocrine therapy, cytotoxic chemotherapy, and immunotherapy in stage II breast cancer: Five year survival. *Breast Canc Res Treat*, 3 (Suppl): 61, 1983.
34. Novaldex Adjuvant Trial Organization: Controlled trial of tamoxifen as adjuvant agent in management of early breast cancer. *Lancet* 1:257, 1983.
35. Knight WA, Livingston RB, Gregory EJ: Estrogen receptor as an independent prognostic factor for early recurrence in breast cancer. *Cancer Res* 37:4669, 2977.
36. Samaan N, Buzdar AU, Aldinger KA: Estrogen receptor. A prognostic factor in breast cancer. *Cancer* 47:554, 1981.
37. McGuire WL, Horwitz KB: Progesterone receptor in breast cancer, in McGuire WL (ed): *Hormones, Receptors, and Breast Cancer*. New York, Raven Press, 1978, p. 31.
38. Bloom N, Tobin E, Degenshein GA: Clinical correlations of endocrine ablation with estrogen and progesterone receptors in advanced breast cancer, in McGuire WL, Raynaud J-P, Baulieu E (eds): *Progesterone Receptors in Normal and Neoplastic Tissue*, vol. 4 in *Progress in Cancer Research and Therapy*. New York, Raven Press, 1977, p. 125.
39. Arafah BM, Manni A, Pearson OH: Effect of hypophysectomy and hormone replacement on hormone receptor levels and the growth of 7,12-dimethylbenza(a)-anthracen-induced mammary tumor in the rat. *Endocrinology* 107:1364, 1980.
40. Ip M, Milholland RJ, Rosen F, Kim U: Mammary cancer: Selective action of the estrogen receptor complex. *Science* 203:361, 1979.
41. Saez S, Martin PM, Chouvet CD: Estradiol and progesterone receptor levels in human breast adenocarcinoma in relation to plasma estrogen and progesterone levels. *Cancer Res* 38:3468, 1973.
42. Bloom ND, Tobin EH, Schreibman B: The role of progesterone receptor in the management of advanced breast cancer. *Cancer* 45:2992, 1980.
43. McGuire WL: Steroid receptors in human breast cancer. *Cancer Res* 38:4289, 1978.
44. Saez S, Chouvet C, Mayer M, Cheix F: Estradiol and progesterone receptors as prognostic factors in human primary breast tumors. *Proc Am Assoc Cancer Res* 21:139, 1980.
45. Pichon M-F, Pallud C, Brunet M, Milgrom F: Relationship of presence of progesterone receptors to prognosis in early breast cancer. *Cancer Res* 40:3357, 1980.
46. Bertuzzi A, Vezzoni P, Ronchi E: Prognostic importance of progesterone receptors alone or in

combination with estrogen receptors in node negative breast carcinoma. *Proc Am Assoc Cancer Res* 22:447, 1981.

47. Clark GM, McGuire WL, Hubay CA, Pearson OH, Marshall JS: Progesterone receptor as a prognostic factor in stage II breast cancer. *N Engl J Med* 309:1343, 1983.
48. Turcot-Lemay L, Kelly PA: Prolactin receptors in human breast tumors. *J Natl Cancer Inst* 68:381, 1982.
49. Pearson OH, Manni A, Chambers M, Brodkey J, Marshall JS: Role of pituitary hormones in the growth of human breast cancer. *Cancer Res* 38:4323, 1978.
50. Pearson OH, Arafah BM, Manni A: Prolactin and mammary cancer, in MacLeod RM, Scapagnini U (eds): *Central and Peripheral Regulation of Prolactin Function*. New York, Raven Press, 1980, p. 237.
51. Persijn JP, Korsten CB, Engelsman E: Oestrogen and androgen receptors in breast cancer and response to endocrine therapy. *Br Med J* 4:503, 1975.
52. Maass H, Engel B, Trams G: Steroid hormone receptors in human breast cancer and the clinical significance. *J Steroid Biochem* 6:743, 1979.
53. Teulings FAG, Vangilse HA: Demonstration of glucocorticoid receptors in human mammary carcinomas. *Horm Res* 8:107, 1977.
54. Allegra JC, Lippman ME, Thompson EB: Distribution, frequency, and quantitative analysis of estrogen, progesterone, androgen, and glucocorticoid receptors in human breast cancer. *Cancer Res* 39:1447, 1979.
55. Allegra JC, Lippman ME, Thompson EB, Simon R, Barlock A, Green L, Huff KK, Do HMT, Aitken SC, Warren R: Relationship between the progesterone, androgen, and glucocorticoid receptor and response rate to endocrine therapy in metastatic breast cancer. *Cancer Res* 39:1973, 1979.

10

Immune Mechanisms: Prognostic, Therapeutic, and Preventive Significance

Maurice M. Black, M.D.
Reinhard E. Zachrau, M.D.

INTRODUCTION

The biological behavior of human breast cancer reflects an interaction between the intrinsic aggressiveness of the primary carcinoma and immunologically mediated tumor-retarding responses of the host.[1-3] In the following presentation we examine data which are pertinent to the development of immunological approaches to treatment and prevention of human breast cancer.

IMMUNOGENICITY OF PREINVASIVE BREAST CANCER

Invasive carcinomas of the breast are commonly associated with coexisting foci of in situ carcinomas (ISCs).[4] Such in situ lesions may also be found in breasts without invasive carcinomas. Since the cytologic appearance of ISC resembles that of invasive carcinomas of the breast, it is probable that invasive breast cancers are derived from ISC. It does not follow, however, that the transition from preinvasive to invasive cancer simply reflects delay in diagnosis. For example, the relative frequencies of in situ and invasive breast cancers vary with ethnic group, age, parity characteristics, and use of oral contraceptives.[5] Thus, the ISC-to-invasive-carcinoma transition cannot be explained by the clinical concept of delay-dependent, stage-wise progression.

In situ carcinomas are commonly associated with a type of host response rarely observed

---

When staging is referred to in our chapter, we are using the following pathological classification system:

Stage 0 is in situ carcinoma (ISC) *without* coexisting foci of invasive carcinoma; *ISC-stage* > *0* refers to foci of ISC *with* coexisting foci of invasive carcinoma.

Stage I is invasive breast carcinoma, regardless of size, *without* microscopic evidence of axillary lymph node metastases and *without* clinical evidence of systemic metastases. *Stage II* is invasive breast carcinoma, regardless of size, *with* regional lymph node metastases, but *without* evidence of systemic metastases.

in association with normotypic duct epithelium, whether normoplastic or hyperplastic. The response in question involves cell-mediated immunity (CMI) which is demonstrable microscopically and can be measured by in vitro and in vivo tests.

Microscopic Observations

Immunological responses involve stimulation of the appropriate lymphoid cells by an immunogenic antigen determinant. The responsive cells then undergo a complex sequence of proliferation and differentiation in the lymphoreticuloendothelial (LRE) system, recognizable as distinctive morphologic patterns in antigen-draining lymph nodes and as focal accumulations of lymphoid cells at the site of the reference antigen. Immunological responses to preinvasive mammary carcinomas would be expected to be associated with microscopically recognizable changes in the regional lymph nodes and in the region of the ISC. The failure to find such changes would indicate either that ISCs are not associated with antigenic changes or that the hosts are immune-incompetent and, therefore, not capable of responding to ISC-associated antigenicity.

Our studies have demonstrated that ISCs are commonly (more than 80 percent) associated with sinus histiocytosis, a distinctive type of regional lymph node reactivity.[4,6] This type of reactivity is characterized by paracortical lymphoid cellular hyperplasia and intrasinusoidal accumulations of large histiocytes whose ultrastructure is similar to that of epithelioid cells.[7] The lymph node changes suggest that the preinvasive phase of breast cancer is associated with antigenic changes which provoke a cell-mediated type of immune response in the host.[1] This interpretation is supported by the findings that approximately 80 percent of patients with stage 0 (no coexisting foci of invasive carcinoma) ISC have lymphoid cellular responses in the regions of their ISC. Such responses (Fig. 10-1) are typically in the form of perivenous lymphoid cellular infiltrates, a reaction which is characteristic of CMI. These perivenous infiltrates may occur with or without simultaneous diffuse lymphoid infiltrations, predominantly of the plasmacytoid type, around the cancerous ducts. The latter type of response is limited to those ISCs whose nuclei are poorly differentiated, i.e., nuclear grade (NG) I, as shown in Fig. 10-2.

While perivenous and/or periductal lymphoid cellular infiltrates are associated with the majority of stage 0 ISCs, such responses are rarely (< 3 percent) seen in association with idiopathic normotypic hyperplasia, lactational hyperplasia, or the pseudolactational changes found with the use of certain medications. However, perivenous lymphocytic infiltrates are demonstrable in approximately one-third of atypical proliferative lesions of the type designated by Black and Chabon as precancerous mastopathy.[5,8,9]

In Vitro Tests

Cell-mediated immunity to specific antigens can be measured by a variety of in vitro test procedures.[10] One such procedure is the leukocyte migration inhibition assay, adapted to measure reactivity of healthy individuals and cancer patients to microscopically characterized areas of breast tissues.[11] These measurements have shown that the majority of stage 0 cancer patients are reactive to autologous and homologous stage 0 ISC within the first three postoperative years.[3,5,9] Such reactivity is not demonstrable in tests against autologous or homologous normotypic breast tissue. These observations confirm the antigenicity of autologous ISC, inferred from the microscopic studies. In addition, simultaneous in vitro tests against autologous and homologous stage 0 ISC indicate that, in the majority of cases, ISCs from different patients have tumor-associated antigens which are similar, if not identical, to one another (Table 10-1). This conclusion is supported by the finding that stage 0 breast cancer patients show a linear correlation between in vitro

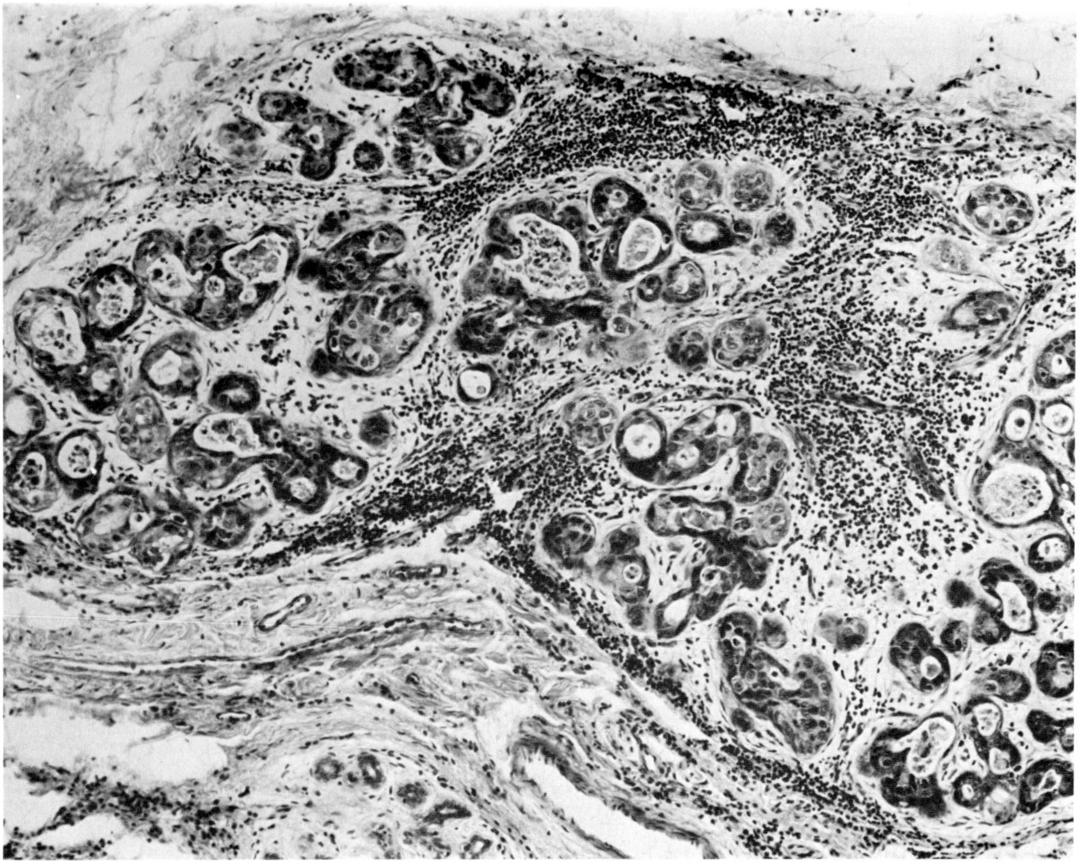

Figure 10-1 Stage 0 ISC, showing intense lymphoid cellular infiltrations around venules within and adjacent to the cancerous lobules. No such reactivity was associated with normotypic, hyperplastic lobules in the same region. (Pat. A.B., 1975; H&E stain, ×255)

reactivity to autologous breast cancer and RIII-gp55.* [12] Such a correlation is not demonstrable in simultaneous tests against diverse non-gp55 protein fractions isolated from the RIII-virus, nor against isolated glycoproteins from A-strain mammary tumor virus and Rauscher leukemia virus.[13] It appears, therefore, that antigenically equivalent, if not identical, CMI determinants are expressed by the majority of ISC and RIII-gp55.

*Gp55 is the major envelope glycoprotein of the RIII-strain murine mammary tumor virus.

In Vivo Tests

Cell-mediated immunity is commonly evaluated by means of skin testing which involves the development of erythema and induration 24 to 48 hours after intradermal injection of an antigen. The skin response reflects the local accumulation of activated mononuclear cells and their liberation of a variety of lymphokines. In vivo measurements of CMI to breast tissue and isolated antigens may also be accomplished by means of a modification of Rebuck's skin window (SW) procedure.[14–16]

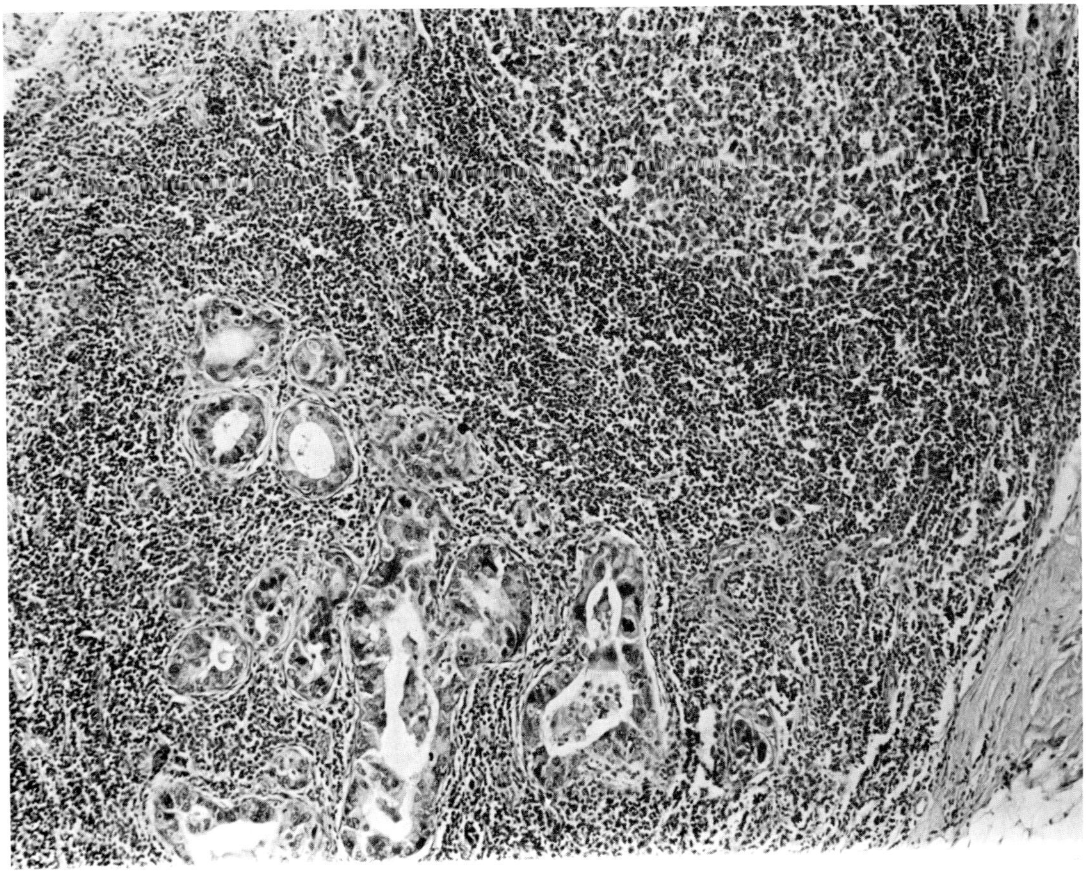

Figure 10-2 In situ carcinoma focus adjacent to invasive breast cancer, showing extensive diffuse plasmacytoid lymphoid cellular infiltration around the cancerous ducts as well as lymph follicular metaplasia in the stroma. Similar responses are also associated with invasive cancer foci. (Pat. V.S., 1972; H&E stain, ×255)

The modification involves the use of specific tumor-related antigens on the SW. To date we have performed approximately 2000 SW tests on several hundred patients over a wide range of postoperative intervals, using cryostat sections of autologous breast cancer and purified gp55 as targets. Response patterns to autologous breast cancer, characterized by prominent, compact accumulations of histiocytic cells and/or aggregates of lymphoblastoid cells, are inversely correlated with the subsequent development of metastatic disease among invasive breast cancer patients.[3] Accordingly, these responses are designated as positive. Positive SW responses were found in the majority of stage 0 breast cancer patients (28/36 = 78 percent), tested against autologous cancer tissue within the first three postoperative years. The SW procedure also demonstrates that stage 0 breast cancer patients typically respond in simultaneous tests to autologous breast cancer and gp55 in a similar fashion, both qualitatively and quantitatively (Fig. 10-3 and Fig. 10-4).

Table 10-1 Relative Frequency of Positive Leukocyte Migration Inhibition Test (LMT) Reactivity of Stage 0 Breast Cancer Patients against Various Types of Homologous Breast Tissue Targets, in Relation to Simultaneous Reactivity against Autologous ISC

Homologous targets	Positive/total LMTs vs. homologous targets, with simultaneous LMTs vs. autologous ISC	
	Positive	Negative
Breast Cancer		
ISC, stage 0	13/19 (68)*,‡	0/5
ISC, stage > 0	8/18 (44)	1/6 (17)
Invasive	26/50 (52)‡	1/16 (6)‡
Normotypic breast parenchyma	0/8‡	0/5

*Numbers in parentheses, percentages.
‡ $p < .005$.

These results confirm the conclusion, based on the microscopic observations and the in vitro measurements, that *the preinvasive phase of mammary carcinogenesis is associated with distinctive immunogenic changes*. This distinctive immunogenicity reflects the expression of an ISC-associated CMI determinant which is common to most, if not all, stage 0 ISCs and also antigenically equivalent to a CMI determinant of RIII-gp55.

IMMUNOGENICITY OF INVASIVE BREAST CANCER

Microscopic Observations

The occurrence and prognostically favorable significance of LRE responses at the site of primary invasive breast cancers and in the regional lymph nodes were reported decades ago.[17,18] Table 10-2 shows that such responses are qualitatively identical to those associated with ISC. However, the relative frequency of LRE responses to invasive breast cancers is lower than that to stage 0 ISC. A more direct comparison of the antigenicity of ISC and invasive breast cancer can be obtained by examining LRE responses to in situ and invasive cancer foci in the same breast. As shown in the table, reactivity to invasive cancer foci appears to be dependent on reactivity to coexisting foci of ISC in the same breast. However, in an appreciable minority of invasive breast cancers, i.e., 66 of 203 (33 percent) in this series, such antigenicity is not expressed. This suggests that the in situ-to-invasive-carcinoma progression may be accompanied by loss of the ISC-associated type of immunogen.

While host responses are demonstrable against both in situ and invasive breast cancers, the critical question is whether such responses are prognostically significant. In addressing this question, it is important to take note of differences in the intrinsic aggressiveness of different breast cancers, a property that correlates inversely with the degree of nuclear differentiation of the cancer cells.[19] Among patients without LRE responses to their carcinomas, prognoses vary with the degree of nuclear differentiation (Table 10-3). Among patients with LRE responses to their carcinomas, survival values are significantly increased in the NG I (poorly differentiated) and NG II (moderately differentiated) series of patients. However, patients with NG III (highly differentiated) carcinomas have such favorable survival characteristics, even in the absence of LRE responses, that only minimal improvement is possible, e.g., 100 percent compared to 84 percent 5-year postoperative

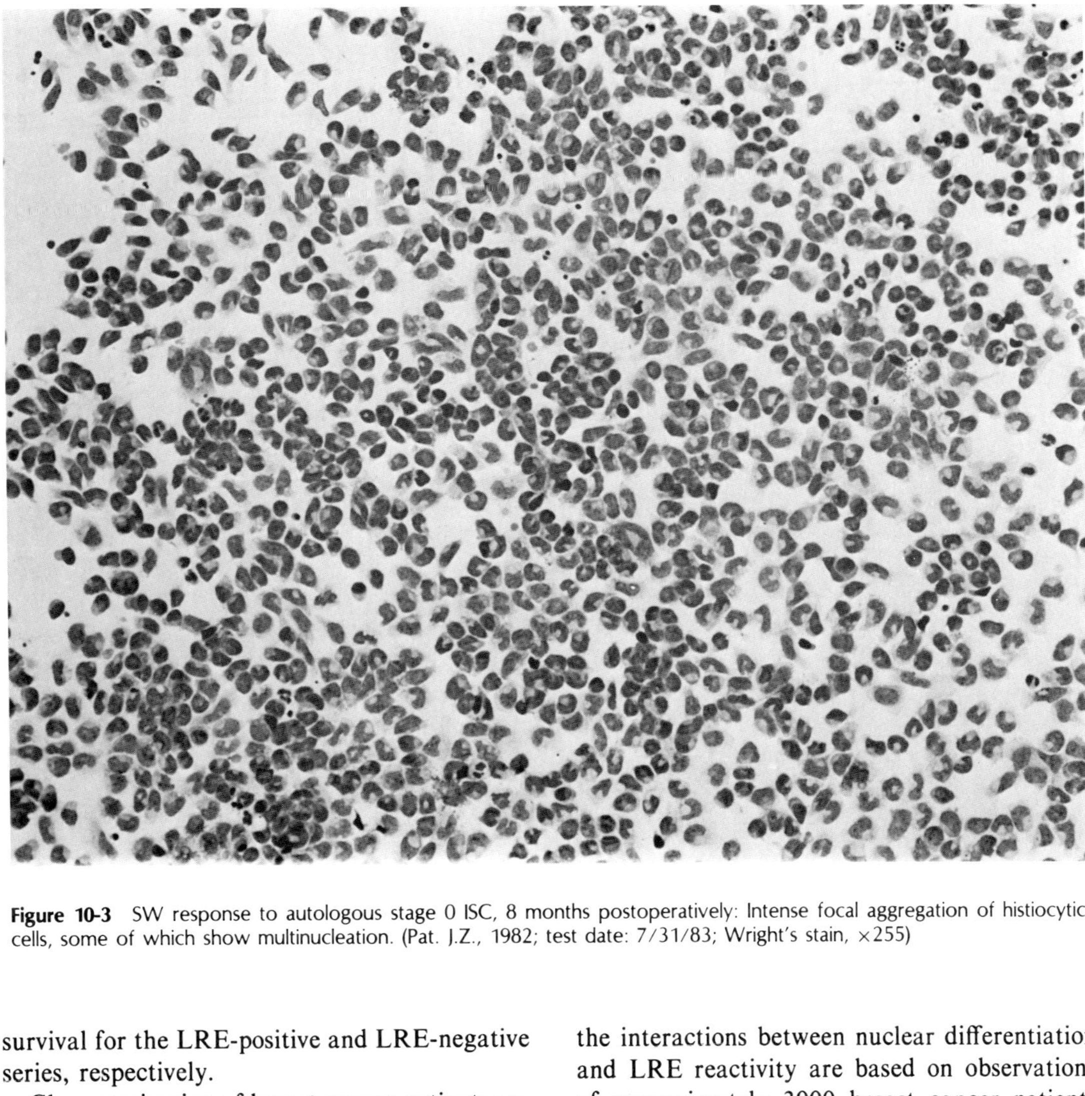

Figure 10-3 SW response to autologous stage 0 ISC, 8 months postoperatively: Intense focal aggregation of histiocytic cells, some of which show multinucleation. (Pat. J.Z., 1982; test date: 7/31/83; Wright's stain, ×255)

survival for the LRE-positive and LRE-negative series, respectively.

Characterization of breast cancer patients according to NG of and LRE reactivity to their tumors reveals a frequently ignored intrastage prognostic heterogeneity.[20] While the prognostically favorable influence of LRE responses to breast cancer is demonstrable even among patients who were unselected as to NG,[21,22] it should be reiterated that this prognostically favorable effect is most apparent among patients with NG I and NG II carcinomas. The conclusions on the prognostic significance of the interactions between nuclear differentiation and LRE reactivity are based on observations of approximately 3000 breast cancer patients who were followed more than 5 years or until death.[2,23–25]

In Vitro Tests

Studies using a leukocyte migration inhibition assay have provided data supporting the conclusion, suggested by the microscopic studies, that CMI to invasive breast cancer tissue is directed against a CMI determinant(s), commonly associated with ISC. Simultaneous tests

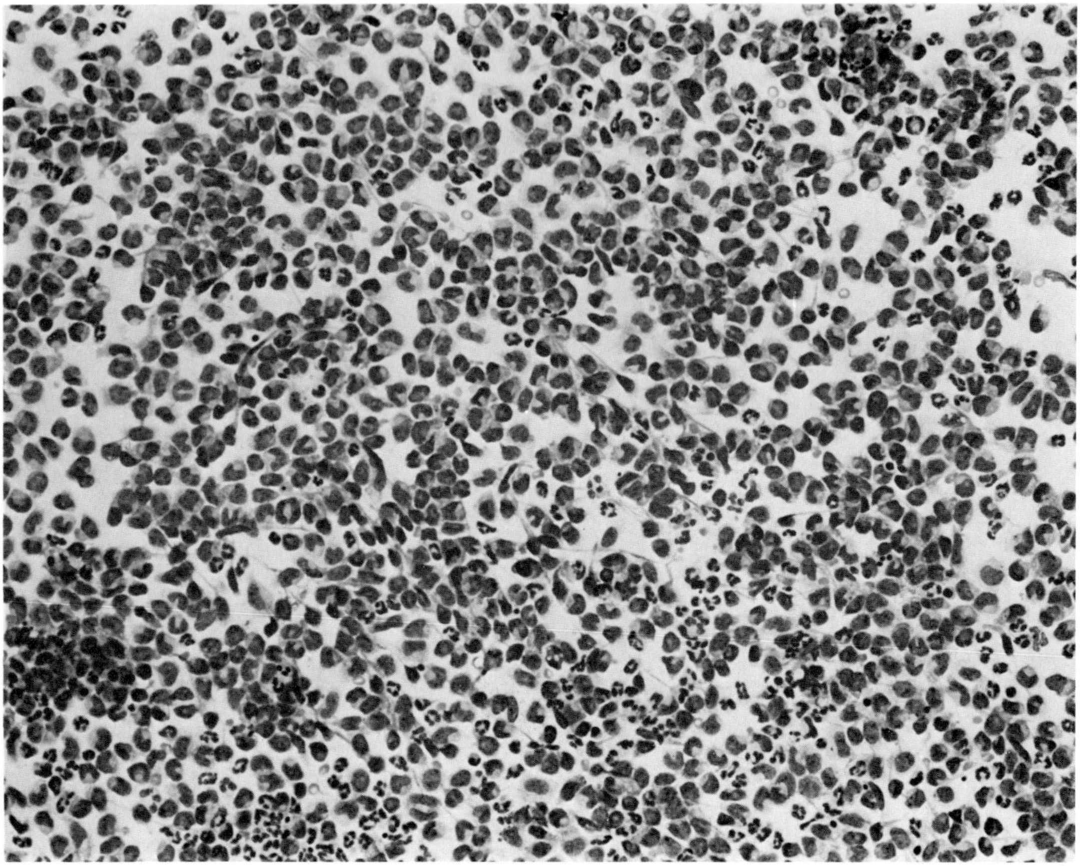

Figure 10-4 SW response to RIII-gp55, simultaneous with SW test against autologous breast cancer, shown in Figure 10-3: Identical pattern of response to that against autologous breast cancer. (Wright's stain, ×255)

of in vitro responses to foci of autologous in situ and invasive cancer from the same breast have demonstrated that reactivity to foci of invasive carcinomas almost universally correlates with reactivity to coexisting foci of ISC.[26] However, reactivity to autologous in situ lesions is not as regularly associated with simultaneous reactivity to coexisting invasive cancer foci. Additional evidence for the ISC-like antigenic characteristics of invasive breast cancers is provided by the observation that stage 0 breast cancer patients who do not react to their autologous ISC rarely react to homologous breast cancers in simultaneous tests. On the other hand, those stage 0 patients who react to autologous ISC, commonly react in simultaneous tests to homologous ISC > LRE-positive >> LRE-negative autologous and homologous invasive breast cancer.[27]

Simultaneous tests against gp55 and invasive breast cancer demonstrate that reactivity to invasive breast cancer is characteristically associated with simultaneous reactivity to gp55. However, reactivity to gp55 is not as regularly associated with simultaneous reactivity to autologous invasive breast cancer.[28] It appears that the immunogenic CMI determinants associated

Table 10-2 Relative Frequency of Positive LRE Reactivity to Precancerous Mastopathy and in Situ and Invasive Carcinoma of the Breast

Target	LRE-positive/total
Precancerous mastopathy, stage 0	24/83 (29)*
In situ carcinoma	
Stage 0	49/62 (79)†
Stage >0	141/217 (65)†
Invasive carcinoma	
with LRE-positive ISC	137/203 (67)‡
with LRE-negative ISC	24/87 (22)‡

*Numbers in parentheses, percentages.
† $p = .053$.
‡ $p < .0005$.

with in situ and invasive breast cancer are antigenically equivalent to a CMI determinant of gp55. This determinant appears to be more regularly expressed by in situ than by invasive breast cancer tissues. The critical issue is that in vitro responses to autologous invasive breast cancer are prognostically significant, i.e., invasive breast cancer patients who manifest postoperative in vitro reactivity to autologous breast cancer are less likely to develop systemic metastases within the subsequent 4 years than NG-matched patients lacking such reactivity.[3,29] A similar prognostic relationship has been reported when in vitro CMI is measured employing a blastogenesis technique.[30]

Table 10-3 Influence of Nuclear Differentiation of and LRE Reactivity to Invasive Breast Cancer on 5-year Postoperative Patient Survival (Unselected Invasive Breast Cancer Patients; Saskatchewan Cancer Registry: 1946, 1951, 1960, and 1968)

Nuclear grade	LRE reactivity: Positive	LRE reactivity: Negative
I	42/67 (63)[a,b]	17/49 (35)[b,c]
II	36/43 (84)[d]	74/129 (57)[c,d,e]
III	16/16 (100)	37/44 (84)[e]
Total	94/126 (75)[f]	128/222 (58)[f]

[a]Patients, surviving 5 years postoperatively/total number of patients; numbers in parentheses, percentages.
[b]$p < .01$.
[c]$p < .02$.
[d,e,f]$p < .005$.

In Vivo Tests

Skin window (SW) responses to autologous invasive breast cancer are qualitatively similar to SW responses to autologous stage 0 ISC. However, as with LRE and in vitro responses, the proportion of patients responding to autologous breast cancer at different postoperative intervals is greater in the stage 0 patient series (Table 10-4). When invasive breast cancer patients are SW-tested against gp55, they manifest the same qualitative range of responses

Table 10-4 Spontaneous Skin Window Responses to RIII-gp55, among Patients with Stage 0 ISC and Patients with Invasive Breast Cancer (INV), at Various Postoperative Intervals

	Months postoperative					
	1–5		6–12		13–36	
Skin window response*	ISC	INV	ISC	INV	ISC	INV
Positive	4 (44)†	4 (13)	8 (62)	12 (39)	7 (54)	13 (38)
Intermediate	0	5	0	5	3	4
Negative	5 (56)	22 (71)	5 (38)	14 (45)	3 (23)	17 (50)
Total	9 (100)	31 (100)	13 (100)	31 (100)	13 (100)	34 (100)

*Maximal response per patient per postoperative interval.
† Numbers in parentheses, percentages.

as that observed in tests of stage 0 patients against gp55. However, the proportion of anti-gp55 SW-positive cases is greater among the stage 0 than the invasive breast cancer patients.

Simultaneous SW tests against gp55 and autologous invasive breast cancer demonstrate that lack of reactivity to gp55 is, in most instances, accompanied by lack of reactivity to the autologous cancer (Table 10-5). In contrast, positive SW reactivity to gp55 is associated with simultaneous reactivity to autologous invasive breast cancer in a significant proportion (58 percent) of the tests, performed during the same postoperative interval. These observations indicate that the antigenicity of invasive breast cancer may vary independently of host CMI and that the CMI determinants of immunogenic invasive breast cancers are similar to those of stage 0 ISC and a CMI determinant of gp55. Moreover, positive SW reactivity to NG-classified autologous breast cancer, 1 to 12 months postoperatively, is associated with a reduced risk of systemic metastases within the succeeding 4 years (Table 10-6). This finding is not dependent on a preselection of patients according to stage at the time of diagnosis.

Gp55-cross-reacting antigens have also been demonstrated by application of anti-gp55 antibodies to microscopic sections of human breast cancer tissues.[31,32] In such studies, gp55-specific antisera prepared in experimental animals reacted selectively with invasive breast cancer cells in approximately 50 percent of the cases. However, in contrast to the findings with CMI tests, anti-gp55 antisera rarely reacted with preinvasive breast cancer cells. Moreover, patients whose invasive breast cancers reacted with anti-gp55 antibodies tended to have an *unfavorable* prognosis. It appears that the gp55 determinant(s) which elicits serological responses is different from the determinant which elicits CMI. We have also found that postoperative breast cancer patients uncommonly have demonstrable circulating antibodies against gp55 or autologous breast cancer, regardless of whether they have spontaneous CMI against these targets or not (unpublished observations). These findings merit consideration in attempts to influence the behavior of breast cancer by stimulation of serological reactivity or by introduction of antibodies against autologous breast cancer.[33]

Table 10-5 Simultaneous Spontaneous Skin Window Responses to RIII-gp55 and Autologous Breast Cancer among Patients with Stage 0 ISC and Patients with Invasive Breast Cancer (INV), 1 to 60 Months Postoperatively

Response to RIII-gp55	Response to autologous breast cancer			
	Positive	Intermediate	Negative	Total
Positive				
ISC	18 (78)*	4	1	23 (100)
INV	18 (58)†	8	5	31 (100)
Intermediate				
ISC	4	8 (52)	1	13 (100)
INV	1	9 (47)	9	19 (100)
Negative				
ISC	1	2	13 (81)	16 (100)
INV	0†	4	75 (95)	79 (100)

*Numbers in parentheses, percentages.
† $p < .0005$.

Table 10-6 Influence of SW Reactivity to Autologous Invasive Breast Cancer (BCa) during the 1-to-12-Month Postoperative Interval on the 5-Year Postoperative Survival Characteristics

SW reactivity to autologous BCa	Nuclear grade of the BCa		
	I	II	III
	Number of patients with/without systemic recurrence (ratio)		
Positive	4/14 (0.29)	0/20	0/13
Negative	30/14 (2.14)	18/18 (1.00)	2/16 (0.13)
	Odds, relative to those of NG I, SW-negative patients[a]		
Positive	0.15 (0.04-0.50)[b,c]	0.01 (0.00-0.21)[d]	0.02 (0.00-0.32)[e]
Negative	*1.00*	0.48 (0.19-1.17)[f]	0.07 (0.02-0.31)[g]

[a] Relative odds of developing systemic recurrent disease < 5 years postoperatively; values corrected for small sample sizes.
[b] In parentheses, 95% confidence limits of the corrected relative odds.
[c] $p < .005$.
[d,e,g] $p < .0005$.
[f] Not significant.

Considered in toto, the presented data lead to the following conclusions:

1 Specific immunogenicity develops during the preinvasive phase of most, if not all, breast cancers.

2 Such ISC-associated immunogenicity is dependent on the presence of CMI determinants which are antigenically equivalent among stage 0 ISC of different patients and equivalent to a CMI determinant of gp55.

3 This ISC-associated, gp55-like CMI determinant provokes CMI in most, if not all, stage 0 breast cancer patients.

4 This ISC-associated, gp55-like CMI determinant is less regularly expressed in invasive than in preinvasive breast cancers.

5 At any postoperative interval, measurable CMI to ISC-associated, gp55-like determinants is more regularly demonstrable in stage 0 than invasive breast cancer patients.

6 In vitro and in vivo measurable CMI to gp55 and autologous breast cancer fades in some stage 0 and invasive breast cancer patients with increasing postoperative intervals.

7 Postoperative survival characteristics of invasive breast cancer patients correlate with the degree of nuclear differentiation of the primary cancer cells and with CMI against autologous cancer.

These phenomena have practical and conceptual implications for the prognosis, treatment, and prevention of human breast cancer.

PROGNOSTIC SIGNIFICANCE

Prognostic classification systems seek to identify variables which correlate with differences in the subsequent clinical behavior of subpopulations of patients having a particular disease. Such classification is necessary to define the natural course of a disease and evaluate the effects of therapeutic procedures. Our studies indicate that prognostically different subpopulations of breast cancer patients can be identified according to *tumor-host interactions* in individual patients. These interactions correlate with the degree of nuclear differentiation of the cancer cells, with tumor antigenicity, and with tumor-specific host CMI. Such a classification is prognostically significant without regard to primary tumor size or stage of the disease. In fact, it reveals intrastage prognostic heterogeneity.

Recognition of this type of heterogeneity is particularly important in evaluating the effects of adjuvant chemotherapy regimens.[20] Patient selection for adjuvant treatment of breast cancer is typically based on the presence of metastases to lymph nodes. To ignore nuclear differentiation in the characterization of cancers to be treated appears inappropriate, since the effects of cytotoxic chemotherapeutic agents tend to vary with the mitotic activity of the target cells.

The evaluation of host CMI against autologous breast cancer and gp55 is pertinent to the assessment of the patients' risk of developing subsequent second primary breast cancers as well as the risk of developing recurrent disease. Patients who are reactive against autologous breast cancer have a reduced risk of developing recurrent disease. In addition, the development and progression of metachronous second primary breast cancers should be impeded in such patients, since CMI against autologous breast cancer is typically directed against a gp55-like antigen and since the development of second primary breast cancers involves an in situ phase which is typically associated with gp55-like antigenicity.

On the other hand, patients who are not reactive against autologous breast cancer will not demonstrate an immunologically mediated delay in the development of recurrent disease. However, some of these patients should be at a reduced risk of development and progression of second primary breast cancers. Such a prognostic dichotomy would be expected in patients who are nonreactive against autologous breast cancer but who are reactive against gp55. In these patients, the lack of reactivity against autologous cancer appears to reflect loss of the prognostically significant ISC-associated, gp55-like tumor antigenicity. Nevertheless, the anti-gp55 CMI should impede development and progression of immunogenic second breast cancers in these patients.

Postoperative monitoring of breast cancer patients' specific CMI by periodic testing provides insight into the changes which occur in the dynamic tumor-host relationships. It is well known that the risks of recurrent disease and second primary breast cancers persist for decades. It is therefore important to identify variables which might influence such risks over a wide range of postoperative intervals. Such information may provide a basis for new approaches to treatment and prevention of breast cancer.

THERAPEUTIC SIGNIFICANCE

Since spontaneous CMI against autologous breast cancer is prognostically favorable, the ability to maintain and/or restore such reactivity should be therapeutically beneficial. It is important to recognize that tumor-specific CMI involves two parameters which may vary independently, namely tumor antigenicity and host reactivity. When patients react against their autologous cancers, these cancers are obviously antigenic. However, failure of patients to react against autologous cancer may be due to lack of tumor antigenicity and/or specific host CMI. Thus, immune stimulation in nonreactive patients can have therapeutic potential only against cancers with prognostically significant antigenicity, i.e., in the case of breast cancer, the ISC-associated, gp55-like antigenicity. Therefore, evaluation of the effects of putative immunotherapeutic agents should include measurements of CMI against gp55 as well as against autologous tumors.[34]

Immunostimulants should effect a negative-to-positive change in the CMI of breast cancer patients against gp55. Such induced reactivity should reduce the risk of metachronous second primary breast cancers as well as that of recurrent disease from those breast cancers which retain the ISC-associated, gp55-like antigenicity. This relationship between immune stimulation and tumor-retarding effects should apply, regardless of the immune stimulatory method employed.[34] Diverse methods have been used, with varying success, to enhance antitumor immune reactivity in cancer patients.[35] The value of such studies would be markedly increased, if all investigators routinely included measurements of specific immunity before and after attempted immune stimulation. In addition, the evaluation of the effects of such stimulatory procedures should take account of the prognostic heterogeneity associated with the different degrees of nuclear differentiation of cancer cells.

In our experience, treatment with high doses of vitamin A and of vitamin E has resulted in negative-to-positive changes in SW reactivity to autologous breast cancer and gp55. Such a stimulation of SW reactivity has been observed in approximately one-half of the patients treated, over a wide range of postoperative intervals.[36] If it can be shown that the induced reactivity is biologically equivalent to spontaneous reactivity, agents which can effect such changes in reactivity should be of value in the adjuvant therapy of breast cancer. This expectation is based on our experience with the prognostic effects of spontaneous tumor-specific CMI of postoperative, clinically disease-free breast cancer patients. We have only limited experience with regard to immune stimulation of patients having overt systemic metastatic disease.

To date, there are no data to support the thesis that the progression of human breast cancer is impeded by spontaneously occurring antibodies. Accordingly, the use of experimentally derived antitumor antibodies differs from conventional immunotherapeutic procedures in that it does not represent an augmentation of a naturally occurring, prognostically significant host response. However, there is increasing interest in the use of monoclonal antibodies as therapeutic agents in the treatment of recurrent cancers. As indicated by Mastrangelo et al., "it is probably unrealistic to anticipate that antibody can reliably effect clinically meaningful tumor regressions."[33]

PREVENTIVE SIGNIFICANCE

One might question how an invasive breast cancer could develop and progress, if a *preinvasive* cancer is immunogenic and elicits an immune response in the host. However, this is no more incongruous than the development of progressive and lethal infection by an antigenic organism. The critical immunoprophylactic expectation in infectious diseases is that subsequent de novo infections will be impeded in an immunized host. Such protective immunity may develop after an episode of infection from which the patient recovered, or after immunization by injection of the infectious agent in attenuated form or of an antigen isolated from the agent.

Table 10-7 Stage and Postoperative Survival Characteristics Associated with Breast Cancers, Arising after Prior Removal of Normotypic Breast Lesions and of Precancerous Mastopathies (PCM) and ISC (Saskatchewan Cancer Registry)

Initial lesion	Characteristics of the subsequent breast cancer	
	Stage 0 ISC	DOD < 5 years*
Normotypic	9/89 (10)†,‡	20/51 (39)§
PCM and ISC	16/64 (25)‡	5/34 (15)§

*Number of patients who died of disseminated breast cancer in less than 5 years after surgery for the subsequent breast cancer, per total number of patients.
†Numbers in parentheses, percentages.
‡,§ $p < .05$.

Immunoprophylaxis of infectious diseases depends on the existence of antigenic determinants which are regularly associated with the infectious agent in question and which provoke immune responses in the host. Our studies have shown that this requisite for immunoprophylaxis is met in the preinvasive phase of breast cancer, as judged by the demonstration of (1) a CMI determinant which is equivalent in most, if not all, preinvasive breast cancers; (2) the development of CMI which is directed against the ISC-associated determinant; and (3) the tumor-retarding influence of such CMI. Furthermore, since a high proportion of postoperative stage 0 breast cancer patients have demonstrable CMI to the ISC-associated antigen, and since subsequent second primary breast cancers must pass through an in situ phase, it can be expected that the development of metachronous second primary breast cancers be impeded in such patients.[5,37] To date, we have two independent tests of this expectation.[38,39]

Table 10-7 demonstrates the unusually favorable stage and survival characteristics associated with breast cancers arising after prior removal of breast cancer precursor lesions, i.e., precancerous mastopathies or stage 0 ISC, in comparison to those associated with breast cancers arising after removal of normotypic lesions. Table 10-8 indicates that the overall incidence ratios of second primary breast cancers were similar in both the stage 0 and invasive breast cancer series. However, invasive second breast cancers were proportionately less common in the former than in the latter series. In short, among postoperative stage 0 breast cancer patients, the preinvasive-to-invasive cancer transition appears to be impeded.

The observations suggest that the development of invasive second primary breast cancers

Table 10-8 Total Number of Metachronous Second Breast Cancers and Proportion of Stage 0 ISC per 100,000 Patient Years at Risk after Removal of the First Breast Cancer; Patients of All Ages and Those Less than 50 Years of Age, by Stage of the Initial Breast Cancer at Time of Diagnosis

Initial breast cancer characteristics	Subsequent breast cancer rates per 100,000 patient years at risk	
	Total	Stage 0 ISC
	All ages	
Stage 0 ISC	668	320 (48)[c,d]
Invasive breast cancer		
Localized[a]	648	88 (14)[d,e]
with regional metastasis[b]	745	89 (12)[e]
	Age < 50 years	
Stage 0 ISC	633	387 (61)[f]
Invasive breast cancer		
Localized[a]	794	137 (17)[f,g]
with regional metastasis[b]	882	85 (10)[g]

[a] Invasive breast cancer without regional lymph node or systemic metastasis.
[b] Invasive breast cancer with regional lymph node metastasis, but without systemic metastasis.
[c] Numbers in parentheses, percentages relative to the total rates.
[d,f,g] $p < .0005$.
[e] Not significant.

would be impeded in individual patients in the presence of spontaneous or induced CMI to the ISC-associated, gp55-like antigen determinant. Accordingly, the demonstration that at any postoperative interval the presence of measurable CMI against the ISC-associated, gp55-like antigen determinant(s) impedes the development of an invasive second primary breast cancer would strongly support the thesis that the induction of such immunity in control women should reduce the risk of a first breast cancer.

CONCLUSION

Determination of the nuclear differentiation of cancer cells and the periodic evaluation of host CMI against autologous cancer and gp55 should be included in the classification of breast cancer patients. Such dynamic prognostic information should be used in the evaluation of all therapeutic procedures, whether primary or adjuvant, radiation, chemo- or immunotherapy. Such evaluation should be specifically related to the development of systemic metastatic disease and of metachronous second primary breast cancers.

The consistent recording of nuclear differentiation and the monitoring of tumor-specific CMI will generate data permitting a more critical assessment of the feasibility of immunotherapy, as well as the prevention of breast cancer by induction of CMI against gp55.

ACKNOWLEDGMENT

Appreciation is expressed to the following individuals who were associated with the authors during various phases of these studies: Roy H. Ashikari, M.D., Thomas H.C. Barclay, M.D., Ada B. Chabon, M.D., Sidney F. Cutler, Sc.D., Arnold S. Dion, Ph.D., Benjamin F. Hankey, Sc.D., Steven C. Kwon, M.D., Henry P. Leis, Jr., M.D., Samuel Pilnik, M.D., and Francis D. Speer, M.D..

REFERENCES

1. Black MM: Human breast cancer. A model for cancer immunology. *Israel J Med Sci* 9:284, 1973.
2. Black MM, Barclay THC, Hankey BF: Prognosis in breast cancer utilizing histologic characteristics of the primary tumor. *Cancer* 36:2048, 1975.
3. Black MM, Zachrau RE: Antitumor immunity in breast cancer patients. *J Reprod Med* 23:21, 1979.
4. Black MM, Chabon AB: In situ carcinoma of the breast. *Pathol Annu* 4:185, 1969.
5. Black MM, Kwon CS: Precancerous Mastopathy: Structural and biological considerations. *Path Res Pract* 166: 491, 1980.
6. Black MM: Cellular and biologic manifestations of immunogenicity in precancerous mastopathy. *Natl Cancer Inst Mongr* 35:73, 1972.
7. Hirschl S, Black MM, Kwon CS: Ultrastructural characteristics of sinus histiocytic reaction in lymph nodes draining various stages of breast cancer. *Cancer* 38:807, 1976.
8. Black MM, Barclay THC, Cutler SJ, Hankey BF, Asire AJ: Association of atypical characteristics of benign breast lesions with subsequent risk of breast cancer. *Cancer* 29: 338, 1972.
9. Black MM: Structural, antigenic and biological characteristics of precancerous mastopathy. *Cancer Res* 36:2596, 1976.
10. Herberman RB: Assessment of cellular immune response to cancer of the breast. *Ann Clin Lab Sci* 9:467, 1979.
11. Black MM, Leis HP Jr, Shore B, Zachrau RE: Cellular hypersensitivity to breast cancer: Assessment by a leukocyte migration procedure. *Cancer* 33:952, 1974.
12. Black MM, Zachrau RE, Shore B, Dion AS, Leis HP Jr: Cellular immunity to autologous breast cancer and RIII-murine mammary tumor virus preparations. *Cancer Res* 38:2068. 1978.
13. Zachrau RE, Black MM, Dion AS, Shore B, Williams CJ, Leis HP Jr: Specificity of the simultaneous cell-mediated immune reactivity to RIII-murine mammary tumor virus glycoprotein 55 and human breast cancer tissues. *Cancer Res* 38:3414, 1978.
14. Rebuck JW: Cytology of acute inflammation in man by two original technical procedures with particular reference to the role of lymphocytes. Doctoral thesis, University of Minnesota, 1947.

15. Black MM, Leis HP Jr: Human breast carcinoma. III. Cellular responses to autologous breast cancer: Skin window procedure. *NY State J Med* 70:2583, 1970.
16. Black MM, Leis HP Jr: Cellular responses to autologous breast cancer tissue: Sequential observations. *Cancer* 32:384, 1973.
17. MacCarty WC, Mahle AE: Relation of differentiation and lymphocytic infiltration to post-operative survival in gastric carcinoma. *J Lab Clin Med* 6:473, 1921.
18. Black MM, Opler SR, Speer FD: Survival in breast cancer cases in relation to the structure of the primary tumor and regional lymph nodes. *Surg Gynecol Obstet* 100: 543, 1955.
19. Black MM, Speer FD: Nuclear structure in cancer tissues. *Surg Gynecol Obstet* 105:97, 1957.
20. Black MM, Hankey BF, Barclay THC: Intrastage prognostic heterogeneity: Implications for adjuvant chemotherapy of breast cancer. *J Natl Cancer Inst* 68:445, 1982.
21. Syrjänen KJ: The lymph nodes. Reactions to experimental and human tumors. *Exp Pathol Suppl* 8:1, 1982.
22. Fisher ER, Kotwal N, Hermann C, Fisher B: Types of tumor lymphoid response and sinus histiocytosis: Relationship to five-year, disease-free survival in patients with breast cancer. *Arch Pathol Lab Med* 107:222, 1983.
23. Black MM, Speer FD, Opler SR: Structural representations of tumor-host relationships in mammary carcinoma. Biologic and prognostic significance. *Am J Clin Pathol* 26:250, 1956.
24. Cutler SJ, Black MM, Goldenberg IS: Prognostic factors in cancer of the female breast. I. An investigation of some interrelations. *Cancer* 16:1589, 1963.
25. Cutler SJ, Black MM, Mork J, Harvei S, Freeman C: Further observations on prognostic factors in cancer of the female breast. *Cancer* 24:653, 1969.
26. Black MM: Immunopathology of breast cancer. *Pathobiol Annu* 7:213, 1977.
27. Black MM, Zachrau RE: Immunoprophylaxis of breast cancer: A conceptual appraisal, in Paterson AHG, Lees AW (eds): *Reviews on Endocrine-Related Cancer: Fundamental Problems in Breast Cancer.* Mississauga, Ontario, ICI Pharma, 1984, p.137.
28. Black MM, Zachrau RE: Stepwise mammary carcinogenesis: Immunological considerations, in Zander J, Blatzer J (eds): *Advances in Early Detection and Treatment of Breast Cancer.* Berlin-Heidelberg, Springer, 1985, p. 64.
29. Akiyoski T, Nakamura Y, Kawaguchi M, Tsuji H: Cellular hypersensitivity to autologous tumor extracts in patients with breast carcinoma. *Jpn J Surg* 8:236, 1978.
30. Cannon GB, Dean JH, Herberman RB, Keets M, Alford C: Lymphoproliferative responses to tumor extracts as prognostic indicators in patients with resected breast cancer. *Int J Cancer* 37:131, 1981.
31. Mesa-Tejada R, Keydar I, Ramanarayanan M, Ohno T, Fenoglio C, Spiegelman S: Immunohistochemical detection of a cross-reacting virus antigen in mouse mammary tumors and human breast carcinomas. *J Histochem Cytochem* 26:532, 1978.
32. Spiegelman S, Mesa-Tejada R, Ohno T, Ramanarayanan M, Nayak R, Bausch J, Fenoglio C, Keydar I: The presence and clinical implications of a virus-related protein in human breast cancer. *Cold Spring Harbor Conf Cell Prolif* 7:1149, 1980.
33. Mastrangelo MJ, Berd D, Maguire HC Jr: Current condition and prognosis of tumor immunotherapy: A second opinion. *Cancer Treat Rep* 68:207, 1984.
34. Black MM, Zachrau RE: Immunotherapy of breast cancer?, in Gallager HS, Leis HP, Jr, Snyderman RK, Urban JA (eds): *The Breast.* St. Louis, CV Mosby, 1978, p. 393.
35. Rosenberg SA: Adoptive immunotherapy of cancer: Accomplishments and prospects. *Cancer Treat Rep* 68:233, 1984.
36. Black MM, Zachrau RE, Dion AS, Katz M: Stimulation of prognostically favorable cell-mediated immunity of breast cancer patients by high dose Vitamin A and Vitamin E, in Prasad KN (ed): *Vitamins, Nutrition and Cancer.* Basel, Karger, 1984, p. 134.
37. Black MM: Human breast cancer. A model for cancer immunology. *Israel J Med Sci* 9:284, 1973.
38. Black MM, Cutler SJ, Barclay THC: Post-biopsy breast carcinoma: A natural experiment in cancer immunology. *Cancer* 29:61, 1972.
39. Black MM, Hankey BF, Aron JL, Prorok PC: Possible immunological implications of an association between the stages of first and second independent breast cancers. *Breast Cancer Res Treat* 4:95, 1984.

Part Four

Detection and Diagnosis of Breast Cancer

11

Mass Screening of Asymptomatic Women

Philip Strax, M.D.

INTRODUCTION

Screening is a procedure to detect disease in a presumably well individual. In the case of breast cancer, screening involves primarily the detection of an abnormality. The physician must then proceed to make the differentiation between a benign and malignant process.

A mass screening program for detection of early breast cancer differs in concept, approach, and techniques from a breast examination in general medical practice. The average woman with signs or symptoms goes to her physician for differential diagnosis and treatment. In mass screening for breast cancer, large numbers of women are involved who presumably have no disease and would not be having the examination were it not for the availability of the screening program. Detection rates may vary from two to three cancers per thousand to as many as 20 per thousand on the initial study. The vast majority of women will have negative results. Since the detection process involves many individuals without serious disease, it should be quick, safe, readily available, economical, and acceptable to the women being screened. It should be able to detect cancer at a stage when it can be treated effectively.

Breast cancer is an insidious disease that may develop over many years without signs or symptoms. If the disease is found and treated when localized to the breast, the cure rate is improved. Such optimum time may be before the woman is aware of the problem or even before a lesion is palpable by the woman or her physician. The incidence of breast cancer is rising, to the point that 1 in 11 women will be affected.[1]

In short, the object of screening for breast cancer is to discover those among the *apparently* well who are in fact suffering from breast cancer. This may afford a better chance for cure.

METHODS FOR SCREENING

The essential ingredients in screening for breast cancer are the interest and dedication of the screener.

The basic procedures used in mass screening are as follows:

1 An interview to develop demographic data, such as ethnic background, education, parity, and menstrual and breast history to develop clues to increased risk.

2 A careful clinical examination by a physician well-versed in the procedure or by a paramedical person after proper training and under the guidance of a clinician.

3 Teaching of breast self-examination and emphasizing its continuing importance.

4 Mammography x-ray examination of the breast. This procedure, which is at least 70 years old, has been considerably refined and brought to a high degree of technical excellence.[2] The radiation dosage is now down to less than about 0.1 rad to the midbreast per complete examination. Other radiologists use their usual x-ray equipment with a Xerox process, producing images on charged selenium-coated aluminum plates, ending with mammograms on special paper. This method (Xeromammography) also produces breast images of excellent quality, although with radiation dosage to the breast of about six times that of modern film-screen combinations. Both methods can produce proper quality.

Two other practical procedures should be mentioned. Mobile screening can make possible examination of large numbers of women in low-income areas to increase motivation in such women.[3] Mobile equipment also makes possible examination of women at their place of work. Another device that can markedly increase the economy of mammography is an automated mammography unit using 105-mm roll film. This makes possible the reduction of cost by at least one-third in film expense, time of examination, and use of personnel.[4]

Women need to be motivated to accept and even demand screening for breast cancer. The American Cancer Society has had excellent input. Organizations such as the United Order of True Sisters are also interested and have been helpful.[5]

In the attempt to make screening more cost-effective, emphasis has been placed on evaluation of high-risk factors for breast cancer, such as positive family history, nulliparity, early menarche, etc. Unfortunately, data from the statisticians of the American Cancer Society indicate that 75 percent of breast cancer is detected in women with no known risk factors—thus, a woman with known high-risk factors should certainly be subjected to periodic screening, but the need for such screening must not be limited to such women, lest only minimal progress be made in control of the disease. All women, at least those over 30, must be considered at risk for developing breast cancer.

RESULTS OF SCREENING

The concept of screening for breast cancer is not new. Before mammography was readily available, far-sighted authorities such as Holleb et al. and Gilbertsen et al. found improved survival results in women followed periodically with palpation and inspection.[6,7] They were, however, confronted with a high percentage of cancers in an "interval" stage, which were detected within a few months of presumably negative findings. We now know that such cancers are often detectable by mammography. In the early 1960s, investigators such as Gershon-Cohen began using mammography as a screening procedure and reported the detection of occult, nonpalpable cancers.[8]

In 1962, when the mass screening program for breast cancer detection was developed by the Health Insurance Plan of Greater New York (HIP) under contract with the National Cancer Institute, there had been a stationary death rate from the disease for 30 years.[9] There was also a generally pessimistic attitude toward improving this rate as exemplified by the so-called doctrine of "biological predeterminism of breast cancer," meaning that mortality could not be reduced by prevailing methods. At this time, too, there had developed a revived interest in mammography as a potentially effective modality to detect the disease in a nonpalpable stage.

The HIP study was set up basically to answer two questions:

1 Would a large-scale screening program using both palpation and mammography result not only in increased survival, but in mortality reduction?

2 What would be the contribution of mammography in such a program?

In this study, 62,000 women aged 40 to 64, chosen as 31,000 carefully matched pairs, were picked at random from medical group lists. One group was the "study group" and the other the "control group." The study group women received clinical examination by the surgeons of the group and mammography initially, and then annually for 3 years. These examinations were done in completely independent fashion so that the surgeon did not know the radiological findings and the radiologist did not know the clinical findings. Two-thirds of the invited women in the study group came at least once. One-third never came in spite of strenuous efforts, but have been continued as part of the study in statistical comparison with the control group to avoid the bias of self-selection. The control group women received their usual medical care and have been followed through records. Data have been and still are being collected.

An important aspect of the program was evaluation of the efficiency of mammography. About one-third of the cancers were detected on mammography alone and were negative on initial clinical examination. At the same time, two-fifths of the cancers were found on clinical examination alone and were negative on mammography. About one-fifth of the cancers were detected on both modalities. It was felt that both modalities were needed for proper yield in screening. The value of mammography was pointed out by the fact that 79 percent of the cancers found on x-ray alone were free of axillary nodal involvement. Cancers found on both modalities were localized in only 48 percent of the cases, comparable to the findings in the control group—45 percent. Obviously, the mammogram was capable of finding substantial numbers of nonpalpable cancers in a localized stage.

After 7 years of follow-up there was a one-third reduction in mortality from breast cancer in the study group compared to the control (70 versus 108). In other words, the screening procedure had apparently resulted in a substantial saving of lives from the disease. The reduction of mortality is persisting after 14 years of follow-up (118 deaths in the study group versus 153 in the control).[10]

These considerations led to the development in 1968 of the Guttman Breast Diagnostic Institute in New York City with the basic objective of developing a mass screening approach that would be feasible and could reach the general population of women. The two major problems to be solved were (1) how to develop a practical, economical, and efficient method that could produce a satisfactory yield of localized cancers; and (2) how to motivate women to accept such a procedure.[11]

Cooperation with the New York City Division of the American Cancer Society has been a key to stimulating women to come for examination. Up to 50,000 examinations per year have been made with such cooperation. Hundreds of cancers have been found in the past 16 years with a large proportion in a localized stage. Film-screen techniques have been developed which use minute amounts of radiation, down to 0.2 to 0.3 rad to the skin per exposure from the 8 rads used in the HIP study, and to less than about 0.1 rad to the midbreast for complete examination. Risk from such a radiation dose has been considered negligible by most authorities, even on a repetitive screening basis and the hazard probably not measurable. Newer techniques have led not only to much reduced radiation compared to that used in the HIP study, but to films of much enhanced quality which lend themselves to greater accuracy and ease in interpretation.

The success of these studies stimulated the large-scale national breast cancer screening program, involving some 280,000 women, the so-called Breast Cancer Detection Demonstration Project, or BCDDP.

The enhanced role of modern mammography is pointed up by comparing the findings of the HIP study with those in the BCDDP screening centers.[12] This is particularly true when comparing results of screening women under 50 years of age. In the HIP study in this age group, 19 percent of the cancers were found on mammography alone compared to 35 percent in the BCDDP groups. Also, 91 percent of all cancers in women under 50 in BCDDP were found on mammography versus 40 percent in HIP; and 14 percent of the cancers found were under 1 cm in size in BCDDP, compared to 4 percent in the HIP study. The improved mammographic techniques have apparently resulted in a substantial increase in cancers found on mammography (Table 11-1).

Enthusiasm for mass screening as a means for detection of early breast cancer was high. In 1976, however, controversy became apparent which led to the first set of guidelines for screening asymptomatic women.[13] The controversy revolved around the combination of two problems. First, the statistician of the HIP study insisted that there was no evidence of significant mortality benefit in that study from screening women under 50 years of age. Second, it was emphasized in medical articles as well as in the media that x-rays were carcinogenic to the breast. Since the BCDDP centers were federally financed, an ethical problem had to be faced by the authorities: Was it proper to permit federal funds to be used to support a medical project which might be producing a hazard without a benefit—such as use of mammography in women under 50? Several committees were set up and several meetings were held which culminated in a consensus meeting at Bethesda in December 1977, at which time guidelines were set up for the BCDDP centers.

1977 Guidelines

1 The guidelines applied only to women who have no symptoms or signs of breast disease whatsoever. This should be emphasized because many misunderstandings have resulted. Symptoms of

Table 11-1 Percentage of Breast Cancers Found by Mammography

	HIP* (%)	BCDDP† (%)
Mammography alone (all ages)	33	42
Negative nodes	79	77
Mammography alone (under age 50)	19	35
Negative nodes	68	73
Minimal cancers under 1 cm in size (mammography and clinical examination)	3.5	13.8‡

HIP: Health Insurance Plan of New York. BCDDP: Breast Cancer Detection Demonstration Project.

* 132 cancers.

† 2379 cancers.

‡ 59% found on mammography alone.

breast disease such as severe pain, tenderness, and nodularity are common. Such women were not involved in these guidelines.

2 Women over 50 should have annual examinations including physical examination as well as mammography, since all agreed that the HIP study indicated a substantial mortality reduction in a screened group versus a control.

3 Women between 40 and 50 years of age should not have mammography unless they have a previous history of breast cancer or a positive family history.

4 Women between 35 and 40 should not have mammography unless they have a previous history of breast cancer.

A new informed consent form was developed. The potential hazard of mammography in women under 50 was strongly emphasized and the possible benefits were minimized considerably.

These guidelines were widely publicized by the media. The net result was, of course, a sudden and marked decrease in the number of women attending the screening centers and, unfortunately, a concomitant substantial drop in detection of early cancers. This commotion and fear of x-radiation hazard has persisted in many circles to this day.

Because the BCDDP data have indicated a remarkable number of cancers found in the nonpalpable stage with a large percentage of no nodal involvement in women under 50, it was deemed important to review the two main obstacles of mass screening.

Further evaluation of the possible carcinogenic risk from x-radiation has led to the general agreement that risk depends on the x-ray dose to the midbreast as well as on the age of the woman. The x-ray dose to the midbreast as generally used today is down to less than about 0.1 rad to the midbreast for complete examination.[14] This is considered negligible and the risk is probably not even measurable. Also, it is now conceded that the risk to the breasts of women past 30 years of age is probably very small, if any. Since screening is done in women over 35 or 40, there is now agreement among radiological authorities that radiation risk from mammography in periodic mass screening, if it exists at all, is far exceeded by the potential benefit.

Table 11-2 Breast Cancer Deaths by Age: 9 Years' Follow-up from Date of Entry

Patients, (Age, years)	Number of Deaths: Study	Control
Age at death		
40 - 49	17	17
50 - 59	40	67
60 and older	34	44
Age at diagnosis		
40 - 49	30	27
50 - 59	40	67
60 and older	12	34
Age at entry		
40 - 49	39	48
50 - 59	40	60
60 - 64	12	20
Total	91	128

The other obstacle to mass screening—the apparent lack of mortality benefit in screening women under 50—has also received some second thoughts. A difference of opinion has developed concerning the questionable mortality benefit demonstrated from screening in the HIP study in women under 50. It is generally agreed that a substantial persistent mortality benefit has been demonstrated in women over 50 years of age. However, when mortality reduction is considered by age groups, the statistician of the HIP study has insisted that no significant change was noted due to the screening process in women under 50. This was determined by noting essentially the same number of deaths from breast cancer when comparing the study and control groups by age at death or age at diagnosis. However, other statisticians, such as Seidman[15] and Dubin[16]

Table 11-3 Breast Cancer Deaths by Date of Entry

	Time Interval from Entry*					
	5 Years		10 Years		14 Years	
	Study	Control	Study	Control	Study	Control
Within 5 years	19	20	39	51	46	61
Within 6 years			45	61	54	72
Within 7 years			54	67	65	82

* Age at entry: 40 to 49.

feel that the proper yardstick is age at entry where the study and control groups could be properly compared, because age at death and age at diagnosis varied within the study itself. When age at entry is used for comparison, a definite reduction in mortality is noted after a 9-year period of follow-up (46 versus 61 deaths). With longer follow-up, the age of entry improvement in the study group compared to the control continues to increase. Considering the marked increase in number of cancers detected in the BCDDP in women under 50, most investigators agree that evidence of mortality benefit in women under 50 years of age in screening is indeed present and should be seriously considered in the future (Tables 11-2 and 11-3).

The latest guidelines for the use of mammography as developed by the American Cancer Society[17] and concurred with by the American College of Radiology and the American Academy of Family Physicians are as follows:

1983 Guidelines

1 All women with signs and symptoms of breast disease should have mammography as well as physical examination as often and whenever needed, regardless of age.*

2 All women should have a baseline mammogram between the ages of 35 and 40, whether symptomatic or not.

3 All women over 40 should have a physical examination annually, and mammography every year or at most every 2 years.

4 All women over 50 should have both a physical examination and mammography on a yearly basis.

**Editors' Note:* The editors believe that a modification of the 1983 Guideline 1 should be made, so that *not all* women with signs and symptoms of breast disease receive mammography: For example, a 17-year-old girl with a typical fibroadenoma does not require mammography.

HORIZONS

Continued attempts are being made to improve the accuracy of mammography as well as to reduce radiation dosage.[18] Use of fiber grids, digital radiography, magnification mammography, and new and faster films and screens are being explored. Other modalities, such as thermography, ultrasonography, diaphanography, and nuclear magnetic resonance are also being evaluated for their potential in detecting the 5 to 10 percent of cancers not being detected at this time with clinical examination and mammography.

Of particular interest are attempts to detect a true high-risk factor which would make mass screenings more efficient.[18] (See Chap. 6.)

CONCLUSIONS

Mass screening for breast cancer offers a practical approach to the reduction of mortality from breast cancer at this time.[19] Concerns over risk in screening women should be allayed. More attention should be paid to remaining problems in screening, such as cost, detection of true high-risk factors, and methods for improving motivation. It is imperative that we move ahead with screening activities by making them more effective, more practical, and more acceptable to women and their physicians.

REFERENCES

1. *Cancer Facts and Figures*. American Cancer Society, 1984.
2. Snyder RE, Masterson MD, Miller DW, Kirch RL, Rothenberg LN, Hammerstein GR, Laughlin JS: Image quality control and radiation exposure in mammography, in Logan WW (ed): *Breast Carcinoma*. New York, John Wiley & Sons, 1977, p. 167.
3. Strax P: Female cancer detection mobile unit. *Preventive Med* 1:422, 1972.
4. Strax P, Malsky S, Strax N: Automated Millirad Mammography. *Proceedings of Third International Symposium on Detection and Prevention of Cancer*. New York, Marcel Dekker, 1976.
   Strax N: Automated Mammography Apparatus for Mass Screening. United States Patent No. 4,104,528, August 1, 1978.
5. Strax P: Strategy (motivation) for detection of early breast cancer. *Cancer* 46:926, 1980.
6. Holleb AI, Venet L, Day E, Hoyt S: Breast cancer detected by routine physical examination. *NY State J Med* 60:823, 1960.
7. Gilbertsen WA, Kfelsberg IM: Detection of breast cancer by periodic utilization of methods of physical diagnosis. *Cancer* 28:1552, 1971.
8. Gershon-Cohen J, Angleby H, Berger SM, Forman M, Curcio B: Mammographic screening for breast cancer. *Radiology* 88:663, 1967.
9. Strax P, Venet L, Shapiro S: Value of mammography in reducing mortality from breast cancer in mass screening. Am J Nat Cancer Inst Rad, 117:686, 1973.
10. Shapiro S, Venet W, Strax P, Venet L, Roeser R: Ten- to fourteen-year effect of screening in breast cancer mortality, J Nat Cancer Inst. 19(2):349, 1982.
11. Strax P: The Guttman Institute Story, in *Control of Breast Cancer through Mass Screening*. Littleton, Mass., PSG Publishing Co., 1979, p. 183.
12. Baker LH: Breast cancer detection demonstration project: Five year summary report. *Cancer* 32:4, 1982.
13. Bailar III, JC: Mammography: A contrary view. *Ann Intern Med* 84:77, 1976.
14. Miller DW, Hammerstein GR, White DR, Masterson ME, Laughlin JS: Radiation Absorbed Dose in Mammography. Presented at annual meeting of American Association of Physicists in Medicine, Cincinnati, Oh., 1977.
15. Seidman H: Lessons from the BCDDP. Possible gains in life expectancy from screening women under 50 for breast cancer, in Strax P (ed): *Control of Breast Cancer Through Mass Screening*. Littleton, Mass., PSG Publishing Co., 1979, p. 37.
16. Dubin N: Analysis of the Benefits of Mammographic Screening for Breast Cancer to Women Under Fifty Years of Age. *Proceedings of the 3rd Annual Conference of the American Society of Preventive Oncology*, New York, 1979.
17. Circular Letter MA-35. American Cancer Society, July 1, 1983.
18. Shore RE, Pasternack BS, Bulbrook RD, Moseson M, Kwa HG, Wang DY, Moore JW, Strax P: Endocrine and environmental factors in breast cancer: The case for prospective studies, in Bulbrook RD, Taylor DJ (eds): *Commentaries in Research in Breast Disease*. New York, Alan R. Liss, 1983.
19. Strax P: Mass screening for control of breast cancer. *Cancer* 53(3):665, 1983.

12

The Role of Mammography in the Diagnosis of Breast Cancer

Herman C. Zuckerman, M.D.

INTRODUCTION

The increasing awareness that micrometastasis frequently occurs early in the course of breast carcinoma continues to alter the approach to early detection. The growth of a cancer to 1 cm size, the accepted threshold of palpability, already represents 30 doubling times; 75 percent of the tumor's life-span has already occurred and only three more doublings will be necessary to increase the size from 1 to 2 cm.[14]

The direction this takes us is toward the recognition that palpation, while very important in avoiding more advanced disease, must not be completely relied upon to distinguish the benign from the malignant breast. At the present time the only consistently proven system for diagnosing earlier carcinoma is by means of routine x-ray mammography, in the hands of a radiologist dedicated to this specialty, and by using only machinery specifically designed for this purpose.

BACKGROUND

The major hurdle in the development of mammography was the difficulty of obtaining sufficient contrasts in the soft tissues of the breast that would define the individual structures. Salomon, a German surgeon, was apparently the first to explore the use of mammography in 1910, when he used the method to determine the extent of carcinoma in breast specimens. Subsequently Warren, Lockwood, Gershon-Cohen,[9] Gros,[6] and Sigrist among others made efforts to increase the contrasts in breast x-rays. In 1953 Leborgne in Uruguay published the first textbook of mammography with superb illustrations accomplished by reducing kilovoltage and increasing milliamperage, and at the same time using breast compression.[11] Egan in 1960 introduced fine-grain industrial film and provoked worldwide interest by presenting a 97 percent accuracy in the diagnosis of breast carcinoma in a tumor institution.[2] Gros improved contrasts with the introduction of a molybdenum anode tube and filter.[6]

Mammography received a temporary setback in 1976 when the radiation hazard was brought into question. The one great contribution of this controversy was the alacrity with which commercial x-ray film companies responded to these pressures by developing a vacuumized screen-film combination[16] that results in approximately 0.1 rad exposure to the midbreast per complete examination—a very acceptable dosage. At present, the availability of a microfocus tube for reducing unsharpness and for image enlargement (Fig. 12-9), and a grid to elicit detail in the denser breasts are indications of continued activity toward improving the modality.

METHOD

The author's experience with mammography has been gained from a large private practice covering a period of 30 years where the number of annual breast examinations totals about 15,000. Clinically obvious carcinoma has never been a significant entry in the statistics, and in the past 3 years the reason for patient referral has been slanted toward routine annual study. Two other reasons are recognized as clinical indecision and high-risk factors. A smaller group is referred for a second opinion.

A technician records the data concerning family history, hormone usage, previous breast operations, previous mammograms, and parity. Skin abnormalities such as scars, keloids, warts, and keratoses are noted, since these may influence the image. Each patient is interviewed and briefly examined by the radiologist, who then develops a commitment to a palpable problem. The size of a palpable lesion may then be recorded to compare with its visual size on x-ray, which is often a valuable criterion in differentiating carcinoma, where the lesion is larger on palpation, from benign lesions. A clinical problem area is marked with an adherent lead marker. If no corresponding x-ray finding appears, supplemental tangential spot film views may become necessary, especially since masses in the axillary tail, upper medial quadrant, or in the region of the inframammary crease may not be adequately represented on the routine study. Since palpation has added a special obligation, it is best that these spot film views be done by the radiologist, who should place the film closer to the area of palpable abnormality for greater detail and with an eye to localization for subsequent surgery.

The films are examined briefly before the patient's departure; if necessary, spot films may be done for greater detail, thereby reducing the need for recall. The films are read with the aid of a magnifying glass, under regular or bright lighting, and often with a minifying glass for better perception of contrasting density and pattern.[23] If the breasts are not too large, similar positions of both breasts are often done on a single film, which is one way to improve detection of asymmetry.[19] When previous films are available for comparison, both accuracy and earlier detection are often enhanced.[13]

The apparatus being used is the Senograph with a dual-focus tube of 0.3 and 0.1 focal spots with pure molybdenum anode and 0.03-mm molybdenum filter. The film used is Eastman Kodak NMB-1 coupled with a rare-earth Minar screen in a vacuum pack. The film is developed automatically at a $3\frac{1}{2}$ min transit time. Three views are employed for each breast: craniocaudal, lateromedial, and a lateral oblique that covers the axillary portion of the breast but is not intended to image axillary nodes.

Compression is always used and serves the following functions: (1) It exaggerates both the distortion produced by attachment of otherwise occult lesions to adjacent tissue as well as the effects of edema; (2) it allows for a more even thickness of breast tissue by converting the cone-shaped breast into a flat unit; (3) it reduces superimposition by distributing breast elements over a wider area; (4) radiation is reduced with the decreased breast thickness; (5) immobilization is improved, even decreasing the effects of the heartbeat; (6) it brings the breast structures closer to the film; (7) it smooths out the skin; and (8) it increases the relative density of lesions which are not compressible.

The use of the spot film is fundamental, especially in demonstrating occult lesions. A superior image is produced with fine coning and more localized pressure. If necessary, small problem areas may be evaluated with AA industrial film for the greatest sharpness and clarity. The secret of good mammography is for the radiologist to overreact to minimal departures from the normal, while exploring the varied armamentarium of mammographic procedure on spot films, such as grid, magnification, and additional projections to explain the problem.

Xeroradiography is an alternative procedure to film-screen mammography and is embraced just as fervently by its adherents. It uses a charged photoconductive selenium plate which is partially discharged by the incident x-ray beam emerging from the breast. A toner powder adheres to the areas of residual charge, forming the image which can then be transferred electrostatically to paper.

ANATOMY

The average adult female breast consists of a cone-shaped mass of connective tissue with the apex at the nipple, within which are 12 to 20 ducts and their lobules which converge toward the nipple. The ducts and their encasing cylindrical sleeves of connective tissue, which also contain vascular and lymphatic elements, are given the inclusive name of trabeculae. The skin and a subcutaneous fatty layer envelop the glandular tissue, and Cooper's ligaments attach the glandular corpus to the skin. As the patient ages, the dense fibrous and glandular breast tissues of early adulthood are gradually replaced by increasing amounts of adipose tissue, which provides the desirable contrast that further facilitates mammographic diagnosis.

DYSPLASIA

Fibrocystic disease is a term most commonly used to cover abnormal proliferative changes in the breast, such as cysts, intraductal epithelial hyperplasia, intraductal papillomatosis, ductal hyperplasia, adenosis, etc. These can all be related to carcinoma, and only duct ectasia is considered unrelated to malignant neoplasia.

Cysts

Cysts are quite common and vary in size from minute to over 7 cm. They are usually smooth, round, or oval, and sharply contoured, unless obscured by adjacent connective tissue, which is of similar density. Not infrequently a thin fat stripe or "security line" separates them from structures nearby, and helps to identify them as noninvasive benign masses. The breast markings in the vicinity are gently displaced, leaving minimal surrounding distortions. Confirmation by needle aspiration or ultrasound may be necessary on occasion to distinguish them from malignant masses such as colloid and medullary carcinomas, the rarer smooth-bordered duct cell carcinomas, intracystic carcinoma, lymphoma, and metastasis. This procedure is encouraged when (1) the density of the cyst-like mass is unusually marked, (2) the adjacent markings are sufficiently disturbed, (3) the size on palpation is greater than the mammographic size (by virtue of surrounding palpable edema and desmoplastic reactions), (4) there is partial irregularity or fuzziness of outline, or (5) the cyst is quite large and is capable of concealing a smaller lesion nearby.

Adenosis

Adenosis is a hyperplasia of lobules, and is recognized on a mammogram as groups of fluffy, flocculent, small, separated, poorly marginated densities which may coalesce and achieve a formless density. A variation of this is *sclerosing adenosis*, where fibrosis is added, and is often associated with numerous, uniform, sharply marginated, well-spaced, rounded microcalcifications. Occasionally these can be smudgy and also occasionally grouped. The degree of separation and bilaterality among other considerations helps to differentiate them from the calcification of carcinoma. Small areas of sclerosing adenosis can occasionally cause scarring and retraction. Calcification may also be present and it may be difficult to differentiate this appearance from a small scirrhous carcinoma. The absence of a central mass and the presence of linear radial streaks of lesser density in the complex help, but biopsy is the safest recommendation (Fig. 12-1).

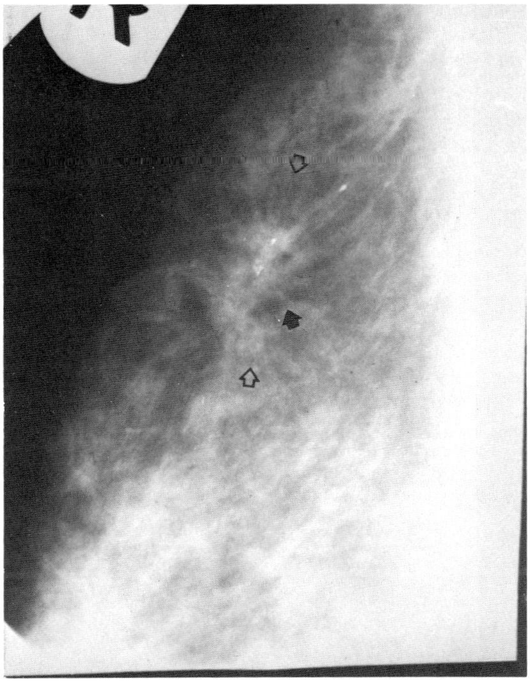

Figure 12-1 Sclerosing adenosis simulating retractile scirrhous carcinoma (between clear arrows). Note black (lucent) radial markings (black arrow) and calcification.

Ductal Hyperplasia

Ductal hyperplasia refers to thickening of the periductal fibrous tissue. When present, ducts can be followed for a greater distance from the nipple into the breast.

Ductal Epithelial Hyperplasia and Papillomatosis

When similar-appearing, rounded, well-formed calcifications are arranged in tandem (Fig. 12-2(A)) in the course of a duct, *ductal epithelial hyperplasia* may be suspected. Pepperings of extremely fine calcification of similar size and density are quite diagnostic of papillomatosis.

Duct Ectasia

Duct ectasia follows inflammatory damage to the duct walls. Secretions are inadequately absorbed and become inspissated. Duct "stones" may appear as rounded or linear calcifications usually with lucent centers. These diseased ducts may rupture and spew their contents into the adjacent tissues, giving rise to a foreign-body reaction and a chemical mastitis. This can cause nipple retraction when healed by fibrosis, but it is easily differentiated from carcinoma on x-ray.

BENIGN SOLID TUMORS

Fibroadenomas

Fibroadenomas are the most common. These may be difficult to distinguish from cysts, since when discrete they have similar densities and sharp margination. A lobulated outline along with coarse calcifications, seen mostly in the postmenopausal years, are helpful. The surrounding lucent "security stripe" is seen more often than in cysts and indicates its noninvasiveness (Fig. 12-3). Aspiration or ultrasound determine its solid nature in difficult cases. Only the coarse calcifications remain as the fleshy portion

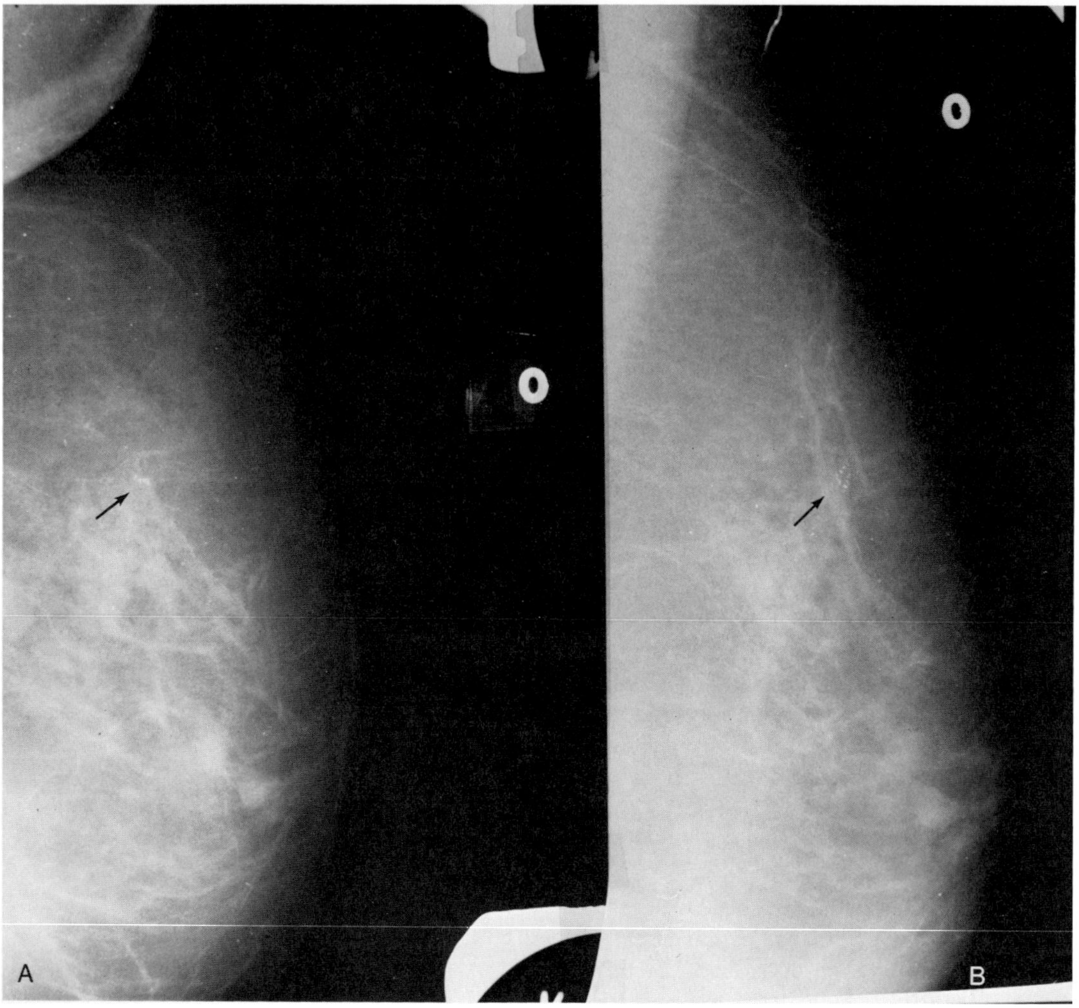

Figure 12-2 A. Four similar calcifications in tandem. Epithelial hyperplasia suggested. B. Thirteen months later. Calcifications have doubled in number. At surgery, intraductal carcinoma in situ.

undergoes absorption. Large fibroadenomas and cystosarcomas may acquire a reticulated form of calcification, but even if malignancy supervenes, it is rarely betrayed on the mammogram. The larger lesions are therefore recommended for excision. Women capable of producing fibroadenomas may have a three times greater risk of developing carcinoma elsewhere in the breasts.

Intraductal Papillomas

Intraductal papillomas are mostly found in the vicinity of the areola, although 25 percent can be found elsewhere in the duct system. These are often difficult to find in two views. A slight increase in density in a sharply marginated small tumor near the areola, or a tiny rosette of calcifications with a barely perceptible rim of soft tissue can sometimes be seen. A bulge

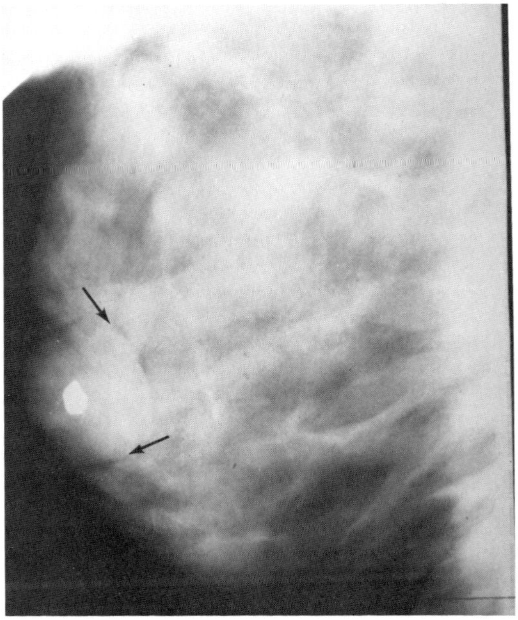

Figure 12-3 Rounded mass surrounded by thin lucent zone (security line). Fibroadenoma.

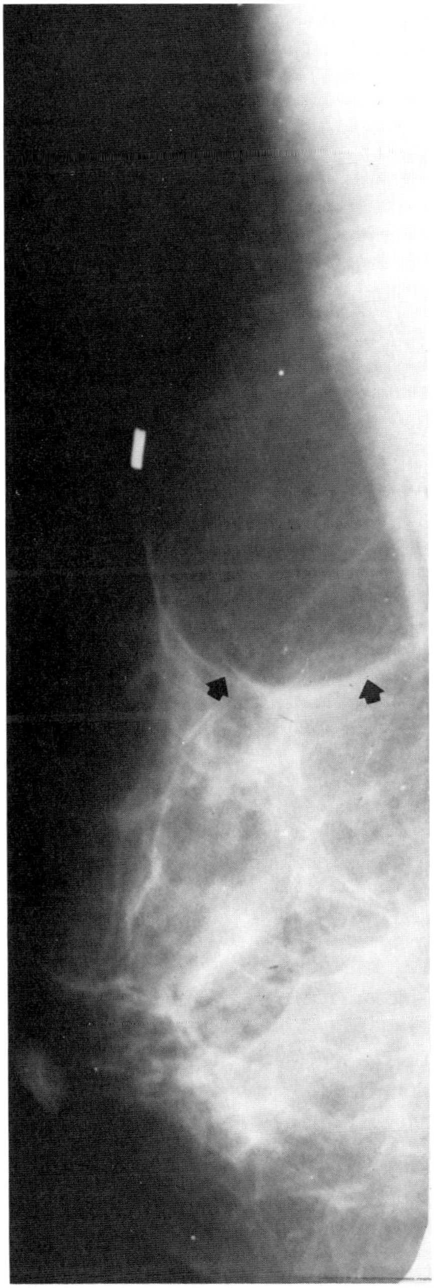

Figure 12-4 Lipoma. Large lucent area (arrows). Note lead marker at site of clinical fullness.

in a visible duct is also suggestive, or a group of similar-appearing nodules in the subareola area.

Galactography, or injection of opaque media into the ducts, can be employed in patients with spontaneous discharge of clear or bloody character. The procedure is somewhat time-consuming and is not generally embraced, since there is a preference for removing the duct system behind the areola along with possible other silent papillomas, and since its ability to localize the nodule is far superior to its ability to distinguish benign from malignant lesions.

Lipomas and Galactocoeles

Lipomas and galactocoeles show a reduced radiographic density (Fig. 12-4). Their importance is simply in explaining palpation findings. Lipomas, when caught between Cooper's ligaments, may sometimes feel like important masses, and galactocoeles can be quite firm and worrisome until x-ray reveals a thin penciled capsule surrounding a lucent center.

Abscesses

Abscesses frequently require differentiation from malignancy, especially with skin thickening. A patch of poorly marginated increased density and skin thickening, coupled with clinical signs of redness, tenderness, and even fever, all of recent development, usually assist in the diagnosis of acute abscess. Most abscesses occur in the vicinity of the areola and occur postpartum, but some are unrelated and problematic. Aspiration and the absence of generalized lymphatic engorgement add further information to differentiate this from inflammatory carcinoma and encourage antibiotics on a temporizing basis for a few weeks.

Fat Necrosis

Fat necrosis will at times suggest a malignant picture, but recent trauma, superficial position, absence of central density, and the presence of oil cysts (Fig. 12-5) all favor waiting for signs of resolution.

With all solid tumors, unless the radiologist can be completely satisfied the lesion is benign, biopsy should be seriously considered (Fig. 12-6). When calcifications of any kind show a preference for this site, or when the surrounding markings are disturbed only in this area, once again this recommendation applies.

MALIGNANT TUMORS

In the demonstration of malignancy the florid lesion was especially favored in earlier texts because of its teaching potential in supplying so many malignant criteria in one illustration. The respect for the dramatic presentation of malignancy is being eroded, however, with growing awareness that sizable malignant lesions do not represent the practical values of mammography. The minimal lesions, on the other hand, have more pertinence, since statistically these patients live longer, have a higher 20-year "cure" rate, and presumably will be more eligible for the newer therapies as these arise. We are therefore oriented toward closer perception of both the point where malignant change supervenes

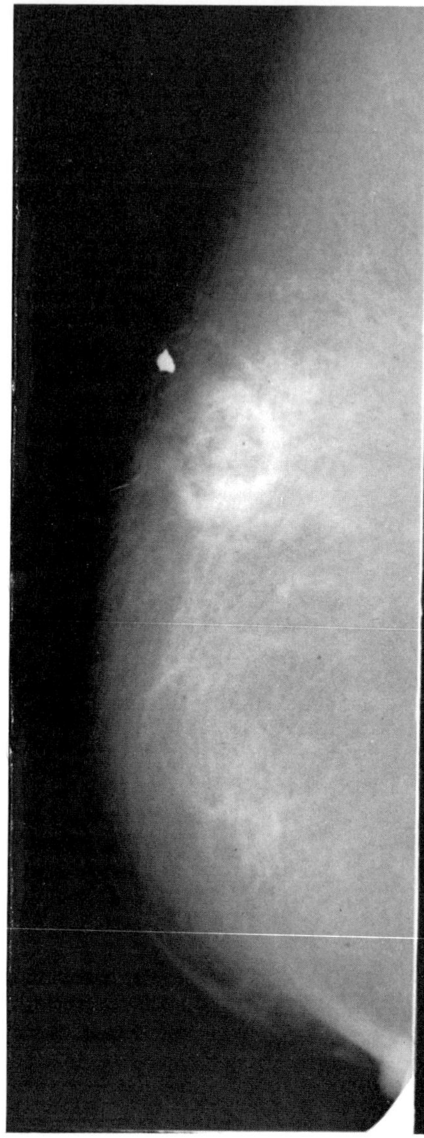

Figure 12-5 Fat necrosis. Note mass with lucent center establishing nonmalignancy. Also, superficial position. History of trauma.

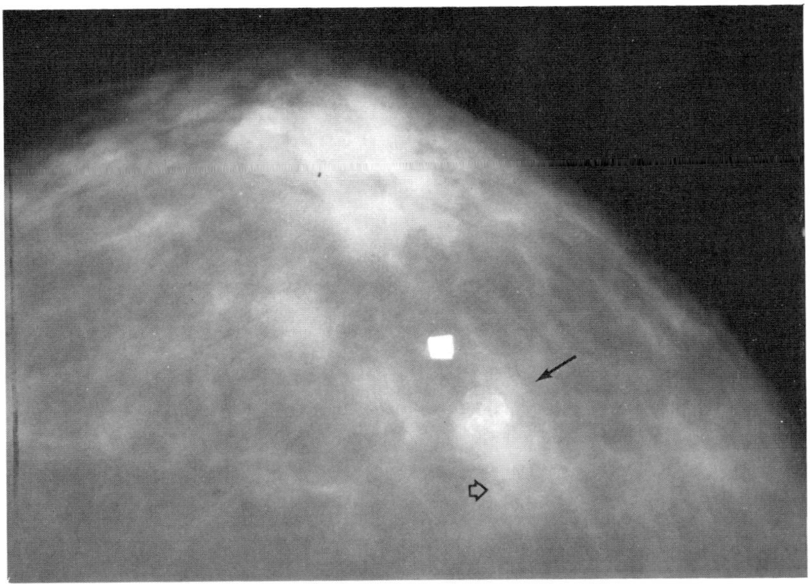

Figure 12-6 Mass with poor margination toward chest wall. Large well-circumscribed calcifications as in fibroadenoma, but lacking appropriate density. Surgery recommended. Osseous metaplasia in duct cell carcinoma.

and to the stages which precede it.[1,8,10,12] An increasing success in the detection of in situ cancer, as well as earlier invasive cancer, occurred (Figs. 12-2 and 12-7). This has necessitated a greater frequency of biopsy with a lower rate of positive findings.

While the radiologist develops some expertise in differentiating duct cell, medullary, colloid, tubular, intracystic, and occasionally lobular cancers, this is not as important as the basic appreciation that malignancy is present. Also, many cancers are of mixed cell type. For this reason the criteria for the diagnosis of malignancy, which have been increasing in numbers over the years, become the all-important consideration. The more this entire armamentarium is learned thoroughly, the more likely any one of these features can trigger sufficient suspicion to set the radiologist on the course for detection. These are related to (1) calcification, (2) increased density, (3) irregularity and indefiniteness of outline, (4) spiculation, (5) edema, (6) retraction, (7) departure from symmetry, (8) altered pattern of adjacent breast markings, (9) neovascularity, (10) smaller visual compared to palpable size, (11) stiffening and displacement of trabeculae, (12) disruption of orderly progression of atrophy, (13) developing density, (14) regrowth of glandular tissue after menopause, (15) solitary duct thickening, (16) blurring of detail, and (17) thickening of skin.

Calcifications

Calcifications in the breast are quite common. Most of these are isolated or well-separated pinpoint rounded entities or considerably larger duct "stones" with a lucent center, following inspissation of duct secretions, or as a result of liponecrosis. These are all considered benign. When microcalcifications become grouped and varied in shape, density, and size, or when frayed, lacking a sharp margin, or filamentous or branching, we become alerted that they may represent malignant change. Rarely do coarse

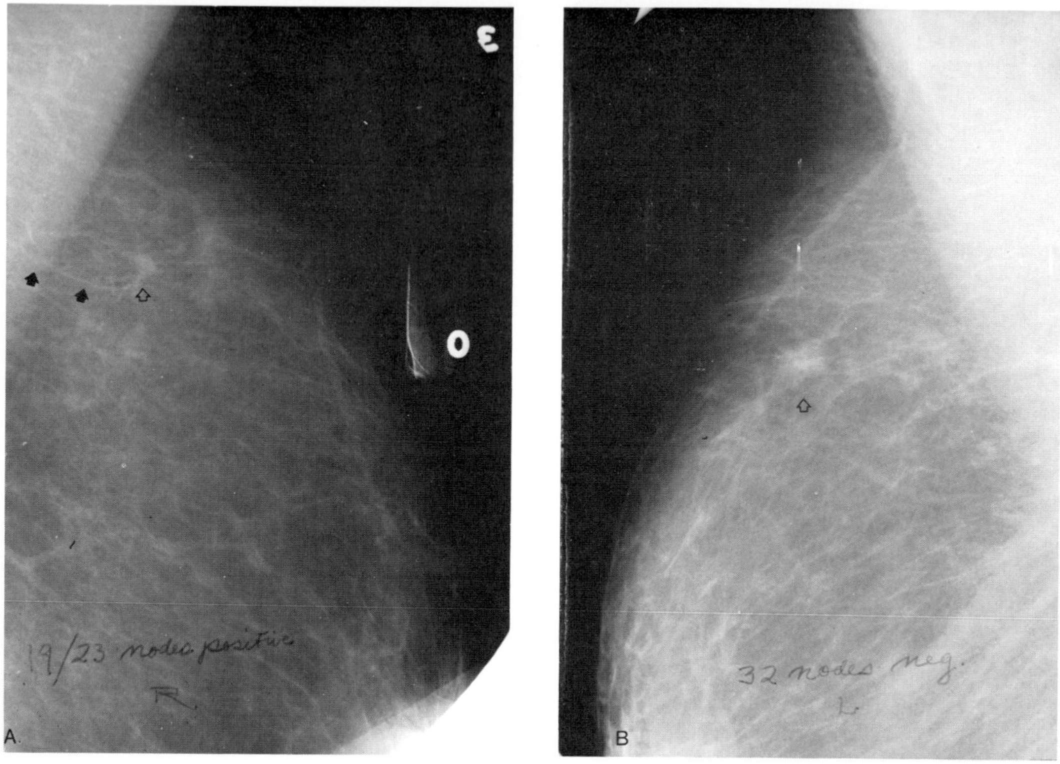

Figure 12-7 Bilateral nonpalpable carcinoma. A. 3-mm carcinoma (clear arrow); 19 out of 23 axillary nodes positive. B. 1-cm carcinoma; 32 axillary nodes negative. Note retracted trabeculum (black arrows) in A.

calcifications occur in malignancy. A certain number of grouped calcification has been stated as necessary for diagnosis, but even this must be discarded, for even a central calcification in a lesion with other leading features may lend assurance to the diagnosis (this central calcification is not produced by the tumor since we have instances of its presence as much as 6 years before the tumor was seen, and it may simply represent malignant transformation in an already diseased duct).

Calcification may also occur a short distance away from the obvious lesion and yet be related to it if occurring nowhere else. The explanation, whether altered tissue alkalinity or other factor, is not known, but the frequency of this association indicates it is not fortuitous. Even arteries crossing the malignant area may acquire calcification localized to this region.[22] Separate calcific groupings in a chain pattern (Fig. 12-8) are particularly diagnostic since they suggest the arborizing feature of ducts. Magnification of these calcific groups, whether done optically or by x-ray or both together, often demonstrates additional calcification not initially appreciated but of smaller size (Fig. 12-9). Malignant calcification may not be associated with visible mass and it is easy to understand how frequently we must be deprived of early diagnosis when the lesion is there but has not developed telltale calcification. When calcification of any kind is limited to an area of disturbed pattern or is in close association with a palpable mass, malignancy is an important consideration. In

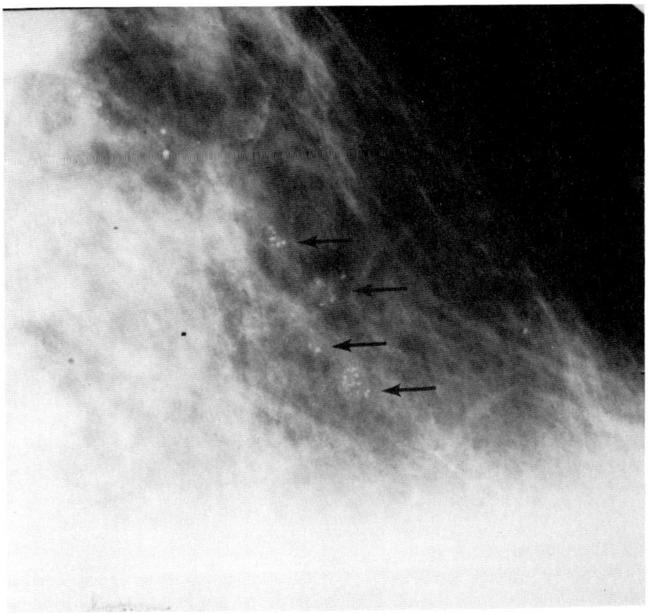

Figure 12-8 Chain arrangement of calcific groupings. Duct carcinoma, comedo type.

Paget's disease that is limited to the nipple and areola, one or two calcifications in the vicinity are not unusual (Fig. 12-10).

Increase in Density

This probably has to do with the lack of fatty elements which occur in normal tissue construction. The use of a minifying glass at different distances can prove remarkably helpful in appreciating relative densities. Colloid carcinoma may be difficult to distinguish from a benign mass because the mucinous factor is quite large and reduces its density (Fig. 12-11).

Irregularity

Irregularity and indefiniteness of outline may at times need careful spot filming for full appreciation. Medullary, colloid, intracystic, and even occasionally duct cell carcinoma may be disconcertingly smooth in outline. Establishing the solid nature of the tumor followed by attention to its influence on adjacent tissues, comparative visual and palpable size, increased density, and presence of calcification in the vicinity may solve the dilemma. Unless there is a great measure of certainty, biopsy is the favored approach (Fig. 12-6).

Spiculation

Spiculation of the tumor periphery deserves special mention, since it is one of the more pathognomonic features of duct cell carcinoma. Here the tumor sends dendritic extensions into the surrounding tissues. In the more equivocal instances of this feature it will be noted that the extension is thickest where it leaves the tumor outline, and tapers distally.[22] On occasion, abscesses, sclerosing adenosis (Fig. 12-1), and fat necrosis can deceive (Fig. 12-5).

Edema

A large halo of lesser density or area of clearing about the lesion occurs with great frequency about malignant tumors and represents edema

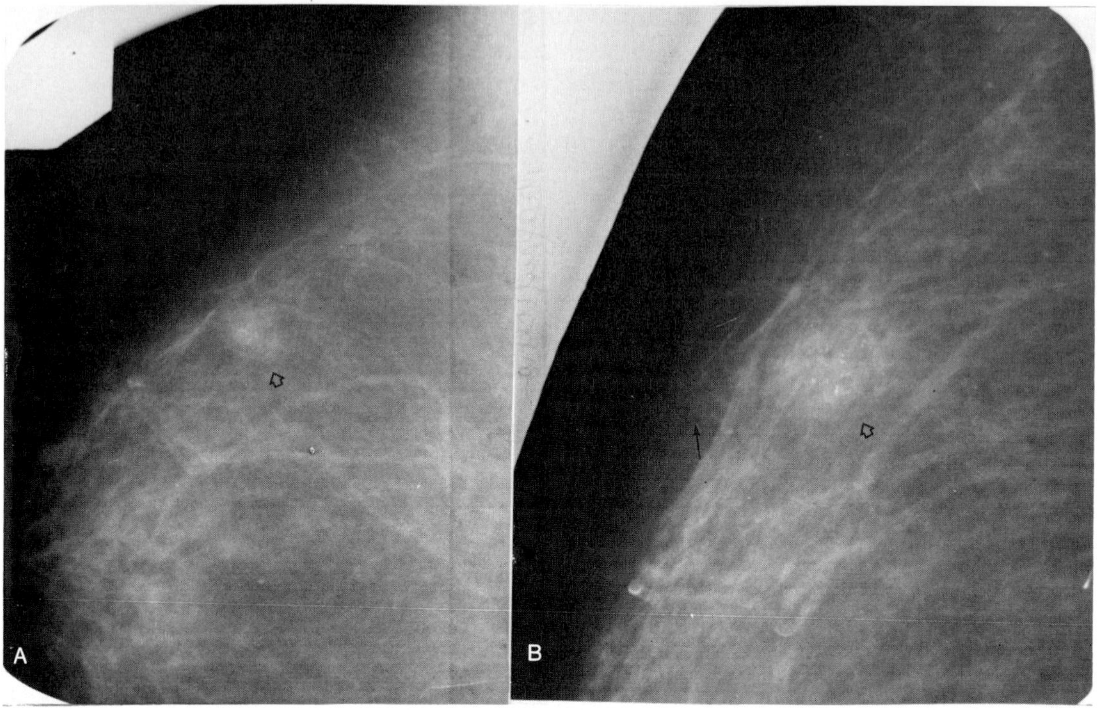

Figure 12-9 A. Magnification. Poorly defined mass with suggestion of calcification. B. X-ray enlargement of *A*. Calcifications, their shape, size, and density clearly seen. Also, margin of mass demonstrated. Note large blood vessels associated in subcutaneous area (black arrow). Hyalinized fibroadenoma (clear arrow).

(Fig. 12-12). This accounts for the larger palpable size as compared with the visual (x-ray) size of the tumor. (A desmoplastic reaction to the presence of malignancy may also increase palpability (Fig. 12-13).) The reducing glass again helps. Parallel convex trabeculae suggesting a ripple effect near the tumor are an expression of pressure of edematous change exaggerated by local spot film pressure (Figs. 12-13 and 12-14). Caution in evaluating the halo is recommended after aspiration since bleeding can also produce it.

Stiffening and Displacement of Trabeculae

Stiffening and displacement of trabeculae are important signs in the earlier detection of breast cancer. There the trabeculum can be bent toward the questionable density (Fig. 12-9A) and at times is clasped to the lesion or, on the other hand, may be displaced away from its normal relaxed course toward the nipple by edema (Figs. 12-13 and 12-14). The thin penciled trabeculum does not call attention to itself very often unless it becomes stiffened and linear (Fig. 12-15), or sharply curved as in palisading about the lesion. This again is probably related to edematous pressure compounded by local spot film pressure.

Retraction

Retraction is very important as the skin, the glandular outline, and even the blood vessels may show obvious displacement toward the lesion.[22]

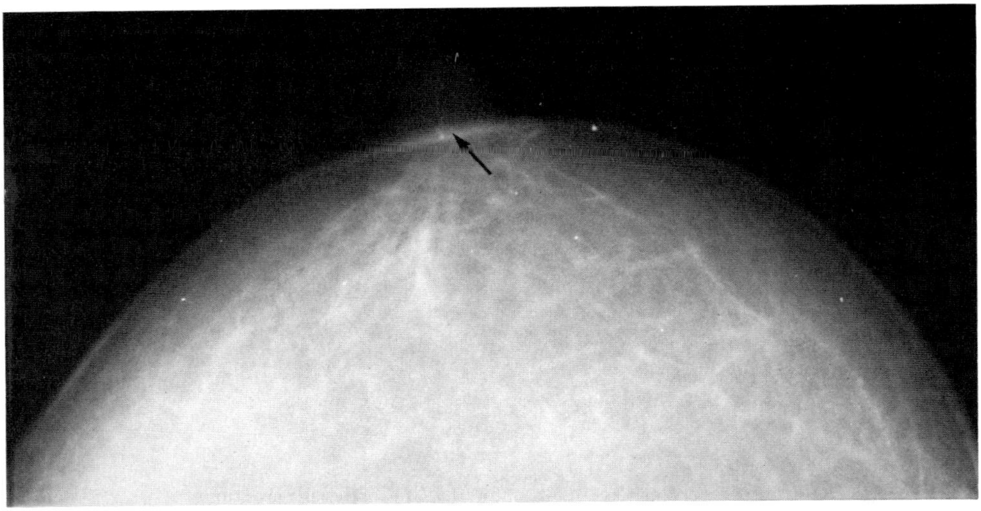

Figure 12-10 Paget's disease. Central nipple calcification (black arrow). Nipple skin erosion clinically.

Neovascularity

The relative size of the blood vessels of the two breasts is not necessarily important, since the normal breast may carry the larger vessels. What is important is the appearance of neovascularity, where a group of small, fine vessels is seen in the usually barren subcutaneous area adjacent to the tumor (Fig. 12-16). Routine and tangential views may supply such clues as to neoplastic activity in the vicinity, and these differ from the larger vessels seen occasionally with fibroadenoma (Fig. 12-9B). For this reason, part of the film reading should recognize the value of scanning the subcutaneous areas of both breasts, dwelling longer where the markings here are "busier."

Size

The size of an invasive malignant mass is usually estimated on palpation to be greater than the size on mammography, due to surrounding edema and desmoplastic reaction. Cysts and fibroadenomas, being somewhat compressible, are usually estimated by palpation to be smaller than they actually are.

Altered Pattern of Breast Markings

An overall altered pattern of breast markings is not infrequent adjacent to a malignant mass. The normal relaxed drift of markings toward the nipple may be replaced at one point by a decided change in pattern (Fig. 12-13). The crispness of markings when compared with the same area of the opposite breast may be quite reduced. A malignant lesion may also produce a fibrous response to its presence, seen particularly well in the fatty breast (Fig. 12-13). The rather homogeneous fibrous density of some breasts may be broken up at one point by the retractile forces of an underlying occult cancer.[22]

Progress of Glandular Atrophy

The general progress of glandular atrophy in the perimenopausal years usually follows a standard course. First the medial half of the breast loses its glandular structure. Then the outer half atrophies, beginning posteriorly and moving toward the nipple. Any glandular deposit that remains behind in the atrophic areas deserves closer attention[22] (Fig. 12-15).

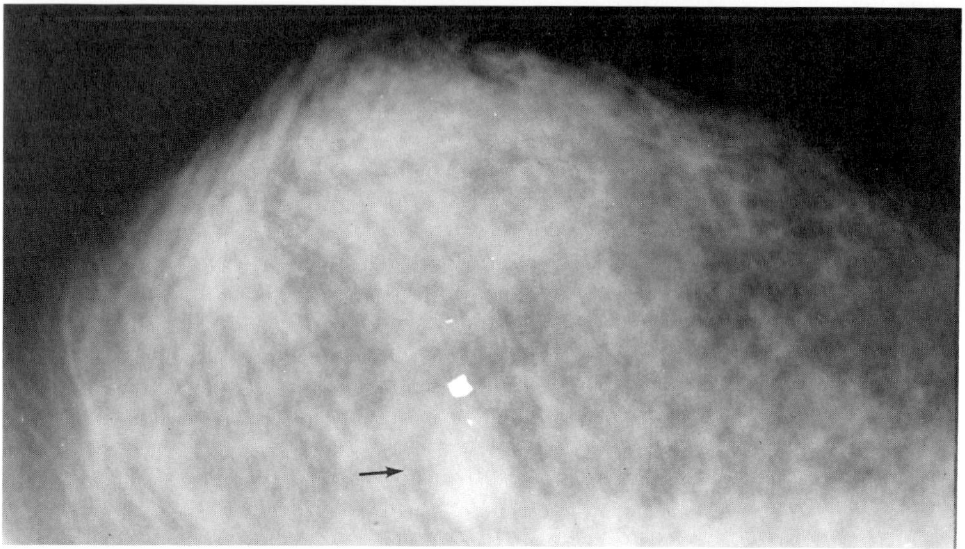

Figure 12-11 Colloid carcinoma (black arrow). Mild densification. To be differentiated from cyst or fibroadenoma.

Regrowth of Glandular Structure

Regrowth of glandular structure in the postmenopausal years in the absence of heavy hormone replacement and glandular tumors elsewhere is almost always an indication of malignant change, and biopsy is recommended.

Solitary Duct Thickening

Solitary duct thickening and prolongation of its visibility into the breast for 2 to 3 cm could be the result of a tumor extending along this conduit, either papilloma or carcinoma.

Skin Thickening

Skin thickening is not always a late sign of cancer, but in the absence of surgery, radiation, scarring, skin excrescences, hemorrhage, infection, fat necrosis, and Pick's syndrome this must be a source of concern. The appearance of thickening may actually be due to flattening of the skin profile as a result of retraction, important for this reason as well. The appreciation of thickening may be limited to the x-ray alone. Tangential views of scars, assisted by application of a lead marker, will often explain the questionably malignant appearance in this area by showing the "mass" to be part of the scar.

Departure from Symmetry

Departure from symmetry is quite important in recognizing the appearance of new structures in one breast or of alterations in glandular contours. Comparison with previous films adds to the possibility of earlier detection here. Developing density also makes use of previous films for comparison and is an alerting sign of possible developing malignant change.

Sarcoma

Sarcoma is rather rare in the female—about 1 percent of breast malignancies. It may be well-circumscribed or poorly marginated and exhibits unusually rapid growth. Retraction and fine calcifications are not present. Giant fibroadenoma, cystosarcoma, medullary and intracystic carcinoma, and metastasis are involved in the differential diagnosis. Given rapid growth

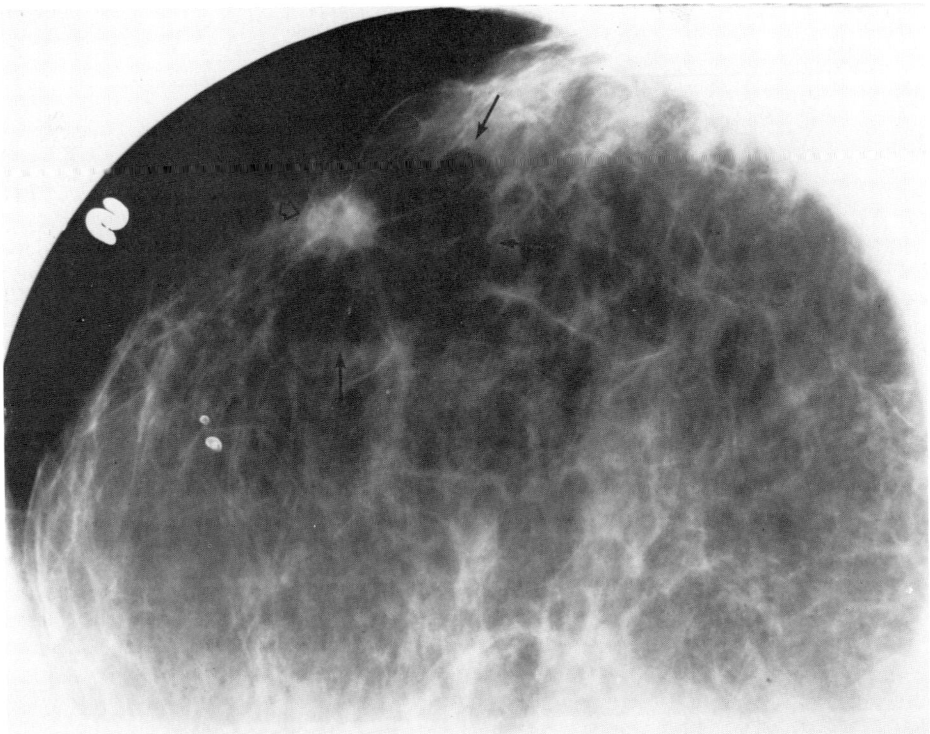

Figure 12-12 Edema. Large lucent halo (black arrows) surrounding 1-cm scirrhous carcinoma (clear arrow).

or history of lymphoma, this entity should be considered.

LOCALIZATION OF NONPALPABLE LESIONS

Guide wires introduced from two directions converging on the lesion with x-ray control and including specimen x-ray has become the most exacting approach to reaching and removing the lesion with minimal sacrifice of adjacent normal tissue. This method and the use of the multiperforated plastic pressure plate, where the individual perforations are identifiable on x-ray for introduction of a needle of measured length through the perforation overlying the lesion, again with x-ray control,[5] are the most popular. A second method makes use of a simultaneous injection of a dye visible to the surgeon and an opaque for the radiologist at the preferred needle position. The needle can then be withdrawn. There are some who still prefer the simple measurements from the nipple. While acknowledging a greater sacrifice of breast tissue, they cite instances where the calcific grouping was some distance from the actual malignant area.[17] (See also Chap. 16.)

FREQUENCY OF MAMMOGRAPHY

When it was learned from the BCDDP series of 270,000 cases that one-third of the breast cancers occurred in women under 50 years, and that 44 percent of these were detected by mammography alone,[15] a significant omission

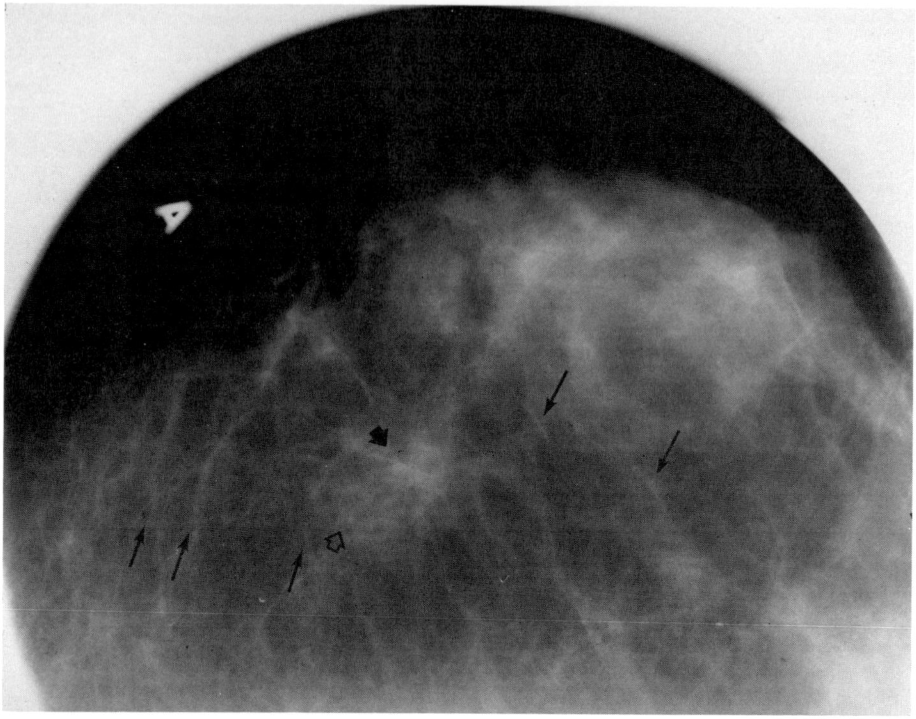

Figure 12-13 Duct cell carcinoma, 8-mm, nonpalpable (small black arrow). Ripple arrangement of trabeculae (long arrows). Fibrous desmoplastic response (clear arrow). Note also disturbance in glandular pattern.

in guidelines for mammography was corrected. This took into consideration the low radiation dose which has been developed.[18] Our present guidelines favor an annual mammography for women over 50 years, for women between 35 to 50 years who have a close or quantitative family history of breast carcinoma or significant premalignancy on previous biopsy, and for everyone after unilateral mastectomy. Otherwise mammography is recommended biannually for women between 40 to 50 years, with a single study as a baseline for women between 35 to 40 years.

Other specific reasons for mammography are

1 examination of voluminous breasts;

2 avoidance of repeated surgery in recurrent benign conditions;

3 evaluation of questionable thickening, usually in women over age 25;

4 evaluation of the same breast in which a dominant mass is present, and of the contralateral breast as well. Every patient undergoing breast surgery should have a preliminary bilateral mammogram for clinically nonapparent carcinoma.*

5 allaying anxiety in cancerophobia;

6 study of women with unexplained enlarged axillary lymph nodes, and in the search for a primary malignancy in the presence of metastatic disease elsewhere;

7 evaluation of breast symptoms without palpatory abnormality (e.g., pain, ecchymosis, nipple discharge, etc.); and

**Editors' Note*: Women under 30 years of age with obviously benign tumors would not require preliminary bilateral mammography before biopsy.

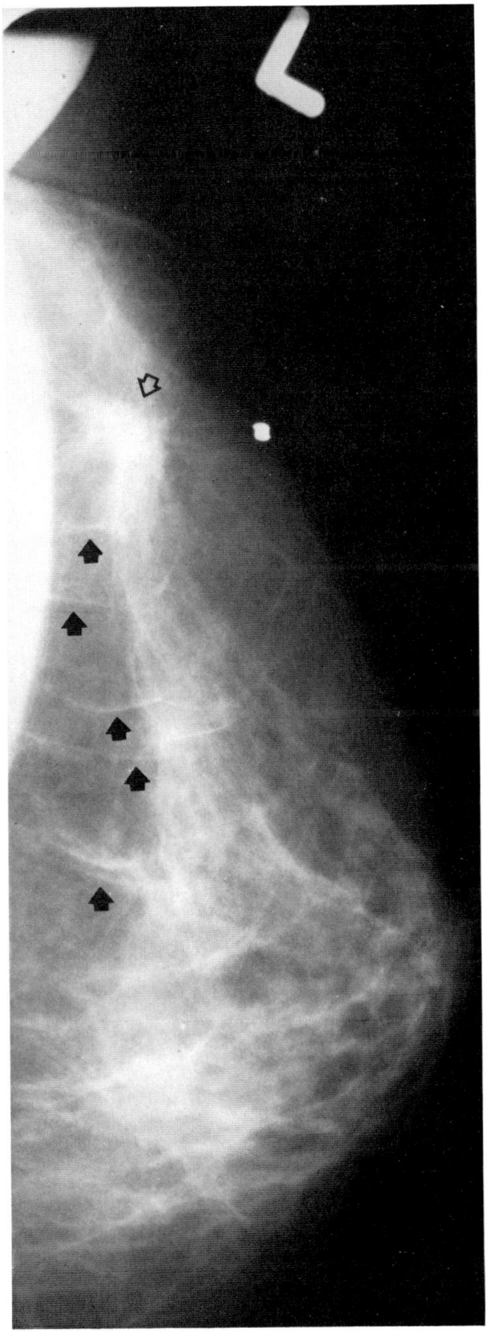

Figure 12-14 Ripple arrangement of trabeculae (black arrows): 1.5-cm palpable duct cell carcinoma (clear arrow).

8 preoperative planning (selection of procedure, approach to biopsy, estimation of operating time).

PERTINENT STATISTICS

In a series of 636 breast cancers seen between January 1974 and June 1976, we reported a 95.3 percent accuracy in the detection of malignancy by mammography.[22] Comparable figures were noted elsewhere and this appeared to be the state of the art.

In the years that followed, there was an increasing awareness that survival statistics did not reflect to any major degree the advantages of this achievement. Our orientation therefore changed to a preoccupation with premalignancy and in situ cancers (Fig. 12-7A), as well as minimally invasive lesions (Fig. 12-17).

In the BCDDP series of 1973 to 1981 involving 270,000 patients, cancer data showed 506 malignant lesions of less than 1 cm in which mammography alone detected 65 percent, mammography and physical examination 30 percent, and physical examination alone 3 percent. In the Jefferson Breast Cancer Screening Project, attention focused on the fact that among cancers measuring less than 0.5 cm, one-half of these had already reached the stage of invasion.[4] It is understandable then that at 1 cm, which represents 8 times the volume of 0.5-cm cancer, 95 percent were already invasive. Survival in minimally invasive cancer, however, has been reported as high as 98 percent at 5 years, 95 percent at 10 years,[21] and 93 percent at 20 years.[3]

Male Breast In the male breast, the main differential lies between gynecomastia and malignancy. Bilaterality favors gynecomastia as does drug intake in adults such as aldactone, phenothiazines, diuretics, digitalis, propranolol, cortisone, and of course hormonal therapy for prostatic cancer. Normally there is no glandular element behind the male nipple.

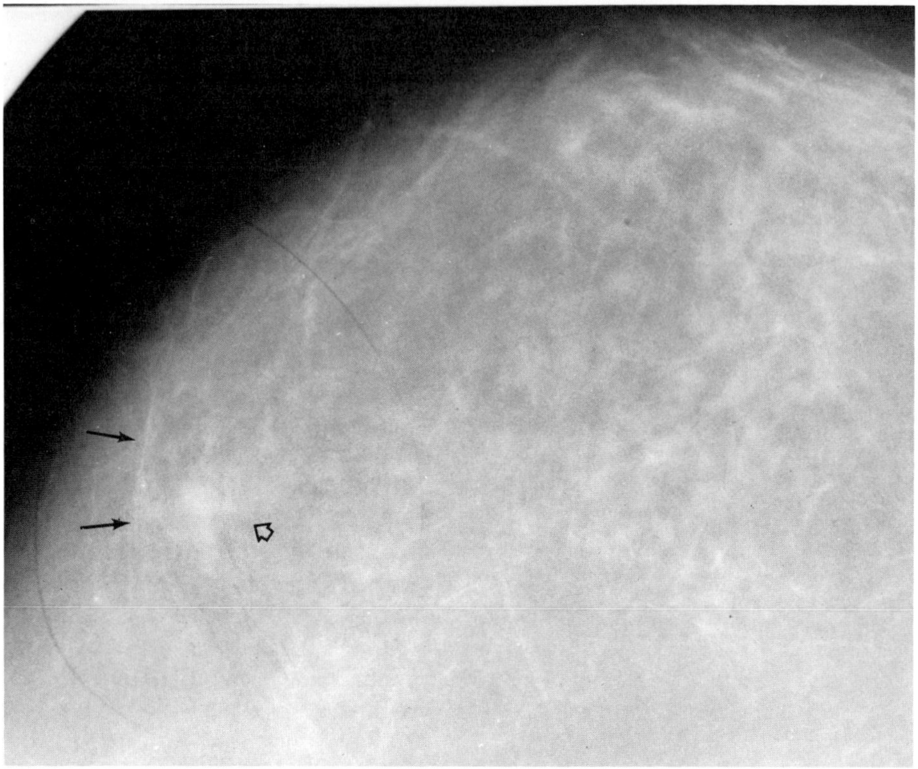

Figure 12-15 Nonpalpable duct cell carcinoma, 5-mm (clear arrow). Stiffened, straightened sentinel trabeculum nearby (long arrow). Note disappearance of glandular elements between lesion and nipple.

An arborizing or nodular density appears in gynecomastia. Benign tumors of the male breast are rarely encountered and appear much as in the female. Malignant tumors occur with a comparative frequency of 1:100 female breast malignancies.

The appearance of carcinoma here is quite similar to its counterpart in the female. A stiffened duct proceeding from the mass may be the earliest sign (Fig. 12-18). Spontaneous bleeding from the nipple is almost invariably due to carcinoma. In our personal experience the mass is most often central rather than eccentric to the nipple, but this differs from the more widespread experiences elsewhere.

SUMMARY

While the focus of this chapter has been the advantages that recent developments in mammography have provided in the earlier diagnosis of malignancy, it would be wrong to overlook the importance of educated palpation. In lesions over 1 cm in size, physical examination in conjunction with mammography, and at times alone, can play a significant part in the diagnosis. The clinician who is well-informed about premalignant dysplasias is sensitized to slight irregularities in palpation and is alerted to the need for some additional tool—in this instance mammography—to complete his or her evaluation.

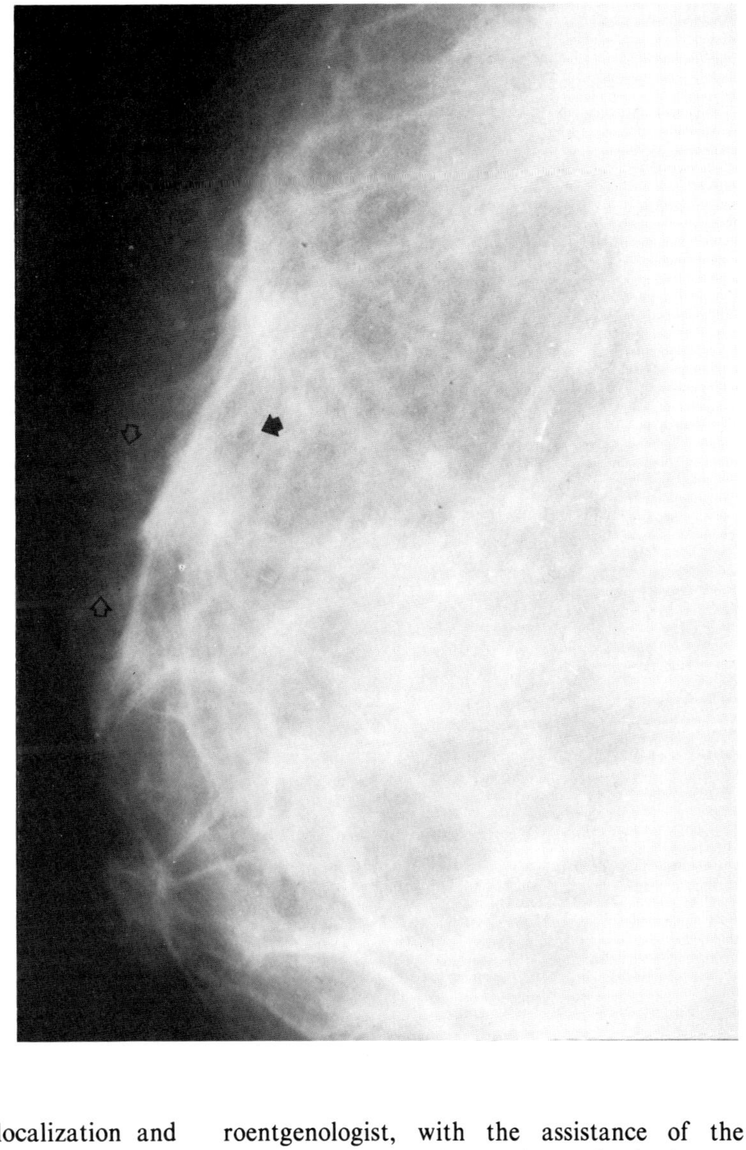

Figure 12-16 Neovascularity. Note cluster of tiny vessels in relatively clear subcutaneous area (clear arrows) adjacent to 1-cm carcinoma (black arrow). Nonpalpable. Photographic enlargement.

With the aid of adequate localization and specimen radiography, the special contributions of the surgeon and the pathologist have been applied to the most deserving areas. Portions of the breast beyond their area of clinical concern, as well as areas in the opposite breast, have been directed advantageously to their otherwise more limited attention.

The criteria for malignant change are continuing to unfold in mammography, and the roentgenologist, with the assistance of the pathologist, is pursuing the hyperplastic changes that seem to give rise to many of the atypias and metaplasias. It would seem unwise, therefore, to assume that mammography has reached the full dimensions of its ability to contribute to the management of breast disease. The dramatic reduction in radiation dosage, the more relaxed guidelines for mammography, the improvement in equipment, and the drift toward

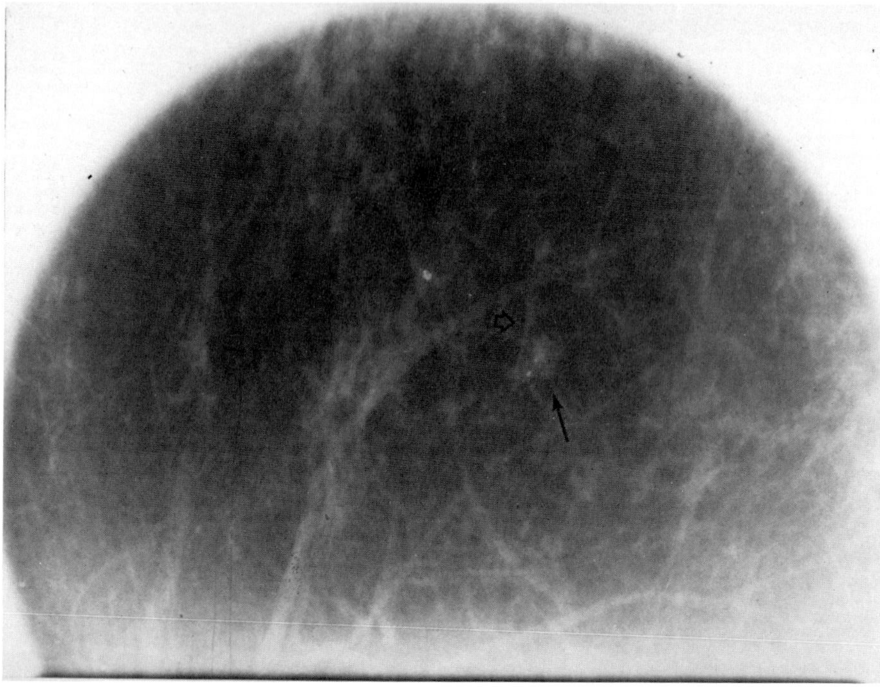

Figure 12-17 A 4-mm lesion (long arrow). Poor margination, calcification. Stiffened trabeculum nearby (clear arrow). Microinvasive duct carcinoma.

specialization in this area of roentgenology continue to favor earlier recognition of breast malignancy and reassessment of its impact on survival.

REFERENCES

1. Black MM, Kwon S: Precancerous mastopathy: Structural and biological considerations. *Path Res Pract* 166:491, 1980.
2. Egan RL: Experience with mammography in a tumor institution. *Radiology* 75:894, 1960.
3. Frazier TG, Copeland EM, Gallager HS, Paulus DD, White EC: Prognosis and treatment in minimal breast cancer. *Am J Surg* 133:697, 1977.
4. Feig SA: Mammographic screening: Benefit and risk, in Feig SA, McLelland R (eds): *Breast Carcinoma.* ACR Chicago, Il., Masson Publishing USA, p.351.
5. Goldberg RP, Hall FM, Simon M: Preoperative localization of non-palpable breast lesions using a wire marker and perforated mammographic grid. *Radiology* 146:833, 1983.
6. Gros M: *Les Maladies du Sein.* Paris, Masson, 1963.
7. Hoeffken WM Lanyi: *Mammography.* Stuttgart, Thieme, 1977.
8. Hutter RVP, Foote FW: Lobular carcinoma in situ: Long term follow-up. *Cancer* 241:1081, 1969.
9. Ingelby H, Gershon-Cohen J: *Comparative Anatomy, Pathology and Roentgenology of the Breast.* Philadelphia, University of Pennsylvania Press, 1960.
10. Lattes R: Lobular neoplasia (lobular carcinoma in situ) of the breast—a histologic entity of controversial clinical significance. *Pathol Res Pract* 166:415, 1980.
11. Leborgne RA: *The Breast in Roentgen Diagnosis.* Montevideo, Impresora Uruguaya, 1953.

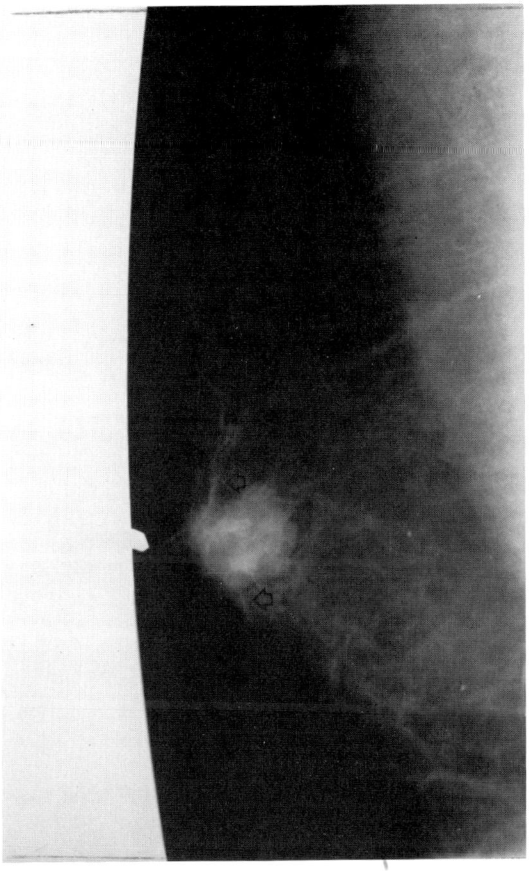

Figure 12-18 Male carcinoma. Note stiffened ducts (clear arrows).

12. Leis HP Jr: Diagnosis of breast cancer: Clinical and pre-clinical. *Compr Therapy* 5:611, November 1979.

13. Logan WW: Screen/film mammography: Technique, in Feig SA, McLelland R (eds): *Breast Carcinoma.* American College of Radiology, Chicago, Il., Masson Publishing USA, 1983, p.141.

14. Marchant DJ: Physical examination and breast self-examination, in Feig SA, McLelland R (eds): *Breast Carcinoma.* 1983, p. 371.

15. Moskowitz M, Gartside PS: Evidence of breast cancer mortality reduction: Aggressive screening in women under age 50. *Am J Roentgen* 138:911, 1982.

16. Ostrum BJ, Becker W, Isard HS: Low-dose mammography. *Radiology* 109:323, 1973.

17. Roses DF, Harris M, Gorstein F: Biopsy for microcalcification detected by mammography. *Surgery* 87:248, 1980.

18. Schecter S, Zuckerman HC: Controversies in mammography. *Cancer Investigation.* 2(2):125, 1984.

19. Tabar/Dean: *Teaching Atlas of Mammography.* New York, Thieme, 1983.

20 Urban JA: Bilaterality of cancer of the breast: Biopsy of the opposite breast. *Cancer* 20:1867, 1967.

21. Wanebo JH, Huvos AG, Urban JA: Treatment of minimal breast cancer. *Cancer* 33:349, 1974.

22. Zuckerman HC: Mammography in diseases of the breast, in Gallager HS, Leis HP Jr, Snyderman RK, Urban JA (eds): *The Breast.* St. Louis, C.V. Mosby, 1979, p. 98.

23. Zuckerman HC: Mammography in the diagnosis of cancer of the breast, Ariel I (ed): *Progress in Clinical Cancer.* New York, Grune and Stratton, 1965, p. 185.

13

Imaging Systems Other than Mammography

Rita F. Girolamo, M.D.

INTRODUCTION

Many methods are available for studying the breast with the goal of approaching the same or better accuracy than x-ray mammography without the disadvantage of ionizing radiation. At the present time the estimated 115,000 carcinomas of the breast diagnosed in 1984 will have been detected in the majority of cases by the patient herself or the examining physician.[1] Other diagnostic techniques consist basically of two types, those that are relatively simple and can be adjuncts to the physical examination, and those procedures with sophisticated, elaborate equipment that require time-consuming studies for the patient and staff. The successful use of x-ray mammography and diagnosis of early-stage cancer was thwarted in 1976 by the Bailer and BEIR reports on the potential of x-ray carcinogenesis.[2,3] This stimulated much interest in the application of other imaging systems which to date have not approached the overall usefulness of x-ray mammography (Table 13-1).

ULTRASOUND

The discipline of ultrasound has grown rapidly since 1951 when Wild and Neal first demonstrated its ability to visualize breast neoplasms by using an A-mode technique.[4] This was the original and simplest method in which the transducer is held in contact with the skin and the amplitude characteristics determine the attenuation values in relationship to the lesion. The problems of immobilization of the breast and coupling of the ultrasound signal to the skin was solved by these researchers in 1954 with the development of a water-filled chamber for the breast. For the next decade this contact scanning technique clearly demonstrated its value in differential diagnosis of cyst from solid mass. Subsequently, specially designed water path tomographic scanners were able to scan the entire

Table 13-1 Chronology of Diagnostic Tests Other than X-Ray Mammography

B.C.	Physicians' fingers
1929	Transillumination[14]
1954	Ultrasonography[4]
1956	Thermography[22]
1969	Tumor-selective radioisotopes
1972	Film diaphanography[15]
1972	Computed tomography
1980	Videodiaphanography–light scanning
1983	Magnetic resonance imaging

breast, which made it possible to correlate ultrasound patterns with histologic findings. Up to the present time, however, the great majority of clinical investigations has been made with B-mode scanning equipment. In this technique, one or more transducers scan the plane to be imaged. The development of gray scale B-mode ultrasonography made it possible to demonstrate echoes of varying strengths with the result that the characteristic internal structure of the breast could be visualized.[5,6] The addition of a multiple transducer technique can provide more complete architectural information.

In Japan, investigators studied ultrasound characteristics and established criteria for differential diagnosis of benign and malignant breast masses. The internal echo content of mass lesions was evaluated by amplitude and distribution, the shape of a lesion's boundaries, and comparison of the echoes posterior to the lesion relative to the adjacent tissue. Using higher frequency transducers, approximately 5 MHz, the dedicated ultrasound equipment can achieve resolution of 2 mm. Static semiautomated and fully automated ultrasound scanners can be used to evaluate parenchymal patterns and internal composition of palpable breast masses (Figs. 13-1 A and B).

Cole-Beuglet et al. described the following criteria for malignant lesions in a series of 104 proven cases of primary breast carcinoma[7]: (1) a solid mass with irregular margins, weak, nonuniformly distributed internal echoes, and great acoustic attenuation; and (2) an alteration in breast architecture manifested as either thickened or retracted Cooper ligaments, or areas of great acoustic attenuation. In the review by Jellins et al. of 1660 ultrasounds using B-scan examination and water path technique, the overall sensitivity was x-ray mammography, 82 percent; ultrasound, 78 percent; and clinical examination, 80 percent.[8] Other investigators reported an ultrasound sensitivity of 71 percent[9] and 58 percent.[10] In Sickles' prospective study of 1000 patients, ultrasound detected only 30 percent of the nonpalpable cancers and 8 percent of lesions smaller than 1 cm. Ultrasound is the procedure of choice in distinguishing a cyst from a solid mass.

The clinical usefulness of ultrasonography of the breast is significantly increased when used in conjunction with physical examination and mammography. The technologic limits of the diagnosis of small carcinomas, microcalcifications, and altered architecture still remain. At the present time its role as a *screening* tool is not documented. It is a time-consuming procedure to visualize the entire breast with dedicated, sophisticated equipment which is very expensive. It may have a preferable role in evaluating younger women as the initial diagnostic test since it is a nonionizing study.[11]

Two other ultrasonic techniques which may improve the overall accuracy of interpretation and diagnosis are currently being investigated. Doppler ultrasound techniques have been used for over 20 years in cerebral vascular and peripheral vascular areas. A characteristic Doppler signal in breast carcinoma has been described by Wells et al.[12] and this has helped to distinguish benign from malignant palpable masses. More sophisticated analyses are being investigated to identify the major supply vessel to a tumor. Schreiman et al. have reported on their preliminary clinical study of ultrasound transmission computed tomography of the breast, a technique based on the speed

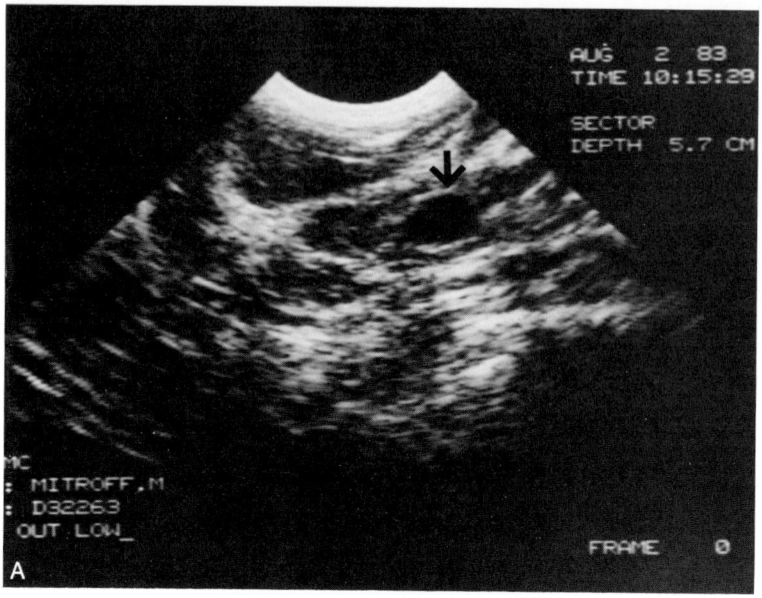

Figure 13-1 A. Fifty-two-year-old premenopausal, high-risk patient with nonpalpable mass in a relatively atrophic breast. Real-time ultrasound clearly identifies a typical cyst (arrow).

of sound wave transmission as well as the attenuation of the waves.[13]

TRANSILLUMINATION

Transillumination of the breast was first described by Cutler in 1929 as a simple method of differentiating cyst from solid mass.[14] It has progressed from the pocket flashlight to the present sophisticated, computerized equipment for breast evaluation. These transillumination systems depend upon detection of light transmitted through the breast using an optimum wavelength from 400 to 1200 nm. Numerous terms are used in the literature to describe transillumination of the breast—diaphanoscopy, diaphanography, videodiaphanography, telediaphanography, and light scanning.

The basic instrumentation consists of a light source and a detector system. The light source is a fiberoptic rod with a slight upward curve and a variable-intensity light. Early diagnosis was based on visual analysis of yellow, red, brown, to black colors transmitted through the breast. The need for a permanent record stimulated the development of the two currently available detector systems. Film diaphanography uses infrared film in a 35-mm single reflex camera which records the visible transmitted light in color.[15] Videodiaphanography views the transilluminated breast on a video monitor and can produce a hard copy on film, or it processes the analog image to digital for storage and/or image processing.[16]

The patient is examined in a semidarkened room with the light source under the breast as the physician palpates and compresses the breast to assure entire visualization to the chest wall. The criteria evaluated are (1) symmetry in overall transillumination of both breasts, (2) detection of focal areas of decreased or increased transillumination, and (3) the vascular

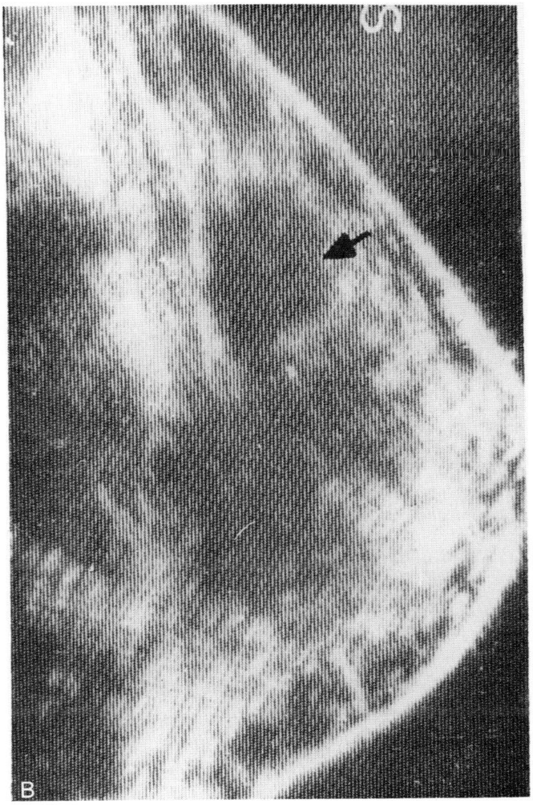

Figure 13-1 B. Forty-four-year-old patient with a palpable mass. Water-path-automated–ultrasound scanner demonstrated the mass (arrow) showing characteristics of a malignancy.

pattern of the superficial veins (Fig. 13-2). The ratio of fibroglandular to adipose tissue determines the amount of light absorbed. Cysts are visualized as discrete, round areas of increased transillumination. Gradations of decreased transillumination of focal areas are noted in benign masses, such as fibroadenomas and papillomas. Poorly defined areas of markedly decreased transillumination are characteristic of malignancy. Modification of the video systems permitting quantitation and transmission of two different wavelength bands can provide important information about differences in tissue characteristics of the breast. One of the major limitations of both the film and video techniques is resolution, which is inherent in light physics. It is difficult to identify deepseated lesions, even with multiple projections. The experience of the observer is another factor in the accuracy of the examination.

Scattered reports using film diaphanography have appeared in the literature since 1977, which indicate wide variation in sensitivity and specificity.* Lesions as small as 6 mm have been reported. The three double-blind studies reported to date have used video light scanning. In 250 asymptomatic women, Brown and Schipper found a specificity of 0.88 for transillumination and 0.62 for mammography. Sensitivity of both modalities was 0.93.[17] Marshall et al. report a series of 1000 patients in whom 29 of the proven 34 carcinomas were diagnosed by mammography. Experienced interpreters of the transillumination video tapes detected 32 carcinomas, whereas interpreters with less than 4 months' experience identified only 26.[18] In a comparison of mammography, ultrasound, and transillumination of 511 women, 23 cancers were diagnosed.[19] Fifteen were by mammography and 16 by transillumination. Twenty-seven percent were not palpable. In a current series of over 1500 cases, there is an equal sensitivity of 0.80 for both modalities in 55 proven cancers. The smallest lesion detected was 5 mm. Carlsen has reported on the largest series of 3293.[20] In 78 carcinomas he demonstrated a sensitivity of 0.92 for light scanning, 0.82 for mammography, and 0.78 for ultrasound.

From the available data, it would seem that transillumination may be approaching the diagnostic accuracy of mammography as the refinements of equipment overcome the problems

*The sensitivity of a test refers to its ability to detect an abnormality; the specificity of a test refers to its ability to separate correctly benign from malignant abnormalities. The more sensitive a test is, the fewer false-negatives there will be; the more specific a test is, the fewer false-positives there will be.

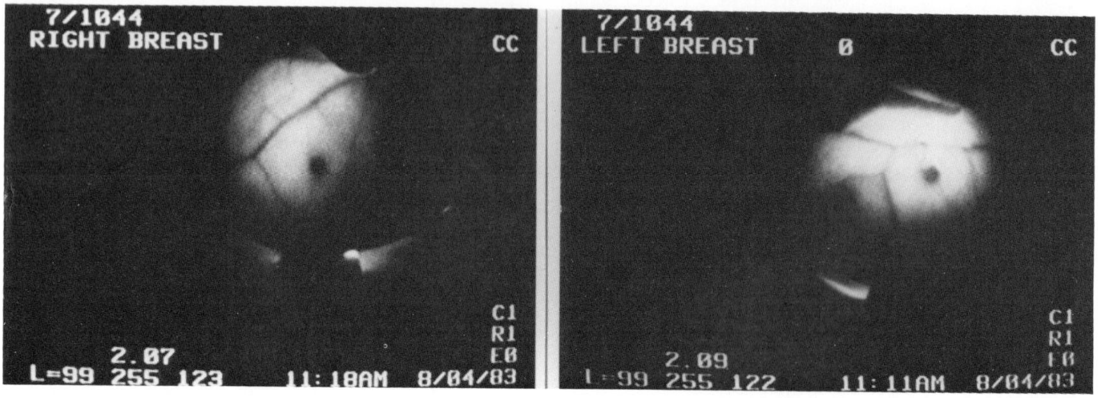

Figure 13-2 Videodiaphanograms of a 37-year-old patient. Asymmetric decrease in transillumination of the lower inner quadrant of the left breast as compared to the right. Xeroradiograms demonstrated a grouping of occult calcifications confirmed on biopsy as carcinoma.

of light scatter and transmission. The detection of microcalcifications has not been addressed in the literature. Transillumination of the breast is currently used as an adjunct to physical examination and mammography. It is helpful in the clinically and mammographically problem breast as another parameter to be used as a baseline follow-up which is nonionizing. At this stage there is no scientific documentation to indicate that it can be used as a screening method.[21]

THERMOGRAPHY

Thermography is a noninvasive, nonionizing technique of measuring the temperature of the breast. In 1956 Lawson was the first to report that the temperature of the breast is elevated in the region of a breast cancer.[22] The temperature changes can be detected by two different techniques: infrared scanning detectors (telethermography) or cholesteric crystals (contact plate thermography).[23,24] Cholesteric crystals are color–temperature sensitive and are encapsulated in the contact plates to produce a color range of red for low temperature through the visual spectrum to blue-violet for high temperatures. Polaroid prints are used for permanent record. Using infrared telethermography, the patient is scanned in front of the detector which then transduces the radiant infrared energy (3 to 14 nm) into an electric signal for display on a cathode ray tube. The data can then be photographed for permanent record in black and white or color and quantitized by computer.

This simple examination is conducted in an ambient temperature of 20°C after cooling for 15 min. Under these conditions, the surface of the breast is about 30°C. Thermograms are analyzed according to vascular or graphic patterns and thermal patterns.[25] Criteria established are (1) vascular symmetry, (2) a localized area of abnormal vascularity, (3) a localized area of temperature increase greater than 1.5°C, (4) a generalized temperature increase of one breast, and (5) a unilateral increase in temperature of one areola greater than 2°C (Fig. 13-3). A modification of this technique, called "graphic stress telethermometry," has been developed which records the thermographic change produced by immersing the patient's hands in ice water. The principle is based on the lack of normal physiologic vasoconstriction in areas of breast cancer.[26]

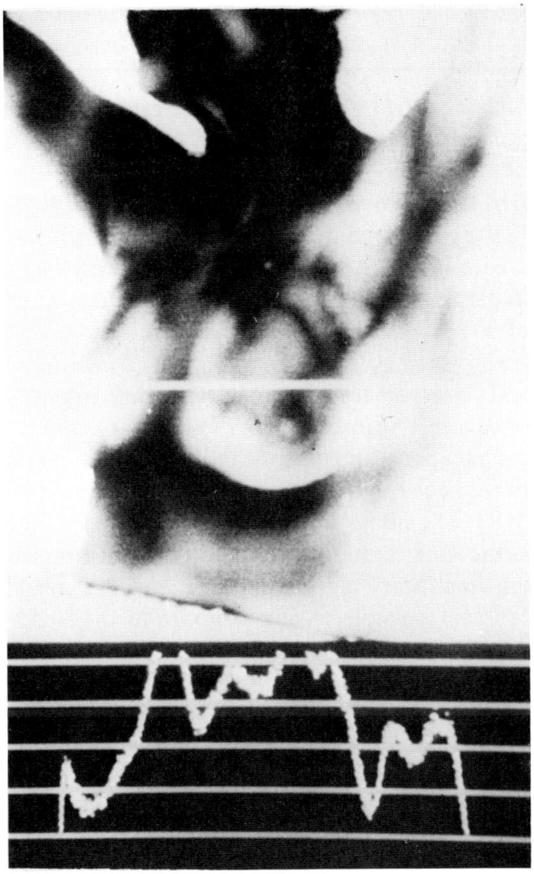

Figure 13-3 Telethermogram of a 57-year-old patient with a dominant area clinically and mammographically in the upper outer quadrant of the left breast. Sitting oblique thermogram demonstrates asymmetric abnormal vessels and increased areolar temperature. Pathologic diagnosis of intraductal carcinoma with positive nodes.

Thermography has both high false-positive and false-negative rates.[27] Cancer detection is more consistently positive with larger tumors (greater than 2 cm) and in rapidly growing tumors with doubling times under 150 days.[28] Experienced thermographers with long patient follow-up have reported that 12 to 20 percent of patients with a positive thermogram as the only abnormal finding have developed carcinoma. The prognosis of cancer patients with abnormal thermograms appears to be less favorable than those with normal studies. The degree of abnormality has been correlated with the predicted response to radiation therapy.[29] Approximately 20 percent of patients with benign disease have abnormal thermograms. Since thermal patterns are unique for each patient and remain unaltered for many years, this completely safe examination can be used at frequent intervals to monitor patients with benign disease and those at "high risk" for cancer. Any persistent abnormal changes would warrant further investigation.

At this time thermography cannot be considered as an effective independent screening technique due to its lack of sensitivity and specificity. In the Breast Cancer Detection Demonstration Project (BCDDP) sponsored by the American Cancer Society and the National Cancer Institute, thermography was discontinued as a screening device after 4 years. Further investigation and evaluation is warranted to assess its role as a useful adjunct to other diagnostic breast examinations and its potential as a risk marker.

COMPUTERIZED TOMOGRAPHIC MAMMOGRAPHY (CTM)

Although this diagnostic technique uses x-ray radiation, it is a specialized examination compared to conventional mammography. Specially designed equipment (General Electric CTM) for the breast using the water path technique is limited to two investigators, Chang and Gisvold.[30,31] In Chang's study of 179 patients, the CTM was superior to mammography for diagnosing cancer in dense parenchyma. His criterion for benign versus malignant is based on the change in density levels (over 25 CT numbers) after intravenous injection of iodinated contrast. This technique decreases false negatives to 5 percent; however, false positives are over 50 percent. Conventional body scanners have demonstrated similar data to that of the dedicated units.[32]

Computerized tomographic mammography may be of value in patients with indeterminate mammograms and dense breasts. It can differentiate soft tissue structures more easily than standard x-ray mammography. The major limitations of CTM are the high entrance dose, which is over 1 rad, and the unwarranted radiation of the entire chest. The limiting factor of thickness of the cross-sectional slice of 5 mm makes it impossible to demonstrate small lesions and calcifications which are of the magnitude of 200 μm. Other disadvantages are length of procedures, need for intravenous contrast medium, and the high cost. This is not a practical clinical diagnostic technique at the present and most unlikely as a screening technique.

MAGNETIC RESONANCE IMAGING

Nuclear magnetic resonance spectroscopy (MRI) has been used by scientists to study atomic and molecular structures since 1945. The application of this technique for tumor detection was introduced in 1971 by Damadian.[33] Since this noninvasive and nonhazardous method of imaging proton distribution (mainly water) on a small scale in animal and human tissues has been extended to the whole body, the terminology of magnetic resonance imaging has been adopted. The basic principle is that the hydrogen nuclei in the body tissues, which are predominately water, will, when immersed in a magnetic field, and then excited with a radio frequency field, absorb and then remit a portion of the energy with a signal that can be detected and analyzed. The spin lattice relaxation time (T_1) can be measured. Goldsmith et al. in 1978 were the first to report on its application to breast carcinoma.[34] They studied 119 breast specimens with a pulse proton magnetic resonance technique and analyzed two parameters of T_1 and T_2. They developed a malignancy index that gave a clear distinction between normal and malignant specimens. El Yousef et al. studied 10 normal volunteers and 45 patients and identified four distinct patterns in breast abnormalities[35]: (1) increased concentration of normal duct tissue with no change in relative signal intensity compatible with dysplasia, (2) tubular dilatation of ducts with relative decrease in signal intensity compatible with cystic hyperplasia, (3) localized oval or rounded areas of low signal intensity—a pattern compatible with cysts and fibroadenoma, and (4) distorted and disorganized area of low signal intensity compatible with carcinoma (Fig. 13-4). Microcalcifications and well-defined calcifications in benign conditions could not be demonstrated on MRI. The limitation of MRI at the present time is the long time of data acquisition with resulting respiratory motion that degrades the image. It is not possible to quantify size of the smallest lesion and the T_1 values for malignant and fibrocystic disease were found to overlap. The current state of the art and principles of MRI are well described by Pykett et al.[36] It would seem that MRI may be useful in identifying malignant versus benign disease. Since detection of early lesions and evaluation of lymph involvement are both important in management, MRI has special potential in preoperatively evaluating axillary lymph nodes with a noninvasive technique. Further studies are needed.

DIGITAL RADIOGRAPHY

Digital radiography utilizes high-efficiency x-ray detectors which can reduce x-ray doses well below that of film/screen and xeromammographic units, probably to the level of yearly background radiation. The photons reaching the detectors are digitized, entered in a computer, and processed into many formats. Pre- and post-contrast studies may enhance the detection of microcalcifications. Preliminary clinical studies have been presented of newly developed digital tomographic radiography which will permit

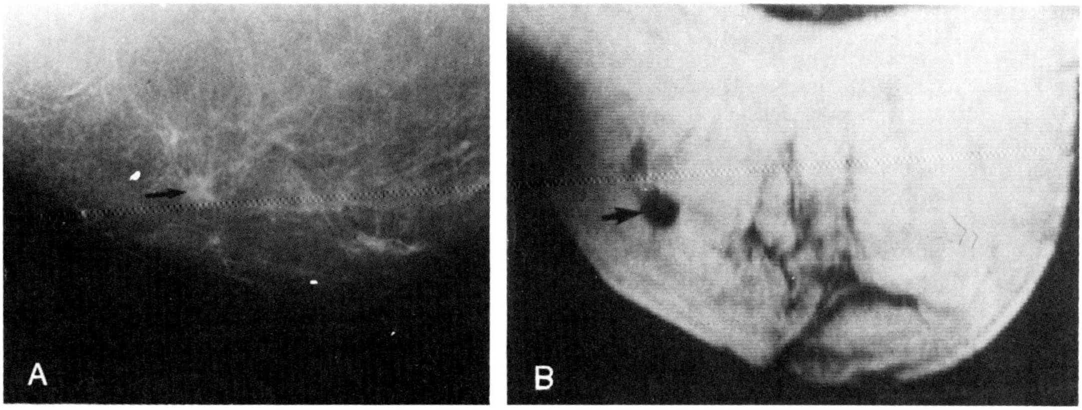

Figure 13-4 A. Film mammogram of a 57-year-old woman demonstrates a stellate mass (arrow) in outer quadrant of left breast, compatible with carcinoma. B. SE 0.03–0.25 sec image obtained with the surface coil demonstrates a small, ill-defined mass in the outer quadrant of the left breast (arrow), suggestive of carcinoma. The finding was confirmed by surgery (*from El Yousef*[35] *by permission of Radiology*).

reconstruction of images in multiple spatial planes with one x-ray exposure.

RADIONUCLIDE STUDIES

Radionuclide Imaging

Nuclear medicine has been a valuable diagnostic technique in the management of cancers since the 1950s as liver, brain, and bone scans have been used for the detection of metastases. Computerized tomography has completely replaced the brain scan, and CT scanning of the liver is more sensitive and specific than ultrasound or radionuclide scanning. Due to the expense and limited availability of CT, liver and spleen scans remain the choice for initial evaluation. Bone radionuclide scanning is definitely superior to plain x-ray films in detecting metastases. The lead time of about 3 months in a positive bone scan is not uncommon before the x-ray becomes abnormal. Lymph node scans using radioactive colloidal compounds for abdominal nodes have an accuracy of 80 to 90 percent.[37] This is a simple, reliable technique compared to the tedious, difficult study of invasive radiographic lymphangiography. More recently, ^{99m} technetium antimony sulfide colloid has been used to visualize the internal mammary lymph node chains. The radionuclide is injected into the posterior rectus sheath at the diaphragmatic insertion at the subcostal site.[38] Axillary lymph nodes can be detected after periareolar injection of the radionuclide. Detection of the lymph nodes by lymphoscintigraphy is useful in improving staging and as a guide for treatment of breast cancer and for possibly detecting metastases.

More advances in equipment and available radioisotopes are being investigated. The sensitivity of detection of liver metastases is significantly increased with the single-photon emission computerized tomogram (SPECT), which provides cross-sectional and three-dimensional imaging. The newer positron emission tomogram (PET) has several advantages over conventional gamma-emitting isotope techniques.[39] It has the ability to quantitate radioactivity in two dimensions, accurately image the biodistribution of positron emitters such as ^{11}C, ^{15}O, and ^{13}N, and can monitor the metabolism of tumors in vivo.

Tumor-Selective Radioisotopes

^{67}Gallium citrate screening has been utilized for tumor imaging since 1969.[40] It has been disappointing since not all tumors concentrate the radionuclide. Many other isotopes, such as ^{32}P, ^{42}K, ^{99m}Tc pertechnetate, and ^{111}In bleomycin, have been tried with little success. Many compounds are localized in breast tumors; however, more than one-third are in non-neoplastic lesions.

Radiolabeled antibodies specific for tumor-associated antigens have the greatest potential for imaging tumors. External scanning has been successful in tumor imaging using tagged antibodies specific for CEA, α-fetoprotein, human chorionic gonadotropin, kidney carcinoma antigen, and ferritin. Tumor-associated monoclonal antibodies tagged with ^{131}I and more recently ^{123}I have been successful in melanoma. Epenetos et al. reported on a survey of 20 patients studied with ^{123}I-tagged antibodies. Six patients with breast cancer had positive localization detected 3 to 15 h after injection.[41] Radiolabeled monoclonal antibodies may be practical in the future for radiation therapy as well as for diagnosis.

CONCLUSION

The imaging techniques that have been reviewed are predominately adjuncts and not replacements for physical examination and x-ray mammography. Ultrasound is the only technique that is more diagnostic than x-ray mammography in the diagnosis of cyst versus solid mass. The others require further evaluation to determine their efficacy in diagnosis and their role in early detection of breast cancer (Table 13-2). Moskowitz has written an excellent review on the evaluation of the rapidly increasing number of diagnostic imaging modalities.[42]

At present, ultrasound has accepted diagnostic applications and CT mammography probable value. Thermography and transillumination have been used for many years without any well-designed study to give a valid evaluation. The promising role of magnetic resonance imaging, digital radiography, Doppler ultrasound, and tumor-seeking radionuclides may provide reliable techniques to detect early breast cancer.

Table 13-2 Present Role of Breast Imaging

Accepted	X-ray mammography
	Ultrasonography (cyst vs solid mass)
Acceptable	Ultrasonography
	Computed tomography
To be determined	Transillumination
	Thermography
	Magnetic resonance imaging
Future	Digital radiography including tomography
	Tumor-selective radioisotopes—monoclonal antibodies

REFERENCES

1. *Cancer Facts and Figures.* New York, American Cancer Society, 1984.
2. Bailer JC III: Mammography. *Ann Int Med* 84:77, 1976.
3. *The Effects on Populations of Exposure to Low Levels of Ionizing Radiation:* 1980. Washington, D.C., National Academy Press, 1980.
4. Wild JJ, Neal D: Further pilot echographic studies of the histologic structure of tumors of the living intact human breast. *Lancet* 1:655, 1951.
5. Jellins J, Kossoff G, Reeve TS: Ultrasonic visualization of the breast. *Med J Aust* 1:305, 1971.
6. Rubin C, Kirtz AB, Goldberg BB: Ultrasonic mammographic parenchymal patterns. A preliminary report. *Radiology* 130:515, 1979.
7. Cole-Beuglet C, Soriano RZ, Kurtz AB, Goldberg BB: Ultrasound analysis of 104 primary breast carcinomas classified according to histopathologic type. *Radiology* 147:191, 1983.
8. Jellins J, Reeve T, Croll J, Kossoff G: Results of breast echographic examinations in Sydney, Australia, 1972–1979. *Semin in Ultrasound* III:58, 1982.

9. Fleischer AC, Muhletaler CA, Reynolds VH, Machin JE, Thieme GA, Bundy AL, Winfield AC, James, Jr AE: Palpable breast masses: Evaluation by high frequency, hand-held real-time sonography and xeromammography. *Radiology* 148:813, 1983.
10. Sickles EA, Filly RA, Callen PW: Breast cancer detection with sonography and mammography: Comparison using state-of-the-art equipment. *AJR* 140:1405, 1983.
11. Egan RL, McSweeney MB, Murphy FB: Breast sonography and the detection of cancer. *Recent Results Cancer Res* 90:90, 1984.
12. Wells PNT, Hallwell M, Skidmore R, Webb AJ, Woodcock JP: Tumor detection by ultrasonic Doppler blood flow signals. *Ultrasonics* 15:231, 1977.
13. Schreiman JS, Gisvold JJ, Greenleaf JF, Bahn RC: Ultrasound transmission computed tomography of the breast. *Radiology* 150:523, 1984.
14. Culter M: Transillumination as an aid in the diagnosis of breast lesions. *Surg Gynecol Obstet* 48:721, 1929.
15. Gros C, Quennville Y, Hummel Y: Diaphanologie mammaire. *J Radiol Electrol* 53:297, 1972.
16. Carlsen E, Transillumination light scanning. *Diagnostic Imaging* 4:28, 1982.
17. Brown R, Schipper H: Electronic diaphanography as an adjunct to the early diagnosis of breast cancer. Presentation at 13th International Cancer Congress, Seattle, Washington, September 1982.
18. Marshal V, Williams D, Smith K: Light scanning: Evaluation of a new modality to screen for breast cancer. Presentation at Radiological Society of North America, 1982.
19. Merritt C, Sullivan M, McKinnon W, Segaloff A: Comparative evaluation of ultrasound, transillumination light scanning and x-ray mammography in benign and malignant disease of the breast. Presentation at Radiological Society of North America, 1982.
20. Carlsen E: Transillumination light scanning. *Diagnostic Imaging* 4:28, 1982.
21. Girolamo RF, Gaythorpe JM: Clinical diaphanography, its present perspective. *CRC Crit Rev Onc/Hem* 2(1):1, 1984.
22. Lawson R: Implications of surface temperatures in the diagnosis of breast cancers. *Can Med Assoc J* 75:309, 1956.
23. Gershon-Cohen J, Berger SM, Haberman JAD, Barnes RB: Thermography of the breast. *AJR* 91:919, 1964.
24. Davison TW, Ewing KL, Ferguson J, Chapman M, Can A, Voorhis CC: Detection of breast cancer by liquid crystal thermography. A preliminary report. *Cancer* 29:1123, 1972.
25. Isard HJ: Breast disease and correlation of images; mammography, thermography, diaphanography. *Proc Clin Biol Res* 107:321, 1982.
26. Gautherie M: Thermopathology of breast cancer: Measurement and analysis of in vivo temperature and blood flow. *Ann NY Acad Sci* 365:383, 1980.
27. Amalric R, Branderne H, Altschuler C: Dynamic telethermography of 2,200 breast cancers. *Acta Thermogr* 3:46, 1978.
28. Fournier VD, Kubli F, Klapp J, Weber E, Schneider-Affeld F: Infra-red thermography and breast cancer doubling time. *Acta Thermogr* 3:107, 1978.
29. Gautherie M, Gros CM: Breast thermography and cancer risk prediction. *Cancer* 45:51, 1980.
30. Chang DHJ, Sibale JL, Gallagher JH: Computed tomography of the breast, a preliminary report. *Radiology* 124:827, 1977.
31. Gisvold JS, Reese DF, Kassell PR: Computed tomographic mammography (CTM). *AJR* 133:1143, 1979.
32. Chang CHJ, Nesbit DE, Fisher DR: Computed tomographic mammography using a conventional body scanner. *AJR* 138:553, 1982.
33. Damadian R: Tumor detection by nuclear magnetic resonance. *Science* 171:1151, 1971.
34. Goldsmith M, Koutcher JA, Damadian R: NMR in cancer, XIII: Application of the NMR malignancy index to human mammary tumors. *Br J Cancer* 38:157, 1978.
35. El Yousef SF, Duchesneau RH, Alfidi RJ, Haaga JR, Bryan PJ, LiPuma JP: Magnetic resonance imaging of the breast. *Radiology* 150:761, 1984.
36. Pykett IL, Newhouse JH, Buonanno FS, Brady TJ, Goldman MF, Kistler JP, Pohost GM: Principle of nuclear magnetic resonance imaging. *Radiology* 143:157, 1982.
37. Costellino RA, Fuks Z, Blank N: Roentgenologic aspects of Hodgkin's disease; repeat lymphography. *Radiology* 109:53, 1973.

38. Ege GN: Lymphoscintigraphy-techniques and application in the management of breast carcinoma. *Semin Nucl Med* XIII(1):26, 1983.
39. Ell PJ, Khan O: Emission computerized tomography: Clinical applications. *Semin Nucl Med* XI:50, 1981.
40. Edwards CL, Hayes RL: Tumor scanning with ^{67}Ga citrate. *J Nucl Med* 10:103, 1969.
41. Epenetos AA, Britton KE, Mather J: Targeting of Iodine-123-labeled tumor associated monoclonal antibodies to ovarian, breast and gastro-intestinal tumors. *Lancet* 2:999, 1982.
42. Moskowitz M, Feig SA, Cole-Beuglet C: Evaluation of new imaging procedures for breast cancer, AJR 140:591, 1983.

14

Biologic Markers

T. Phillip Waalkes, M.D., Ph.D.
Joel H. Shaper, Ph.D.
Martin D. Abeloff, M.D.

INTRODUCTION

Several reviews of biologic markers (biomarkers) for breast cancer have recently been published. [1-4] No attempt will be made to cover the entire subject in this chapter, but specific areas regarding biomarkers will be briefly reviewed, including problems in the interpretation of results, the use of combinations of biomarkers, and the analysis of biomarkers in tumor tissue. The application and possible clinical utility of a biomarker will be demonstrated using carcinoembryonic antigen (CEA) as the example (Table 14-1). Finally, the potential for developing more specific biomarkers for breast cancer through the application of monoclonal antibody technology will be reviewed.

Despite modern instrumentation and radiological scanning techniques to detect or measure a tumor mass, more practical and sensitive laboratory methods are needed to detect the presence of any neoplasm and provide a quantitative estimate of changes associated with growth or dissemination, or response to therapy.

A *biomarker* may be simply defined as a material found in increased amounts in the body fluids of patients with cancer. An ideal biomarker would have both specificity and sensitivity, with a positive role in detection, diagnosis, staging, and for monitoring tumor volume changes in patients during the course of their illness. To date, no biomarker, unique or specific to breast carcinoma, has been found. At present, all nonspecific biomarkers relevant to breast carcinoma also lack the required sensitivity to identify a small, localized mammary tumor or to show when only micrometastases are present. Numerous studies demonstrate that these latter nonspecific biomarkers are normal constituents of body fluids, which for obscure reasons are abnormally elevated as a result of the neoplastic state.

Table 14-1 CEA Levels Over Normal Range—Number of Patients/Total (%)

		Stage at primary surgery nodal status		
Reference	Operable	N^-	N^+	Metastatic
Disease				
8	80/333 (24%)			
8		68/451 (15%)	102/403 (25%)	
17				1011/1714 (59%)*

*Range for metastatic disease, from 34% reported by Haagensen et al.[30] using, however, 10 ng/mL as a discriminant by the CEA-Roche method to 100%.

PROBLEMS IN THE INTERPRETATION OF BIOMARKER RESULTS

The perplexing problem with the biomarkers available for breast carcinoma is the lack of elevated levels in all patients, even in those with advanced, disseminated disease. This variability tends to emphasize that although all breast neoplasms have certain characteristics in common, their expression may differ both qualitatively and quantitatively. At times, apparent discordant results can occur which appear contrary to clinical evidence. The lack of sensitivity and specificity and on occasion the lack of correlation of results with measurable tumor changes have been major disappointments in the field of biomarker research. In clinical application such results can cause obvious problems in interpretation, and caution may be necessary in interpreting biomarker data. An understanding of some of the problems, and the circumstances under which they may occur, is helpful in the clinical evaluation of biomarkers. Much has been learned regarding the behavior of biomarkers through the study of carcinoembryonic antigen (CEA) in breast carcinoma as well as in other neoplastic diseases.

Low Levels

Lack of specificity causes very real difficulties. Thus, all biomarkers now under investigation have a range of values which constitutes normal variation. Levels which are just above this normal range may be due to the tumor or simply be caused by analytical variability or error. Appropriate quality control and precision studies are needed to know the reproducibility and variation of the analytical method. A repeat analysis and/or serial samples at intervals will help to evaluate whether an elevation may be secondary to progressive tumor growth. When immunologic methods for oncofetal proteins are used, normally occurring cross-reacting materials can cause spurious elevated levels, e.g., CEA. Diseases other than cancer may or may not cause a rise in level and for CEA, heavy cigarette smoking must be considered a factor when such an elevation occurs.

Lack of Synthesis

On occasion, actual levels of a biomarker measured in the tumor and in the normal tissue of origin may be the same, suggesting that the tumor cells do not synthesize the material in abnormal amounts.[5] Thus, tissue analysis of the primary tumor could be helpful prior to the contemplated use of a specific biomarker in patients. For some patients, the primary tumor may produce the marker but metastatic lesions may not.[6,7]

Lack of Transfer to the Systemic Circulation

Although a biomarker may be found in abnormally elevated amounts in tumor tissue, the level in the blood of the same patient may fall within the normal limits, suggesting a lack of transfer from tumor tissue to the systemic circulation.[8]

Effect of Surgery Immediate postsurgical levels of a biomarker are frequently elevated. The duration of this elevation varies depending in part on the nature of the biochemical material and, apparently, on the extent of the surgical procedure. For some markers the period of elevation may be prolonged beyond that anticipated by simple excretion studies. In evaluating a breast cancer patient postoperatively for evidence of residual disease using a marker level, it is important to repeat such measurements at intervals to determine the true level after surgery.

Effect of Chemotherapy CEA levels may rise after the initial course of antitumor drugs for patients with small-cell carcinoma of the lung,[9] and remain elevated at least 1 to 2 months afterward despite clinical evidence of tumor response to therapy. For other biomarkers[10] this elevation may even last several months during repeated 28-day courses of the drugs before falling. Preliminary evidence suggests this occurs on occasion but only for those patients whose pretreatment levels are within the normal range or only slightly elevated. The reasons for this discordant result with a transient rise in level is not clear but several factors may be in effect, including lysis of tumor cells as a consequence of treatment, change in the kinetic behavior of the tumor due to the chemotherapy, or simply variation in and near the normal range. Other investigators have noted similar changes in biomarker levels , e.g., CEA, for patients with breast carcinoma when undergoing chemotherapy.[11,12]

In the remainder of this chapter we will concentrate on research areas of biomarkers for breast cancer. In doing so, stages in the progression of breast carcinoma will be considered, periods where available data, though limited, may suggest biomarkers could have a potential role in the total management of patients. Representative results using CEA will be cited.

COMBINATIONS OF BIOMARKERS

Many investigators have turned to the study of combinations of biomarkers because of the lack of a single specific and sensitive biomarker for breast carcinoma. Most such combinations were initially considered on the basis of their ability to select out a majority of patients with advanced disease. Summary data from various studies in which from three to ten biomarkers in combination were measured in the same patients with advanced metastatic disease indicated that one or more biomarkers may be elevated 75 to 100 percent of the time. Obvious overlap between biomarkers occurs, but in all such combinations, each individual biomarker was exclusively elevated in only a small percentage of the patients. Not uncommonly, at least for some markers the degree of elevation above the normal range was low and consequently could compromise potential clinical use. In such instances the elevation of multiple markers measured in the same sample might provide a greater element of confidence.

Carcinoembryonic antigen has been one of the biomarkers included in all multiple marker (combination) studies. Under the condition of the trials, i.e., frequency of elevation for patients with advanced breast carcinoma, CEA has been equal or superior to other markers, although the extent to which most other candidates have been studied has been limited. Carcinoembryonic antigen, despite inherent failings, remains a biomarker which must be included when any consideration is given to using multiple biomarkers in breast carcinoma. The normal range for CEA and elevated levels are based on the conclusions stated by the various authors. These data clearly emphasize that CEA is too insensitive to detect more than a small proportion of patients with primary disease and does not even identify all those with metastatic disease. In the former group, however, excluding false-positive factors, elevations may well indicate clinically undetected tumor or micrometastases. In the latter group, a lack of elevation may indicate little or no involvement of bone or liver, since metastases to these sites usually are associated with elevated levels.[13,14] The data demonstrate the general direct increase in incidence of elevated CEA levels related to increasing tumor burden or extent of disease. The lack of sufficient data for other biomarkers for breast carcinoma precludes a similar summary. Preliminary results provide evidence that the low incidence of elevations in primary disease or at time of recurrence is a common problem with all biomarkers.

PRIMARY DISEASE AND RECURRENCE

Preoperative Biomarker Levels

Preoperative studies of biomarkers have largely been limited to CEA. Most observers[13–17] have shown that preoperative CEA levels for breast cancer patients are not significantly different from normal or disease control subjects and do not identify those patients most likely to have a recurrence. This is in contrast to similar studies with colorectal carcinoma which indicate that CEA can be a useful prognostic test.[18–20]

Immediate Postoperative Levels

Wang et al.[15] found that primary breast cancer patients with 10-day postmastectomy levels for CEA above 2.5 ng/mL had a significantly faster recurrence rate than similar patients below this level. At 2 years, 65 percent of the former group in contrast to 20 percent of the latter had a recurrence. In this study, patients were not separated based on stage of disease or nodal status at operation. However, Myers et al.[21] confirmed these findings and in addition noted a correlation between elevated postoperative CEA levels, different clinical stages of disease, and nodal status (N^+, 25.3 percent elevated; N^-, 13.9 percent).

Correlation with Recurrence (CEA)

Varnavides et al.[16] (seven patients) and Neville et al.[22] (89 patients) have compared a rising CEA level to time of recurrence. In the latter study, 10 of the 89 (11 percent) patients had a rise in CEA preceding recurrence, 40 (45 percent) had a simultaneous rise, and 39 (44 percent) had no change. Haagensen et al.[23] reported 14 of 46 (30 percent) patients with the onset of recurrent disease after surgery developed CEA levels above 10 ng/mL. More recently, Lee[24] reported on 243 patients after mastectomy. Of these, 50 patients developed recurrent disease; 48 percent had elevated CEA levels (i.e., greater than 5 ng/mL). Among the 193 patients who remained disease-free, 10 percent had apparent falsely elevated CEA levels. However, these latter patients had disease conditions other than cancer in which CEA may be elevated. Lang et al.[25] reported that for over 40 percent of patients who had a recurrence, a rise in CEA levels occurred 4 to 14 months before clinical detection. Falkson et al.[26] followed patients with serial CEA analyses at intervals of 3 months or less. All these patients had been N^+ at mastectomy and were receiving adjuvant chemotherapy. These investigators were able to divide the patients into five groups depending upon their patterns of serial CEA levels during an observation period of 1 to 3 years. The results obtained provide suggestive prognostic indications for separating patients into such groups based on CEA patterns. The possible practical application of this approach should be considered.

Multiple Biomarkers for Recurrence

Coombes et al.,[27] studying 19 different biomarkers in combination, found that 7 of 16 patients with a poor prognosis (based on histology and involvement of axillary nodes) had abnormalities of at least one of those biomarkers found most frequently elevated in their patients with metastatic disease (CEA, ferritin, C-reactive protein, acid glycoprotein, alkaline phosphatase, sialyltransferase and urinary hydroxyproline/creatinine ratio). Three of these seven patients relapsed within 1 year. More recently, Coombes et al.,[28] in studying 10 biomarkers, reported that three, including CEA, alkaline phosphatase, and γ-glutamyltranspeptidase, appeared most useful in detecting recurrence. These three biomarkers identified approximately half of 23 patients who developed metastases with a lead time of about 3 months. In combination with chest x-ray and physical examination, these three biomarkers also identified 40 of 47 patients who developed recurrent disease. In 94 patients who remained disease-free, abnormalities were found at a frequency of 3.5 percent and were transient. Subsequently, these investigators[29] have stated their discouragement with attempting to find simple and practical biochemical methods for monitoring patients and suggest that available tests have little role in management. They maintain that the most sensitive means for routine screening for metastases in patients with breast cancer is to use chest x-ray and clinical examination, supplemented with liver function tests and CEA measurements.

Haagensen et al.[30] reported that the combination of CEA (above 10 ng/mL) and gross cystic disease fluid protein (GCDFP) was abnormal in 22 of 46 (48 percent) patients who developed metastases, with only 1 of 22 having elevations of both materials.

Recently, Anderson et al.[31] compared pregnancy-associated α-glycoprotein (PAM) and CEA for detecting recurrence or metastases after mastectomy. Following 30 patients postoperatively, PAM was reported to be superior, with a rise in 10 of 11 patients who developed clinically detectable lesions. This is in contrast to CEA, for which a sustained rise was seen in only 2 of the 11 patients.

METASTATIC CANCER

Elevations of a variety of possible biomarkers have been reported for patients with metastatic disease.[1–4,27,30,32] Few, however, have been thoroughly studied or compared as to their ability to parallel changes in disease status, i.e., with clinically measured regression or progression of tumor. Many investigators,[11–14,23,33] however, have evaluated CEA from this viewpoint. The majority of these found CEA levels to correlate generally (i.e., over 80 percent) with objective changes in tumor measurement or tumor burden, although exceptions were found.[12] Of potential prognostic value, Tormey et al.[14] found a higher response rate for patients with low CEA levels, i.e., less than 5 ng/mL. Similar findings and conclusions have been made by Varnavides et al.[16] Lokich et al.[11] reported that a 20 percent or greater change in CEA level was needed to correlate with a measurable tumor response or progression. Silva et al.[34] confirmed these findings for response and also noted that those patients with greater than 50 percent reduction in plasma CEA level had significantly longer responses than other patients. Using slope analysis of serial CEA determinations, Koch et al.[35] found that 65 percent of patients with metastatic breast carcinoma responding to chemotherapy had negative slopes; most failing therapy had positive slopes. More recently, Silva et al.[34] reported that a negative slope for either CEA or GCDFP correlated with response to therapy for 90 percent of patients. In contrast, a positive slope indicated therapy failure and lack of response for 90 percent using CEA and for 80 percent when GCDFP was used.

BIOMARKERS IN TUMOR TISSUE

Tissue Studies

Qualitative or quantitative analysis for biomarkers in primary breast tumor and in comparison to normal breast tissue could serve several objectives: (1) to determine whether the biomarker is possibly or probably derived from the tumor or elsewhere, (2) to gain an appreciation of the synthetic potential of the tumor cells to make the biomarker as the disease progresses, (3) to compare with blood levels in order to determine the efficiency of transfer or release from the primary tumor to the systemic circulation, and (4) to define possible additional staging and prognostic factors. Similar studies of metastatic tumors could determine changes in synthetic ability of the cells when lodged in different organs or tissues. Investigations to date have involved primarily CEA.[36] Wahren et al.[37] demonstrated a positive correlation between tumor and plasma CEA content but suggested that the biomarker may not always be released in measurable or elevated amounts. Shousha and Lyssiotis,[38] employing an immunoperoxidase technique, showed a positive correlation between the presence of CEA in sections of breast carcinoma and the presence of lymph node metastases. Of singular interest and possible importance, these investigators[39] also found a direct correlation between 5- and 10-year survival and the presence or absence of tumor CEA. A significantly higher proportion of patients with tumors lacking in CEA survived 5 ($p < .001$) and 10 years ($p < .01$). It should be noted that studies using the indirect immunoperoxidase technique to detect CEA in histologic sections of breast cancer have provided conflicting results. For example, the incidence of positivity in reported studies has ranged from 2 to 83 percent. The reasons for these differences are not clear, but could be due to variations in technique coupled with the repeated observation of marked heterogeneity of CEA staining with positivity ranging from region to region and even cell to cell.[40]

Menendez-Botet et al.,[41] in cytosols prepared from breast carcinoma tissues, demonstrated that 70 percent of primary tumors in contrast to 51 percent of metastases had increased amounts of CEA. Several reports[41–43] have compared the presence of CEA in primary and metastatic tumors with estrogen receptors (ER), without finding a consistent or complete concordance, e.g., 66 percent in primary tumors and 51 percent in metastatic lesions, and no correlation with plasma CEA levels.[42] Persijn and Lorsten[42] separated neoplastic breast tumors based on a level of 1.5 μg of CEA per gram of protein. Tumors with a CEA level over 1.5 μg/g included a significantly larger proportion of ER-positive tumors than the group with lower CEA content. Walker [44] studied potential biomarkers, including CEA. One or more were found in 84 percent of tumors, two or more in 60 percent and three or more in 32 percent. Of interest, 75 percent of primary breast carcinomas with no markers had no evidence of axillary lymph node metastases while 72 percent with four or five markers had node metastases. Savlov et al.[45] analyzed primary breast tissue for several enzymes. Patients who failed therapy had tumors with significantly lower enzymatic activity than those who showed no evidence of recurrence during a stated observation period. Monsour et al.[46] combined analysis of plasma and breast cancer tissues for CEA to determine if these results for an individual patient might have prognostic value at the time of primary surgery. These studies were also correlated with estrogen receptor data. When the recurrences were analyzed with respect to CEA, estrogen receptor, and nodal status, only in the CEA-positive versus CEA-negative group was there a significant difference. Their preliminary data suggested that patients with positive tissue and/or plasma CEA had higher recurrence rate with probable poor prognosis. The latter correlated better with CEA status than ER or nodal status. These overall results indicate the possible importance of the further study of selected biomarkers or other biochemical parameters in primary and metastatic tumor tissue. The findings of Shousha et al.,[38,39] using CEA, for example, suggest a further subset of breast cancer patients which can be defined as to prognostic implications of recurrence and survival. This work needs additional confirmation.

AREAS FOR FURTHER EXPLORATION

Various research directions are still being pursued in an effort to improve the current status of biomarkers for breast carcinoma. The development and assessment of new biomarker candidates, varied approaches to evaluation, including provocative tests and analysis of postchemotherapy lysed tumor cell products, improved analytical methodology, and correlation of body fluid-tissue relationships are all areas of interest. However, of greatest current interest is the potential for the development of more specific and sensitive biomarkers for breast carcinoma through the production of monoclonal antibodies.

Specific Biomarkers for Breast Carcinoma

Monoclonal Antibodies

A number of studies have been published detailing the detection of human breast tumor-associated antigens with conventional hyperimmune heteroantisera. These have been reviewed by Colcher et al.[49] For a variety of reasons, ranging from low titer to limited availability of specific heteroantisera, the efficacy of these tumor-associated antigens as clinically useful biomarkers has not been established. With the introduction of hybridoma technology by Kohler and Milstein,[47] it is theoretically possible to develop unlimited quantities of monoclonal antibodies of defined specificity against each cellular antigen from both normal mammary cells and mammary carcinoma cells. Thus, in addition to clinical application, hybridoma technology has the potential to shed light on the current debate concerning the existence of tumor-specific antigens, in contrast to tissue-specific or tumor-associated antigens.

Development of Murine Monoclonal Antibodies against Human Breast Carcinoma Cells

Thompson et al.[48] have reported the development of two murine monoclonal antibodies against the human breast carcinoma cell line MCF-7. One antibody detects a 100-kD antigen which is distinct from the well-characterized protein antigens of normal breast tissue, including casein, α-lactalbumin, and milk fat globulin protein. Histological localization studies indicate that the antibody detects a human breast *tissue-associated* antigen found in malignant breast epithelium, the epithelium of gynecomastia, normal breast epithelium, and the epithelium of the respiratory tract. Interestingly, this tissue-associated antigen is also found in the serum of patients with breast carcinoma. However, the usefulness of serum levels of this antigen as a biomarker has not been reported.

Schlom and colleagues have reported the development of a spectrum of murine monoclonal antibodies against membrane-enriched fractions of metastatic human mammary carcinoma tissue.[49] The screening of over 4000 primary hybridoma cultures resulted in the identification of 11 monoclonal antibodies which reacted with human mammary tumor cells and not with normal human tissue. Of these 11 monoclonal antibodies, several have been extensively analyzed. One antibody (B6.2) has been shown to detect a cell surface tumor-associated antigen of 90 kD on 75 percent of the primary and metastatic breast lesions examined.[49–51] Significantly, this antibody (B6.2) did not bind to the cell surface of noncarcinoma cells examined using the immunoperoxidase technique. In addition, this antibody has been exploited to radiolocalize human mammary tumor in athymic mice[49] and to demonstrate antigenic heterogeneity in human mammary carcinoma cell populations.[52] Clearly these apparent tumor-associated antigens are potentially strong candidates for biomarkers.

Development of Human Monoclonal Antibodies against Human Mammary Carcinoma Cells

Schlom et al.[53] have introduced a novel approach for the production of human monoclonal antibodies against human mammary carcinoma cells. Reasoning that lymphocytes in the axillary nodes of patients with primary breast tumors or metastatic disease may be primed to synthesize antibodies against tumor cells, human-mouse hybrids were produced and screened for their ability to produce human monoclonal antibodies against the mammary carcinoma cell. In spite of the technical problems of obtaining stable human-mouse hybridoma cultures, more than 50 stable cultures have been produced. One human monoclonal antibody (MBE 6) has been analyzed in detail by immunohistological techniques.[54] Eighty-one percent (54/67) of primary malignant mammary tumors, 100 percent (20/20) of metastatic breast lesions, and 14 percent (3/32) of benign breast tumors were identified by this method. Interestingly, positive staining was also observed with some carcinomas of nonbreast origin. In contrast, no staining was observed with normal epithelium or other normal human tissue.

Multiple Biomarkers—Mathematical Models and Quantitative Assessment

Previous results[55] in the treatment of metastatic breast cancer patients suggest that patterns of multiple biomarkers have the capability of defining specific response characteristics better than any single biomarker alone when assessed by multivariate regression analysis. Application of these principles to serial points in time during the course of the illness, whether from primary disease to recurrence or during the therapy of advanced disease, could aid in the practical evaluation of disease status.

Biomarker candidates in combination for such studies would include CEA and other materials of promise from published results. More recent publications suggest additional candidates of merit such as gross cystic disease fluid protein (GCDFP), which, although not new, appears to be in this category.[32,56] The glycosyltransferases, both sialyl-[57,58] and galactosyltransferase,[59,60] merit additional attention. More recently, studies of lipid-associated sialic acid have indicated it has potential for use in patients with breast cancer.[61] Carefully derived criteria are needed for inclusion of a subset of biomarkers in a final combination for study and evaluation.

Despite problems in the development of appropriate mathematical models and their practical approach, the possibility of utilizing multiple markers to define disease or tumor status more clearly remains promising. The practicality of this approach depends upon the analytical laboratory methods involved, adherence to a planned protocol for sequential sample acquisition, and automation of the data.

CONCLUSION

In summary, although a variety of materials may be increased in the body fluids of patients with breast cancer, the lack of elevated levels early in the disease course or with small tumor burden, severely limits the usefulness of biomarkers for this neoplasm. In addition, discordant results occur which appear to be related to the inherent biologic nature of some breast tumors and/or through the influence of therapy. To date, no specific biomarker for breast cancer exists although attempts to identify such markers through the use of monoclonal antibodies appears promising. The measurement of biomarkers in tumor tissue, as well as in blood, in both primary and metastatic disease, may aid in defining prognostic factors in patient subsets.

REFERENCES

1. Herberman RB: Biological markers in breast cancer, in McGuire WL (ed): *Breast Cancer*. New York. Plenum Press, vol. 2., 1978, p. 205.
2. McIntire KR: Use of multiple immunoassays for circulating tumor markers, in Herberman RB and McIntire KR (eds.). *Immunoassays for Cancer*. New York, Marcel Dekker, Inc., 1979, p. 521.
3. Haagensen DE: Tumor markers for breast carcinoma. *Clin Lab Med* 2:543, 1982.
4. Statland BE, Winkel P: Usefulness of clinical chemistry measurements in classifying patients with breast cancer. *ERC Crit Rev Clin Lab Sci* 16:255, 1982.
5. Ravry M, Moertel CG, Schutt AV, Go VLM: Usefulness of serial serum carcinoembryonic antigen determinations during anti-cancer therapy or longterm follow-up of gastrointestinal cancer. *Cancer* 34:1230, 1979.
6. Baylin SB, Abeloff MD, Tomford JW, Wieman KC, Ettinger DS: Elevated histaminase (diamine oxidase) activity in small cell carcinoma of the lung. *N Engl J Med* 293:1286, 1975.
7. Bayling SB, Wesiberger WR, Eggleston JC, Abeloff MD: Variable content of histaminase, L-dopadecarboxylase, and calcitonin in small cell carcinoma of the lung. *N Engl J Med* 299:105, 1978.
8. Livingstone AS, Hampson LG, Shuster S, Gold P, Hinchey EJ: Carcinoembryonic antigen in the diagnosis and management of colorectal carcinoma. *Arch Surg* 109:259, 1974.
9. Waalkes TP, Abeloff MD, Woo KB, Ettinger DS, Ruddon RW, Aldenderfer P: Carcinoembryonic antigen for monitoring patients with small cell carcinoma of the lung during treatment. *Cancer* 40:4420, 1980.
10. Waalkes TP, Ableoff MD, Ettinger DS, Woo KB, Kuo KC, Gehrke CW: Serum protein-bound carbohydrates and small cell carcinoma of the lung. *Cancer* 52:131, 1983.
11. Lokich JL, Zamcheck N, Lowenstein M: Sequential carcinoembryonic antigen levels in the therapy of metastatic breast cancer. *Ann Intern Med* 89:902, 1978.
12. Mughal AB, Hortobagyi GN, Fritsche HA: Serial plasma CEA measurements during treatment of metastatic breast cancer. *JAMA* 249:1881, 1983.
13. Chu TM, Nemoto T: Evaluation of carcinoembryonic antigen in human mammary carcinoma. *J Natl Cancer Inst* 51:1119, 1973.
14. Tormey DC, Waalkes TP, Snyder JJ, Simon RM: Biological markers in breast carcinoma. III: Clinical with correlations with carcinoembryonic antigen. *Cancer* 39:2397, 1977.
15. Wang DY, Bulbrook RD, Hayward JL, Hendrick JC, Franchimont P: Relationship between plasma carcinoembryonic antigen and prognosis in women with breast cancer. *Eur J Cancer* 11:615, 1975.
16. Varnavides LA, O'Higgins NJ, Clark CG: Carcinoembryonic antigen (CEA) in mammary disease: A clinical appraisal. *Clin Oncol* 4:329, 1978.
17. Rimsten A, Adami HO, Wahren B, Nordin B: Carcinoembryonic antigen in serum of unselected breast cancer patients and of non-hospitalized controls. *Br J Cancer* 39:109, 1979.
18. Dhar P, Moore T, Zamcheck N, Kupchick HZ: Carcinoembryonic antigen (CEA) in colon cancer. Use in preoperative and postoperative diagnosis and prognosis. *JAMA* 221:31, 1972.
19. Wanebo HJ, Bhaskar R, Pinsky CM: Preoperative carcinoembryonic antigen level as a prognostic indication in colorectal carcinoma. *N Engl J Med* 299:498, 1978.
20. Stater G, Paptestas AE, Anfses AH: Preoperative carcinoembryonic antigen levels in colorectal carcinoma. *Arch Surg* 114:52, 1979.
21. Myers RE, Sutherland DJ, Meakin JW, Kellen JA, Malkin DG, Malkin A: Carcinoembryonic antigen in breast cancer. *Cancer* 42:1520, 1978.
22. Neville AM, Patel S, Capp M: The monitoring role of plasma CEA alone and in association with other tumor markers in colorectal and mammary carcinoma. *Cancer* 42:1448, 1978.
23. Haagensen DE, Kister SJ, Vandevoorde J: Evaluation of carcinoembryonic antigen as a plasma monitor for human breast carcinoma. *Cancer* 42:1512, 1978.
24. Lee M: Carcinoembryonic antigen as a monitor of recurrent breast cancer. *J Surg Oncol* 20:109, 1982.
25. Lang BA, Korent A, Nekulava M, Hlavkova J: Three-year follow up of carcinoembryonic antigen levels in the serum of patients with breast cancer. *Neoplasma* 31:79, 1984.
26. Falkson HC, Falkson G, Protugal MA, Van Derwatt JJ, Schoeman HS: Carcinoembryonic antigen as a marker in patients with breast cancer

receiving postsurgical adjuvant chemotherapy. *Cancer* 49:1859, 1982.

27. Coombes RC, Gazet JC, Sloane JP: Biochemical markers in breast cancer. *Lancet* 2:132, 1977.
28. Coombes RC, Gazet JC, Fort HT: Assessment of biochemical tests to screen for metastases in patients with breast cancer. *Lancet* 1:296, 1980.
29. Coombes RC, Dearnally DP, Ellison ML, Neville AM: Markers in breast and lung cancer. *Ann Clin Biochem* 19:263, 1982.
30. Haagensen DE, Kister SJ, Panick J, Giannola J, Hansen HJ, Wells S: Comparative evaluation of carcinoembryonic antigen and gross cystic disease fluid protein as plasma markers for human breast carcinoma. *Cancer* 42:710, 1979.
31. Anderson JM, Stimson WH, Gettinby G, Jhunjhunwala SK, Burt RW: Detection of mammary micrometastases by pregnancy-associated glycoprotein (PAG or PAM) and carcinoembryonic antigen (CEA). *Eur J Cancer* 15:709, 1979.
32. Waalkes TP, Gehrke CW, Tormey DC: Biological markers in breast carcinoma. IV: Serum fucose-protein ratio; comparison with carcinoembryonic antigen and human chorionic gonadotrophin. *Cancer* 41:1871, 1978.
33. Steward AM, Dixson D, Zamcheck N, Aisenberg A: Carcinoembryonic antigen in breast cancer patients: Serum levels and disease progress. *Cancer* 33:1246, 1974.
34. Silva JS, Leight GS, Haagensen DE: Quantitation of response to therapy in patients with metastatic breast carcinoma by serial analysis of plasma gross cystic disease fluid protein and carcinoembryonic antigen. *Cancer* 49:1236, 1982.
35. Koch M, Paterson AHG, McPherson TA: Slope analysis of plasma carcinoembryonic antigen levels in monitoring response to treatment in patients with metastatic carcinoma of the breast. *Clin Oncol* 6:323, 1980.
36. MacSween JM, Anderson GH; The quantitative relationship of carcinoembryonic antigen to tumor cells of different organs. *Cancer* 40:808, 1977.
37. Wahren B, Lidbrink F, Waalgren A, Eneroth P, Zajicek J; Carcinoembryonic antigen and other tumor markers in tissue and serum or plasma of patients with primary mammary carcinoma. *Cancer* 42:1870, 1978.
38. Shousha S, Lyssiotis T: Correlation of carcinoembryonic antigen in tissue with spread of mammary carcinoma. *Histology* 2:433, 1978.
39. Shousha S, Lyssiotis T, Godfrey VM, Schever PJ: Carcinoembryonic antigen in breast cancer tissue: A useful prognostic indicator. *Br Med J* 1:777, 1979.
40. Kuhajda FP, Offutt LE, Mendelsohn G: The distribution of carcinoembryonic antigen in breast carcinoma. *Cancer* 52:1257, 1983.
41. Menendez-Botet CV, Nisselbaum JS, Fleisher M: Correlation between estrogen receptor protein and carcinoembryonic human antigen in normal and carcinomatous human breast tissue. *Clin Chem* 22:1366, 1976.
42. Persijn JP, Korsten CB: Carcinoembryonic human antigen in normal and carcinomatous human breast tissue. *Clin Chem* 22:1366, 1976.
43. Schwartz MK: Estrogen receptors and tumor associated antigens in breast cancer. *Ann Clin Lab Sci* 9:258, 1979.
44. Walker RA: Biological markers in human breast carcinoma. *J Pathol* 137:109, 1982.
45. Savlov ED, Hilf R, Libson SL, Felstein M: Low tissue enzyme activity seen in breast cancers of patients who fail adjuvant chemotherapy. *Cancer* 47:2214, 1981.
46. Monsour EG, Hastert M, Park CH: Tissue and plasma CEA in early breast cancer. A prognostic factor. *Cancer* 51:1243, 1983.
47. Kohler G, Milstein C: Continuous cultures of fused cells secreting antibody of predefined specificity. *Nature* 256:494, 1975.
48. Thompson CH, Jones SL, Whitehead RH, McKenzie IFC: A human breast tissue-associated antigen detected by a monoclonal antibody. *J Natl Cancer Inst* 70:409, 1983.
49. Colcher D, Zalutsky M, Kaplan W, Kufe D, Austin F, Schlom J: Radiolocalization of human mammary tumors in athymic mice by a monoclonal antibody. *Cancer Res* 43:736, 1983.
50. Kufe DW, Nadler L, Sargent L: Biological behavior of human breast carcinoma-associated antigens expressed during cellular proliferation. *Cancer Res* 43:851, 1983.
51. Nuti M, Colcher D, Hand PH, Austin F, Schlom J: Generation and characterization of monoclonal antibodies reactive with human primary and metastatic mammary tumor cells, in Albertin

A, Elkins R (eds.): *Monoclonal Antibodies and Developments in Immunoassay*. Elsevier/North Holland Biomedical Press, 1981, p. 87.

52. Hand PH, Nuti M, Colcher D, Schlom J: Definition of antigenic heterogeneity and modulation among human mammary carcinoma cell populations using monoclonal antibodies to tumor-associated antigens. *Cancer Res* 43:728, 1983.
53. Schlom J, Wunderlich D, Termoto A: Generation of human monoclonal antibodies reactive with human mammary carcinoma cells. *Proc Natl Acad Sci* 77:6841, 1980.
54. Teramoto A, Mariani D, Wunderlich D, Schlom J: The immunohistochemical reactivity of a human monoclonal antibody with tissue sections of human mammary tumors. *Cancer* 50:241, 1982.
55. Woo KB, Waalkes TP, Ahmann DL, Tormey DC, Gehrke CW, Oliverio VT: A quantitative approach to determining disease response during therapy using multiple biologic markers. Application to carcinoma of the breast. *Cancer* 41:1685, 1978.
56. Haagensen DE, Barry WF, McCook TA, Giannola J, Amimirata S, Wells S: The value of serial plasma levels of CEA and gross cyst disease fluid protein in patients with breast carcinoma and osseous metastases. *Ann Surg* 191:599, 1980.
57. Dao TL, Ip C, Patel J: Serum sialytransferase and 5 nucleotidase as reliable biomarkers in women with breast cancer. *J Natl Cancer Inst* 65:529, 1980.
58. Stewart JF, Rubens RD, Hoare S, Bulbrook RD, Kessel D: Serum sialyltransferase levels in patients with metastatic breast cancer treated by chemotherapy. *Br J Cancer* 46:208, 1982.
59. Paone JF, Waalkes TP, Baker RR, Shaper JH: Serum UDP-galactosyltransferase as a potential biomarker for breast carcinoma. *J Surg Oncol* 15:59, 1980.
60. Paone JD, Baker RR, Waalkes TP, Shaper JH: Sequential galactosyltransferase and CEA levels in advanced breast cancer. *J Surg Res* 31:269, 1982.
61. Dnistrian AM, Schwartz MK, Katopodis N, Fracchia AA, Stock CC: Serum lipidbound sialic acid as a marker in breast cancer. *Cancer* 50:1815, 1982.

15

Breast Biopsy

Joseph B. Cleary, M.D.

INTRODUCTION

Breast biopsy is required when the benign or malignant nature of a breast abnormality must be determined. The indications for biopsy are as follows:

1 The presence of a dominant mass or area of thickening, including a mass in the axilla.

2 Nipple discharge of the bloody, serous, or clear type. There may or may not be an associated palpable mass.

3 Mammogram detected, nonpalpable mass or area of suspicious calcifications.

4 Persistent encrustation or eczema over the surface of the nipple (possible Paget's disease of the breast).

5 Persistent redness of the skin of the breast, not attributable to infection (possible inflammatory carcinoma).

6 Other signs suggestive of cancer, which are often found in association with one or more of the above conditions, such as skin dimpling, skin edema (*peau d'orange*), or significant nipple retraction.

Biopsy may be done by the *open* or *closed method. Open biopsy* removes the entire mass (*excision*) or just a part of the mass (*incision biopsy*). Definitive surgical treatment may follow immediately after biopsy—a one-stage approach—or it may be delayed for several days after biopsy, becoming a two-stage approach.

Closed biopsy is done with a needle, and may be either an *aspiration* or a *core biopsy.* In the needle aspiration technique, individual cells or cell clusters are obtained for cytologic examination, and may be prepared as a Papanicolaou smear; in the core biopsy technique, a fragment of tissue is sought for histologic examination, which may be done via a frozen section and permanent paraffin section (Fig. 15-1).

The current TNM system of classification is used throughout.

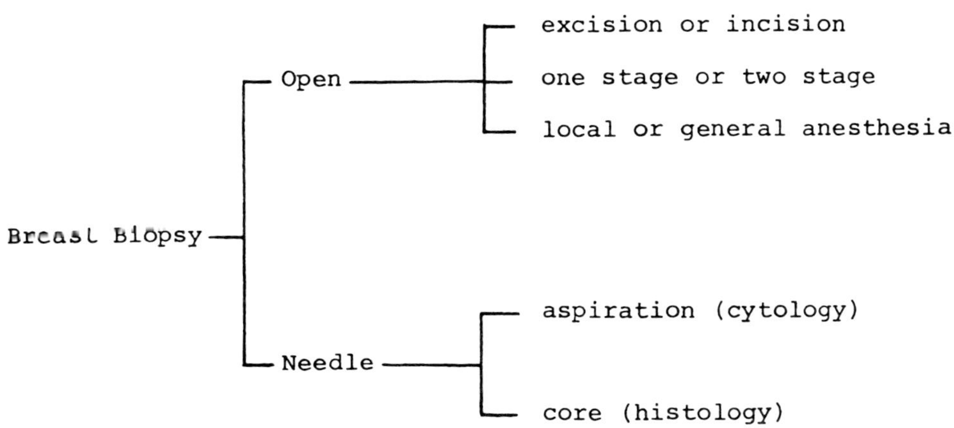

Figure 15-1 Options in diagnostic breast biopsy.

This chapter will discuss the approach to a palpable breast abnormality. Mammogram-detected nonpalpable lesions, nipple conditions, and inflammatory carcinoma are discussed in separate chapters.

PALPABLE BREAST MASS OR THICKENING

A dominant mass or dominant area of thickening in the breast is the most common reason for biopsy. One must *not* depend on mammogram or other diagnostic aids to determine the benign or malignant nature of a clinically dominant lesion. Only microscopic examination of tissue obtained by biopsy can conclusively indicate a benign or malignant condition. The various diagnostic aids may be used to add certain information, such as the presence of separate nonpalpable lesions in one or both breasts. In addition, a positive mammogram can substantiate a clinical impression of malignancy, and by so doing aid in choosing a particular biopsy method.

As with overdependence on diagnostic aids, one must also guard against overdependence on "clinical impression" to determine the benign or malignant nature of a mass. Although with experience the benign or malignant nature of a lump can often be predicted, clinical impression is no substitute for definitive tissue diagnosis. It is sufficient for the examining physician to detect and confirm the presence of an abnormality; the definitive answer as to whether or not the abnormality is malignant rests only with microscopic examination, not with the fingertips.

A dominant mass may feel cystic on examination. Often, more than one cyst is present in the same or both breasts. In such a case, fluid aspiration from the cyst is the procedure of choice. This may be done as a simple office procedure, using a no. 20 or 22 gauge needle attached to a 10- or 20-mL syringe. With the patient supine, the skin is prepared with alcohol and the cyst is immobilized between the fingers of one hand, while the needle is directed toward the cyst with the other. The fluid withdrawn varies greatly in color and clarity, usually being greenish or brownish, and either clear or turbid. After aspiration, a small pressure dressing is applied. Bloody fluid is a serious sign, and a formal biopsy should be undertaken. Following aspiration, the mass (cyst) should be gone; if there is a residual mass or thickening in the area, biopsy is required.

The aspirated fluid may be preserved in 95 percent alcohol, and submitted for cytologic examination, bearing in mind that a negative report does not exclude the possibility of cancer. Positive cytology from cyst fluid is rare.[1,2] In 1979, a series of 3545 cases of fine-needle aspiration of breast masses was reported; 1015 of these were cysts, and of these, 8 (0.7 percent) subsequently proven malignancies were diagnosed based on the cyst fluid examination. Of the eight malignant cases, three had cyst fluid which was *not* bloody.[1]

A mammogram should be obtained (in patients over 30 years of age) to determine the presence of any radiologically suspicious area around the cyst. Finally, the patient is examined at regular intervals to check for recurrence. If the cyst recurs, aspiration is repeated. If there is recurrence after three aspirations, open biopsy should be considered.

Excision Biopsy

Excision biopsy is preferable to incision biopsy in most cases. It provides a complete specimen from which the pathologist can select representative areas for microscopic study. When possible, the skin incision for this procedure should be a gently curving one, paralleling the curved areolar margin. If a mastectomy is likely to follow, the direction and length of the skin incision should be such that it will be contained within the planned elliptical mastectomy incision.

Incision Biopsy

Incision biopsy is useful under certain conditions:

1 To confirm the diagnosis of cancer in an advanced case, and to provide tissue for hormone receptor determination.

2 To obtain the diagnosis of cancer in a case where it is technically preferable to let a large tumor remain as part of the mastectomy specimen. It is advisable to do the hormone receptor studies on the biopsy specimen, since a period of decreased vascularity to the tumor mass during mastectomy dissection may result in loss of receptor activity.

3 Incision biopsy may be of help in confirming the benign nature of what is clinically and radiographically considered to be a broad area of prominent fibrocystic breast parenchyma, which, because it has no similar counterpart in the same or opposite breast, causes some diagnostic question.

In cases of inoperable stage III and stage IV cancer, excision biopsy of a representative tumor mass is still preferable, provided the mass is not too large. If a single primary lesion is extensive or fixed to the chest wall, incision biopsy is utilized. General anesthesia has the advantage of avoiding infiltration of the tumor mass with anesthesia solution, as well as allowing for ease of placement of suture ligatures if required for hemostasis. In view of the neck movement associated with general anesthesia, local-standby should be considered for primary lesion biopsy in a patient with known marked cervical spine metastases. If incision biopsy is used for an advanced primary lesion, effort is made to sample a portion of the tumor that lies below a layer of skin, as closure of skin over the biopsy site provides for better wound healing. If the tumor is completely ulcerated, needle biopsy is preferred.

Mass in the Axilla

The presence of a mass in the axillary region may represent lymph node metastases from an ipsilateral breast cancer, even when the breast is clinically and mammographically normal.[3–10] In 1907 Halsted described three patients with clinically normal breasts and metastatic carcinoma in the axillary nodes. Overt breast cancer subsequently developed in each patient.[3] Since then, many such cases have been reported. The axillary mass is excised and frozen section examination obtained to determine the presence of metastatic cancer. If cancer is present, a portion of the specimen is immediately preserved for hormone receptor studies. The permanent paraffin section is awaited, which may suggest breast as the origin. In any event, if clinical and mammographic breast examination is negative, search for an extramammary primary site must be planned. The following organs are possible primary sites giving rise to axillary lymph node metastases: breast, first and foremost; also, thyroid, lung, stomach, colon, pancreas, liver, genitourinary tract, and skin. In regard to skin, it is important to question the patient about any previous removal or cauterization of moles or other lesions. If no extramammary site can be found as the source of the metastatic axillary tumor, then the ipsilateral breast is treated as the primary site. Mastectomy has been the most common treatment; however, breast preservation, utilizing radiotherapy, has been recently reported.[10] When mastectomy is performed, a small focus of carcinoma is usually found on serial sectioning of the breast. These cancers are often lobular carcinoma in situ, intraductal carcinoma, or intraductal carcinoma with early invasion.[7] In some cases, even after serial sectioning of the breast specimen, no focus of cancer can be found.[4,7,9] The prognosis in this condition is as good or better than that for palpable breast cancer with axillary metastases.[5–10]

Breast Biopsy as an Outpatient Procedure

Breast biopsy as an outpatient procedure under local anesthesia has been advocated in numerous reports.[11–18] A primary impetus for this approach is the fact that the majority of breast lesions which require biopsy turns out to be benign.[11,12,14]

In some reports, outpatient-local anesthesia biopsy is reserved for those cases where the breast mass is clinically benign,[11,12,14] while in others this approach is practiced for all undiagnosed, palpable, solid breast masses.[13,15] Opinion also varies in regard to details of technique. Reports have described the use of a main operating suite, along with an intravenous line in place, plus anesthesia standby;[17] others have utilized an operating suite in the surgery outpatient clinic,[18] and some see no need for either premedication or an intravenous line.[15] In view of the possibility of a reaction to the local anesthetic or the occurrence of a nonspecific vasovagal reaction with bradycardia, the surgeon should choose a technique which makes adequate provision for these rare but potential situations.

Reported complications have been few, except for an infrequent hematoma or stitch abscess. Of significance is a report by Leis of 17 patients on whom he reoperated for residual masses; there were three cancers that had not been detected by outpatient-local anesthesia biopsy done at other institutions.[19] Urban has stated that there is a great tendency to limit the extent of excisional biopsy when it is performed under local anesthesia.[20]

The following is a list of conditions which, in most circumstances, are considered unsuitable for outpatient-local anesthesia biopsy:

1 Small mass located deep in a large breast.

2 Nipple discharges requiring a central duct excision procedure, particularly in the absence of a palpable mass.

3 Nonpalpable mammogram-detected abnormality. Although with proper technique the area of suspicion is readily removed in the initial tissue excision and demonstrated in the specimen mammogram, there is a potential need for repeat tissue sampling in this condition.

4 A large mass or multiple lesions, where the amount of local anesthetic solution required may reach the maximum allowable dosage.

5 A patient who is resistant to local anesthesia and to the idea of being awake during a procedure; or a patient who has a medical condition which might become exacerbated during a period of stress.

Also open to question would be those patients who have lesions which are clinically suspicious for cancer. In general, a case of probable malignancy is best admitted to the hospital, where, after agreement is reached regarding treatment options, biopsy and definitive surgery may be carried out. The ongoing expansion of ambulatory surgery programs provides the opportunity to utilize general anesthesia for excision biopsy on an outpatient basis.

One-Stage versus Two-Stage Method

A one-stage method utilizes immediate frozen section diagnosis of the biopsy specimen, followed by immediate surgery. The two-stage method consists of performing only the biopsy at one procedure, awaiting microscopic diagnosis by paraffin section, and then proceeding with surgery at a later date. Both these approaches require appropriate discussion of treatment options with the patient. In the case of the two-stage method, however, discussion may be delayed until after the diagnosis is confirmed.

Frozen section examination of tissue excised from the breast provides reliable diagnosis.[21–23] The technique was first described in 1905 by Wilson.[24] A recent analysis of the technique was reported by Rosen in 1978.[21] In his study 556 consecutive breast biopsies were examined; 145 (26 percent) were interpreted as cancer, and on subsequent paraffin section, there were no errors; 381 (68.6 percent) were interpreted as benign, and on subsequent paraffin section, 8 cancers were found (3 percent false-negative rate); in 30 instances (5.4 percent) the frozen section diagnosis was deferred, and 10 of the 30 proved to have cancer on the subsequent permanent section. The cases where frozen section diagnosis was deferred were usually lesions in which the distinction had to be made between ductal hyperplasia versus carcinoma. In cases where the frozen section was reported as benign, and the permanent section found cancer, the carcinoma was found in a portion of the specimen other than the one selected for frozen section analysis. The majority of these cancers was noninvasive.[21]

If frozen section diagnosis is to be utilized in an accurate and reliable manner, the pathologist must not be pressed for diagnosis. In cases where there is any doubt regarding the nature of the lesion, diagnosis must be deferred for permanent section. When a benign report is received on frozen section, unless the case is obviously benign from a clinical standpoint, it is best to await the permanent paraffin report before conveying definitive statements to the patient.

Consideration must be given to the utilization of frozen section for the diagnosis of small, occult breast lesions found by mammography. It may be advisable to bypass frozen section altogether on this type of lesion, and utilize the available tissue for paraffin section.[23] Obtaining a representative portion of the biopsy for hormone receptor study is a concern; approximately 500 to 1000 mg of tumor tissue is needed for hormone receptor assay by standard techniques.

The two-stage approach to biopsy and treatment has been recommended by the 1979 National Institutes of Health Consensus Development Conference.[25] This panel indicated that the two-stage procedure allows time for detailed pathologic examination of biopsied tissue, and an opportunity to discuss with the patient subsequent diagnostic and therapeutic procedures. Kinne states that this recommendation was primarily an attempt to encourage patients to enter more clinical trials exploring alternatives to standard mastectomy.[26] Delay between biopsy and subsequent mastectomy (if mastectomy is decided upon) has no apparent adverse effect on prognosis.[27–29] Some authors contend that delay beyond 2 weeks[20] or 4 weeks[30] is accompanied by a decreased overall survival rate in those cases where regional lymph nodes prove to contain metastases.

It is clear that the two-stage approach is applicable in many cases, particularly when the probability exists that the lesion is benign, with small lesions, or when there is doubt regarding a frozen section diagnosis. With large tumors, however, where there is a strong clinical suspicion of carcinoma, it is advisable to consider a one-stage approach.[26,31]

Needle Biopsy

Needle biopsy for the diagnosis of breast lesions is being used more frequently.[1,32–37,47–53] This technique was described in detail by Martin and Ellis in 1930.[38] They stated that the indication for needle puncture and aspiration is a tumor mass which lies below the surface of normal tissue where surgical exposure is deemed contraindicated for any reason.

Needle aspiration biopsy utilizes a no. 20 to 22 gauge needle, attached to a 10- or 20-mL syringe. The needle is advanced toward the mass, and when it has entered, suction is applied via the syringe. With suction maintained, the needle is advanced; to obtain sufficient tissue the needle is directed to different areas of the mass, maintaining vacuum on the syringe at all times. The vacuum should be slowly released before withdrawing the needle from the mass, to prevent a sudden aspiration of needle contents into the barrel of the syringe, making collection difficult. The contents of the needle are then discharged onto a glass slide after the syringe has been disconnected from the needle, filled with air, and reconnected. A smear is made, and the material prepared for staining.[37,38] Alternatively, fixative solution may be aspirated to mix with the cells, to be followed by centrifugation and staining.[48,49]

Zajicek et al. in 1970 reported on 4700 consecutive mammary aspiration biopsies for both cystic and solid lesions done from 1955 through 1964. In 2111 cases (45 percent) surgery was performed after needle biopsy and the excised tissues were histologically examined. Invasive cancer was histologically observed in 1068 cases; in 90 percent of the cases, the cytologic report was carcinoma or suspected carcinoma; in 8.3 percent (89 of 1068 cases) the cytologic examination did not suggest malignancy—a false-negative rate of 8.3 percent. Benign histology was observed in 1009 cases; in 28 of these cases (2.8 percent) the cytologic examination indicated "carcinoma suspected," while in 41 (4.1 percent) the cytology report indicated "cellular atypia."[32] Kline et al. in 1979 reported the results of 3545 breast aspirations for both cystic and solid lesions, done over an 8-year period.[1] There were 368 cancers; in 9.6 percent (35 of the 368 cases) the cytologic examination did not suggest malignancy—a false-negative rate of 9.6 percent. Of 3177 benign cases, 60 (1.9 percent) were cytologically diagnosed as "positive for malignancy"—demonstrating, as in the previous series, the occurrence of false positives.

Abramson in 1981 reported results of fine-needle aspiration biopsy and cutting-edge core needle biopsy. In the latter technique, a core of tissue is obtained for histologic (not cytologic) examination, utilizing a Vim-Silverman type instrument. Of 19 patients, 15 had cancer; fine-needle aspiration cytology was positive in 7 of the 15; core biopsy histologic examination on frozen section was positive in 6 of the 15, while core biopsy on paraffin section was positive in 11 of the 15. There were no false positives.[35] These reports indicate that open biopsy should be done on any clinically suspicious mass, regardless of a negative cytologic report.

The *sensitivity* of fine-needle aspiration (i.e., the probability that the test will be positive when cancer is present) varies from 74 percent[47] to 96 percent.[50] This reemphasizes that a negative cytologic report must not be accepted for a dominant solid mass, and open biopsy should follow. The *specificity* of fine-needle aspiration (i.e., the probability that the test will be negative when cancer is absent) varies from 79 percent[48] to 100 percent.[47,49] This is a crucial area, where treatment based on a false positive can result in unnecessary surgery. Sensitivity will increase if "atypical" and "suspicious" lesions are included as positive; however, such relaxed criteria will reduce specificity. Conversely, specificity can be enhanced by including as positive only those lesions which are "definitely malignant."

The sensitivity of cutting-edge core needle biopsy varies from 67 percent[52] to 90 percent.[51] It has been more frequently utilized when a breast mass shows clinical evidence of malignancy. Accuracy is related to tumor size, with the larger tumors being more amenable to diagnosis by this technique,[52,53] particularly those over 5 cm.[52]

Treatment Based on Needle Biopsy The question arises as to whether radical surgery may be done based on the results of needle biopsy, without first obtaining an open biopsy and complete specimen examination. This obviously depends to a great extent on the experience of the pathologist. Radical surgery has been done based on cytologic examination alone[34,37,47]; other reports indicate it may be done based on core biopsy paraffin section.[35,51–53] Nevertheless, the *standard* approach under most circumstances for the diagnosis of a solid breast tumor prior to treatment should be open biopsy and histologic examination by frozen section and/or paraffin section. Certain benign lesions, such as sclerosing adenosis, bear a very close resemblance to cancer, both grossly and microscopically.[39–41] They are best diagnosed when a complete excisional biopsy specimen is submitted for pathologic study. A complete specimen also allows for the discernment of histopathologic variables which influence treatment and prognosis, such as specific histologic type, presence or absence of lymph and vascular channel invasion, and presence or absence of contiguous foci of in situ carcinoma. Uncommon tumors, such as sarcomas, may pose difficulty in diagnosis when specimen sampling is limited. In addition, evaluation of the gross specimen is often as important as examining the microscopic picture.[46]

Possible Dissemination of Tumor Attention must be given to the possibility of enhancing local or distant dissemination of tumor cells as a result of the trauma caused by the needle passage. There are reported cases of needle tract implantation in various types of tumors.[42,43] Some specify that a wide-bore core biopsy needle was used, others do not specify needle size. Engzell et al. in 1971 reported on experimental laboratory work to investigate this question. They collected efferent blood and lymph samples after aspiration biopsy (no. 18 gauge needle) of a tumor-bearing lymph node in the experimental animal. Also, leakage of cells from the puncture site on the surface of the lymph node was studied. While it was unusual to find the efferent blood and lymph to contain malignant cells, the fluid material which escaped through the needle punctures in the lymph node capsule was found to contain malignant cells in 10 out of 12 instances. In conjunction with the experimental work, the records of 626 patients were reviewed, each of whom had undergone primary diagnosis of a tumor by fine-needle biopsy. These authors concluded that "... although it is likely that tumor cells spread along needle tracks of aspiration biopsy, this possible spread lacks practical clinical implications."[44]

Berg and Robbins in 1962 reported on the question of whether or not aspiration biopsy of breast lesions was detrimental to the prognosis of the patient.[45] Each of 370 patients who had aspiration biopsy was matched with a patient who had the diagnosis determined in some other way. Fifteen-year actuarial survival rates were the same, as were 15-year crude survival rates. In 106 cases, the patient with aspiration biopsy died of breast cancer while the control was still alive; in 116 cases, the matched control patient had died while the other was still alive. It is concluded, within the limits imposed by attempting to match cases with multiple variables, that aspiration biopsy does no harm.

CONCLUSION

There are several variations in the approach to diagnostic breast biopsy. No single procedure will be ideal for all cases. Only after evaluating the patient thoroughly, and having considered the advantages and disadvantages of the various methods, can a biopsy plan best suited to a particular patient be selected.

REFERENCES

1. Kline TS, Lalita JP, Hunter NS: Fine-needle aspiration of the breast: Diagnoses and pitfalls. *Cancer* 44:1458, 1979.
2. Abramson DJ: Clinical evaluation of aspiration of cysts of the breast. *Surg Gynecol Obstet* 139:531, 1974.
3. Halsted WS: Results of radical operation for cure of carcinoma of breast. *Ann Surg* 46:1, 1907.
4. Fienerman L, Attie JN, Rosenberg B: Carcinoma in axillary lymph nodes as an indicator of breast cancer. *Surg Gynecol Obstet* 114:5, 1962.
5. Larsen RR, Sawyer KC, Sawyer RB, Torres RC: Occult carcinoma of the breast. *Am J Surg* 107:553, 1964.
6. Ximenes J, Brown HW, Goodsitt E: Occult carcinoma of the breast: Two case reports and review of the literature. *Int Surg* 47:159, 1967.
7. Westbrook KC, Gallager HS: Breast carcinoma presenting as an axillary mass. *Am J Surg* 122:607, 1971.
8. Copeland EM, McBride CM: Axillary metastases from unknown primary site. *Ann Surg* 178:25, 1973.
9. Ashikari R, Rosen PP, Urban JA, Senoo T: Breast cancer presenting as an axillary mass. *Ann Surg* 183:415, 1976.
10. Vilcoq JR, Calle R, Ferme F, Veith F: Conservative treatment of axillary adenopathy due to probable subclinical breast cancer. *Arch Surg* 117:1136, 1982.
11. Abramson DJ: 857 Breast biopsies as an outpatient procedure: Delayed mastectomy in 41 malignant cases. *Ann Surg* 163:478, 1966.
12. Abramson DJ: Delayed mastectomy after outpatient breast biopsy. Long-term survival study. *Am J Surg* 132:596, 1976.
13. Saltzstein EC, Mann RW, Chua TY, DeCosse JJ: Outpatient breast biopsy. *Arch Surg* 109:287, 1974.
14. Scher KS: Outpatient breast biopsies: A selective approach. *Milit Med* 144:823, 1979.
15. Baker RR: Out-patient breast biopsies. *Ann Surg* 185:543, 1977.
16. Caffee HH, Benfield JR: Data favoring biopsy of the breast under local anesthesia. *Surg Gynecol Obstet* 140:88, 1975.
17. Lou MA Sr, Mandal AK, Alexander JL: The pros and cons of outpatient breast biopsy. *Arch Surg* 111:668, 1976.
18. Hunt TK, Crass RA: Breast biopsies on outpatients. *Surg Gynecol Obstet* 141:591, 1975.
19. Leis HP: Breast biopsy: Indications and techniques. *Breast* 6(3):2, 1980.
20. Urban JA: Guest editorial: The case against delayed operation for breast cancer. *CA* 21–22:132, 1971–1972.
21. Rosen PP: Frozen section diagnosis of breast lesions. Recent experience with 556 consecutive biopsies. *Ann Surg* 187:17, 1978.
22. Horn RC: What can be expected of the surgical pathologist from frozen section examinations. *Surg Clin North Am* 42:443, 1962.
23. Sparkman RS: Reliability of frozen section in the diagnosis of breast lesions. *Ann Surg* 155:924, 1962.
24. Wilson LB: A method for the rapid preparation of fresh tissues for the microscope. *JAMA* 45:1737, 1905.
25. Moxley JH III, Allegra JC, Henney J, Muggia F: Treatment of primary breast cancer: Summary of the National Institutes of Health Consensus Development Conference. *JAMA* 244:797, 1980.
26. Kinne DW: Opinion: The case for the one-step biopsy procedure for breast cancer. *CA* 32:46, 1982.
27. Margolese RG: Response: The case for the two-step biopsy procedure for breast cancer. *CA* 32:51, 1982.
28. Pierce EH, Clagett OT, McDonald JR, Gage RP: Biopsy of the breast followed by delayed radical mastectomy. *Surg Gynecol Obstet* 103:559, 1956.
29. Jackson PP, Pitts HH: Biopsy with delayed radical mastectomy for carcinoma of the breast. *Am J Surg* 98:184, 1959.
30. Sayago C, Sirebrenik D: Surgical biopsy as a disseminating factor in breast cancer. *Acta Unio Internationalis Contra Cancrum* 15:1161, 1959.
31. Urban JA: Treatment of primary breast cancer; management of local disease: Minority report. *JAMA* 244:800, 1980.

32. Zajicek J, Casperson T, Jakobson P, Kudynowski J, Linsk J, Us-Krasovec M: Cytologic diagnosis of mammary tumors from aspiration biopsy smears. Comparison of cytologic and histologic findings in 2111 lesions and diagnostic use of cytophotometry. *Acta Cytol* 14:370, 1970.
33. Abele JS, Miller TR, Goodson WH III, Hunt TK, Hohn DC: Fine-needle aspiration of palpable breast masses. A program for staged implementation. *Arch Surg* 118:859, 1983.
34. Innes DJ, Feldman PS: Comparison of diagnostic results obtained by fine needle aspiration cytology and Tru-Cut® or open biopsies. *Acta Cytol* 27:350, 1983.
35. Abramson DJ: The needle biopsy in diagnosis of breast masses. *Breast* 7:9, 1981.
36. Hennig K, Johansson H, Rimsten A, Stenkvist B: X-ray and fine needle biopsy in diagnosis of nonpalpable breast lesions. *Acta Cytol* 19:7, 1975.
37. Zajicek J: Fine-needle aspiration biopsy of palpable breast lesions, in Logan WW (ed): *Breast Carcinoma, The Radiologist's Expanded Role*. New York, John Wiley & Sons, Inc., 1977, p. 319.
38. Martin HE, Ellis EB: Biopsy by needle puncture and aspiration. *Ann Surg* 92:169, 1930.
39. Pack GT, Ariel IM: Introduction 1: Classification, principles of treatment, and prognosis of tumors of the breast, in Pack GT, Ariel IM (eds): *Treatment of Cancer and Allied Diseases*, vol. IV. New York, Hoeber, Harper & Row, 1964, p. 11.
40. McDivitt RW, Stewart FW, Berg JW: *Atlas of Tumor Pathology. Second Series: Tumors of the Breast*. Washington, D.C., Armed Forces Institute of Pathology, 1968, p. 133.
41. Raff LJ: Frozen section needle biopsy of the breast: A technique of limited usefulness. *Breast* 8(3):11, 1982.
42. Ackerman LV, Wheat MW Jr: The implantation of cancer—an avoidable surgical risk? *Surgery* 37:341, 1955.
43. Burkholder GV, Kaufman JJ: Local implantation of carcinoma of the prostate with percutaneous needle biopsy. *J Urol* 95:801, 1966.
44. Engzell U, Esposti PL, Rubio C, Sigurdson A, Zajicek J: Investigation on tumor spread in connection with aspiration biopsy. *Acta Radiol* 10:385, 1971.
45. Berg JW, Robbins GF: A late look at the safety of aspiration biopsy. *Cancer* 15:826, 1962.
46. Azzopardi JG: *Problems in Breast Pathology*. Philadelphia, W.B. Saunders Co., 1979.
47. Wanebo HJ, Feldman PS, Wilhelm MC, Covell JL, Binns RL: Fine-needle aspiration cytology in lieu of open biopsy in management of primary breast cancer. *Ann Surg* 199:569, 1984.
48. Norton LW, David JR, Wiens LC, Trego DC, Dunnington GL: Accuracy of aspiration cytology in detecting breast cancer. *Surgery* 96:806, 1984.
49. Somers RG, Young GP, Kaplan MJ, Bernhard VM, Rosenberg M, Somers D: Fine needle aspiration biopsy in the management of solid breast tumors. *Arch Surg* 120:673, 1985.
50. Shabot MM, Goldberg JM, Shick P, Nieberg R, Pilch YH: Aspiration cytology is superior to Tru-Cut® needle biopsy in establishing the diagnosis of clinically suspicious breast masses. *Ann Surg* 196:122, 1982.
51. Foster RS Jr: Core-cutting needle biopsy for the diagnosis of breast cancer. *Am J Surg* 143:622, 1982.
52. Roberts JG, Preece PE, Bolton PM, Baum M, Hughes LE: The "tru-cut" biopsy in breast cancer. *Clin Oncol* 1:297, 1975.
53. George WD, Burn JI: Drill biopsy in the diagnosis of breast cancer. *Clin Oncol* 1:291, 1975.

Part Five

Treatment of Potentially Curable Breast Cancer

16

The Management of Clinically Nonpalpable Breast Cancer

Henry P. Leis, Jr., M.D.
Angelo Cammarata, M.D.
Raymond D. LaRaja, M.D.

INTRODUCTION

Ever-increasing numbers of breast cancers are being detected before they can be clinically detected by the use of diagnostic aids, especially breast x-rays (mammography and xerography).[5] This accounts for the largest yield. Breast cancers are also being found by (1) careful histologic studies of the surrounding tissue removed when performing a wide excisional biopsy of a benign lesion, (2) by histologic studies of the tissue removed in random biopsies of the other breast when the first is found to have cancer, (3) by histologic studies of the tissues obtained in reduction mammoplasties, and (4) in prophylactic mastectomies performed in carefully selected cases. Early diagnosis of these clinically nondetectable breast cancers is of paramount importance, resulting in better cure and long-term survival rates, less extensive surgery, less adjuvant therapy, and easier reconstruction as well as decreased need for it.

When staging is referred to, the TNM classification is used but with modification as described in Table 16-1.

Meaning of Truly Early Diagnosis

In the past, "early diagnosis" meant the finding of a small lump in the breast. Based on the pioneer work of Gershon-Cohen and associates,[37] in their classic paper on "biological predeterminism" in 1963, regarding the doubling time of breast cancers, it was found that the average breast cancer doubles at about the rate of once every 110 days, so that it probably has been present for about 9 years before it reaches the size of 1 cm. This is the size that is usually needed for clinical palpation.

Truly early diagnosis, where the prognosis for cure is excellent with appropriate therapy, means the finding of cancers in this nonpalpable stage.[58] In the past there was no way of

Table 16-1 Staging System (Potentially Curable Breast Cancers)

Stage 0			
In situ (Noninvasive)	T_{IS}		
Invasive			
a (Not fixed to pectoral muscle or fascia)			
b (Fixed to pectoral muscle or fascia)			
Tumor up to 0.5 cm	T_{1ai} T_{1bi}	N_0	M_0
Tumor 0.5 –0.9 cm	T_{1aii} T_{1bii}	N_0	M_0
Stage I			
Tumor 1.0 –1.9 cm	T_{1aiii} T_{1biii}	N_0	M_0
Tumor 2.0 –5.0 cm	T_{2a} T_{2b}	N_0	M_0
Tumor over 5 cm	T_{3a} T_{3b}	N_0	M_0
Stage II			
No evidence of primary tumor	T_0	N_{1a} or N_{1b}	M_0
N_{1a} (Micrometastasis)	T_{1a} or T_{1b}	N_{1a} or N_{1b}	M_0
N_{1b} (Gross metastasis	T_{2a} or T_{2b}	N_{1a} or N_{1b}	M_0
to nonfixed, homolateral axillary nodes)	T_{3a} or T_{3b}	N_{1a} or N_{1b}	M_0

finding these nonpalpable cancers except when they were found incidentally in tissue specimens obtained from surgery performed for other reasons. The term *occult carcinoma* was first used by Halsted[43] in 1907 when he described three patients who had axillary masses that proved to be metastatic breast cancer on histological examination, in which no mass could be palpated in the breast.

Terminology for Clinically Undetected Cancers

Many terms have been used to designate lesions that cannot be detected by clinical examination. Gallager and Martin[34,35] coined the term *minimal breast cancer* to designate highly curable forms of breast cancer, including lobular carcinoma in situ, intraductal carcinoma, and invasive carcinoma, either lobular or ductular, that formed a mass no greater than 0.5 cm in diameter.

Wanebo, Huvos, and Urban[111] included under this term of minimal breast cancer in situ lobular carcinoma, intraductal carcinoma, minimal Paget's disease, small infiltrating breast cancers arising in the outer one-half of the breast and measuring 1 cm or less in diameter, and low-grade infiltrating cancers including intracystic, papillary, tubular, and adenoid cystic and malignant cystosarcoma phyllodes.

We refer to cancers that are less than 1 cm in size, both invasive and noninvasive, as occult, presymptomatic, or preclinical cancers.[24,59,61,64,67] We classify them as stage 0 cancers. Under the TNM classification this would include T_{IS} (in situ cancers), T_0 (no evidence of primary tumor), T_{1ai} and T_{1bi} (tumors less than 0.5 cm), and T_{1aii} and T_{1bii} (tumors 0.5 cm to 1 cm)(see Table 16-1). Even though they are less than 1 cm in size, some of these invasive cancers can have axillary metastases. This occurred in 15.8 percent of our cases, but the number of metastases was usually minimal.[67]

It must be emphasized that there are cancers larger than 1 cm in size, usually found by mammography, that are clinically nondetectable and their management must also be considered. They are most often seen in patients with large breasts, with multinodular breasts, or with very dense breasts where palpation is difficult.

The various types of aids for detection include the following:

1 Breast x-rays, both xerography[117,118] and mammography[8,11,40,47,80,100,106,120]
2 Thermography[19,36]
3 Ultrasonography (sonography or echography)[10,91,102]
4 Breast CT scanning or computerized axial tomography[22,93]
5 Heavy-ion mammography[14,105]
6 Magnetic resonance imaging (MRI) or nuclear magnetic resonance (NMR)[25,73,75]
7 Diaphanography or transillumination recording of the breast on infrared films[39,41a,83]

Breast x-rays,[40,106,117,118,120] despite their formerly publicized oncogenic risk[3,8] (which is now realized to be minimal if it exists at all with current low-dose techniques especially as related to mammography)[4] are the only aids that can detect any appreciable number of preclinical cancers. Mammography must be combined with a clinical examination since certain cancers cannot be detected by x-rays. It is also of paramount importance to never defer doing a biopsy of a clinically suspicious lesion because of a negative mammogram, since there may be false-negative mammograms.

Thermography is a risk indicator of considerable value[19] and may also be a worthwhile indicator of prognosis in breast cancer,[36] but its ability to detect occult cancers in the breast is practically nil and it cannot localize the area of concern for biopsy.

Ultrasonography[10,91,102] is valuable in differentiating cysts from solid lesions and as such is helpful in a combined use with mammography, although simple needle aspiration can be utilized to identify cysts easily.[56,58] Breast CT scanning,[22,93] heavy-ion mammography,[14,105] magnetic resonance imaging,[25,73,75] and diaphanography[39,41a,83] are still in the experimental stage.

OCCULT LESIONS

Finding Occult Lesions by Mammography

Biopsies are recommended for any of the following radiographic findings (Fig. 16-1):

1 Breast calcifications suspicious for malignancy because of their size (less than 2 mm), shape (punctate, microlinear, or branching), distribution (clustered, grouped, along ducts), or concentration (more than five calcifications per centimeter).

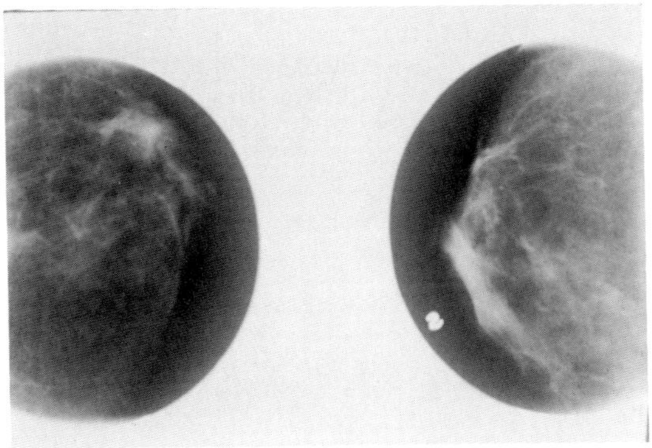

Figure 16-1 Cephalocaudal and lateral mammograms showing occult microcalcifications.

2 Stellate-shape breast masses.

3 Breast masses with ill-defined borders or nodular contours.

4 Dominant, well-circumscribed, smooth. masses which are larger than any other mass in the breast

5 Areas of increased tissue density or distorted breast architecture.[27,99] (See also Chap. 12.)

Biopsy of Occult Lesions

It is our opinion, as well as that of Shingelton,[101] that occult lesions are best biopsied under general anesthesia, after localization, as an inpatient, two-step procedure. These lesions are small and are usually best studied by multiple sections of permanently fixed material so that there is no room for doubt about the diagnosis. However, in a survey of hospitals Homer[50] found that a considerable number of surgeons did these under local anesthesia on an outpatient basis. Specimen radiography (x-ray of the tissue removed)[17] is always done to ensure that the area of concern is in the biopsy specimen; this area is then marked for the pathologist. Frozen sections should always be done if possible. This allows retrieval of nonfixed tissue to determine the status of estrogen and progesterone receptors if a cancer is found.

Preoperative localization of occult lesions can be done by obtaining specific measurements from the radiologist,[16] by tape grid radiopaque markers in numbers and figures,[30] by radiopaque dye injection just prior to surgery,[103] or by needle localization, which is the technique that we prefer.[21,62] Muhlow[79] and Taber and Dean[107] have reported on the use of a multiperforated plexiglass compression plate for needle localization.

Needle Localization

Needle localization can be done by utilizing regular $1\frac{1}{2}$-in to $3\frac{1}{2}$-in no. 22 gauge needles, or heavier needles if the breast tissue is dense. Needle length is based on the size of the breast and the depth of the lesion.[89] There are also hooked needles,[46] spring hooked needles,[54,76] flat-head needles,[53] and plastic needles with removable metal stylets such as the Longdwel Teflon needle.[52] Novak[82] has described a technique utilizing mammography control of needle aspiration biopsies for occult lesions. Homer,[50] in a questionnaire sent to 100 hospitals, reported that localizations were most commonly done either by dye injection or by needle localization, the latter being the most often used method.

Procedure We have utilized the simple method of needle localization with a no. 22 gauge needle, which was found to be easy, requiring no special equipment. After the patient has been prepared for biopsy, she is brought to the radiology department and craniocaudal and lateral mammograms are done. Previous films, if satisfactory, may also be used for this

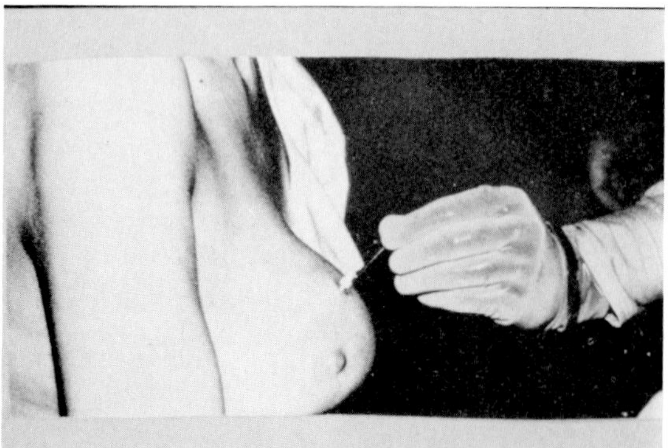

Figure 16-2 Needle insertion for localization.

purpose. Using nipple-to-lesion measurements in both views, a site on the skin surface that is in the same vertical and horizontal plane as the lesion can be determined. Feig and Schwartz[27] prefer to use an arc method of measurement in certain patients instead of a linear measurement; they use a compensation mammographic magnification compression technique as well. We have not found this necessary.

Using 1% lidocaine under aseptic technique, a disposable no. 22 gauge needle of appropriate length is inserted into the breast and directed toward the expected site of the lesion (see Figs. 16-2, 16-3). Mammograms are repeated in both directions to ascertain the position of the needle tip in relation to the lesion. If the needle tip is farther from the lesion than desired, then it is adjusted if only depth is involved; if this is not possible, a second needle, using the first as a guide, is put in and the mammogram repeated (Figs. 16-4, 16-5, 16-6). The needle is taped in place and the patient is given her preoperative medication and sent directly to the operating room. One would like to have the needle tip within 1 cm of the lesion.

The biopsy incision is made along the natural dynamic wrinkle lines of Kraissl,[55] which are concentric circles radiating out from the nipple and areola, in order to get the best possible cosmetic results. A small ellipse of skin is taken around the needle and the tissue is incised about

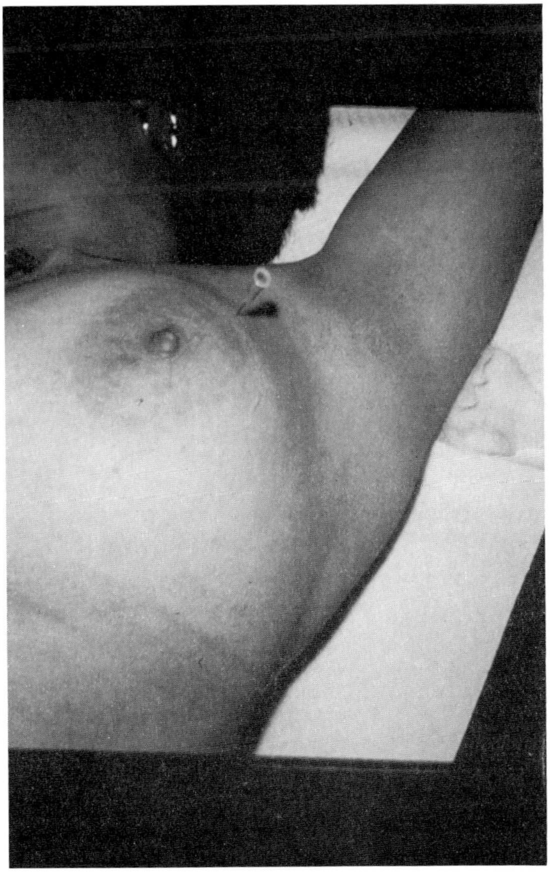

Figure 16-3 Needle in position.

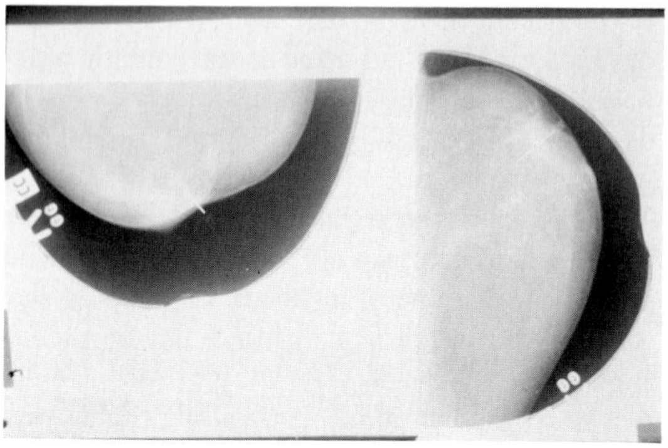

Figure 16-4 Cephalocaudal and lateral mammograms showing needle in position localizing area of microcalcifications.

the needle down to the area of the tip, where an adequate amount of tissue is removed to ensure that the area containing the occult lesion has been removed. Specimen radiography is then done and, if the area of concern is in the specimen, it is marked and taken to the pathologist.[17] If not, additional tissue is excised until the area of concern is removed (Figs. 16-7, 16-8).

Results Using this needle localization technique in a series of 387 patients with occult lesions, 239 (61.8 percent) were found to have benign lesions and 148 (38.2 percent) to have cancers. Of the cancers, 80 (54.1 percent) were invasive and 68 (45.9 percent) were noninvasive. Of these noninvasive cancers, 46 (76.6 percent) were noninvasive intraductular and 22 (32.4 percent) were lobular carcinoma in situ. Of the 239 benign lesions, 137 (57.3 percent) were fibrocystic disease without atypia, 56 (23.4 percent) were fibrocystic disease with atypia, 35 (14.7 percent) were fibroadenomas, 7 (2.9 percent) were intraductal papillomata, and 4 (1.7 percent) were intramammary nodes.

We have recently used a hook-wire needle,[46] which anchors in the region of the lesion and does away with the "backing out" that sometimes occurs with the plain no. 22 gauge needle. However, one disadvantage with this needle was found, inasmuch as the needle cannot be repositioned if it is not in the right location. Kopans and Meyer[54] and Meyer and Kopans[76] have developed a spring hook-wire needle to overcome the immediate anchoring of the plain hook-wire needle

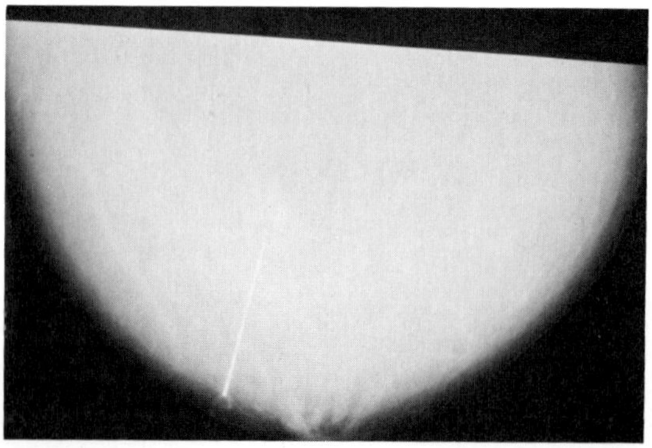

Figure 16-5 Cephalocaudal mammogram of solid occult tumor with needle localization.

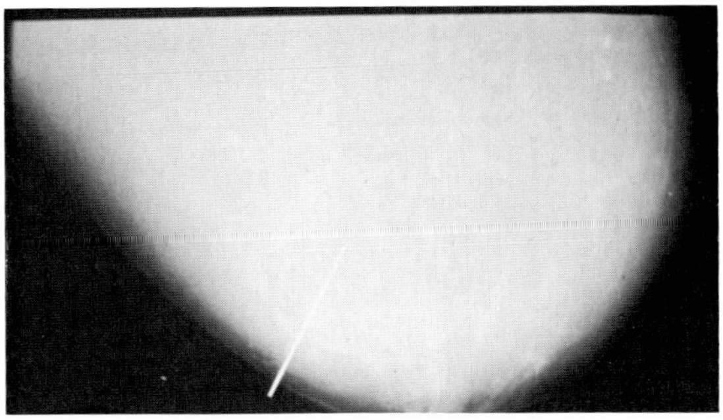

Figure 16-6 Lateral mammogram of solid occult tumor with needle localization.

after it is inserted, thus making repositioning possible.*

Incidence

Noninvasive cancers were considered to be rarities in the past, but they are much more common than is generally appreciated.[72] The American College of Surgeons conducted a national survey on this subject, which indicated an incidence rate of 1.4 percent.[98] In smaller collected series from specific centers, Nevin et al.[81] found that the incidence rates ranged from 5 to 10 percent. Farrow[26] credits noninvasive cancers as accounting for over 5 percent of all breast cancers. In our series, the percentage of noninvasive cancers was 7.4 percent.

Treatment of Occult Cancers

Once the clinically undetected lesion has been localized and a biopsy and histological examination[21,62] have indicated that there is a carcinoma, then a course of definitive therapy must be decided on.[57,59,61,64,67,68,71] Prognostic parameters should be available in order to make a proper choice as to the type of therapy needed.[15,60,65a,67]

No one form of therapy is applicable to or best for every patient with breast cancer.[48,49,59,70,108] Using prognostic parameters and a careful evaluation of the physical and mental status of the patient, the physician must select and tailor a form of therapy to fit each individual case.[15,60,65a,67] The primary goal must always be cure. Cosmetic appearance and functional results, while of serious import, must be subordinate to attempting to achieve a cure.

Concepts regarding the treatment of breast cancer have changed a great deal over the past decade.[63,64] Because of the well-known multicentricity of breast cancer,[34,97] a true cancer operation entails removal of all breast tissue; procedures such as segmental or partial mastectomies, where two-thirds to three-quarters of the breast is left behind, are unsatisfactory in our opinion. Likewise, subcutaneous mastectomies, where all the breast tissue cannot be removed, are also unsatisfactory.[67] It has been shown that even when radiotherapy is combined with limited surgery there are recurrences in breast tissue.[45,84] To rely on the hope that the removal of a primary focus of cancer (the tumor load) would stimulate immune competence, triggering an autoimmune mechanism allowing for the control of any pathologic breast tissue in the remainder of the ipsilateral breast or in the contralateral one is not a safe or logical conclusion.

Definition of Noninvasive Cancer

Noninvasive cancer, defined as cancer of the breast confined within the basement membrane in light microscopy, may be lobular carcinoma in situ arising from the epithelium of

*The needles are now commercially available through Cook, Inc., Box 489, Bloomington, Indiana.

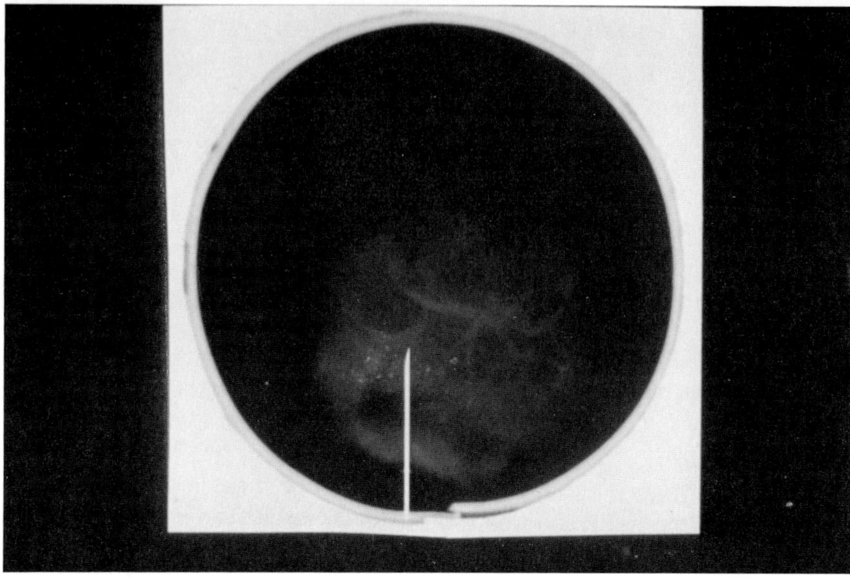

Figure 16-7 Specimen radiography of excised specimen showing area of microcalcifications with needle localization.

the lobules, or intraductal arising from ductal epithelium. The latter may be cribriform, intracystic, noninvasive Paget's, papillary, or solid (comedo).[114]

LOBULAR CARCINOMA IN SITU

Since Foote and Stewart[29] first described the entity of lobular carcinoma in situ in 1941, it has remained an enigma. There is some debate as to whether it is a true noninvasive cancer or a premalignant lesion. Reports as to its exact rates of incidence, multicentricity, bilaterality, and potential for invasive cancer transformation potential, as well as the time frame for this are at variance. Furthermore, there are several different procedures recommended for its treatment.

The time of onset of lobular carcinoma in situ is about 5 to 10 years before that of invasive breast cancer.[72] Since there is no lobular structure in the male breast, it only occurs in the female[26] unless there has been exogenous hormonal treatment. These lobular carcinomas in situ usually present without a mass and are most often discovered by histologic examination of the tissue removed around benign breast biopsies, random biopsies of the other breast, prophylactic mastectomies, and reduction mammoplasties. While they can be diagnosed by mammography, this is certainly not as common as it is in intraductal carcinomas where microcalcifications are frequently seen.

Most authorities feel that lobular carcinomas in situ are true noninvasive cancers, but Haagensen[42] classifies them as premalignant lesions and calls them *lobular neoplasias*, although admitting that they do have a substantial invasive malignant transformation potential in the same breast or the opposite one.

Incidence

In a series of 2227 mastectomies performed for patients with primary potentially curable breast cancers at the New York Medical College Affiliated Hospitals between 1950 and 1980,[67]

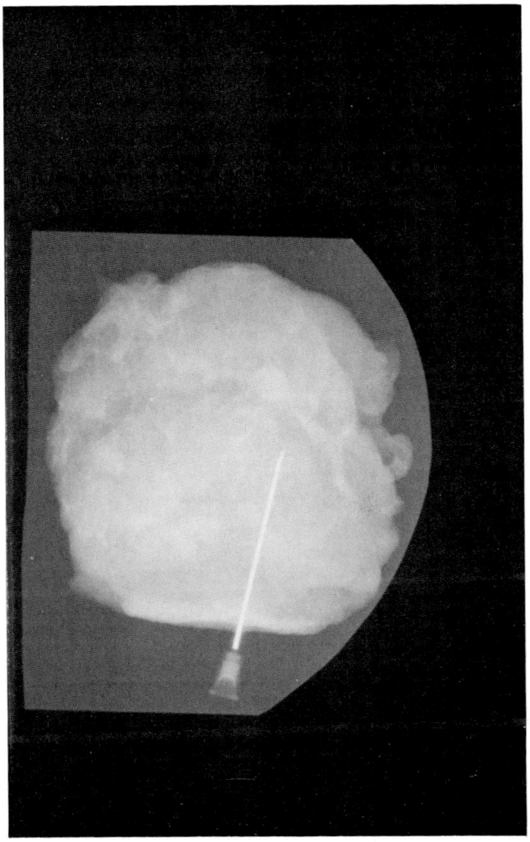

Figure 16-8 Specimen radiography of excised specimen showing solid occult lesion with needle localization.

1147 patients have been followed for 10 or more years. Of these, 157 (13.7 percent) were stage 0, preclinical cancers, smaller than 1 cm in size. This included invasive and noninvasive cancers. Eighty-five (7.4 percent) were noninvasive, of which 40 (47.1 percent) were lobular carcinomas in situ, and 45 (52.9 percent) were intraductal carcinomas.[67]

In a review of 403 noninvasive breast cancers reported by Farrow[26] in 1968 from the Memorial Sloan-Kettering Cancer Center and collected over a 16-year period, 197 (48.8 percent) were lobular carcinomas in situ, and 206 (51.2 percent) were noninvasive intraductal carcinomas.

Montague et al.[78] in 1983 reported on a series of 132 noninvasive cancers collected between 1948 and 1977 at the University of Texas Medical Center–M.D. Anderson Hospital. Forty-one (31.1 percent) were lobular carcinomas in situ, and 91 (68.9 percent) were intraductal carcinomas.

In our series, in which 148 cancers were found by mammography alone, 22 (32.4 percent) were lobular carcinomas in situ, and 46 (67.6 percent) were noninvasive intraductal carcinomas.

This seeming increase in the relative percentage of intraductal carcinomas as compared to lobular carcinomas in situ is probably due to the fact that intraductal carcinomas not uncommonly produce masses, while lobular carcinomas in situ do not. In addition, intraductal carcinomas are more easily recognized by mammography.

Lobular carcinomas in situ are probably multifocal in more than 30 percent of patients and bilateral in at least another 30 percent.[28,113] In a review of nearly 500 reported cases by Warner,[112] 70 percent were found to be multicentric and 35 to 59 percent were bilateral.

Invasive breast cancers will eventually develop over a 20-year period in about 30 to 40 percent of patients treated by excisional biopsy only, and nearly half of these will develop in the other breast.[95,96,113,115] The invasive transformation potential has been emphasized in studies by Gallager and Hutter,[33] and by Hutter and Foote.[51] In the former report, it is stated that when lobular carcinoma in situ is treated by local excision only, the long-term risk for ipsilateral invasive carcinoma is high—on the order of 50 percent within 22 years. Furthermore, within the same period some 30 percent of patients develop contralateral invasive carcinomas. It is of interest that some 70 percent of the invasive carcinomas found in patients with previous lobular carcinomas in situ were of the duct cell type.

McDivitt et al.[74] in a study of cumulative patient risk for the development of invasive carcinomas following only an excision of lobular carcinoma in situ calculated the risk at 5 years to be 8 percent, at 10 years to be 15 percent, at 15 years to be 22 percent, and at 20 years to be 35 percent.

Treatment

Treatment modalities for patients with lobular carcinomas in situ are at considerable variance. These include (1) simple to wide local excision,[2,42] (2) subcutaneous mastectomy,[32] (3) simple or total mastectomy with lower axillary node sampling and preferably with a random biopsy of the other breast,[96] (4) bilateral simple or total mastectomies with axillary node sampling,[13,57,59,64–67] and (5) conservative modified radical mastectomy.[108,111] Rarely is more extensive surgery done since lesser forms of treatment control the disease quite well. Because of the high incidence of bilaterality a random biopsy of the other breast should be done. We prefer doing bilateral total mastectomies with axillary node samplings followed by breast reconstructions.[61,104,119] We feel that this procedure offers the only truly safe guarantee and that it offers a good cosmetic appearance and functional results.

It would seem that those who recommend only follow-up after simple excisional biopsy[2,42] do so in the face of the information that there is at least a 33 percent risk that an invasive cancer will develop in the same or opposite breast. We also feel that subcutaneous mastectomy[32] is not an adequate answer, since all breast tissue cannot be removed with this technique. Simply doing a random biopsy of the other breast[96] is not adequate treatment, since cancer can develop in the breast tissue left behind and the random biopsy may not have removed an appropriate area of importance. On the other hand, doing a conservative modified radical mastectomy[108,111] for this lesion seems to be more surgery than is necessary. However, when doing a simple or total mastectomy, axillary node sampling should be done. Occasionally a focus of invasive cancer is found when multiple sections are done on the removed breast. Also, while rare, there can be nodal metastases at lower levels because of an unknown occult invasive cancer.

INTRADUCTAL CARCINOMA

The other type of noninvasive carcinoma, intraductal, has different subtypes and differs from lobular carcinoma in situ in other aspects. Unlike lobular carcinoma in situ, this lesion often presents with a mass but it may only be picked up by an abnormal mammogram with no clinical findings whatsoever or by nipple symptoms.[6,18,114]

Incidence

The incidence of intraductal carcinoma was found to be 52.9 percent of 85 noninvasive cancers.[67] In the 403 noninvasive cancers collected by Farrow,[26] 51.2 percent were noninvasive intraductal carcinomas. Montague et al.[78] in their 132 noninvasive cancers reported 68.9 percent of them to be intraductal carcinomas. With respect to our needle localization series of occult cancers found by mammography alone, there were 68 noninvasive cancers, of which 67.6 percent were intraductal carcinomas. The increasing use of mammography is responsible for finding a larger number of these occult lesions because of the characteristic punctate microcalcifications they often display.

Intraductal carcinomas are multicentric in over 30 percent of patients.[6,18,114] Von Rueden and Wilson[110] reported an incidence rate of multicentricity from several series of 30 to 38 percent. There seems to be general agreement that bilaterality is not as common as it is in lobular carcinoma in situ, but von Rueden and Wilson[110] reported that its incidence of bilaterality approached 15 percent.

Treatment

There are not too many reports in the literature concerning noninvasive intraductal carcinomas treated by biopsy only and the percentages of invasive cancers developing in these patients. Page et al.,[85] in a review of 11,760 breast biopsies, found that in those patients with intraductal carcinomas who were treated by biopsy only, 28 percent developed invasive breast cancers within 10 years in the ipsilateral breast. Westbrook[113] feels that probably 30 to 40 percent of patients treated by biopsy only will develop invasive duct cell carcinoma of the ipsilateral breast within 10 years.

Since intraductal carcinomas are commonly multicentric but infrequently bilateral, we advise a simple or total mastectomy with axillary node sampling. We do not advise a contralateral mastectomy as in lobular carcinoma in situ, but we do advise a random biopsy of the other breast. Breast reconstruction is also recommended with appropriate management of the other breast for symmetry if it is large or ptotic.[61,104,119] We prefer this to simple excision, to subcutaneous mastectomy, and to conservative modified radical mastectomy, although we do not object to a limited lower axillary dissection.[67]

Radiation Therapy

Despite the paucity of information concerning the treatment of these cancers with primary radiotherapy, there are a few publications from which some inferences can be drawn. Connolly et al.[24] noted a significantly higher risk of local failures in patients receiving primary radiotherapy after excision of an invasive tumor if there were areas of noninvasive carcinomas adjacent to the primary invasive tumor than for those patients in which noninvasive cancers were absent in tissue adjacent to the invasive tumor. This would raise the possibility of the lack of destruction of these noninvasive carcinomas by radiotherapy and open to question whether one should use simple excision and primary radiotherapy as a treatment for noninvasive cancers. It must be recalled that both lobular carcinoma in situ and intraductal carcinoma are known to be very multicentric.[113]

Montague et al.,[78] however, reported on a small number of noninvasive breast cancers treated by radiotherapy in which the results were good. They did admit that, at the time of their report, theirs was the only reported series that they were aware of, listing the results of such treatment. Between 1958 and 1977, 132 patients (2 of which were dropped from the report because they only had local excisions) who had noninvasive carcinomas, either lobular in situ or intraductal, were treated by two modes of therapy. Patients in group 1 were treated by surgery alone. These 101 patients had either simple mastectomy or modified radical mastectomy. The remaining 29 patients in group 2 received excision and irradiation. The irradiation was given only to the breast for patients with lobular carcinoma in situ, and to the breast and axilla for those with intraductal carcinomas. They reported a 100-percent free-of-disease, 10-year survival rate for these patients. There was only one recurrence in the breast in this group, which was subsequently managed by mastectomy. They further reported that there was no statistical difference in the 10-year survival rates of the 101 patients treated by mastectomies as compared to the 29 treated by primary radiotherapy.

Since the series ran from 1958 through 1977 the question must be raised as to whether all cases had at least a 10-year follow-up. Ten years would not be adequate to evaluate patients with lobular carcinomas in situ who were treated by any other method other than total removal of the breast. Patients treated by simple excision alone continue to develop invasive cancers over a 20-plus year period.[74] In addition, a significant number of local-regional recurrences after treatment with radiotherapy do not occur for prolonged periods.[45,84]

Finally, the recurrences with radiotherapy are more frequent in patients with multicentric cancers,which is a well-known characteristic of both lobular carcinoma in situ and intraductal carcinoma.[114] Montague et al.[78] did emphasize the need for the collection of data from a larger series of patients over a long period of time in order to confirm the results reported in their small series. Recently, Fisher et al.[28a] reported good results with lumpectomy and radiation for patients with intraductal carcinomas but there was only a 39-month average follow-up.

MANAGEMENT OF SMALL INVASIVE CANCERS

We advise a modified radical mastectomy with preservation of both pectoral muscles and removal of the axillary nodes lateral to the border of the pectoralis minor muscle.[67] A random biopsy of the other breast is also advised.[65,66] If the invasive cancer is larger than 1 cm but not palpable clinically, then appropriate surgery is advised based on prognostic parameters.[60,67] The operations most commonly used are the conservative modified radical mastectomy with removal of the second or pectoral level of nodes if indicated, or the full modified radical mastectomy with removal of all the structures, as in the classical radical mastectomy except for the pectoralis major muscle. Radical mastectomies are seldom used.[67] Again, if possible, a random biopsy of the other breast is done.[65,66] If the cancer is close to the chest wall a portion of the pectoralis major muscle is removed.[67]

In our series of 561 random biopsies of the other breast in which there were no adverse clinical or mammogram findings, 7.3 percent unsuspected occult carcinomas were found. In addition, another 15.8 percent of patients showed histologic atypia for a combined figure of 21.4 percent.[66] The reported yield of cancers from random biopsies ranges from 4.5 to 12.5 percent. The rate of detection seems to correlate with the diligence of the examining pathologist and the size of the specimen. It will also depend on whether or not areas of clinical or mammographic changes are excluded, in order to have a true random biopsy.[65,66]

As to prophylactic contralateral simple mastectomies in patients with a high risk for having cancer develop in the second breast,[65,66] we have performed 127 with a yield of 19.7 percent unsuspected occult carcinomas. Another 22 percent of patients showed histologic atypia for a combined yield of 41.7 percent in patients who had no clinical or mammogram adverse findings in the other breast.[65,66]

Primary Radiotherapy

Primary radiotherapy[1,7,9,12,20,23] is being tried as an alternative to mastectomy in a number of centers throughout the world for early invasive cancers, both clinically detectable and occult.[38,41,44,45,70,77,78,84,86,87,90,92,94,109,116]

It must be preceded by limited surgery ranging from tumorectomy to tylectomy to segmental mastectomy, with or without axillary node sampling or full dissection. When segmental mastectomy is combined with a complete axillary dissection,[109] there can be some deformity, often aggravated by the added radiotherapy.

The time period for therapy is rather long, requiring treatments daily for 5 days a week over a period of about 6 to 8 weeks. Adequate dosage of at least 6000 rads and careful techniques are currently being recommended as being of vital importance, as are booster doses of radiation to the tumor area of about 2000 rads using interstitial radioactive implants or an external beam of radiation.

Results

Reports of end results are at considerable variance. Some[44,70,90,109] indicate that survival and recurrence rates are on a par with those obtained by mastectomies in patients with early breast cancers that are not multicentric. However, actuarial rather than crude or absolute survival rates are often used, making for better survival statistics. In some reports, the number of patients with long-term follow-ups is too small for statistical evaluation.

Current reports[41,45,84] regarding primary radiotherapy indicate that a significant proportion of local-regional recurrences do not occur for prolonged periods of time after therapy, unlike those after mastectomies in which about 85 percent of local recurrences are identified within 5 years.[41] The percentage of local recurrences is also higher than with mastectomies.[41,45,84]

Goodson[41] reported that radiation therapy does lengthen the time interval before local recurrences, but it does not reduce the incidence, which is higher than it is in patients treated by mastectomies. After mastectomy he noted that 85 percent of local recurrences are identified within 5 years. In contrast, French and Canadian data show that, after radiation therapy, only 50 to 66 percent are identified at 5 years.

Harris et al.,[45] in a 15-year follow-up of 152 patients treated by primary radiotherapy for early breast cancers (T_1 and T_2 lesions, with the majority being T_1 and with 145 patients having negative nodes), reported a crude 15-year local recurrence rate of 22 percent. Of 30 patients who developed an isolated local recurrence and who had a secondary mastectomy, the 10-year freedom from disease relapse rate was 50 percent.

In a study of 263 patients by Osborne et al.[84] with unilateral primary breast cancer treated by local excision of the tumor and radiotherapy, the local-regional recurrence rate was 22 percent at 10 years for those patients with T_1 or T_2, N_0 or N_{1a} lesions, and 52 percent for those with T_1 and T_2, N_{1b} tumors. Salvage mastectomy for radiation failure produced only a 42 percent crude-relapse-free, 5-year survival rate.

In order to determine if primary radiotherapy with adequate radiation is a justifiable alternative to selective mastectomies followed by reconstructions, its efficacy and safety must be evaluated by statistics derived from a large collected series of patients, with detailed prognostic parameters available for evaluation.[41] The end results reported must be on a basis of at least 10 or more years and should include (1) crude or absolute survival rates, with no evidence of disease; (2) local and regional recurrences; (3) percentages of required secondary mastectomies because of radiation failures; (4) cosmetic and functional results; (5) complications both local and regional, including the effects of spray radiation on the opposite breast;[41] and (6) the numbers and types of radiation-induced cancers over a 20-to-30-year period.

Complications

Complications now are less with supervoltage radiotherapy than they were with kilovoltage, but they occur and some are not manifested for many years. Complications include (1) breast atrophy; (2) fibrotic bands and thickening of the breast; (3) lung damage; (4) supraclavicular thickening; (5) telangiectasis; (6) pigmentation changes; (7) severe radiation dermatitis, even ulcers, breast, and arm swelling (edema); and (8) various types of bone and joint damage, especially rib fractures. Supervoltage therapy has also resulted in some additional subtle changes which occur at later dates that were not seen with kilovoltage, including damage to nerves, especially the brachial plexus, to large blood vessels, and to the myocardium. Finally, there is the inherent risk of spray radiation to the opposite breast, and of radiation-induced cancers at a later date, which cannot be evaluated for many years.

It must also be noted that certain patients with breast cancers are not good candidates for primary radiotherapy. These include patients with small breasts, those with tumors located in the upper inner quadrant or central area of the breast, those with relatively large tumors, and those with multicentric tumors.

PROGNOSIS FOR PRECLINICAL CANCERS

Gallager and Martin[34,35] predicted, after defining minimal breast cancers, that cure rates with conventional treatment modalities would exceed 90 percent at 10 years. Subsequent clinical investigations by Frazier et al.[31] and by Peters et al.[88] have shown that 10-year survival rates of 90 to 96 percent are in fact obtained.

Wanebo, Huvos, and Urban,[111] with their more liberal meaning reported on 162 patients treated by modified radical mastectomies in which the absolute or crude survival rate, free of disease, was 93 of 95 patients (98 percent) at 5 years and 42 of 49 patients (95 percent) at 10 years.

Leis and Cammarata[67] reported a series of 157 patients with stage 0, preclinical cancers, both invasive and noninvasive, which were smaller than 1 cm. The absolute (no evidence of disease) 10-year survival rate was 151 of 157 patients (96.2 percent). It was 84 of 85 patients (98.8 percent) with noninvasive cancers, and 67 of 72 patients (93.1 percent) with invasive cancers. Patients with noninvasive cancers were treated by total mastectomies and axillary node sampling, and those with invasive cancers by conservative modified radical mastectomies. There were no local recurrences.

This emphasizes the importance of early preclinical diagnosis of breast cancers. It is very impressive when compared to the 10-year absolute, no-evidence-of-disease survival rates reported by the same authors[67] for stage I and stage II cancers. These were 403 of 552 patients (73 percent) with stage I cancers, and 189 of 438 patients (43.1 percent) with stage II cancers.

CONCLUSION

The esthetic value of the breasts and the variance in therapy recommendations for patients with breast cancers, especially for those with cancers that cannot be clinically detected, make it mandatory for the physician to discuss in detail the different therapeutic modalities available with patients and also their families if possible, so that patients can make an intelligent, informed decision concerning their therapy.[68]

The physician must recommend the procedure that he or she feels is best suited for the individual patient. For a proper informed consent he or she must cover a number of necessary disclosures, such as (1) the clinical diagnosis and the various methods of biopsy used in determining the exact diagnosis; (2) the probable prognosis without any definitive therapy and with various forms of therapy; (3) the nature of these various therapeutic modalities; and (4) the possible complications, risks, and results related to these different types of treatment.[68]

REFERENCES

1. Alpert AB, Ghossein NA, Stacey P, et al: Primary management of operable breast cancer by minimal surgery and radiotherapy. *Cancer* 42:2054, 1978.
2. Anderson JA: Lobular carcinoma in situ: A long-term follow-up in 52 cases. *Acta Pathol Microbiol Scand* 82:519, 1974.
3. Advisory Committee on the Biological Effects of Ionizing Radiations, National Academy of Sciences—National Research Council, Division of Medical Science, 1972.
4. American Cancer Society, National Task Force on Breast Cancer Control: Recommendations of the National Advisory Committee on cancer detection regarding breast cancer detection in asymptomatic women. American Cancer Society, Inc., New York, 1983.
5. American Cancer Society: *Cancer Facts and Figures 1984*. American Cancer Society, Inc., New York, 1984.
6. Ashikari R, Huvos A, Snyder RE: Prospective study of non-infiltrating carcinomas of the breast. *Cancer* 39:435, 1977.
7. Atkins H, Hayward JL, Klugman DJ, et al: Treatment of early breast cancer: A report after ten years of clinical trial. *Br Med J* 2:423, 1972.
8. Bailer JC: Mammography: A contrary view, *Ann Intern Med* 84:77, 1976.
9. Bataini JP, Picco C, Martin M, et al: Relationship between time-dose and local control of operable breast cancer treated by tumorectomy and radiotherapy or by radical radiotherapy alone. *Cancer* 42:2059, 1978.
10. Baum G: Ultrasound mammography. *Radiology* 122:199, 1977.
11. Bears OH, Shapiro S, Smart C: Report of the working group to review the National Cancer Institute—American Cancer Society Breast Cancer Detection Project. *J Natl Cancer Inst* 62:640, 1979.
12. Bedwinek JM, Brady L, Perez CA, et al: Irradiation as the primary management of stages I and II adenocarcinoma of the breast. Analysis of the RTOG Breast Registry. *Cancer Clin Trials* 3:11, 1980.
13. Benfield JR, Fingerhut AG, Warner NE: Lobular carcinoma of the breast. *Arch Surg* 99:129, 1969.
14. Benton EV, Henke RP, Tobias CA: Heavy particle radiography. *Science* 182: 474, 1973.
15. Berg JW, Robbins GF: Factors influencing short and long term survival of breast cancer patients. *Surg Gynecol Obst* 122:1311, 1966.
16. Berger SM, Curcio BM, Gershon-Cohen J, et al: Mammographic localization of unsuspected breast cancer. *Am J Roentgenol* 96:1046, 1966.
17. Bremond A, Frappart AB: Radiography of the excised tissue in breast surgery. *Int J Breast Mammary Pathol (Senolgia)* 1:281, 1982.
18. Brown PW, Silverman J, Owens E, et al: Intraductal non-infiltrating cancer of the breast. *Arch Surg* 111:1063, 1976.
19. Byrne, R: Utilization of thermography as a risk indicator in breast cancer. *Breast, Diseases of the Breast* 2:43, 1976.
20. Calle R, Pilleron JP, Schlienger P et al: Conservative management of operable breast cancer by primary radiotherapy. *Cancer* 42:2045, 1978.
21. Cammarata A, Rosen PP, Leis HP Jr: Breast biopsy, surgical aspects, role of frozen section and specimen radiography, in (eds) Gallager HS, Leis HP Jr, Snyderman RK, Urban JA, *The Breast*. St. Louis, C.V. Mosby Co., 1978.
22. Chang CH, Sibala JL, Fritz SL, et al: Computed tomography in detection and diagnosis of breast cancer. *Cancer* 46:939, 1980.
23. Cohen AM: Time for a balanced approach to the local treatment of operable carcinoma of the breast. *Surg Gynecol Obstet* 150:891, 1980.
24. Connolly JL, Schnitt SJ, Harris JR, et al: Pathologic correlates of local tumor control following primary radiation therapy in patients with early breast cancer, in Harris JR, Hellman S, Silen W (eds), *Conservative Management of Breast Cancer*. Philadelphia, J. P. Lippincott, Co., 1983.
25. Damadian R: Tumor detection by nuclear magnetic resonance. *Science* 171:1151, 1971.
26. Farrow JH: Clinical considerations and treatment of in-situ lobular breast cancer. *J Roentgenol Radium Therapy Nucl Med* 102:652, 1968.
27. Feig SA, Schwartz GF: Radiologic technique for biopsy of non-palpable breast lesions, in Feig S A, McLelland R (eds): *Breast Carcinoma: Current Diagnosis and Treatment*. New York, Masson Publishing, USA, Inc., 1983.

28. Fisher ER, Fisher B: Lobular carcinoma of the breast; An overview. *Ann Surg* 185:377, 1977.
28a. Fisher ER, Sass R, Fisher B, et al: Pathologic findings from the National Surgical Adjuvant Breast Project (Protocol 6) 1. Intraductal carcinoma (DCIS). *Cancer* 57:197, 1986.
29. Foote FW Jr, Stewart FW: Lobular carcinoma in-situ. *Am J Pathol* 17:491, 1941.
30. Frankel G, Rosenfeld DD: Xeroradiographic detection of occult breast cancer. *Cancer* 35:542, 1975.
31. Frazier TG, Copeland EM, Gallagher HS, et al: Prognosis and treatment in minimal breast cancer. *Am J Surg* 132:697, 1977.
32. Freeman BS: Technique of subcutaneous mastectomy with replacement. *Br J Plast Surg* 22:161, 1969.
33. Gallager HS, Hutter RVP: Pathology and pathogenesis of breast cancer, in Gallager HS, Leis HP Jr, Snyderman RK, Urban JA (eds): *The Breast.* St. Louis, C.V. Mosby Co., 1978.
34. Gallager HS, Martin JE: The study of mammary carcinoma by correlated mammography and subserial whole organ sectioning. *Cancer* 23:855, 1969.
35. Gallager HS, Martin JE: An orientation to the concept of minimal breast cancer. *Cancer* 28:1505, 1971.
36. Gautherie M, Gros CM: Breast thermography and cancer risk prediction. *Cancer* 45:51, 1980.
37. Gershon-Cohen J, Berger SM, Klickstein HS: Roentgenography of breast cancer moderating concept of "Biologic Predeterminism." *Cancer* 16:961, 1963.
38. Ghossein NA, Vilcog JR, Stacey P, et al: Conservative surgery and radiotherapy in the treatment of localized breast cancer. A retrograde analysis, in Vaeth J M (ed): *Frontiers of Radiation Therapy and Oncology.* Basel, Switzerland, S. Karger, Publisher, vol. 17, 1983.
39. Girolamo RF, Leis HP Jr: Diaphanography: A fourth dimension in the diagnosis of breast cancer? *Breast, Diseases of the Breast* 8:16, 1982.
40. Gold RH, Bassett LW: Mammography: History and state of the art, in Feig SA, McLelland R (eds): *Breast Carcinoma: Current Diagnosis and Treatment.* New York, Masson Publishing, Inc., USA, 1983.
41. Goodson WH III: The next big question in the treatment of carcinoma of the breast. *Surg Gynecol Obstet* 156:795, 1983.
41a. Greene FL, Hicks C, Eddy V, et al: Mammography, sonomammography and diaphanography. *Am Surg* 51:59, 1985.
42. Haagensen CD: *Diseases of the Breast.* Philadelphia, W. B. Saunders, Co., 1971.
43. Halsted WS: The results of radical operation for the cure of cancer of the breast. *Ann Surg* 46:80, 1907.
44. Harris JR, Hellman S: The results of primary radiotherapy for early breast cancer at the Joint Center for Radiation Therapy, in Harris JR, Hellman S, Silen W (eds): *Conservative Management of Breast Cancer.* Philadelphia, J. B. Lippincott, 1983.
45. Harris JR, Recht A, Amalric R, et al: Time course and prognosis of local recurrence following primary radiation therapy for early breast cancer. *J Clin Oncology* 2:37, 1984.
46. Hoen JL, Williams GH: Localization of nonpalpable breast lesions. *Breast, Diseases of the Breast* 5:28, 1979.
47. Holland R, Hendriks JHCL, Mravunac M: Mammographically occult breast cancer: A pathologic and radiologic study. *Cancer* 52:1810, 1983.
48. Hermann RE: Selective conservative operations for cancer of the breast. *Breast, Diseases of the Breast* 2:41, 1976.
49. Hermann RE, Esselstyn CB, Crile G Jr: Conservative surgical treatment of potentially curable breast cancer, in Gallager HS, Leis HP Jr, Snyderman RK, Urban JA (eds): *The Breast.* St. Louis, C. V. Mosby Co., 1978.
50. Homer MJ: Localization of nonpalpable breast lesions: State of the art. *Int J Breast Mammary Pathol (Senolgia)* 1:215, 1982.
51. Hutter RVP, Foote FW: Lobular carcinoma in situ: Long term follow-up. *Cancer* 24:1081, 1969.
52. Inlow PM: Localization of occult breast cancer. *Appl Radiol* 1:91, 1979.
53. Kalisher L: An improved needle for localization of nonpalpable breast lesions. *Radiology* 128:815, 1978.
54. Kopans CB, Meyer JE: Versatile spring hookwire breast lesion localizer. *Am J Radiol* 138:586, 1982.

55. Kraissl CJ: The selection of appropriate lines for elective surgical incisions. *Plast Reconstr Surg* 8:1, 1951.
56. Leis HP Jr: *Diagnosis and Treatment of Breast Lesions*. Flushing, New York, Medical Examination Publishing Co., Inc., 1970.
57. Leis HP Jr: Minimal breast cancer. *Mod Med* 75:58, 1975.
58. Leis HP Jr: The diagnosis of breast cancer. *CA* 27:209, 1977.
59. Leis HP Jr: Selective moderate surgical approach for potentially curable breast cancer, in Gallager HS, Leis HP Jr, Snyderman RK, Urban JA (eds): *The Breast*. St. Louis, C. V. Mosby Co., 1978.
60. Leis HP Jr: Criteria and standards for evaluation of treatment results, in Gallager HS, Leis HP Jr, Snyderman RK, Urban JA (eds): *The Breast*. St. Louis, C. V. Mosby Co., 1978.
61. Leis HP Jr: Selective and reconstructive surgical procedures for cancer of the breast. *Surg Gynecol Obstet* 148:17, 1979.
62. Leis HP Jr: Breast biopsy: Indications and techniques. *Breast, Diseases of the Breast* 6:2, 1980.
63. Leis HP Jr: Current trends in breast cancer surgery in the United States and Canada. *Int Surg* 65:3, 1980.
64. Leis HP Jr: The surgeon's role in breast cancer: Changing concepts. *Breast Cancer Research and Treatment* 1:5, 1981.
65. Leis HP Jr: Managing the remaining breast. *Cancer* 46:1068, 1980.
65a. Leis HP Jr: Prognosis in breast cancer, in Strombeck JO, Rosato FE (eds): *Surgery of the Breast*. Stuttgart and New York, Georg Theime Verlag, 1986.
66. Leis HP Jr, Cammarata A, LaRaja R, Reed L, Cleary J, Makoon S: Bilateral breast cancer. *Breast, Diseases of the Breast* 7:13, 1981.
67. Leis HP Jr, Cammarata A: Modified radical mastectomy: The moderate selective surgical approach, in Feig Sa, McLelland R (eds): *Breast Carcinoma: Current Diagnosis and Treatment*. New York, Masson Publishing, USA, Inc., 1983.
68. Leis HP Jr, Cammarata A, LaRaja R: Informed consent in breast surgery. *Breast, Diseases of the Breast* 10:2, 1984.
69. Leis HP Jr, Urban JA, Snyderman RK: Management of potentially malignant breast lesions, in Gallager HS, Leis HP Jr, Snyderman RK, Urban JA (eds): *The Breast*. St. Louis, C. V. Mosby Co., 1978.
70. Leslie NT, Harris JR, Hellman S: The current status of radiotherapy in the treatment of early breast cancer. *Breast Cancer Research and Treatment* 2:213, 1982.
71. Letton AH, Mason EM: The treatment of nonpalpable carcinoma of the breast. *Cancer* 46:980, 1980.
72. Lewison EF, Finney GG: Lobular carcinoma in-situ of the breast. *Surg Gynecol Obstet* 126:1280, 1968.
73. Mansfield P, Morris PG, Ordidge R, et al: Carcinoma of the breast imaged by nuclear magnetic resonance (NMR). *Br J Radiol* 52:242, 1979.
74. McDivitt RW, Hutter RVP, Foote FW Jr, et al: In-situ lobular carcinoma: A prospective follow-up study indicating cumulative patient risks. *JAMA* 201:82, 1967.
75. Medina D: Nuclear magnetic resonance studies on human breast dysplasia and neoplasms. *J Natl Cancer Inst* 54:813, 1975.
76. Meyer JE, Kopans DB: Preoperative roentgenographically guided percutaneous localization of occult breast lesions. *Arch Surg* 117:65, 1982.
77. Montague E: Radiotherapy as primary modality in treatment of curable breast cancer, in Gallager HS, Leis HP Jr, Snyderman RK, Urban JA (eds): *The Breast*. St. Louis, C. V. Mosby Co., 1978.
78. Montague E, Spanos WJ Jr, Ames FC, et al: Conservative treatment of noninvasive and small-volume invasive breast cancer, in Feig SA, McLelland R (eds): *Breast Cancer: Current Diagnosis and Treatment*. New York, Masson Publishing, USA, Inc., 1983.
79. Muhlow A: A device for precision needle biopsy of the breast at mammography. *Am J Roentgenol* 121:843, 1974.
80. National Cancer Institute: Consensus Development Meeting on Breast Cancer Screening, Bethesda, Maryland, 1977.
81. Nevin JF, Pinzon G, Morgan TJ, et al: Minimal breast cancer. *Am J Surg* 1339:357, 1980.
82. Novak R: Position controlled needle aspiration biopsy mammography. *Fortschr Geb Roentgenstr Nukleamed* 131:659, 1979.

83. Ohlsson B, Gunderson J, Nilsson DM: Diaphanography: A method for evaluation of the female breast. *World J Surg* 14:701, 1980.
84. Osborne MP, Ormiston N, Harmer CL, et al: Breast conservation in the treatment of early breast cancer. *Cancer* 53:349, 1984.
85. Page DL, Dupont WD, Rogers LW, et al: Intraductal carcinoma of the breast: Follow-up after biopsy only. *Cancer* 49:751, 1982.
86. Pantoja E, Frede T, Kunchala S: Complications of postoperative radiation in breast cancer. *J Breast, Diseases of the Breast* 4:4, 1979.
87. Peters V: Wedge resection with or without radiation in early breast cancer. *Int J Radiol Oncol Biol Phys* 6:17, 1980.
88. Peters TG, Donegan WL, Burg EA: Minimal breast cancer: A clinical appraisal. *Ann Surg* 186: 704, 1977.
89. Peysta RG: Needle localization of nonpalpable lesions of the breast. *Surg Gynecol Obstet* 148:703, 1979.
90. Pierquin B: Conservative treatment of carcinoma of the breast: Experience of Creteil—ten year results, in Harris JR, Hellman S, Silen W (eds): *Conservative Management of Breast Cancer.* Philadelphia, J. B. Lippincott, 1983.
91. Pluygers E, Rombaut M: Ultrasonic diagnosis of breast diseases. *Tumor Diagn* 4:187, 1980.
92. Prosnitz LR, Goldenberg IS, Packard RA, et al: Radiation therapy as initial treatment for early stage cancer of the breast without mastectomy. *Cancer* 39:917, 1977.
93. Reese DF, Carney JA, Gisvald JJ, et al: Computerized reconstructive tomography applied to breast pathology. *Am J Roentgenol* 126:406, 1976.
94. Rissanen PM: Comparison of conservative and radical surgery combined with radiotherapy in the treatment of stage I carcinoma of the breast. *Br J Radiol* 42:423, 1969.
95. Rosen PP, Braun DW Jr, Kinne DE: The clinical significance of pre-invasive breast cancer. *Cancer* 46:919, 1980.
96. Rosen PP, Braun DW, Lyngholms B, et al: Lobular carcinoma in situ of the breast: Preliminary results and treatment by ipsilateral mastectomy and contralateral breast biopsy. *Cancer* 47:813, 1981.
97. Rosen PP, Frachia AA, Urban JA, et al: "Residual" mammary carcinoma following simulated partial mastectomy. *Cancer* 35:739, 1975.
98. Rosner D, Ramez B, Vana J, et al: Non-invasive breast carcinoma: Results of a national survey by the American College of Surgeons. *Ann Surg* 192:139, 1980.
99. Schwartz GF, Feig SA, Patchefsky AS: Clinicopathologic correlation and significance of clinically occult mammary lesions. *Cancer* 41:1147, 1978.
100. Shapiro S, Strax P, Venet L, et al: Change in 5 year breast cancer mortality in breast cancer screening program, in Proceedings of the 7th National Cancer Conference, Philadelphia, J. B. Lippincott, Co., 1973.
101. Shingelton WW: Breast biopsy techniques, in Feig SA, McLelland R (eds): *Breast Carcinoma: Current Diagnosis and Treatment.* New York, Masson Publishing, USA, Inc., 1983.
102. Sickles E, Filly RA, Callen PW: Breast ultrasonography, in Feig SA, McLelland R (eds): *Breast Carcinoma: Current Diagnosis and Treatment.* New York, Masson Publishing, USA, Inc., 1983.
103. Simon N, Lesnick GI, Luer WN, et al: Roentgenographic localization of small lesions of the breast by spot method. *Surg Gynecol Obstet* 134:572, 1971.
104. Snyderman RK: Breast reconstruction today. *Breast Cancer Research and Treatment* 3:5, 1983.
105. Sommer FG, Capp MP, Tobias CA, et al: Heavy-ion radiography: Density resolution and specimen radiography. *Invest Radiol* 13:163, 1978.
106. Strax P: Screening for breast cancer: Role of the primary physician, in Gallager HS, Leis HP Jr, Snyderman RK, Urban JA (eds): *The Breast.* St. Louis, C. V. Mosby Co., 1978.
107. Taber L, Dean PB: Interventional radiologic procedure in the investigation of lesions of the breast. *Radiol Clin North Am* XVII, 1979.
108. Urban JA: Selective radical surgical treatment for primary breast cancer, in Gallager HS, Leis HP Jr, Snyderman RK, Urban JA (eds): *The Breast.* St. Louis, C. V. Mosby Co., 1978.
109. Veronesi U, DelVecchio M, Greco M, et al: Results of quadranectomy, axillary dissection and radiotherapy (QUART), in TINO patients in conservative management of breast cancer, in Harris J, Hellman S, Silen W (eds): *Conservative*

Management of Breast Cancer. Philadelphia, J. B. Lippincott, 1983.

110. von Rueden DG, Wilson RE: Intraductal carcinoma of the breast. *Surg Gynecol Obstet* 158:105, 1984.
111. Wanebo HJ, Huvos AG, Urban JA: Treatment of minimal breast cancer. *Cancer* 349, 1974.
112. Warner NE: Lobular carcinoma of the breast. *Cancer* 2:840, 1969.
113. Westbrook KC: Management of noninvasive carcinoma of the breast, in *Postgraduate Manual, Course No, 10*, 68th Annual Clinical Congress, American College of Surgeons, Chicago, 1982.
114. Westbrook KC, Gallager HS: Intraductal carcinoma of the breast, a comparative study. *Am J Surg* 130:667, 1975.
115. Wheeler J, Enterline H, Roseman J: Lobular carcinoma in-situ of the breast: Long term follow-up. *Cancer*. 34:554, 1974.
116. Wisenberg JJ: Carcinoma of the breast. *Surg Gynecol Obstet* 142:321, 1979.
117. Wolf JN: Risk for breast cancer development determined by mammography parenchymal patterns. *Cancer* 37:2486, 1976.
118. Wolf JN: Xeroradiography of the breast, in Gallager HS, Leis HP Jr, Snyderman RK, Urban JA (eds): *The Breast*. St. Lous, C. V. Mosby Co., 1978.
119. Woods JE: Breast reconstruction after mastectomy. *Surg Gynecol Obstet* 150:869, 1980.
120. Zuckerman HC: Mammography in diseases of the breast, in Gallager HS, Leis HP Jr, Snyderman RK, Urban JA (eds): *The Breast*. St. Louis, C. V. Mosby Co., 1978.

17

Breast-Preserving Operations

Mary Ann Tinker, M.D.
Leslie Wise, M.D.

INTRODUCTION

In spite of all the alternatives in the surgical management of breast cancer, the mortality rates (deaths/100,000 population) have not changed significantly in the the past 50 years. For 1978 through 1979, the age-adjusted breast cancer death rate in the United States was 27.1 per 100,000 population.[8] Variations in surgery and/or radiotherapy have failed to have a significant impact on the mortality rates.

While there has been a slight improvement in the relative 5-year survival rate in the past three decades,[8] when patients are compared stage for stage, this must be viewed with caution in light of the continuing stability of the mortality rates. The improvement in relative 5-year survival rates may be due in part to the detection of more cancers in a "localized" stage which includes more patients in the preclinical phase of their disease. It has been suggested that some lesions called breast cancer may be histologically malignant but biologically behave in a benign fashion, which would artificially improve the survival rates for patients with localized disease.[15,27] This is similar to the situation that exists with carcinoma of the prostate. Hopefully, the apparent improvement in survival in patients with regional disease in recent years does reflect a real effect on survival.

Even on theoretical grounds, radical mastectomy, which has served as the "gold standard" to which other forms of treatment have been compared, is not a complete cancer operation. It does not address the internal mammary lymph nodes which have been shown to be involved with metastastic disease in approximately one-third of the patients who are considered potentially curable.[17] The extended radical mastectomy was designed with the hope of improving survival rates by removing all regional lymph nodes.[9,20,24]

Staging classification varies in references.

The muscle-sparing operations such as the modified radical mastectomy and its variations were devised to improve cosmetic and functional results. They have achieved this goal and have been widely adopted without any apparent detrimental effect on survival.[33,48] Simple mastectomy, when combined with radiotherapy, has also been shown to provide adequate local control of breast cancer with survival results similar to the more radical procedures.[13,28]

The arguments for and against a given technique abound in the literature. These arguments involve the details of surgical technique, the limit and extent of resection, the advisability and efficacy of radiotherapy, the validity of study design, patient selection, and even the methods of statistical analysis and the interpretation of results. Implicit in the arguments was the belief that the means of attaining local control of the disease could influence outcome and ultimate survival. What was not focused on was the fact that the vast majority of breast cancer patients do not die of local disease but they die from systemic disease with or without local recurrence.[14,31,32,47]

It was not until the "early" dissemination of breast cancer was recognized and the classical halstedian concepts of cancer spread were challenged[4,14,22,25,26] that the modern era of breast cancer treatment began. If, then, the real threat to the survival of patients with breast cancer is metastatic systemic disease, then the least mutilating procedure which provides adequate local control without jeopardizing survival should be offered to these patients.

Despite the current publicity about local excision for the therapy of breast cancer, the concept of breast conservation in the management of breast cancers is not new. As early as 1928, Keynes published his results using radium needles in 42 patients with and without excisional biopsy.[21] Since then, multiple publications have appeared which reported the use of local excision with a variety of radiotherapy techniques to provide local control of the primary cancer. Data from about 8000 patients suggest that the results compare favorably with mastectomy with respect to survival.[45] We have been offering local excision with radiotherapy as an alternative to mastectomy to most of our patients for the past 20 years. In our opinion, the vast majority of patients who present with a primary carcinoma of the breast are suitable candidates for a breast-conserving operation.

CONTRAINDICATIONS TO BREAST CONSERVATION

Size of the Primary Lesion

We do not regard size per se as a limiting factor which precludes local excision. However, if the primary lesion is so large in relationship to the size of the breast that a local resection would result in an unacceptable cosmetic result, then a mastectomy, with the possibility of breast reconstruction, might be a preferable alternative. The key here is that the wishes of the patient must be considered. We have been surprised by how many women are happy with a result which we would consider cosmetically poor. This has also been noted by other investigators.[5,18]

Location of the Primary Lesion

Until recently, we felt that a lesion under the nipple was not amenable to local resection when it necessitated removal of the nipple areolar complex. Again, our reasons were based primarily on cosmesis. Some patients have themselves questioned this and requested such procedures with subsequent nipple reconstruction. We have performed a few of these excisions and as yet have no evidence to suggest that the chances for survival are impaired.

Multicentricity

Two lesions which are close to each other can be resected together by a wider local excision or quadrant resection and an acceptable cosmetic result can still be achieved. It is unlikely that two or more dominant lesions, widely separated in the same breast, can each be resected with a good cosmetic result unless the lesions are quite small. In addition, such obvious multicentricity would also imply that the breast is prone to the development of subsequent cancer. Therefore, for breasts with two or more independent dominant cancers, we advise mastectomy. For patients with one dominant mass and microscopic evidence of multifocal noninvasive carcinoma, we rely on radiotherapy following local excision. There are no good long-term studies on the results and we use careful surveillance to identify lesions which may subsequently arise in the same or opposite breast.

Margins of the Primary Lesion

Rarely, a primary lesion diffusely infiltrates the breast and neither gross nor microscopically clear margins can be obtained. Mastectomy is advised in this instance.

SURGICAL APPROACHES TO BREAST CONSERVATION

Excision of the Primary Lesion

Whether the differences in extent or technique of local resection will have an effect on either local recurrence or survival remains unknown. There have been no prospective randomized trials to compare their relative effectiveness. While surgical wisdom holds that local failure is due to inadequate surgery, the fact may be that local failure is more a reflection of the biology of the cancer than not enough surgery.[30]

Patients who have an excision of their primary lesion fare better than patients who are diagnosed by aspiration or needle or drill biopsy and treated by radical radiotherapy only.[2,36,42] Moreover, excision of the tumor provides tissue for hormone receptor analysis.

There are three types of local resection of the primary lesion. The first, *excisional biopsy*, involves removal of the primary cancer with only a small rim of what grossly appears to be normal breast tissue. The second, a *wide local excision or tylectomy*, involves the removal of a 1-to-2-cm margin of apparently normal breast tissue around the primary lesion with an ellipse of overlying skin. The third, a *segmental mastectomy or quadrantectomy*, implies the removal of approximately one-quarter of the breast substance surrounding the primary lesion. Deformity of the breast is more likely to occur with this last option, especially if the lesion is in the upper inner quadrant.[5] Frozen sections may be used with any of the three types of local resection, to confirm tumor-free margins. If, on permanent sections, the margins are shown to be involved with cancer, either an external beam booster dose of radiation or ^{192}Ir interstitial implants are used to control the residual microscopic tumor in addition to the whole breast irradiation.

Our operative technique consists of excising the tumor with a small margin of grossly normal breast tissue around it in all dimensions. A 2-cm margin is no longer considered necessary as it often sacrifices cosmesis in moderate-sized breasts. The skin incision is oriented with respect to Langer's lines, radial incisions are avoided, and an ellipse of skin is removed with the tumor if it is superficial. When the primary tumor is in the outer upper quadrant, adjacent to the axilla, a single incision is used to include removal of the primary tumor in-continuity with the axillary dissection. When the primary tumor is in another quadrant of the breast, two separate incisions are made. Electrocautery is avoided during resection so that denaturation of steroid receptor protein does not occur. We believe that the margins of resection should be clear of involvement by tumor. This requires a team approach. The specimen is tagged with sutures for orientation and a pathologist is available in the operating room to handle it, both for diagnostic frozen sections and to harvest tissue for estrogen and progesterone receptor analysis. The surgical margins of the specimen are painted with india ink for identification. Frozen sections of all grossly suspicious margins are performed. If a margin is found to be involved with tumor, further resection of the corresponding portion of the biopsy site is carried out until the frozen section confirms the margins to be free of involvement by tumor. In most cases, after irrigation with sterile water used to lyse free cancer cells, the breast tissue is approximated with 2-0 chromic catgut sutures and the skin is closed with interrupted 3-0 nylon sutures. Closed suction drainage is provided for 24 to 48 h to avoid hematoma formation.

Axillary Dissection

The three types of axillary dissection can be accurately described by the anatomic extent of the resection.

The first, *blind axillary sampling*, is carried out through a small transverse incision between the anterior and posterior axillary folds which gains limited access to the lower portion of the axilla. Easily accessible nodes are removed. The axillary vein and the nerves to the serratus anterior and latissimus dorsi are not exposed. Blind sampling is to be condemned because the number of nodes removed is unlikely to be sufficient to assess adequately axillary node metastases and, therefore, pathologic staging on which subsequent adjuvant therapy is based may be inaccurate.

The second, *open axillary node dissection*, provides full exposure of the axillary vein and the nerves to the serratus anterior and latissimus dorsi muscles. With this technique, all level I and some level II nodes can be removed, usually yielding about 20 axillary nodes for examination. This procedure provides adequate material for accurate pathologic staging in over 95 percent of the patients.[16]

The third, *total axillary clearance*, implies a complete dissection and removal of the axillary contents from all three levels of the axilla including the apex or level III nodes, medial to the pectoralis minor muscle. The pectoralis minor muscle is either transsected or resected in order to accomplish the procedure. Total axillary clearance has been advocated in the past for its therapeutic value and it obviates the need to radiate the axilla. We believe, however, that a complete axillary dissection is not only unnecessary, but is more likely to result in significant lymphedema of the arm. In our view, axillary dissection is performed for pathologic staging, rather than for therapeutic considerations.

Our technique of axillary dissection is as follows: The incision through which the local excision was performed is closed, the breast is reprepped and draped and the surgeons change their gowns and gloves before the axillary incision is made. The axillary incision is made either transversely between the anterior and posterior axillary folds or lies parallel and lateral to the anterior axillary fold. We no longer divide the pectoralis major tendon but rather retract the muscle in order to provide access to the lower portion of the axilla (level I). Retraction of the pectoralis minor muscle provides access to level II. The axillary vein is exposed and the nerves to the latissimus dorsi and serratus anterior are always identified. All level I and most level II nodes are removed. This technique provides 15 to 20 lymph nodes for pathologic staging. Closed suction drainage is provided for 24 to 48 h and the wound is closed with interrupted 3-0 nylon sutures.

RADIATION TECHNIQUES

Our patients receive external beam radiation from a 10-MV linear accelerator source beginning at least 10 days after operation. No bolus is used. The radiation is given in divided doses via tangential fields at a rate of 180 rads per day, 5 days a week for 5 to $5\frac{1}{2}$ weeks for a total of 4500 to 5000 rads to the entire breast. Wedges are used to create a homogeneous distribution throughout the entire tumor volume treated. A boost to the primary site of 1500 to 2000 rads is given with an electron beam. Patients who have proven axillary metastases receive radiation not only to the breast, but also to the apical axillary lymph nodes and the supraclavicular lymph nodes through anterior fields to a depth of 3 to 4 cm for a calculated midaxillary plane dose of 4500 to 5000 rad. Patients with histologically negative axillary nodes do not receive the apical axillary or supraclavicular radiation. For patients with medial or central lesions, the internal mammary nodes are treated by extending the medial border of the tangential breast fields 3 cm across the midline.

The complications of radiotherapy include some thickening of the skin, mild *peau d'orange*, and occasional telangiectasia. Fibrosis and contracture of the breast is very infrequent but does tend to increase over time. While in the past radiation has almost always complemented local excision in order to provide local control, the recently published opinions of a prominent radiotherapist question whether or not routine radiotherapy is indeed a necessary and beneficial component of the initial treatment of certain primary breast cancers (T_1 N_0 and T_2 N_0).[35]

SYSTEMIC ADJUVANT THERAPY

The adjuvant chemotherapy protocols followed by us are based on the chemotherapy studies reported in patients treated by radical mastectomy.[3] Thus, if the axillary lymph nodes are not involved by metastatic cancer, then no adjuvant chemotherapy is employed. If one to three nodes are involved, six cycles of CMF (cyclophosphamide, methotrexate, and 5-fluorouracil) are given. If four or more nodes are involved, six cycles of CMF plus vincristine and prednisone,[39] or four cycles of cyclophosphamide, doxorubicin, and 5-fluorouracil are used.[7] In the past, we had elected not to give radiotherapy and chemotherapy simultaneously. A "sandwich" schedule was used so that three cycles of chemotherapy, for a 3-month period, were given before the radiotherapy was initiated. Upon completion of the radiotherapy, the final three cycles of chemotherapy were given.[49] Although there are no long-term results reported, based on the reports of Botnick et al.[6] we no longer rigidly adhere to the "sandwich" technique, but have been giving concomitant radiotherapy and chemotherapy to some patients, allowing breaks in the chemotherapy schedule if myelosuppression is noted. All postmenopausal node-positive, estrogen-receptor-positive patients receive tamoxifen for 2 years.

SURVEILLANCE

An especially careful and frequent routine surveillance schedule is mandatory following any breast-conserving operation. This is not just to follow the patients for the appearance of asymptomatic metastastic disease, but is of particular importance so that a local recurrence can be identified and treated as early as possible. Patients are seen every 3 months for the first 2 years, every 4 months for the next 2 years, and every 6 months thereafter. A yearly chest x-ray and mammogram of both breasts are obtained in all patients. Those patients who were node-positive at the time of their initial therapy have annual liver and bone scans, even though the yield may be small and the potential advantages of treatment for subclinical disease before the patient is symptomatic has been questioned.

The most important reason for the frequency of the follow-up examinations is to identify, as early as possible, evidence of local recurrence so that it may be treated promptly.

LOCAL RECURRENCE

The issue of local recurrence is of particular importance when considering a breast-conserving operation. The rate is approximately 10 percent at 10 years[1,10] and, although most recurrences are manifest in the first 3 to 5 years, they continue to appear at a rate approaching 1 percent per year. Therefore, patients with breast-conserving operations must be advised that a local recurrence may appear. It is important to emphasize the different prognostic significance of local relapse following local excision and radiotherapy as compared to mastectomy. A local recurrence following radical surgery usually heralds or coincides with the appearance of widespread metastatic disease and is generally a predictor of the rapid demise of the patient.[12,19] Local recurrence[1,11] following a breast-conserving operation is amenable to local treatment and does not carry the same grave prognosis, as it does not seem to significantly jeopardize the survival of the patient.[1,42]

It is our practice to recommend a mastectomy for a true local recurrence. On occasion, in consultation with the patient, further local excision only is carried out. Not all apparent local recurrences are true recurrences of cancer. Pseudorecurrences do occur, such as fibrotic tissue or suture granulomas. Therefore, excisional biopsy and frozen sections of the suspected recurrence must be performed for tissue confirmation before embarking on a mastectomy.

RESULTS

Cosmetic results are excellent in 90 percent of the patients. For patients with stage I disease, the survival rates at 5 years for patients treated by local excision and radiotherapy range roughly from 80 to 90 percent, and at 10 years from 70 to 80 percent. For stage II patients, the survival rates are approximately 70 to 80 percent at 5 years, and 60 to 70 percent at 10 years.[1,29,34,37,38] These results are comparable to those following radical mastectomy. The prospective randomized trials currently in progress have again showed no difference in survival for patients treated either by radical mastectomy or local excision and radiotherapy.[41,46] Long-term retrospective studies also suggest no difference in the 5- and 10-year survival rates when patients treated by mastectomy and patients treated by local excision with radiotherapy are compared.[37,50]

Psychological Sequelae

It has been the clinical impression of a number of investigators that serious psychological sequelae exist in many patients who have had mastectomy. The symptoms noted include depression, anxiety, and sexual dysfunction; the adjustment problems relate primarily to concerns about body image and femininity.[43] The early proponents of breast conservation had postulated that the fear of losing the breast led many patients to delay in seeking treatment. They hoped to entice patients to seek earlier treatment by offering a breast-conserving alternative which would remove the fear of breast amputation.[22] Only in recent years have scientific investigations of the psychological sequelae of mastectomy been studied.[23,40] In a recent study,[44] we have interviewed, at intervals up to 14 months after surgery, 21 patients treated by local excision and 46 patients treated by mastectomy. There was clear evidence that patients who had undergone mastectomy have real concerns about body image. They experience feelings of decreased femininity and attractiveness. The patients who had local excision had fewer long-term psychological side-effects and demonstrated better overall adaptation to their operations. It has been suggested by some that patients who have had local excision might have an inordinate fear of recurrence of their cancers. We have not found this to be so.

CONCLUSION

When the results of the various primary treatments for potentially curable breast cancer are compared, variations in local therapy do not materially affect survival rates; therefore, the least mutilating surgical procedure may appropriately be offered to most patients.

REFERENCES

1. Amalric R, Santamaria F, Robert F, et al: Conservative therapy in operable breast cancer—results at 5, 10, and 15 years in 2216 conservative cases, in Harris JR, Hellman S, Silen, W (eds): *Conservative Management of Breast Cancer*. Philadelphia, J. B. Lippincott Co., 1983, p. 15.
2. Bataini JP, Picco C, Martin M, Calle R: Relation between time-dose and local control of operable breast cancer treated by tumorectomy and radiotherapy or by radical radiotherapy alone. *Cancer* 42:2059, 1978.
3. Bonnadona G, Rosi A, Tancini G, et al: Adjuvant chemotherapy trials in resectable breast cancer with positive axillary nodes. The experience of the Milan Cancer Institute, in Jones SE, Salmon SE (eds): *Adjuvant Therapy of Cancer IV*. New York, Grune & Stratton, 1984, p. 195.
4. Baum M: The curability of breast cancer. *Br Med J* 1:439, 1976.
5. Bosworth JL, Ghossein MD: Limited surgery and radiotherapy in the treatment of localized breast cancer. An overview. *Surg Clin North Am* 64:1115, 1984.
6. Botnick LE, Cane S, Christopher MR, et al: Primary breast irradiation and concomitant adjuvant chemotherapy, in Harris JR, Hellman S, Silen, W (eds.): *Conservative Management of Breast Cancer*. Philadelphia, J. B. Lippincott Co., 1983, p. 321.
7. Buzdar AU, Smith TL, Blummenschien GR, et al: Breast cancer adjuvant therapy trials of M.D. Anderson Hospital: Results of two studies, in Jones SE, Salmon SE (eds.): *Adjuvant Therapy of Cancer IV*. New York, Grune & Stratton, 1984, p. 217.
8. *CA—A Journal for Clinicians*. 35(1):24, 1985. American Cancer Society Publishers.
9. Caceres E: An evaluation of radical mastectomy and extended radical mastectomy for cancer of the breast. *Surg Gynecol Obstet* 125:337, 1967.
10. Calle R, Vilcoo JR, Pilleron JP, et al: Conservative treatment of operable breast carcinoma by irradiation with or without limited surgery—ten year results, in Harris JR, Hellman S, Silen, W (eds.): *Conservative Management of Breast Cancer*. Philadelphia, J. B. Lippincott Co., 1983, p. 3.
11. Clark RM: Alternatives to mastectomy—the Princess Margaret hospital experience, in Harris JR, Hellman S, Silen, W (eds.): *Conservative Management of Breast Cancer*. Philadelphia, J. B. Lippincott Co., 1983, p. 35.
12. Donegan WL, Perez-Mesa CM, Watson FR: A biostatistical study of locally recurrent breast carcinoma. *Surg Gynecol Obstet* 122:529, 1966.
13. Fisher B, Redmond C, Fisher ER, et al: Ten-year results of a randomized clinical trial comparing radical mastectomy and total mastectomy with or without radiation. *N Engl J Med* 312:674, 1985.
14. Fitzwilliams DCL: A plea for a more local operation in really early breast carcinoma. *Br Med J* 28:405, 1940.
15. Fox MS: On the diagnosis and treatment of breast cancer. *JAMA* 241:489, 1979.
16. Gazet JC: Surgical management of breast cancer, in Coombs RC, Pooles TJ, Ford JC, et al (eds.): *Breast Cancer Management*. New York, Grune & Stratton, 1981, p. 97.
17. Haagensen CD: *Diseases of the Breast*, 2d ed. Philadelphia, London, Toronto, W. B. Saunders Co., 1971.
18. Harris JR, Beadle GF, Hellman S: Clinical studies on the use of radiation therapy as primary treatment of early breast cancer. *Cancer* 53:705, 1984.
19. Harris JR, Hellman S, Silen, W (eds.): *Conservative Management of Breast Cancer*. Philadelphia, J. B. Lippincott Co., 1983, p. 72.
20. Kaae S, Johansen H: Simple mastectomy plus postoperative irradiation by the method of McWhirter for mammary carcinoma. *Ann Surg* 170:895, 1969.
21. Keynes G: Radium treatment of primary carcinoma of the breast. *Lancet* 2:108, 1928.
22. Keynes G: Conservative treatment of cancer of the breast. *Br Med J* Oct. 2, 1937, p. 643.
23. Kohn J: Psychological impact of two types of breast surgery. *JAMA* 248:1800, 1982.
24. Lacour J, Bucalossi P, Caceres E, Jacobelli G, Koszarowski T, Le M, Rumeau-Roquette C, Veronesi U: Radical mastectomy versus radical mastectomy plus internal mammary dissection. *Cancer* 37:206, 1976.
25. MacDonald IG: Biological predeterminism in human cancer. *Surg Gynecol Obstet* 92:443, 1951.
26. McKinnon NE: Cancer of breast: Invalid evidence for patients in early treatment. *Can J Public Health* 42:218, 1951.
27. McKinnon NE: Limitations in diagnosis and treatment of breast and other cancers. A review. *Can Med Assoc J* 72:614, 1955.

28. McWhirter R: The value of simple mastectomy and radiotherapy in the treatment of cancer of the breast. *Br J Radiol* 21:599, 1948.
29. Montague ED: Conservative surgery and radiation therapy in the treatment of operable breast cancer. *Cancer* 53:700, 1984.
30. Mueller CB: Surgery for breast cancer, less may be more. *New Engl J Med* 312:712, 1985.
31. Mustakallio S: Treatment of breast cancer by tumor extirpation and roentgen therapy instead of radical operations. *J Fac Radiol* 6:23, 1954.
32. Mustakallio S: Conservative treatment of breast carcinoma—review of 25 years follow-up. *Clin Radiol* 23:110, 1972.
33. Nemoto T, Vana J, Bedwani RN, Baker HW, McGregor FH, Murphy, GP: Management and survival of female breast cancer: Results of a national survey by the American College of Surgeons. *Cancer* 45:2917, 1980.
34. Papillon J, Montbarbon J, Ingels J, Gerard JP, Boisson M: L'association tumorectomie—irradiation dans le treatment du cancer du sein operable, in Masson C (ed): *Conservative Treatments of Breast Cancers Symposium International*. Strasbourg, June 1972, p. 255.
35. Peters MV: "Local" treatment of early breast cancer. *Surg Clin North Am* 64:1151, 1984.
36. Pierquin B: Conservative treatment for carcinoma of the breast: Experience of Creteil—ten year results, in Harris JR, Hellman S, Silen, W (eds.): *Conservative Management of Breast Cancer*. Philadelphia, J. B. Lippincott Co., 1983, p. 11.
37. Rissensen PM: A comparison of conservative and radical surgery combined with radiotherapy in the treatment of stage I carcinoma of the breast. *Br J Radiol* 42:423, 1969.
38. Rissenen PM, Holsti P: Vergleich zwischen konservativer und radikaler chiurgie, combiniert mit strahlentherapie, gie der behandlung des brustkrebses in stadium I eine untersuchung an 866 patient en im zeitraun von 10 jahren. *Strahlentherapie* 147:370, 1974.
39. Rivkin SE, Glucksberg H, Foulkes M: Adjuvant chemotherapy for operable breast cancer with positive axillary nodes: A comparison of CMFVP versus L-Pam (Southwest Oncology Group Study), in Jones SE, Salmon SE (eds.): *Adjuvant Therapy of Cancer IV*. New York, Grune & Stratton, 1984, p. 209.
40. Sanger CK, Reznekoff M: A comparison of the psychological effects of breast saving procedures with the modified radical mastectomy. *Cancer* 48:2341, 1981.
41. Sarazin D, Le M, Fontaine MF, Arriadada R: Conservative treatment versus mastectomy in T_1 or T_2 breast cancer. A randomized clinical trial, in Harris JR, Hellman S, Silen, W (eds.): *Conservative Management of Breast Cancer*. Philadelphia, J. B. Lippincott Co., 1983, p. 101.
42. Spitalier J, Brandone YA, Amalric R, Santamaria F, Seigle J: Cesium therapy of breast cancer. A five-year report on 400 consecutive patients. *Int J Radiat Oncol Biol Phys* 2:231, 1977.
43. Stehlin JS, Gutierrez AE, Greeff PJ: Treatment of carcinoma of the breast. *Surg Gynecol Obstet* 149:911, 1979.
44. Steinberg MD, Wise LW, Juliano MA: Psychological outcome of lumpectomy compared to mastectomy in the treatment of breast cancer. *Am J Psychiatry* 142:34, 1985.
45. Tinker MA, Wise L: The conservative management of breast cancer, in Neyhus, L(ed.): *Surgery Annual*. New York, Appelton Century Croft, 1986.
46. Veronesi U, Saccozzi R, DelVecchio M, et al: Comparing radical mastectomy with quadrantectomy, axillary dissection and radiotherapy in patients with small cancers of the breast. *N Engl J Med* 305:6, 1981.
47. Williams IG, Murley RS, Curwen MP: Carcinoma of the female breast: Conservation and radical surgery. *Br Med J* October 10:788, 1953.
48. Wilson RE, Donegan WL, Mettlin C, Smart CR, Murphy GP: The 1982 National Survey of carcinoma of the breast in the United States by the American College of Surgeons. *Surg Gynecol Obstet* 159:309, 1984.
49. Wise L: Techniques of surgery—local excision, in Harris JR, Hellman S, Silen, W (eds.): *Conservative Management of Breast Cancer*. Philadelphia, J. B. Lippincott Co., 1983, p. 141.
50. Wise L, Mason AY, Ackerman LV: Local excision and irradiation: An alternative method for the treatment of early mammary cancer. *Ann Surg* 174:392, 1971.

18

Radiation Therapy Following Local Excision or Partial Mastectomy

Florence F. C. Chu, M.D.

INTRODUCTION

An alternative to mastectomy has become available in recent years for the management of early breast cancer, which consists of a combination of limited surgery (local excision or partial mastectomy) and radical radiation therapy. The goal of this approach is to achieve satisfactory local tumor control and survival while preserving the breast.

REVIEW OF STUDIES

Treatment of patients with early breast cancer by local excision and radiation therapy was started in Europe and Canada in the 1930s.[23,29,31] Initial results have shown some long-term survivals. There was, however, a high local recurrence rate due to the use of orthovoltage radiation and its inability to deliver adequate tumor doses without severe normal tissue reactions.

In the 1960s, many investigators began to use megavoltage radiation to treat early breast cancer.[1,6,12,33,42] Not only were high survival rates observed, but local recurrence rates were reduced significantly, Further, cosmetic results improved. The satisfactory results obtained have convinced many surgeons, radiation therapists, and other oncologists to use limited surgery and radiation therapy as an alternative to mastectomy. Physician's recommendations, coupled with women's desire for an alternative treatment, have made breast-conserving surgery and radiation therapy an increasingly used procedure.

Retrospective Studies

Keynes, a British surgeon at the St. Bartholomew's Hospital, London, England, began to treat breast cancer with local excision and

The specific meaning of the stages used will be indicated at each point.

Table 18-1 Results of Local Excision and Radiation Therapy

Number of cases	5-Year relative survival rate	Number of cases with 10-year follow-up	10-Year relative survival rate	10-Year recurrence rate
702 (T_1T_2)	87%	418	75%	25%

Source: From Mustakallio, 1972.[30]

implantation of radium needles in the early 1930s. He reported in 1937 that the 3- and 5-year survival results of 250 patients treated by conservative surgery and radium implant were identical to those of a comparable series of patients treated by another surgeon employing mastectomy.[23]

Mustakallio[29] of the Helsinki Radiotherapy Clinic, Finland, was among the pioneers who strongly advocated the approach of local excision and external beam radiation therapy. In the late 1930s he treated a small number of patients who refused radical mastectomy. When satisfactory results were observed, he continued to practice this method and in 1972 he reported a series of 702 patients treated with local excision and radiation therapy.[30] Of these, 418 were followed for 10 or more years. All patients had a T_1 or T_2 primary tumor, with no clinical evidence of axillary lymph node enlargement. These patients were treated during the orthovoltage era and were given a modest dose of radiation therapy in the range of 2500 to 3500 rad to the breast and regional lymph node areas, over a period of 2 weeks. He reported a 5-year relative survival rate* of 87 percent and 10-year relative survival rates of 75 percent. The observed 10-year survival rate was 61 percent (257/418). The local or regional recurrence rate was about 25 percent at 10 years (Table 18-1).

Rissanen, who succeeded Mustakallio at the Helsinki Clinic, made subsequent reports.[37,38]

*Relative survival rate is obtained by dividing the observed survival rate by the expected survival rate.

Of particular interest was a presentation on the 20-year results at the 1977 International Radiological Conference.[39] Rissanen and Holsti analyzed the 20-year data on patients with T_1 N_0 lesions who were less than 50 years of age when the treatment was started, in order to minimize the influence of other causes of death. These patients were treated during the period 1936 to 1956. There were 51 cases in the radical mastectomy group and 40 in the excision group. The absolute 20-year survival rates of the two groups were similar; 78 percent for radical mastectomy and 73 percent for local excision and radiation therapy. The local recurrence rate was higher in the excision group as compared with that of the mastectomy group (20 percent versus 8 percent) (Table 18-2). Since the use of megavoltage therapy in 1969, they have observed a significant reduction in the recurrence rates.

Another early proponent for conservative surgery and radiation therapy is Peters[31] at the Princess Margaret Hospital in Toronto, Canada. Peters, in 1977, reported a study matching each patient treated by local excision with three patients treated by radical mastectomy according to age, tumor size, and year treated.[32] These patients were treated between the years 1939 and 1972. There were 203 patients with T_1 N_0 M_0 or T_2 N_0 M_0 lesions treated by excision (184 with radiation therapy and 19 without), and 609 treated by radical mastectomy (552 with radiation therapy and 57 without). Up to 30-year follow-up, the survival without evidence

Table 18-2 Local Excision and Radiation Therapy: 20-Year Results, $T_1N_0M_0$, Age under 50 Years

	Radical mastectomy (%)	Local excision (%)
Absolute 20-year survival	78	73
Died of cancer	20	20
Local recurrence	8	20
Swelling of arm	22	8
Regional recurrence	6	10
Died of cancer after 10 years	8	13

Source: From Rissanen and Holsti, 1977.[39]

of disease was identical in the two groups (Fig. 18-1).*

Data are now being accumulated on the results of treatment by more modern radiation techniques using megavoltage therapy. Calle and his colleagues at the Foundation Curie in Paris, France, used local excision and cobalt therapy to treat patients with tumors less than 3 cm in diameter (T_1 and small T_2's) without clinical evidence of axillary lymph node involvement (N_0 N_{1a}). They delivered a 5000-rad tumor dose over a 5 to 6 week period to the breast and regional lymph node areas. An additional dose of 1500 rads in 1 week was delivered to the lumpectomy site through a small field. Patients with tumors larger than 3 cm and all patients with clinically significant axillary lymph nodes (N_{1b}) were treated exclusively by radiation therapy.[6-9]

Calle, in 1983, updated their results.[9] There were 140 patients treated with local excision and cobalt therapy who were followed for 10 years. Of these, 111 (78 percent) survived without evidence of cancer. One important aspect to be emphasized is that of these 111 patients who survived, 99 (89 percent) had their breasts preserved. (Table 18-3). Their 10-year recurrence rate (breast and/or axillae) was 14 percent (20/140). Eighteen of the 20 patients had salvage surgery and 72 percent (13/18) were alive and free of cancer with a minimum follow-up of 4 years after surgery.

In an earlier report in 1978, Calle and his associates[6] compared their 10-year results with the data from Memorial Sloan-Kettering

Editors' Note: Only 83 patients in each series were followed for 10 years or longer; the results are reported by actuarial methods.

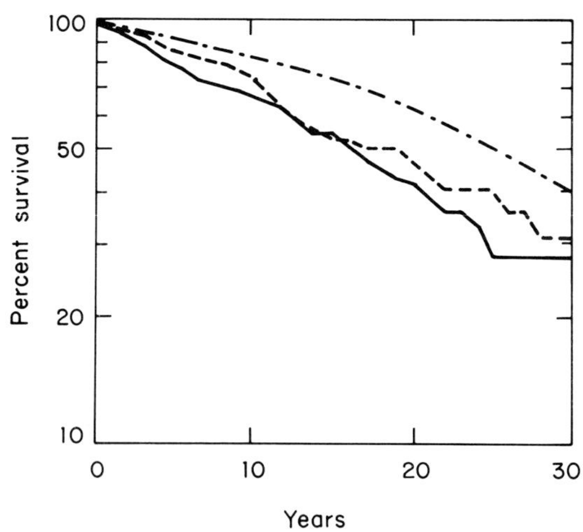

Figure 18-1 Survival to 30 years. Excision plus radiation (E + R) versus mastectomy plus radiation (M + R) (E + R included 19 patients without radiation therapy, and M + R included 57 patients without radiation therapy). Excluding dead from extraneous disease under 10 years. E + R (203 patients): — —; M + R (609 patients): —; normal survival: ———. ———.) (*From Peters, 1977.*[32])

Table 18-3 Lumpectomy and Irradiation (1960–1971): Ten-year Results According to the Extent of Primary Disease

	Number of patients	Absolute survival, NED* (%)	Alive NED with breasts preserved (%)
T_1 N_0 N_{1a}	87	73/87 (84)	66/73 (90)
T_2 ($\leq$3 cm) N_0 N_{1a}	56	38/56 (68)	33/38 (86)
Total	143	111/143 (78)	99/111 (89)

*NED = No evidence of disease.
Source: From Calle et al., 1983.[9]

Cancer Center in New York City, published by Schottenfeld and colleagues.[41] For T_1 N_0 or N_{1a} lesions, Memorial Hospital's 10-year disease-free survival with radical or modified radical mastectomy, was 90 percent (59/66). At the Foundation Curie the 10-year disease-free survival of patients treated by local excision and radiation therapy was 90 percent (36/40) (Table 18-4). The survival results were equally excellent.

Amalric et al.[1,2,42] of the Marseilles Cancer Institute, France, have treated more than 4000 patients, with or without local excision, using similar radiation factors and dose as the Foundation Curie. There were 274 patients who had local excision and radiation therapy and were followed for 10 years. The 10-year disease-free survival was 74 percent and of these, 86 percent had preservation of the breast (Table 18-5). The local-regional recurrence rate at 10 years was 13.9 percent (7.9 percent breast only, 4.1 percent breast and axilla and 1.9 percent axilla only) (Table 18-6.)

In the United States, Prosnitz et al.[35] in 1977 had to pool material from four institutions to report on the preliminary results of the treatment of 150 patients. In recent years, however, there has been a rapid increase in the number of patients treated with breast-conserving

Table 18-4 Operable Breast Cancer: Comparison of Surgical and Radiotherapeutic Results at 10 Years

	Memorial Hospital[41]		Foundation Curie	
	Number of cases	Alive, NED* (%)	Number of cases	Alive, NED* (%)
T_1, N_0, N_{1a}	66	59 (89)	40	36 (90)
T_2 N_0, T_1/T_2 N_{1b}	176	92 (52)	129	69 (53)
T_3 N_0, T_3 N_{1b}	62	18 (29)	89	67 (30)
Total	304	169 (55)	258	132 (51)

*NED = No evidence of disease.
Note: Only T_1 N_0 N_{1a} group was treated entirely by local excision and radiation therapy. The remainder had radiation therapy, with or without local excision, depending on tumor size and axillary node status. See text.
Source: From Calle, 1978.[6]

Table 18-5 Radiation Therapy with Primary Limited Surgery: NED* Survival and Breast Preservation

	5 Years			10 Years			15 Years		
	N†	% NED	%PB‡	N	% NED	%PB	N	% NED	% PB
T_1N_0	309	92	94	111	81	83	23	61	71
T_1N_1	79	82	95	28	79	82	2	50	50
T_2N_0	259	82	95	84	71	92	11	54	100
T_2N_1	133	74	92	51	61	90	4	50	100
Overall	780	85	94	274	74	86	40	57	74

*NED = No evidence of disease.
†Includes 26 patients with nonpalpable tumors.
‡% PB = Proportion of NED patients with preserved breasts.
Source: From Amalric et al., 1983.[2]

surgery and radiation therapy as an alternative to mastectomy.

Hellman, Harris, Levene, and their colleagues at the Harvard Joint Center, Boston, Massachusetts, have been strong proponents for primary radiation therapy.[16,19,25] In 1984 they gave their overall experience of treating 357 patients with International Union Against Cancer (UICC) clinical stages I and II (T_1 T_2 N_0) and II (T_1 T_2 N_1) breast cancer.[15] A total of 366 breasts were treated because nine patients had bilateral cancers. The minimal follow-up was 24 months, the median 52 months. The great majority of patients received a boost to the primary tumor area by interstitial implantation of ^{192}Ir delivering an additional dose of 1500 to 2500 rads.

It was concluded that the local tumor control rate was dependent on two important factors: (1) complete excision of the tumor, and (2) the primary tumor area would be boosted to at least 6000 rads. The 6-year local tumor control for patients treated by total excision and adequate radiation therapy was 96 percent for stage I and 90 percent for stage II breast cancer (Fig. 18-2). The 6-year local recurrence rate was 6 percent for patients who received a boost dose as compared to 12 percent for patients who did not.

An evaluation of the cosmetic results showed that at 5 years following treatment, 73 percent of patients were judged to have excellent cosmetic results (essentially no detectable effects present), 8 percent as good (slight but definite

Table 18-6 Radiation Therapy with Primary Limited Surgery* — Local-Regional Failures at 10 Years

	Breast only (%)	Breast and axilla (%)	Axilla only (%)	Total (%)
$T_{1\text{-}2}N_0$	19/202 (9.4)	7/202 (3.5)	2/202 (1.0)	28/202 (13.9)
$T_{1\text{-}2}N_1$	2/64 (3.1)	4/64 (6.3)	3/64 (4.7)	9/64 (14.1)
Overall	21/266 (7.9)	11/266 (4.1)	5/266 (1.9)	37/266 (13.9)

*Excludes 17 patients who had axillary dissection. Only those failures in which the first relapse is local-regional are scored.
Source: From Amalric et al., 1983.[2]

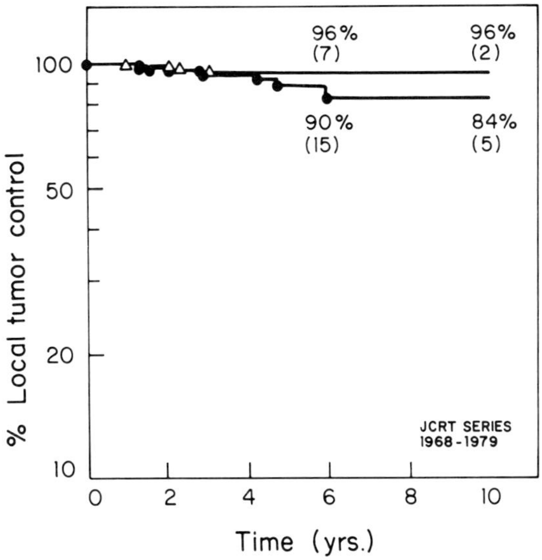

Figure 18-2 Local control for patients treated with excisional biopsy, whole-breast irradiation, and the use of a boost to the primary tumor area. Δ, Stage I (107); •, Stage II (146). Excisional biopsy and boost to primary (≥ 6000 rads). (*From Harris et al, 1984.*[15])

effects present), and 15 percent as fair (obvious effects of treatment present). Only 4 percent had poor results (marked effects of treatment present).

The Joint Center group also did a clinical pathological study which was reported in 1983.[17] They identified a subgroup which was characterized by the presence of a constellation of histological features in the biopsy specimen. These features included (1) poor nuclear grade or extensive mitosis, (2) extensive intraductal carcinoma within the primary tumor, and (3) extensive intraductal carcinoma in the adjacent tissue. All these features were present in 18 percent of patients, and their local control rate was 61 percent at 5 years, as compared with a 5-year local control rate of 96 percent for those patients having none, one, or two of these features. The authors recommend a slightly higher tumor dose, about 6500 rads in $6\frac{1}{2}$ weeks instead of the usual 6000 rads in 6 weeks, for treatment of this type of tumor. Additional follow-up is needed for final judgment. The surgical treatment consisted of excisional biopsy in 344 cases and needle or incisional biopsy in the remaining 22 cases. All patients received external beam radiation therapy using 4-MV linear accelerator. The breast usually received 4600 to 5000 rads in $4\frac{1}{2}$ to 5 weeks, and the dose to the upper axillary and supraclavicular areas was 4500 rads at a depth of 5 cm.

Montague[28] in 1984 reported on a study analyzing 1073 patients with clinically favorable breast cancer treated at the M.D. Anderson Hospital, Houston, Texas, from 1955 to 1980. Seven-hundred and twenty-eight patients were treated with radical or modified radical mastectomy alone and 345 were treated with conservative surgery and radiation.

Their results of treatment according to the stage of disease indicated no significant difference in the recurrence rates in patients treated with conservative surgery and radiation therapy when compared with radical or modified radical mastectomy alone (Table 18-7). The overall actuarial survival rates of the two groups of patients were identical. The 5-year and 10-year survival rates according to the stage of the disease were also similar in the two groups (Table 18-8).

There have been reports from other authors discussing various aspects of primary radiation therapy after a local excision or partial mastectomy.[4,5,10,27,34,36]

Prospective Randomized Studies

In addition to retrospective studies there have been several randomized clinical trials to determine the efficacy of breast-conserving surgery combined with radiation therapy.

The first prospective randomized study to compare limited surgery with radical mastectomy was by Atkins, Hayward, and their colleagues at the Guy's Hospital, London, England.[3] Between 1961 and 1971 a total of

Table 18-7 Local-Regional Recurrences, 1955–1980

	Conservation surgery + irradiation (345 patients) (%)	Radical or modified radical mastectomy (728 patients) (%)
Minimal breast cancer*	1/54 (1.9)	1/134 (.75)
Stage I (T_1 N_0)	8/134 (5.9)	11/224 (4.9)
Stage II (T_1 N_1) (T_2 N_0 N_1)	8/157 (5.1)	29/370 (7.8)

Analysis, March 1983.

*Minimal breast cancer: 20 patients with microinvasion (<5 mm) and 34 with noninvasive intraductal carcinoma.

Source: From Montague, 1984.[28]

370 operable breast cancer patients over age 50 entered the trial. Manchester stages I and II were used (stage I included T_1, T_2 or T_{3a}, N_0, N_{1a} and stage II included T_1, T_2, T_3, N_{1b}). Patients were randomized into radical mastectomy plus postoperative radiation therapy or wide excision (tylectomy) plus radiation therapy.

Those who had radical mastectomies were given radiation treatment to the axilla, supraclavicular area, and internal mammary chain. A total dose of 2500 to 2700 rads was given over a period of 18 days. Those patients who had extended tylectomy were given 2500 to 2700 rads to the supraclavicular and axillary areas over a period of 12 days. In addition, the breast, including the internal mammary chain, received a tumor dose of 3500 to 3800 rads in 3 weeks through tangential fields using a 6-MV linear accelerator with bolus.

For patients with clinically uninvolved axillary lymph nodes (Manchester stage I), the actuarial survival rate of patients who had a wide excision was similar to those having a

Table 18-8 Five-year and 10-Year Disease-Free Survival Rates, 1955–1980

	Conservation surgery + irradiation		Radical or modified radical mastectomy alone	
	5 year (%)	10 year (%)	5 year (%)	10 year (%)
Minimal breast cancer*	97	92	97	95
Stage I				
T_1 N_0	85	78	88	80
Stage II				
T_1 N_1				
T_2 N_0 N_1	78	73	77	65

Analysis March, 1983. No statistical significance between any group.

*Minimal breast cancer: 20 patients with microinvasion (< 5mm) and 34 with noninvasive intraductal carcinoma.

Source: From Montague, 1984.[28]

radical mastectomy. For patients with clinically positive axilla (Manchester stage II), however, the survival of patients having a wide excision was significantly less than those who had a radical mastectomy. Local and regional recurrence rates were higher in the group of patients who had wide excision, and most occurred in the axilla. The high recurrence rates were definitely due to the low radiation doses given.

Hayward apparently was not satisfied with the finding that a high incidence of local recurrence did not affect distant metastasis or survival rates in patients with clinically negative axilla. He studied a second series of 253 patients who had clinically uninvolved axillae. These patients were randomly allocated to either wide excision or radical mastectomy; both groups received radiation therapy. The radiation dosages given were the same as that for the first series, *even though these dosages were known to be inadequate.* He reported in 1981[21] that the local and distant recurrence rates were significantly higher and the survival was lower in the wide excision group.

It is difficult to understand why there was a discrepancy of findings from the two series of patients done in the same hospital. It is also unfortunate that in the second series the same inadequate radiation dosages were used. Hayward, in a subsequent paper,[22] stated that the first series was carried out before the establishment of their Breast Unit. Mastectomies were performed by a heterogeneous group of surgeons, including trainees. In the second series all mastectomies were performed by a few full-time experienced breast surgeons. This implied that they were comparing improved mastectomies with antiquated radiation therapy in the second series.

In 1972, a randomized trial was started at the Institute Gustave Roussy, Villejuif, France, in response to a proposal made by the World Health Organization. Patients with unilateral breast cancer of 2 cm or less, with or without palpable axillary lymph nodes, were accepted for the trial. The patients were randomized to be treated either by mastectomy or by local excision plus radiation. In both groups low axillary dissections were performed. If one or more positive nodes were found, a complete axillary dissection was carried out.

The radiation therapy technique utilized included the use of cobalt 60 to irradiate the breast and nodal areas. The breast received 4500 rads in 18 fractions over 1 month, plus a boost dose of 1500 rads given to the tumor bed in 6 fractions. The lymph node areas received 4500 rads over a period of 1 month.

From 1972 to 1980 a total of 179 patients were entered into the study. The results were published by Sarrazin and his coinvestigators in 1984.[40] No significant difference was found in either relapse-free survival or overall survival between the two groups, although the conservatively treated group showed slightly better results at 5 years (Figs. 18-3 and 18-4). The cosmetic results of conservative treatment were satisfactory in 92 percent of the cases. In view of the satisfactory results with conservative surgery, these investigators have abandoned mastectomy in the treatment of tumors *2 cm or less.*

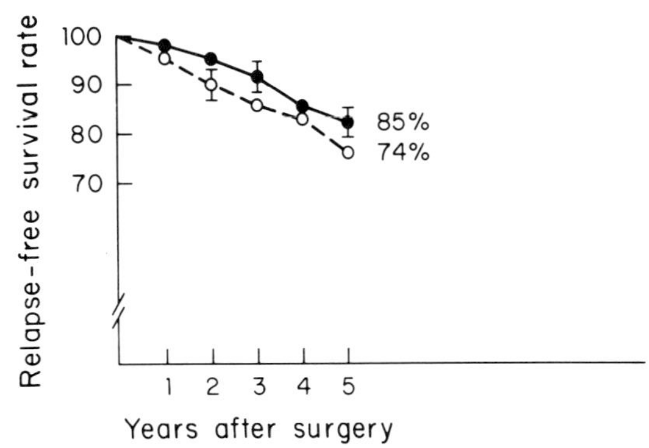

Figure 18-3 Relapse-free survival according to surgical treatment: tumorectomy–88 patients, 17 relapses or deaths; mastectomy–91 patients, 23 relapses or deaths. •, tumorectomy; 0- - -0, mastectomy. (*From Sarrazin et al., 1984.*[40])

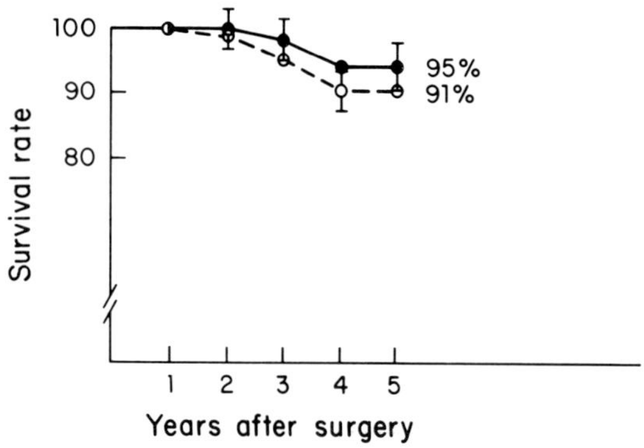

Figure 18-4 Survival curves according to surgical treatment: tumorectomy–88 patients, 6 deaths; mastectomy–91 patients, 12 deaths. •–•, tumorectomy; 0- - -0, mastectomy. (*From Sarrazin et al., 1984.*[40])

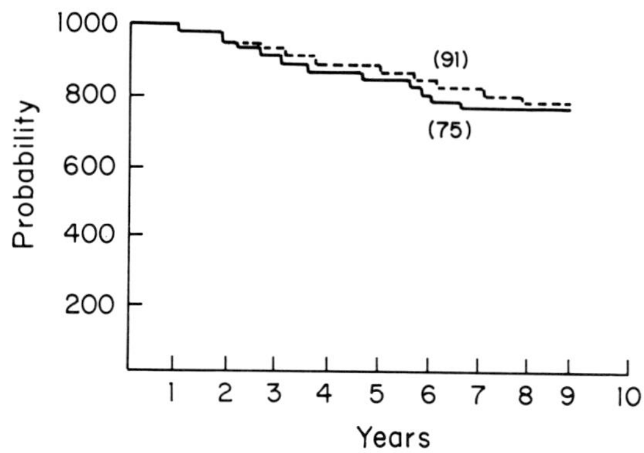

Figure 18-5 Actuarial disease-free survival in patients treated with Halsted mastectomy or with quadrantectomy, axillary dissection, and radiation therapy (QUART). —, Halsted (349); — —, QUART (352). (Loq rank test p = .29.) (*From Veronesi et al., 1983.*[45])

An important randomized trial was started in 1973 at the National Cancer Institute of Milan, Italy. This trial has accrued a large number of patients and was conducted to compare radical mastectomy with quadrantectomy (resection of an entire quadrant of the breast) plus axillary dissection plus radiation therapy. Radiation therapy was given to the breast; 5000 rads in 5 weeks through tangential fields using ^{60}Co, plus a boost dose of 1000 rads to the area of the scar, using orthovoltage therapy. The trial was limited to cases with tumors less than 2 cm and no palpable axillary nodes (T_1 N_0 M_0.) Since 1976 all patients with histologically positive nodes were treated with 12 cycles of chemotherapy with a CMF regimen.[43–45]

A total of 701 evaluative patients was entered into the trial from 1973 to 1980; 349 were treated with a Halsted mastectomy and 352 with quadrantectomy. The two series appear completely comparable in all parameters such as age, menopausal status, tumor site by quadrant, dimension of the primary cancer, incidence of axillary metastasis, or previous biopsy. Actuarial survival curves showed no difference between the two groups in disease-free survival (Fig. 18-5) or overall survival (Fig. 18-6). The incidence of local and distant recurrences was also similar in both groups. Since 1982, the quadrantectomy technique has become the treatment of choice at the National Cancer Institute in Milan for breast carcinoma less than 2 cm without clinical evidence of metastasis.

In the United States a three-arm randomized study was initiated by the National Surgical Adjuvant Breast Project (NSABP) in 1978. Patients with primary tumors up to 4 cm in diameter, with or without axillary lymph node enlargement, were randomized to receive (1) total mastectomy, (2) segmental mastectomy plus radiation therapy, or (3) segmental mastectomy alone. An axillary dissection was performed in all three treatment arms. All patients with histologically positive axillary lymph nodes were given adjuvant chemotherapy. This study not only compares the relative efficacies of total mastectomy and segmental mastectomy plus radiation therapy, but also investigates the biological question of the significance of multicentric breast disease by including a third arm of segmental mastectomy alone.

The 5-year results of this study have been published by Fisher and his colleagues in

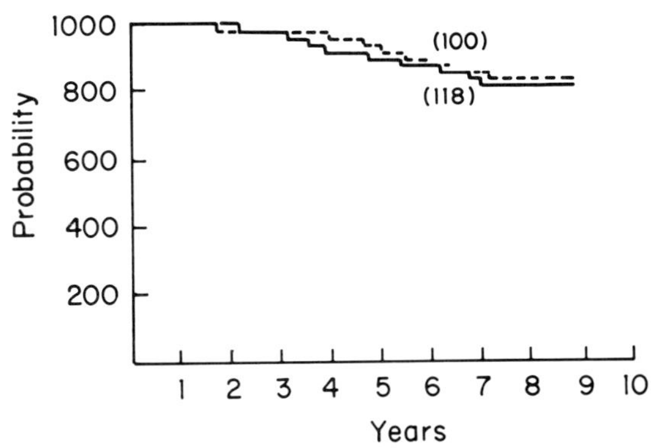

Figure 18-6 Actuarial overall survival in patients with Halsted mastectomy or with quadrantectomy, axillary dissection, and radiation therapy (QUART). —, Halsted (349); — —, QUART (352). (Loq rank test $p = .35$.) (*From Veronesi et al., 1983.*[45])

March 1985.[14] Based on the life-table analysis of 1843 patients, the major findings are as follows:

1 Preservation of the breast has not resulted in an adverse effect on disease-free survival, distant disease-free survival, and overall survival, as determined by actuarial projection to 5 years.

2 Segmental mastectomy plus radiation therapy offers better local tumor control than segmental mastectomy alone, 92.3 percent as compared with 72.1 percent at 5 years ($p < .001$). In other words, only 7.7 percent of patients receiving radiation therapy had a recurrence of tumor in the breast at 5 years, as compared with 27.9 percent of those treated by segmental mastectomy without radiation.

3 In patients with positive lymph nodes, 97.9 percent of patients treated with radiation and 63.8 percent of those receiving no radiation remained tumor-free ($p < .001$), although both groups received the same chemotherapy.

It is to be noted that fewer tumors developed in the breast after segmental mastectomy and radiation therapy in patients with positive nodes (all of whom received a course of chemotherapy before starting radiation therapy) than in those with negative nodes (who received no chemotherapy). The authors suggest that radiation therapy and chemotherapy may be additive, if not synergistic, in their effects.

The authors concluded that segmental mastectomy followed by breast irradiation in all patients and adjuvant chemotherapy in women with positive nodes is appropriate therapy for stages I and II breast tumors equal or less than 4 cm, provided that margins of resected specimen are free of tumor.

INDICATIONS

Based on the accumulated data both from retrospective studies and randomized clinical trials, it appears clear that limited surgery and radiation therapy can accomplish excellent results in the treatment of early breast cancer. This approach is not to replace radical or modified radical mastectomy, but is used to offer patients an alternative to mastectomy. There are many women who have a strong desire to keep their breasts. The fact that there is an alternative available means a great deal to them.[27]

Since the combination of breast-conserving surgery and radiation therapy is a relatively new approach compared to many decades of traditional treatment of radical or modified radical mastectomy, the indications for this method of treatment are not too well defined at present. Undoubtedly there will be changes as more knowledge and experience are gained in the future. It does appear clear that patients with T_1 or small T_2 tumors without palpable axillary nodes are probably the best candidates for local excision and radiation therapy. However, primary radiation therapy has been applied to patients with tumor sizes up to 5 cm in diameter and also to patients with palpable axillary lymph nodes, with uncertain results.

The surgical procedure should be at least a total excision of the primary tumor with a clear margin. An axillary lymph node dissection is also recommended for the following reasons: (1) histological examination of the nodes will provide information on the patient's prognosis, (2) removal of the nodes will minimize the need for intensive radiation to the axilla, and (3) patients with positive lymph nodes should receive adjuvant chemotherapy.

The extent of the axillary dissection ranges from sampling of a few lymph nodes to a complete axillary dissection. Sampling of nodes is not preferred because it might not yield adequate information and also when the sampled nodes are positive, the whole axilla will have to be irradiated. A full axillary dissection, up to the apex of the axilla (level III) has the advantage of complete removal of all axillary lymph nodes. However, it is usually associated with a higher incidence of breast and arm edema. Most radiation therapists and surgeons prefer a thorough dissection of lymph nodes in the lower and middle axilla (levels I and II). If positive lymph nodes are found, the apex of the axilla (level III) can be easily irradiated together with the supraclavicular nodes in one field.

CONTRAINDICATIONS

Contraindications for the approach of breast-conserving surgery and radiation therapy are still to be clearly defined as more experience is gained. There are two situations in which limited surgery and radiation therapy appeared to be contraindicated. Patients with two or more primaries, particularly in different quadrants of the breast, should not be considered for radiation therapy because the procedure will involve more than one local excision and more than one area for the boost treatment. The other situation involves patients with extensive multifocal disease with widespread calcifications demonstrated on mammogram. These patients are probably better treated with mastectomy.

RADIATION THERAPY TECHNIQUE

The major reasons for achieving improved local tumor control and cosmetic results of primary radiation therapy in recent years include the use of megavoltage therapy and the continuous refinement of treatment techniques.

Primary radiation therapy requires skillful, meticulous planning and execution of the course of treatment. The basic technique was derived from the irradiation of primary inoperable breast cancer but with two important modifications. First, in the case of inoperable cancer the local disease is advanced and the skin of the breast is often involved. Therefore, the skin should receive an adequate radiation dose mainly with the application of bolus. In early breast cancer, however, the skin is not involved by cancer and should be spared as much as possible in order to accomplish good cosmetic results. Therefore, the use of bolus should be avoided and instead, wedge compensators are to be applied to achieve a homogeneous dose in the breast without delivering an excessive dose to the skin. Second, the radiation dose required to eradicate the residual disease in the breast after tumor excision is less than the dose needed for a locally advanced, bulky tumor.

The areas to be irradiated depend on the location of the primary tumor and the axillary status. The techniques recommended are as follows.

Patients without an Axillary Dissection

For a patient who has had a local excision or partial mastectomy without an axillary dissection, the entire breast, axilla, internal mammary, and supraclavicular lymph node areas should be irradiated. The breast is usually treated with medial and lateral tangential fields using wedged filters to compensate for the irregular shape of the breast and to achieve a homogeneous radiation dose within the breast.

The dose given to the breast is usually between 4500 to 5000 rads delivered over a period of $4\frac{1}{2}$ to 5 weeks. This is followed by a boost dose of about 1500 rads in $1\frac{1}{2}$ weeks to the original tumor site. The boost dose may be delivered either by an interstitial implant of ^{192}Ir or by external beam therapy using photon or electron beam, depending on the patient's situation and the radiation therapist's preference. The ultimate results should be equally good.

A separate anterior field is used to irradiate the supraclavicular and axillary areas. The axilla may be boosted through a small posterior field. The internal mammary nodes should be incorporated in the tangential fields whenever possible. Occasionally a separate internal mammary field is used when the patient's chest is large, and it is not possible to include the internal mammary nodes in the tangential fields without underdosing the center of the breast. Whenever separate fields are used, however, extreme care must be exercised to avoid overdosage or underdosage at the adjoining fields. Overlapping of the fields, for example, can produce match line fibrosis.

The radiation dose given to the lymph node areas is usually about 4500 to 5000 rads in 4 to 5 weeks. Any palpable axillary lymph node should receive an additional dose of about 1000 rads in 1 week.

Patients with Axillary Dissection

For those patients who have had an axillary dissection, the treatment policy varies according to the location of the primary tumor and the extent of the dissection, as well as the axillary findings.

Negative Axillary Lymph Nodes

A patient with an outer quadrant primary tumor and negative axillary lymph nodes needs only to be treated to the breast. For a patient who had an inner quadrant lesion and negative axilla, the breast and internal mammary chain should be treated because there is a chance of medial metastasis to these lymph nodes, even though the axilla is negative.

Positive Axillary Lymph Nodes

Radiation therapy should be given to the breast and its regional lymph node areas. When axillary sampling only was performed and the nodes were positive, the whole axilla needs to be treated. When a thorough dissection was carried out to remove all nodes in the lower and middle axilla (levels I and II), only the apex of the axilla needs to be irradiated. The apex of the axilla is usually incorporated in the supraclavicular field.

In a patient who has had a complete dissection of nodes up to the apex of the axilla (levels I, II, and III), it is not necessary to irradiate the axilla at all.

Adjuvant chemotherapy should be considered for patients with positive axillary lymph nodes.[13,26]

Complications

Any treatment method is usually associated with some side effects. Primary radiation therapy for early breast cancer is no exception. With the use of modern techniques and careful treatment planning, undesirable side effects can be kept to a minimum. Possible complications associated with aggressive radiation therapy include radiation pneumonitis, rib fracture, late skin changes, and breast fibrosis. All of these occur rarely, below 5 percent of cases treated. There is also a possibility of breast or arm edema, particularly in patients who had an axillary dissection performed.

There is some concern regarding the possibility of radiation-induced secondary malignancy. Long-term follow-ups of many patients treated by primary radiation therapy, however, have shown no evidence of increased incidence of radiation-induced cancers.

RECURRENCE AND SALVAGE SURGERY

It is difficult to assess accurately the recurrence rates following limited surgery and radiation therapy because of different case materials and different reporting methods used by various authors. When orthovoltage therapy and modest radiation doses were used, the local-regional recurrence rate was about 25 percent at 10 years for patients with T_1, T_2, N_0 tumors.[30] Since the advent of modern radiation therapy techniques delivering higher tumor doses, the recurrence rates have shown a significant decrease. Based on some of the representative series reported, the overall recurrence rates, including patients with T_1, T_2, N_0, N_1 lesions, are about 5 to 6 percent at 5 years,[16,34,40] 13 to 14 percent at 10 years,[2,9] and 22 percent at 15 years.[20] The 22 percent 15-year recurrence rate was reported by Harris et al.[20] who did a collaborative study using materials from three institutions: Princess Margaret Hospital, Toronto, Canada; the Marseilles Cancer Institute, Marseilles, France; and the Institute Curie in Paris, France, to determine the time, course, and prognosis of local recurrence following primary radiation therapy. A total of 152 patients with early breast cancer treated before 1967 were examined. There were 35 local recurrences in the 158 breast cancers treated, for a crude 15-year rate of 22 percent. The authors pointed out that the techniques used in these three institutions before 1967 have since substantially improved and that recent radiation techniques have resulted in better local tumor control rates.

It has been emphasized by most authors who presented their experiences on limited surgery and radiation therapy that local-regional recurrences can be effectively treated by salvage surgery. It appears clear from many studies that recurrence in the breast or axilla after treatment by limited surgery and radiation therapy carries a different biological behavior in contrast to recurrence developed after a mastectomy. The majority of local or regional recurrences after a radical or modified mastectomy occurs within 3 years of surgery and usually signifies a poor prognosis, as many patients develop distant metastases and succumb to the breast cancer disease.[11] In the case of limited surgery and radiation therapy, local recurrence usually occurs at a later date and does not necessarily carry a poor prognosis. Most of these patients are still suitable for a mastectomy with reasonable expectation of long-term tumor control and survival. In general, the 5-year survival rates after a salvage surgery range from 60 to 70 percent.[2,9,20,28] It has also been reported that the overall survival rates of patients who had salvage mastectomy are similar to those who did not have breast or axillary recurrence.[6,24]

COSMETIC RESULTS

The cosmetic results of limited surgery and radiation therapy depend on the surgical and radiation therapy techniques. Skillful surgery in performing local excision and axillary dissection leave minimal or no deformity. Similarly, radiation therapy, when skillfully administered, produces minimal or no residual changes.

During the orthovoltage era, the irradiation of the breast with a moderate tumor dose frequently resulted in moist skin reactions, tanning, telangiectasia, and fibrosis. Megavoltage therapy has the advantage of deeper penetration and skin sparing. It is possible to deliver a higher tumor dose with minimal side effects. The cosmetic results of radiation therapy have shown significant improvement in recent years due to the use of megavoltage therapy, coupled with the continuous refinement of treatment techniques.

With the use of modern radiation techniques, excellent to good cosmetic results can be expected in over 90 percent of the patients treated.

SUMMARY

Surgery and radiation therapy are the two most effective local treatment methods for early carcinoma of the breast. A relatively new approach combining limited surgery and aggressive radiation therapy has evolved to treat patients with early cancer in order to achieve satisfactory tumor control and survival results without the loss of the breast.

The tumor control and cosmetic results depend on the combined skills of the surgeon and the radiation oncologist who manage the patient. Skillful surgery in performing tumor excision and axillary dissection will minimize deformities and lymph edema of the breast and arm. One of the major reasons contributing to the increasing use of primary radiation therapy in recent years is the improved radiation techniques utilizing megavoltage therapy and meticulous treatment planning. A high dose can be delivered to tumor-bearing areas with minimal side effects.

At the present time it appears safe to offer patients with early breast cancer the choice of breast-conserving surgery and primary radiation therapy as an alternative to mastectomy. This approach is relatively new,* therefore, there undoubtedly will be further refinements of treatment techniques based on the knowledge and experience gained from treating a greater number of patients.

REFERENCES

1. Amalric R, Santamaria F, Robert F, Seigle J, Altschuler C, Kurtz JM, Spitalier JM, Brandone H, Ayme Y, Pollet JF, Burmeister R, Abed R: Radiation therapy with or without primary limited surgery for operable breast cancer: A 20-year experience at the Marseilles Cancer Institute. *Cancer* 49:30, 1982.
2. Amalric R, Santamaria F, Robert F, Seigle J, Altshuler C, Pietra JC, Amalric F, Kurtz JM, Spitalier JM, Brandone H, Ayme Y, Pollet JF, Bressac C, Fondarai J: Conservation therapy of operable breast cancer—results at 5, 10, 15 years in 2216 consecutive cases, in Harris JR, Hellman S, Silen W. (eds.): *Conservative Management of Breast Cancer—New Surgical and Radiotherapeutic Techniques*. Philadelphia, J. B. Lippincott, 1983, p. 15.
3. Atkins H, Hayward JL, Klugman DJ, Wayte AB: Treatment of early breast cancer: A report after 10 years of a clinical trial. *Br Med J* 2:423, 1972.
4. Bedwinek JM, Perez CA, Kramer S, Brady LW, Goodman R, Grundy G: Irradiation as the primary management of stages I and II adenocarcinoma of the breast: Analysis of the RTOG breast registry. *Can Clin Trials* 3:11, 1980.
5. Bedwinek J: Treatment of stages I and II adenocarcinoma of the breast by tumor excision and irradiation. *Int J Radiat Oncol Biol Phys* 7:1553, 1981.
6. Calle R, Pilleron JP, Schlienger P, Vilcoq JR: Conservative management of operable breast cancer: Ten years experience at the Foundation Curie. *Cancer* 42:2045, 1978.
7. Calle R, Pilleron JP: Radiation therapy with and without lumpectomy for operable breast cancer: Ten year results. *Breast* 5:2, 1979.
8. Calle R, Vilcoq JR, Stacey P, Ghossein NA: The outcome of treatment by tumorectomy and radiotherapy of patients with operable breast cancer. *Int J Radiat Oncol Biol Phys* 5:124, 1979.
9. Calle R, Vilcoq JR, Pilleron JP, Schlienger P, Durand JP: Conservative treatment of operable breast carcinoma by irradiation with or without limited surgery—ten year results, in Harris JR, Hellman S, Silen W (eds.): *Conservative Management of Breast Cancer—New Surgical and Radiotherapeutic Techniques*. Philadelphia, J. B. Lippincott, 1983, p. 3.
10. Chu AM, Cope O, Russo R, Wang CC, Schulz MD, Wang C, Rodkey G: Treatment of early stage breast cancer by limited surgery and radical irradiation. *Int J Radiat Oncol Biol Phys* 6:25, 1980.
11. Chu FCH, Lin FJ, Kim JH, Huh SH, Garmatis GJ: Locally recurrent carcinoma of the breast—results of radiation therapy. *Cancer* 37:2677, 1976.
12. Clark RM, Wilkinson RH, Mahoney LJ, Reid JG, Macdonald WD: Breast cancer: A 21 year experience with conservative surgery and radiation. *Int J Radiat Oncol Biol Phys* 8:967, 1982.
13. Danoff BF, Goodman RL, Glick JH, Haller DG, Pajak TF: The effect of adjuvant chemotherapy

**Editors' Note:* Longer follow-up is necessary to determine the exact role of this form of treatment in the curative treatment of breast cancer.

on cosmesis and complications in patients with breast cancer treated by definitive irradiation. *Int J Radiat Oncol Biol Phys* 9:1625, 1983.

14. Fisher B, Bauer M, Margolese R, Poisson R, Pilch Y, et al: Five-year results of a randomized clinical trial comparing total mastectomy and segmental mastectomy with or without radiation in the treatment of breast cancer. *N Engl J Med* 312:665, 1985.
15. Harris JR, Goeffrey F, Beadle MBBS, Hellman S: Clinical studies on the use of radiation therapy as primary treatment of early breast cancer. *Cancer* 53:705, 1984.
16. Harris JR, Botnick L, Bloomer WB, Chaffey JT, Hellman S: Primary radiation therapy for early breast cancer—the experience at the Joint Center for Radiation Therapy. *Int J Radiat Oncol Biol Phys* 7:1549, 1981.
17. Harris JR, Connolly JL, Schnitt SJ, Cohen RB, Hellman S: Clinical-pathologic study of early breast cancer treated by primary radiation therapy. *J Clin Oncol* 1:184, 1983.
18. Harris JR, Hellman S, Silen W: *Conservative Management of Breast Cancer: New Surgical and Radiotherapeutic Techniques.* Philadelphia, J. B. Lippincott, 1983.
19. Harris, JR, Levene MG, Svensson G, Hellman S: Analysis of cosmetic results following primary radiation therapy for stages I and II carcinoma of the breast. *Int J Radiat Oncol Biol Phys* 5:257, 1979.
20. Harris JR, Recht A, Amalric R, Calle R, Clark M, Reid JG, Spitalier JM, Vilcoq FR, Hellman S: Time course and prognosis of local recurrence following primary radiation therapy for early breast cancer. *J Clin Oncol* 2:37, 1984.
21. Hayward J: The surgeon's role in primary breast cancer. *Breast Cancer Res Treat* 1:27, 1981.
22. Hayward JL: The Guy's Hospital trials on breast conservation, in Harris JR, Hellman S, Silen W (eds.): *Conservative Management of Breast Cancer—New Surgical and Radiotherapeutic Techniques.* Philadelphia, J. B. Lippincott, 1983, p. 77.
23. Keynes G: Conservative treatment of breast cancer. *Br Med J* 2:643, 1937.
24. Kurtz JM, Spitalier JM, Amalric R: Results of salvage surgery for local recurrence following primary radiation therapy of operable breast cancer. *Int J Radiat Oncol Biol Phys* 7:1221, 1981.
25. Levene MB, Harris JR, Hellman S: Treatment of carcinoma of the breast by radiation therapy. *Cancer* 39:2840, 1977.
26. Lippmann ME, Lichter AS, Edwards BK, Gorrell CR, d'Angelo T, DeMoss EV: The impact of primary irradiation treatment of localized breast cancer on the ability to administer systemic adjuvant chemotherapy. *J Clin Oncol* 2:21, 1984.
27. Margolis GJ, Carabell SC, Goodman RL: Psychological aspect of primary radiation therapy for breast carcinoma. *Am J Clin Oncol* 6:533, 1983.
28. Montague ED: Conservation surgery and radiation therapy in the treatment of operable breast cancer. *Cancer* 53:700, 1984.
29. Mustakallio S: Treatment of breast cancer by tumor extirpation and roentgen therapy instead of radical operation. *J Fac Radiol* 16:23, 1954.
30. Mustakallio S: Conservative treatment of breast cancer review of 25 years follow up. *Clin Radiol* 23:110, 1972.
31. Peters MV: Wedge resection and irradiation: An effective treatment of early breast cancer. *JAMA* 200:144, 1967.
32. Peters MV: Wedge resection with and without radiation in early breast cancer. *Int J Radiat Oncol Biol Phys* 2:1151, 1977.
33. Pierquin B, Own R, Maylin C, Ptmezguine Y, Raynal M, Meuller W, Hannoun S: Radical radiation therapy of breast cancer. *Int J Radiat Oncol Biol Phys* 6:17, 1980.
34. Pierquin B: Conservative treatment for carcinoma of the breast—Experience of Cretail-ten year results, in Harris JR, Hellman S, Silen W (eds.): *Conservative Managment of Breast Cancer—New Surgical and Radiotherapeutic Techniques.* Philadelphia, J. B. Lippincott, 1983, p. 11.
35. Prosnitz L, Goldenberg IS, Harris J, Levene M, Hellman S, Wailner PE, Brady LW: Primary radiotherapy for stages I and II breast cancer: Follow-up report from four east coast university hospitals. *Int J Radiat Oncol Biol Phys* 6:1339, 1980.
36. Prosnitz LR, Goldenberg IS, Weshler Z, Lawrence R: Radiotherapy instead of mastectomy for breast cancer—The Yale experience, in Harris JR, Hellman S, Silen W (eds.): *Conservative Management of Breast Cancer—New Surgical and Radiotherapeutic Techniques.* Philadelphia, J. B. Lippincott, 1983, p. 61.

37. Rissanen PM: A comparison of conservative and radical surgery combined with radiotherapy in the treatment of stage I carcinoma of the breast. *Br J Radiol* 42:423, 1969.
38. Rissanen PM, Holsti P: A comparison between conservative and radical surgery combined with radiotherapy in the treatment of breast cancer stage I—a 10-year follow up study on 866 patients. *Strahlentherapie* 147:370, 1974.
39. Rissanen P, Holsti P: Late results of local excision combined with radiotherapy in the treatment of early breast cancer—twenty year follow up—effect of megavoltage therapy in incident of local recurrences. Presented at the International Congress of Radiology, Rio de Janeiro, Brazil, October 1977.
40. Sarrazin D, Le M, Rouesse J, Contesso G, Petit J, Lacour J, Viguir J, Hill C: Conservative treatment versus mastectomy in breast cancer tumors with macroscopic diameter of 20 millimeters or less—the experience of the Institut Gustave-Roussy. *Cancer* 53:1209, 1984.
41. Schottenfeld D, Nash AG, Robbins GF, Beattie EJ: Ten-year results of the treatment of primary operable breast cancer: A summary of 304 patients evaluated by the TNM system. *Cancer* 38:1001, 1976.
42. Spitalier J, Brandone H, Ayme Y, Amalric R, Santamaria F, Seigels J: Cesium therapy of breast cancer—a five-year report on 400 consecutive patients. *Int J Radiat Oncol Biol Phys* 2:231, 1977.
43. Veronesi U, Banfi A, Saccozzi R, Salvadori B, Zucali R, Uselghi C, Greco M, Luini A, Rilke F, Sultan L: Conservative treatment of breast cancer: A trial in progress at the Cancer Institute of Milan. *Cancer* 39:2822, 1977.
44. Veronesi U, Saccozzi R, Del Vecchio M: Comparison of radical mastectomy with quadrantectomy, axillary dissection and radiotherapy in patients with small cancers of the breast. *N Engl J Med* 305:6, 1981.
45. Veronesi U, Del Vecchio M, Greco M, Luini A, Muscolino G, Responi A, Saccozzi R, Zucali R: Results of quadrantectomy, axillary dissection and radiotherapy (QUART) in T_1 N_0 patients, in Harris JR, Hellman S, Silen W. (eds.): *Conservative Management of Breast Cancer—New Surgical and Radiotherapeutic Techniques*. Philadelphia, J. B. Lippincott, 1983, p. 91.

19

Modified Radical Mastectomy

Gerson Lesnick, M.D.

INTRODUCTION

The radical mastectomy operation was devised at a time when most patients with breast cancer sought care only after a large tumor deforming the breast had already developed. Prior to the era of aseptic surgery, all operations on the breast for cancer were associated with a frightful mortality from overwhelming sepsis, and patients who survived that experienced rapid local and regional recurrence. Halsted, in 1894,[1] reported his results in the first 50 cases of what he called the complete operation for breast cancer, now known as the radical mastectomy or Halsted operation. His local recurrence rate at that time was 6 percent (although he considered the appearance of skin nodules away from the scar as evidence of a regional rather than local recurrence), while the local recurrence rates were 60 to 85 percent in cases treated by other surgeons. Combining local and regional recurrences, his total local-regional recurrence rate was 24 percent.[2] This was a dramatic improvement over the earlier results and was responsible for the rapid acceptance of the radical mastectomy as the standard treatment for all operable breast cancer. Although there was already evidence[3] that less extensive procedures, in which the pectoralis major was not removed and in which axillary dissection was not as complete, had postoperative survival superior to that with the more radical operation, the authors could not believe their own statistics; they reasoned that the improved survival after less extensive procedures must have been due to selecting more severe or more extensive cases for the more extensive operative procedure. Shortly thereafter, the newly discovered roentgen ray was used to supplement the surgical procedure. For 50 years after these developments, radical

The current TNM system of classification is used throughout.

mastectomy supplemented by x-radiation remained the standard treatment for operable breast cancer.

MODIFICATION OF RADICAL MASTECTOMY

Persistently high mortality and recurrence rates, as well as dissatisfaction with the disability following the radical operation, led to reconsideration. Patients were being seen earlier in the course of their disease with smaller tumors. It seemed illogical that these small tumors required the same sort of therapy as larger ones. Patey and Dyson,[4] influenced by the anatomical studies of Gray, which showed that the pectoral fascia was relatively free of lymphatic channels and so was an unlikely route for spread of cancer, devised an operative procedure leaving the pectoralis major muscle intact but removing the breast, pectoralis minor, and axillary contents. In 1948 they compared the results in 42 of their patients treated by standard radical mastectomy with 40 of their patients treated by modified radical mastectomy. There was no difference in 3-year survival rates after either operation in the patients with axillary node involvement and in those without such involvement. There was also no difference in local recurrence rates.

The several advantages of this surgical approach to the treatment of breast cancer were compelling. The improved results in appearance and function after modified mastectomy with preservation of the pectoralis muscles were obvious. The muscle provided a better bed for skin graft should this be necessary. It also provided a better cover for a prosthesis in any attempted reconstruction. Preservation of the muscle improved arm function and permitted active participation in sports. Prostheses were more easily fitted, and normal clothing could be worn. In retrospective studies, results from this operation compared favorably with those from the standard radical mastectomy.

The Patey Operation

The modification of the radical mastectomy proposed and practiced by Patey and Dyson and reported by them in 1948[4] was based on the same concept of spread of cancer as that which led to the Halsted radical mastectomy. The modification was prompted by anatomical studies which showed the skin to be particularly rich in lymphatics and the pectoral fascia to be practically devoid of lymphatics and, therefore, an unlikely route for spread of cancer. They noted that resection and axillary dissection following the modified procedure was just as thorough as that following the radical operation provided that the pectoralis minor muscle was divided. They had noted also that the major nerve supply and blood supply of the pectoralis major could be preserved with this dissection. The modified operation yielded substantially improved appearance and function of the arm. It was followed by atrophy of the lateral third of the pectoralis major muscle caused by division of the medial pectoral nerves secondary to division of the pectoralis minor muscle. They commented that there was no additional deformity if the lateral part of the pectoralis major was widely excised when the tumor was close to it. Handley in 1965 described the operation in detail.[5]

The Auchincloss–Madden Operation

In 1963 Auchincloss,[6] basing his recommendations on Pickren's[7] findings indicating the extreme infrequency of involvement of apical lymph nodes in the absence of extensive lymph node metastasis, suggested that breast cancer could be controlled by removing the breast and axillary nodes from a point opposite approximately the middle of the posterior surface of the pectoralis minor laterally to the subscapular vessels. Madden in 1972 described a similar operation.[8]

Dissection of the extreme apex of the axilla is more difficult when the pectoralis minor is to be preserved. It can be accomplished, however, if the vessels and lymphatics entering the apical nodes are controlled with hemostatic clips. The pectoralis minor and major are elevated together with flat retractors to permit this access. Preservation of the pectoralis minor and its nerve supply controls the tendency of the shoulder on the affected side to be elevated following either modified or radical mastectomy. Injury to the medial pectoral nerve, which is inevitable if the pectoralis minor is divided, results, as above, in atrophy of a varying amount of the lateral and inferior part of the pectoralis major. The consequent deformity may mimic that following a radical mastectomy, but will not be as severe as when the lateral pectoral nerve is injured in addition. It is possible to identify and preserve the medial pectoral nerve. The nerve reaches the pectoralis minor from the brachial plexus at a point lateral to the insertion of the pectoralis minor into the coracoid process. It runs along the lateral edge of this muscle for a variable distance before penetrating the muscle. Branches to the pectoralis major traverse the pectoralis minor and then cross the interpectoral space to enter the pectoralis major on the lateral aspects of its deep surface. There may be one or more such branches of the pectoral and lateral thoracic vessels. The pectoralis major is also innervated by the lateral pectoral nerve. Careful dissection of the interpectoral space will permit division of the vessels and preservation of the small nerves which can then be retracted superiorly during dissection of the fat and lymph nodes in the interpectoral space (Fig. 19-1).

Branches of the medial pectoral nerve may also proceed directly from the lateral edge of

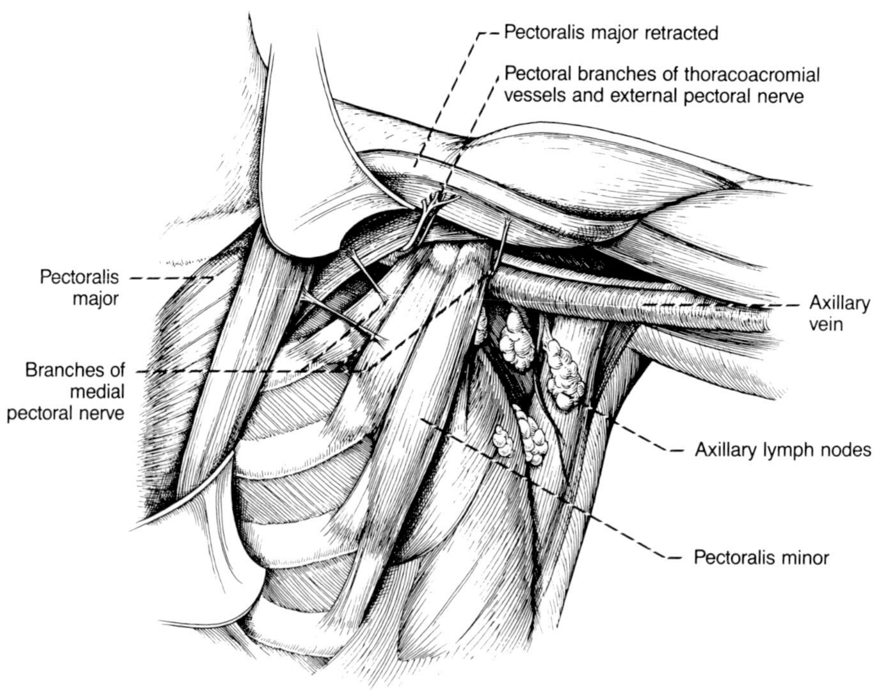

Figure 19-1 Anatomy of axilla after retracting the pectoralis major demonstrating the external and medial pectoral nerves.

the pectoralis minor to the superior part of the lateral edge of the pectoralis major where they accompany branches of the lateral thoracic vessels. With care, these medial pectoral branches also can be identified and preserved without interfering with the subsequent axillary dissection. Preservation of these nerves results in a more normal contour of the anterior axillary fold and of the chest wall.

PRESENT TECHNIQUE OF MODIFIED MASTECTOMY

The incision is an oblique ellipse surrounding the breast and extends from the region of the xiphoid process to the lower axilla. The incision should be placed to clear the biopsy incision and the tumor by 4 cm in all directions. Skin flaps are then raised to the level of the first rib superiorly, the midline medially, to a line approximately 2 cm below the inframammary fold inferiorly, and to the anterior edge of the latissimus dorsi muscle laterally. The dissection is performed in a plane between the dermis and the membranous layer of the superficial fascia.

At the superior and medial limits of flap dissection the incision is carried to and then through the pectoral fascia. The breast is separated from the pectoral muscle by sharp dissection in this plane. The perforating branches from the internal thoracic and intercostal vessels can be identified and clamped before they are divided. Dissection is continued to the lateral edge of the pectoralis major. During this dissection any ecchymosis or hematoma from the biopsy incision can be seen if the tumor had been located deep in the breast near the pectoral fascia. At such points a portion of the pectoralis major muscle underlying the tumor can be excised. This is done, although all the surgeons who have reported their results with operations preserving the pectoralis major muscle have indicated that recurrences in this muscle are extremely infrequent.

The dissection of the pectoral fascia continues on the undersurface of the pectoralis major and the interpectoral space is entered. Branches of the pectoral and lateral thoracic vessels cross this space, as do branches of the medial pectoral nerve. The vascular branches can be divided but if the medial pectoral nerve is preserved, it will avoid atrophy of the lateral third of the pectoralis major muscle.

Dissection of the Interpectoral Nodes (Rotter's Nodes)

Although division of the pectoralis minor facilitates dissection of the apex of the axilla, it does not assist in dissection of the interpectoral space or in removal of Rotter's nodes. The latter accompany the pectoral branches of the thoracoacromial vessels and the lateral pectoral nerve as they run on the deep surface of the pectoralis major and are closely adherent to this muscle. The nodes, which are small, can be felt on the deep surface of the muscle. They are more readily palpable if they are involved with metastatic cancer. In excising them care must be taken to avoid damage to the accompanying neural and vascular structures, the lateral pectoral nerve, and the pectoral branches of the thoracoacromial vessels. Preservation of these structures is essential to survival of the pectoralis major muscle. This neurovascular bundle attains the undersurface of the pectoralis major at the medial edge of the tendon of the pectoralis minor.

The interpectoral nodes should always be searched for and excised. In approximately 1 percent of patients with breast carcinoma, Rotter's nodes are the only nodes involved. Identification of these patients for postoperative adjuvant therapy is worthwhile.[9]

Dissection of the Axilla

Dissection of the axilla is continued from the apex to the subscapular vessels. The lateral thoracic vessels are ligated close to their origins and insertions into the axillary vessels. The subscapular vessels are preserved, but the anterior circumflex humeral is divided. The long thoracic and the thoracodorsal nerves are identified. The nodes in the subscapular space between these nerves are excised together with the subscapular fat pad. Small vessels crossing through the fat pad are ligated and divided, freeing the entire specimen.

To minimize any tendency toward edema of the arm, care should be taken to avoid dissection superior to the axillary vein. The dissection of the nodes should stop laterally at the subscapular vessels. Nodes lateral to these vessels drain lymphatics from the arm. They are involved by metastatic breast cancer only when axillary involvement is massive.

The operation is completed by dividing the lateral branches of the intercostal vessels and nerves from the second to the fifth interspaces, where they emerge through the serratus muscle. When it is unlikely that axillary nodes are involved with tumor, it is possible to spare the intercostobrachial nerve. Preservation of this nerve preserves sensation to the medial aspect of the dorsum of the upper arm and eliminates annoying paresthesia in this region which otherwise frequently follows axillary dissection. Catheters are placed into the axilla and medial part of the wound for postoperative suction drainage. It is almost always possible to close the wound primarily without tension. A dressing is placed on the wound on the chest wall but the arm is left free so that its motion is not restricted.

The patient is encouraged to use her arm normally from the first day. If the nerves are spared there is no need for any structured exercise regimen. Vigorous exercise leads only to excess serum accumulation in the wound. Motion is usually complete within about 6 weeks without any special care. At this time any residual limitation responds readily and completely to a little encouragement of active use of the arm.

RESULTS AFTER MODIFIED MASTECTOMY

All comparisons of modified radical mastectomy and radical mastectomy have shown no differences in survival or recurrence rates. In 1948 Patey and Dyson,[4] in their original description of the operation, reported the experience of patients operated upon by Dr. Patey. He had treated 40 patients by modified radical mastectomy and followed them up for 3 to 9 years. Their survival was compared to that of 42 patients whom he had treated by radical mastectomy during the same time interval. There was no difference in survival in either patients with involved axillary lymph nodes or in those without such involvement (Table 19-1).

In 1963 Handley and Thackray,[10,11] in a comparative international study reported their results from modified mastectomy. These results were compared with survival following radical mastectomy at several other institutions. Cases were staged by the Columbia clinical classification described by Haagensen.[11] Handley and Thackray noted 75 percent survival

Table 19-1 Three-Year Survival following Standard Radical and Modified Radical Mastectomy

	Standard radical mastectomy	Modified radical mastectomy
Survival with axillary involvement, %	46	45
Survival without axillary involvement, %	78	83

Source: Patey and Dyson.[4]

in stage A cases, 57 percent in stage B, and 25 percent in stage C. (These stages correspond roughly to stages I, II, and III of the International TNM staging system.) For stage A and stage B cases these results were almost identical to those reported by Butcher after radical mastectomy[11] and Dahl-Iversen and Tobiassen after extended radical mastectomy[11] (Table 19-2). Haagensen and Cooley reported improved survival of 84 percent in stage A cases, 59 percent in stage B cases, 43 percent in stage C, and 16 percent in stage D. In interpreting these findings one must consider Haagensen's very strict application of criteria of operability.[11] In 1969,[12] the 10-year results for these same series also yielded only small differences, which might well have been due to differences in the populations studied.

In 1975 Papatestas and Lesnick[13] reported a comparative evaluation of results obtained in patients treated by conventional radical mastectomy and modified mastectomy performed by Lesnick during the years 1965 through 1968. During this time assignment to one or the other treatment group was dictated by circumstances; generally, patients who expressed an aversion to radical mastectomy and elderly and poor-risk patients were assigned to the group which underwent modified mastectomy. From December 1964 to December 1968 164 patients with carcinoma of the breast apparently localized to the breast and regional lymph nodes had been treated. Of these patients, 105 were treated by conventional radical mastectomy, 56 by modified mastectomy, 2 by simple mastectomy, and 1 by segmental resection. During this time interval, radical mastectomy was the procedure of choice in operable carcinoma of the breast. Modified radical mastectomy was offered to patients with stage I or II tumors who were poor operative risks due to illness or age or who expressed aversion to radical mastectomy. The simple mastectomies and the partial mastectomy were used for extremely elderly, poor-risk patients. In order to obtain a meaningful comparison of the two operative procedures, patients previously treated for other cancers were excluded from the study as were patients presenting with simultaneous bilateral carcinomas. In addition, all patients with stage III tumors were excluded; staging was by the International TNM System. There remained 134 patients with clinical stage I and stage II tumors, of whom 51 were treated by modified radical mastectomy and 83 by conventional radical mastectomy. Of these patients, 132 (99 percent) completed a 5-year follow-up study. The remaining patients were considered as dying of disease at the time of the last visit. There was 81 percent 5-year survival in patients treated by radical mastectomy and 84 percent in those treated by modified radical mastectomy. Among patients who did not have palpable axillary adenopathy, survival was identical in both

Table 19-2 Results of Treatment in Mammary Carcinoma: 5-Year Survival Columbia Clinical Classification

Columbia Clinical Classification	Handley–Thackray, conservative radical mastectomy		Butcher, radical mastectomy		Haagensen–Cooley, radical mastectomy		Dahl-Iversen–Tobiassen, super radical	
	Patients	Surviving, %	Patients	Surviving, %	Patients	Surviving, %	Patients	Surviving, %
A	77	75	216	76	344	84	277	77
B	58	57	135	48	138	59	61	48
C	8	25	48	48	63	43	20	50
D	0		26	11	11	18	8	37
Total	143	65	425	60	556	72	366	70

Source: Haagensen, Cooley et al.[11]

groups, 83 percent. When nodes were histologically negative, 5-year survival of 86 percent was noted for both groups. When nodes were positive, there was 73 percent survival after radical mastectomy and 80 percent after modified mastectomy. There were few local or regional recurrences in the 5-year period. They occurred in three patients treated by modified mastectomy and in six of those treated by radical mastectomy.

In 1979 the series was extended to include all patients treated through June 1972.[14] By then, there were 107 patients treated by modified radical mastectomy and 208 by Halsted radical. The results again were essentially identical after modified and radical mastectomy (Table 19-3). Local recurrences were also infrequent (Table 19-4).

Ten-Year Survival

Ten-year survival data are now available on 148 patients treated by modified radical mastectomy from 1966 through 1973. Their survival can be compared with that observed in 221 patients treated by radical mastectomy during the same years. At the beginning of this period radical mastectomy was considered the treatment of choice for operable breast cancer. During this period of time increasing numbers of patients were treated by modified mastectomy. After 1974 modified mastectomy was used for most patients with stages I and II breast cancer.

Patients were clinically staged by the TNM staging system of the Union International Contre Cancer (UICC) and the American Joint Committee for Cancer Staging and End Results Reporting. Results in patients with stage I tumors, that is, tumors less than 2 cm in diameter (T_1) without palpable axillary adenopathy (N_0), were compared after modified and radical mastectomy. Patients with stage II tumors (tumors 2 to 5 cm in diameter (T_2) without palpable axillary adenopathy (N_0) or with mobile axillary nodes (N_1) and tumors less than 2 cm in diameter (T_1) with palpable mobile axillary nodes (N_1) were compared with stage II tumors treated by radical mastectomy.

Patients with larger tumors, more than 5 cm in diameter, with tumors invading skin or fascia (T_3) and (T_4), as well as patients with axillary nodes adherent to each other or to fascia (N_2) were eliminated from this analysis. Patients previously treated for breast cancer or other cancers (except skin cancers) and patients

Table 19-3 Five-Year Survival Rates Radical and Modified Radical Mastectomy, January 1967 through June 1972

	107 Modified radical		208 Radical	
Category	Stage I (%)	Stage II (%)	Stage I (%)	Stage II (%)
Clinical staging*				
Living without recurrence	85	64	86	65
Living	91	69	91	75
Died of breast cancer	2	18	6	21
Histologic staging T_1 and T_2 tumors				
Living without recurrence	79	52	78	59
Living	81	65	85	74
Died of breast cancer	8	22	12	24

*Clinical staging UICC (Union International Contre Cancer) TNM system. Stage I T_1N_0, Stage II T_1N_1, T_2N_0 and N_1.

Source: Lesnick.[14]

Table 19-4 Five-Year Local Recurrence Rates, January 1967 through June 1972 (%)*

Category	Modified	Radical
$T_1\ N_0$,† $T_1\ N_1$	1.9	2.7
$T_2\ N_0$, $T_2\ N_1$	5.5	9
All cases	3.7	6.7

*Total series 5.7.
†N_0: No palpable axillary nodes.
Source: Lesnick.[14]

with bilateral breast cancer were also eliminated from the analysis.

Since many of the patients were elderly and died from causes unrelated to their breast cancer without having displayed any evidence of recurrent disease, mortality from breast cancer is given as well as overall mortality. These results are shown graphically in Figs. 19-2 and 19-3 as survival curves calculated by the method of Berkson and Gage.[15] Five- and ten-year survival rates are also shown in Table 19-5.

The survival following either radical or modified radical mastectomy for stage I tumors again shows virtual identity. However, the results in stage II cases show some differences. As time progressed and modified mastectomy was used more frequently, the case distribution of those treated with modified or radical mastectomy changed. Increasing numbers of the more favorable stage II cases received modified mastectomy, leaving a larger proportion of more advanced cases in the radical group. Thus, although there was no difference in survival in stage I patients, the stage II patients show a decreased survival from breast cancer after radical mastectomy. On the other hand, this increased mortality from breast cancer was balanced by an increased mortality from non-cancer-related causes in the group treated by modified mastectomy which contained more patients over 70 years of age (Fig. 19-4). There were no significant differences in absolute survival after either modified or radical mastectomy.

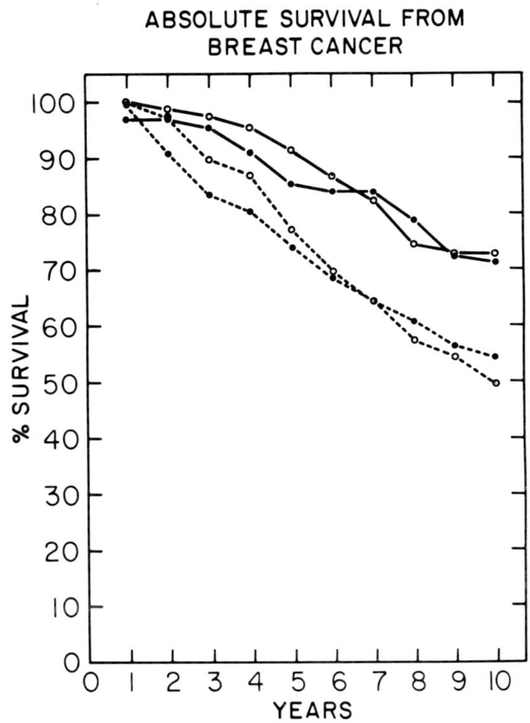

Figure 19-2 Ten-year absolute survival of patients with breast cancer after radical or modified mastectomy. Stage I: Modified (o—); radical (•—), Stage II: Modified (o---); radical (•---). (*Source: Patients of G. Lesnick, operations 1966 through 1973.*)

The survival curves demonstrate that deaths from breast cancer continue throughout the period of observation (Fig. 19-3). Seventeen of the 206 patients living at the end of this 10-year period had evidence of recurrent cancer at that time.

Local and Regional Recurrences

Local and regional recurrences were infrequent. They occurred in 7 of the 148 patients treated by modified mastectomy (4.7 percent) and 17 of the 221 patients treated by radical mastectomy (7.7 percent). They occurred most frequently in the patients with larger tumors. The most common site was the supraclavicular region, which had 45 percent of the recurrences.

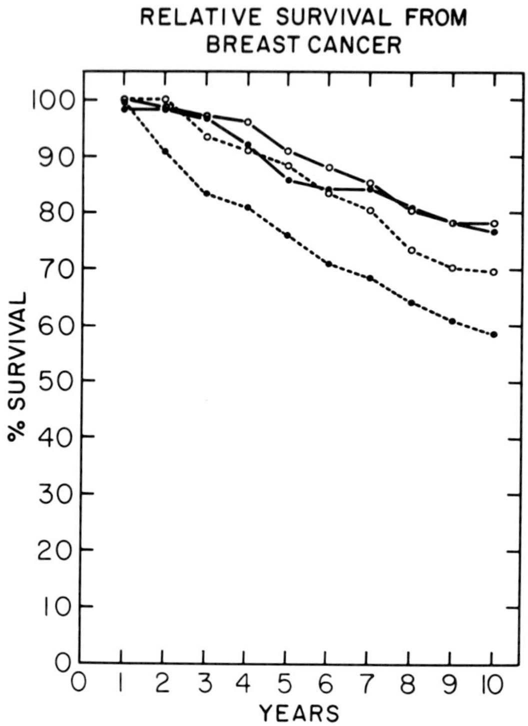

Figure 19-3 Survival from breast cancer after radical or modified mastectomy. Stage I: modified (o—); radical (•—). Stage II: modified (o---); radical (•---). Losses from noncancer deaths in patients with no evidence of recurrence of cancer censored at time of death. (*Source: Patients of G. Lesnick, operations 1966 through 1973.*)

There is some question as to whether this should be considered a local recurrence or whether it is really evidence of systemic dissemination. The tissues of the chest wall on the operated side was the second commonest site, with 40 percent of the recurrences. The axillary and parasternal regions were responsible for the remaining instances. Two-thirds of the recurrences appeared within 5 years after operation. The remainder occurred thereafter, some as late as 10 or more years after operation.

Similar results have been reported by Robinson et al. from the Mayo Clinic,[16] Baker et al. from The Johns Hopkins Hospital,[17] and Mendes Da Costa et al. from the Institute Jules Bordet in Brussels.[18]

Results of Prospective Randomized Trials

In 1981 the first report of a prospective randomized trial was reported by Turner et al.[19] The trial included 534 patients with stages I and II breast cancer treated between October 1969 and September 1976 by five participating surgeons. The data presented included a median follow-up of 5 years range, 1 to 128 months. Actuarial curves were prepared for total survival, local recurrence, distant metastases, and disease-free interval. There was no statistically significant difference in any of the variables. The curves for radical and modified mastectomy were superimposable for the greater part of the 10 years.

Another multiauthored trial from the University of Alabama in Birmingham was reported in 1983.[20] Three-hundred-and-eleven patients were treated by 91 surgeons between 1975 and 1978 in a surgical and adjunctive chemotherapy trial. After 5.5 years median follow-up there was no significant difference in disease-free survival or overall survival. There was, however, a trend toward improved survival in the radical mastectomy group and a statistically insignificant increased incidence of local recurrence in patients treated by modified mastectomy.

CONCLUSION

All these reports indicate the equal effectiveness of modified mastectomy and the standard Halsted radical mastectomy in the treatment of T_1, T_2, N_0, and N_1 breast cancer. Before any controlled trial, modified radical mastectomy had become the operation of choice for operable breast cancer. Pattern-of-care studies of the American College of Surgeons Commission on Cancer showed that in 1972, 50 percent of women surveyed who had breast cancer had a Halsted mastectomy and only 28 percent

Table 19-5 Five- and 10-Year Survival Rates following Modified Radical and Standard Radical Mastectomy

	5-Year survival, %		10-Year survival, %	
	Modified	Standard	Modified	Standard
Stage I T_1 N_0				
Number of patients	69	69	69	69
Survival from breast cancer, %	91	86	79	76
Absolute survival, %	91	85	73	71
Stage II T_1 N_1 + T_2 N_0 + T_2 N_1				
Number of patients	79	154	79	154
Survival from breast cancer, %	88	76	68	58
Absolute survival, %	77	74	49	54

Source: Patients of G. Lesnick—operations performed between January 1, 1966, and December 31, 1973.

had a modified radical mastectomy. In 1976, 55 percent underwent modified radical mastectomy and 28 percent had a Halsted operation. In 1981 only 3 percent of the women treated had the Halsted operation and 78 percent had undergone a modified radical mastectomy.[21]

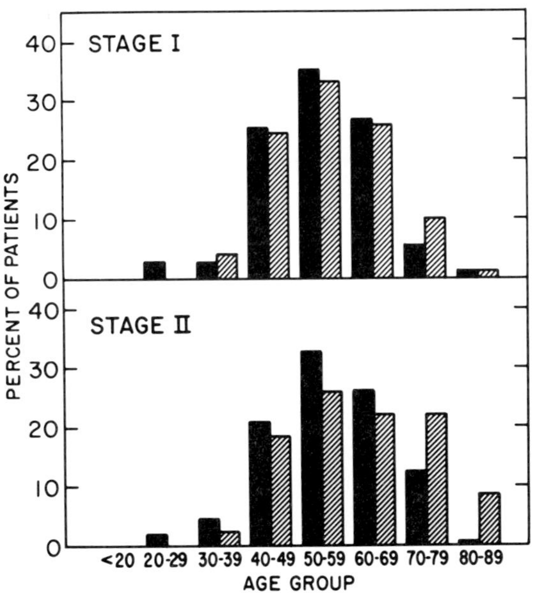

Figure 19-4 Age distribution of patients treated by modified and radical mastectomy. Stage I mastectomy: Radical, ■; modified, □. (*Source: Patients of G. Lesnick, operations 1966 through 1973.*)

REFERENCES

1. Halsted WS: The results of operations for the cure of cancer of the breast performed at The Johns Hopkins Hospital from June 1889 to January 1894. *Johns Hopkins Hosp Rep* 4:297, 1894–95.
2. Halsted WS: A clinical and histologic study of certain adenocarcinomas of the breast and a brief consideration of the supraclavicular operation and of the results of operations for cancer of the breast from 1889 to 1898 at the Johns Hopkins Hospital. *Tr Am SA* 16:44, 1898.
3. Greenough RB, Simmons CC, Barney JD: The results of operations for cancer of the breast at the Massachusetts General Hospital from 1894 to 1904. *Tr Am SA* 25:80, 1907.
4. Patey DH, Dyson WH: The prognosis of carcinoma of the breast in relation to the type of operation performed. *Br J Cancer* 2:7, 1948.
5. Handley RS: The technique and results of conservative radical mastectomy (Patey's operation). *Prog Clin Cancer* 1:462, 1965.
6. Auchincloss H: Significance of location and number of axillary metastases in carcinoma of the breast. *Ann Surg* 158:37, 1963.

7. Pickren JW, Rube J, Auchincloss H: Modification of conventional radical mastectomy. A detailed study of lymph node involvement and follow-up information to show its practicality. *Cancer* 18:942, 1965.
8. Madden JL, Kandalaft S, Bourque RA: Modified radical mastectomy. *Ann Surg* 175:624, 1972.
9. Kay S: Evaluation of Rotter's lymph nodes in radical mastectomy specimens as a guide to prognosis. *Cancer* 18:1441, 1965.
10. Handley RS, Thackray AC: Conservative radical mastectomy (Patey's operation). *Ann Surg* 157:162, 1963.
11. Haagensen CD, Cooley E, Kennedy CS, Miller E, Handley RS, Thackray AC, Butcher HR, Dahl-Iversen E, Tobiassen T, Williams IG, Curwen MP, Kaae S, Johansen H: Treatment of early mammary carcinoma. A cooperative international study. *Ann Surg* 157:157, 1963.
12. Haagensen CD, Cooley E, Kennedy CS, Miller E, Handley RS, Thackray AC, Butcher HR, Dahl-Iversen E, Tobiassen T, Williams IG, Curwen MP, Kaae S, Johansen H: Treatment of early mammary carcinoma. A cooperative international study. *Ann Surg* 170:875, 1969.
13. Papatestas AE, Lesnick GJ: Treatment of carcinoma of the breast by modified radical mastectomy. *Surg Gynecol Obstet* 140:22, 1975.
14. Lesnick G: Surgical treatment of breast cancer. *NY State J Med* 79:211, 1979.
15. Berkson J, Gage RP: Calculation of survival rates for cancer. *Proc Staff Meetings of the Mayo Clinic* 25:270, 1950.
16. Robinson GN, Van Heerden JA, Payne WS, Taylor WF, Gaffey TA: The primary surgical treatment of carcinoma of the breast. A changing trend toward modified radical mastectomy. *Mayo Clin Proc* 51:433, 1976.
17. Baker RR, Montague CW, Childs JN: A comparison of modified radical mastectomy to radical mastectomy in the treatment of operable breast cancer. *Ann Surg* 189:553, 1979.
18. Mendes Da Costa P, Mattheiem W, Andry G: Mastectomie radicale modifiée. Experience de L'Institute Bordet. *Acta Chir Belg* 4:423, 1977.
19. Turner L, Swindell R, Bell WFT, Hartley RC, Tasker JH, Wilson WW, Anderson MR, Leck IM: Radical versus modified radical mastectomy. *Ann R Coll Surg Engl* 63:239, 1981.
20. Maddox WA, Carpenter JT Jr, Laws HL, Soong SJ, Cloud G, Urist MM, Balch M: A randomized prospective trial of radical (Halsted) mastectomy versus modified radical mastectomy in 311 breast cancer patients. *Ann Surg* 198:207, 1983.
21. Wilson RE: Progress in breast cancer treatment, today and tomorrow. *Am Coll Surg Bull* 68:2, 1983.

20

Adequate Surgery Including Radical Mastectomy

Hiram S. Cody III, M.D.
Jerome A. Urban, M.D.

INTRODUCTION

No treatment for early breast cancer has ever yielded better local control of disease or long-term survival than radical mastectomy and extended radical mastectomy. Despite a recent hypothesis that breast cancer is already a systemic disease at the time of clinical presentation,[1] the greatest survivals have been observed after meticulous and thorough local therapies, even among patients felt to be at highest risk for occult systemic disease. Over the last two decades, increasing public awareness and advances in breast cancer screening (especially through the use of mammography) have allowed earlier diagnosis and the gradual adoption of more conservative regional treatments.

In the best studies[2] of breast-conserving approaches early survival compares favorably to that seen after radical mastectomy or modified radical mastectomy, while local control is poorer. Longer follow-up will be required to determine the ultimate value of these methods.

METHODS AND RESULTS

The following is a summary of treatment results of 544 patients treated by the senior author (JAU) between 1965 and 1970.[3] All patients were felt to have operable breast carcinoma. The only criteria for inoperability were supraclavicular or distant metastases, arm edema, inflammatory carcinoma, or medical contraindications. A selective operative approach was used, applying modified radical mastectomy (MRM), extended radical mastectomy (ERM), and radical mastectomy (RM) to appropriate patients. MRM was performed in patients with clinically negative axillae and small laterally placed cancers (mean size 1.2 cm), 15 percent of the entire group. ERM was performed for medially placed

---

The staging system used is clearly specified at each point.

larger cancers (mean size 3.0 cm), 19 percent of the patients. The remainder, 66 percent, had RM (mean tumor size 2.4 cm).

Forty-eight patients had noninfiltrating carcinoma (intraductal or lobular carcinoma in situ) and are excluded from the survival calculations. Eight-three percent of this group underwent MRM and 10-year, no evidence of disease (NED) survival was 94 percent.

Contralateral breast biopsy was done in most patients. These results are presented in detail in Chapter 36. Ninety percent of axillary node-positive patients received postoperative radiotherapy, most often about 4500 rads (^{60}Co) given through a "hockey stick" portal. *No patient received postoperative systemic adjuvant chemotherapy.*

At 10 years of follow-up, local recurrence developed in 3 percent of patients as the first sign of treatment failure, and in 3 percent of patients coincided with or occurred after distant metastases. For the 496 patients with infiltrating cancer, survival according to type of operation, axillary node status, clinical stage (Columbia and AJC–UICC) and pathologic stage (AJC–UICC) is reported in Tables 20-1 and 20-2. A detailed comparison of results for RM and ERM is given in Table 20-3, and analysis of survival according to axillary and internal mammary nodal status in Table 20-4.

DISCUSSION

Modified Radical Mastectomy

In this study, MRM consisted of a total mastectomy and axillary node dissection with preservation of the pectoralis major muscle. For noninfiltrating cancers, the pectoralis minor was preserved and a low axillary node dissection done (95 percent of intraductal and 99 percent of lobular carcinomas in situ are axillary node-negative). For infiltrating cancers a full axillary node dissection with excision of the pectoralis minor was done (anticipating the 27.5 percent rate of false-negative clinical examination of the axillary nodes observed in this study). Whether the increasing use of MRM throughout the 1970s will yield 10-year survival and local recurrence rates comparable to more extensive operations is not clear. In our experience (Table 20-5), use of MRM has increased from 15 percent (1965 to 1970) to 24 percent (1971 to 1974) to 51 percent (1975 to 1978), without seeming to compromise systemic or local control. Nevertheless, a recent prospective randomized study from the University of Alabama,[4] comparing RM to MRM in 311 patients with stages I to III operable breast cancer (with a median 5.5 year follow-up), demonstrates a trend toward improved survival (84 percent versus 76 percent, $p = .14$) and decreased local recurrence (3 percent versus

Table 20-1 Primary Operable Breast Cancer, 1965–1970. Infiltrating Cancer Survival by Operation

		5-year %		10-year %	
	No.	Alive	NED*	Alive	NED
RM	351	80	72	70	63
ERM	105	80	69	67	60
MRM	40	92	90	89	86
Axilla −	276	88	82	81	75
Axilla +	220	71	62	58	50
Total	496	81	73	71	64

*NED = No evidence of disease.

Table 20-2 Primary Operable Breast Cancer, 1965–1970. Infiltrating Cancer Survival by Stage

System	Stage	No.	5-year % Alive	NED*	10-year % Alive	NED
Columbia	A	374	88	82	80	74
Clinical	B	116	59	47	41	35
	C	6	(4/6)	(3/6)	(3/6)	(2/6)
AJC–UICC	I	223	91	86	85	78
Clinical	II	250	73	63	59	52
	III	23	64	55	64	50
AJC–UICC	I	160	92	87	87	82
	II	313	76	67	63	55
	III	23	64	55	64	50
Total		496	81	73	71	64

*NED = No evidence of disease.

10 percent, $p = .09$) in patients treated by RM. While neither difference was "statistically significant," the results suggest a policy of selectivity in the use of MRM, particularly as local failure was more frequent when MRM was applied to patients with more clinically advanced disease.

A potential flaw in the MRM procedure is the failure to excise the interpectoral (Rotter's) lymph nodes. Although studies by Haagensen and his associates[5] have shown interpectoral node involvement in as many as 19 percent of operable breast cancers, a study by the present authors[6] of 500 consecutive MRMs performed for *early* (T_1 and T_0) breast cancer found positive interpectoral nodes in only 4 percent of patients. Rotter's nodes were the only site of a nodal metastases in only 0.5 percent of axillary node-negative patients. The figures would certainly be higher if MRM were applied indiscriminately for all breast cancers. Our present policy is to perform MRM for patients with stage I and early stage II disease, reserving RM for patients

Table 20-3 Primary Operable Breast Cancer, 1965–1970. RM versus ERM Survival

		No.	5-year % Alive	NED*	10-year % Alive	NED
RM						
	Axilla −	176	89	82	83	75
	Axilla +	175	70	62	57	50
	Total	351	80	72	70	63
ERM						
	Axilla −	64	82	75	73	66
	Axilla +	41	78	61	59	49
	Total	105	80	69	67	60

*NED = No evidence of disease.

Table 20-4 Primary Operable Breast Cancer, 1965–1970. ERM Survival by Nodal Status

Nodes	No.	5-year % Alive	NED*	10-year % Alive	NED
All negative	54	84	78	78	70
Axilla +/IM–	24	87	75	68	60
Axilla –/IM+	10	68	59	45	45
Axilla +/IM+	17	65	41	47	35
Total	105	80	69	67	60

*NED = No evidence of disease.

with large cancers and extensive axillary node involvement.

Extended Radical Mastectomy

Extended radical mastectomy was devised to eradicate all possible sites of local nodal metastases by removing en bloc with the RM specimen the parasternal chest wall and internal mammary nodes.[7] The procedure has been used by the senior author (JAU) selectively in patients with large inner quadrant tumors felt to be at high risk for internal mammary nodal metastases. Indeed, these nodes were positive in 35.4 percent of patients treated by ERM in the early 1950s. Among 507 patients treated between 1955 and 1964,[8] a 10-year NED survival advantage of 9 percent was noted comparing ERM to RM, 60 percent versus 51 percent. The present data show comparable survivals between ERM and RM, 60 percent versus 63 percent, perhaps because different statistical methods were used (previously crude survival, currently life table analysis), and perhaps because no effort was made to choose comparable patients for each operation. Lacour et al.,[9] in a prospective randomized study comparing RM to ERM in 1580 patients, found no 5-year survival advantage for ERM *except* in axillary node-positive patients with inner quadrant tumors, 71 percent for ERM versus 52 percent for RM. This, of course, is the group of patients most likely to have positive internal mammary nodes. Veronesi and Valagussa,[10] reanalyzing a subgroup of 737 patients from the above trial, found no survival advantage for ERM in any subgroup of patients.

The most interesting result of the experience with ERM is the demonstration of a high salvage rate in patients with positive internal mammary and negative axillary nodes, 45 percent 10-year NED survival in our experience (Table 20-4), and 45.8 percent in that of Veronesi.[10] This demonstrates first that internal mammary metastases do not indicate unsalvageable inoperable disease (as previously asserted by Haagensen[11]), and second, that internal mammary metastases (present in 16 percent of our axillary node-negative patients) do indicate increased risk of relapse compared to patients with all nodes negative, yet would remain *unidentified* by conventional techniques of RM and MRM. Accordingly, based on the above findings and a steadily decreasing rate of internal mammary nodal metastases (18 percent in our most recent experience), our current practice is to perform extrapleural biopsy of the internal mammary nodes as a staging procedure in all patients with inner quadrant breast

Table 20-5 Primary Operable Breast Cancer: Changing Patterns of Surgery

	1965–1970	1971–1974	1975–1978
RM,%	66	63	39
MRM,%	15	24	51
ERM,%	19	12	10

cancers. If positive nodes are found, either ERM is performed or postoperative radiotherapy is given to the area, followed in either case by systemic adjuvant chemotherapy. Blind irradiation of the internal mammary nodes not only overtreats the 80 percent of patients with negative nodes, but risks overlooking the internal mammary positive/axilla-negative subgroup of patients, for whom adjuvant chemotherapy may be indicated.

Radical Mastectomy

The survival data cited for the 66 percent of patients who had RM form a basis for evaluating other breast cancer therapies. While MRM appears increasingly satisfactory for managing patients with stage I and early stage II disease, many breast cancer patients still present with large cancers and/or gross axillary nodal involvement. For this group RM ensures the most complete removal of all local disease, including the interpectoral lymph nodes normally left behind at MRM. As noted above, consistent excisional biopsy of the interpectoral nodes in patients with early breast cancer found positive nodes in only 4 percent of patients sampled; this figure would certainly be higher in patients with T_2 to T_3, N_1 to N_2 breast cancers, a group in which MRM is increasingly being performed. We are seeing in consultation increasing numbers of patients with early local recurrence in whom a stage II to III breast cancer was inappropriately treated elsewhere by MRM. For more locally advanced breast cancers RM should remain the operation of choice.

A significant finding in our data is a 50 percent 10-year NED survival rate for all axillary node-positive patients, none of whom received systemic adjuvant chemotherapy. If, in fact, all breast cancers are systemic at the time of their clinical presentation, as Fisher[1] and his colleagues have hypothesized, one certainly would not expect a 50 percent salvage rate for local therapies alone. Clearly, regional lymph nodes do not function consistently as a simple filter for tumor cells. Equally clearly, the high salvage rate after meticulous, thorough excision of the pathologically positive nodes suggests that the cancer indeed was localized in many patients. As Osborne[12] has pointed out, no single hypothesis is adequate to explain the behavior of a disease as complex and heterogeneous as breast cancer. Local therapies must continue to be emphasized until systemic agents with *curative* potential are developed: none currently exist.

Alternatives to Mastectomy

Increasing experience with radical radiotherapy for early breast cancer is yielding long-term survival results which compare favorably to mastectomy.[13–14] A brief summary of the inherent limitations of radiotherapy follows.

1 *Radiotherapy is ineffective in managing preinvasive breast cancers*, either intraductal or lobular carcinoma in situ, presumably because the biology of preinvasive breast cancers more closely approximates that of normal breast tissue. Harris and his associates,[15] in a study of early breast cancers treated by radiotherapy, found that intraductal carcinoma in and adjacent to the primary cancer (together with high nuclear grade) was associated with a 5-year local failure rate of 39 percent, versus 4 percent local failure for patients with none of these characteristics.

2 *Radiotherapy is inferior to adequate surgery for local control of large breast cancers.* In the experience of the Foundation Curie,[13] 60 percent of patients with tumors larger than 3 cm required subsequent salvage surgery for either immediate or subsequent local failure. At the Marseilles Cancer Institute,[14] local failure was 10.5 percent for stage I, 25 percent for stage II, and 34 percent for patients not treated by prior surgical excision. About half of these failures are salvageable by mastectomy; however, the claim that local failure after radiotherapy does not adversely affect overall survival remains unproven.

3 *Radiotherapy is inferior to surgery in preventing local and distant relapse for larger breast cancers.* A prospective randomized study from Guy's Hospital[16] compared RM with wide local excision and radiotherapy (3500 to 3800 rads, less than would currently be given): Both local recurrence and 10-year survival were quite similar for patients with stage I disease. For stage II patients, local control and survival were markedly inferior for the patients treated by wide excision and radiotherapy. More distressing is the same finding in a later group of randomized stage I patients subsequently reported by Hayward,[17] in which both local control and survival were inferior in the group treated by radiotherapy, despite selection for this trial of patients with the most prognostically favorable disease.

4 *Radiotherapy requires long and frequent follow-up.* After RM, local failures occur most frequently in the early years following treatment. After radiotherapy, local failures occur at a constant rate over at least 15 years (about 2 percent per year in the collective series of Harris et al.[18]) Surgical scarring and radiation fibrosis may necessitate more frequent physical examination, mammography, needle aspiration, and biopsy than would otherwise be required.

5 *Local excision and radiotherapy offer no advantage over radical mastectomy in terms of postoperative physical or emotional problems.* Patients should be aware that the *only* advantage of breast-preserving therapies is preservation of the breast. In a careful analysis by Schain et al.[19] of physical and psychosocial sequelae in patients randomized to either mastectomy or wide local excision/ axillary dissection/ radiotherapy, the only significant differences found in the numerous factors examined were better body image and more frequent shoulder stiffness in the patients with intact breasts.

Thus patients most suitable for local excision and radiotherapy are those with small tumors (less than 2 cm), clinically negative axillae, favorable histology (with minimal in situ disease), and a relatively easy to examine breast, who are willing and able to remain under close follow-up indefinitely. A most important therapeutic trial currently under way is a prospective randomized study comparing radical mastectomy with wide local excision, full axillary node dissection, and radiotherapy for patients with clinical stage I (T_1 N_0) breast cancers.[2] Patients were enrolled between 1973 and 1975, and no survival differences are apparent at present. Nevertheless, in the initial report of this trial, follow-up only ranged from 1 to 7 years. Thus, the final requirement for a breast-preserving therapy is that the patient be willing to accept an element of uncertainty as to the long-term results of this particular approach. Clearly, for the majority of early breast cancer patients who do not satisfy all the above criteria, adequate surgery must remain the treatment of choice.

CONCLUSION

Our present clinical approach to operable breast carcinoma is briefly summarized.

1 *Preoperative evaluation*: All patients undergo a complete history and physical examination, bilateral mammography (primarily to rule out the presence of occult lesions of the contralateral breast), needle aspiration cytology (which, if unequivocally positive, would eliminate the need for incisional biopsy intraoperatively), chest x-ray, and blood chemistries. Bone and liver scans are not done routinely, but reserved for patients with locally advanced cancers, symptoms, suspicious physical findings, or abnormal blood chemistries.

2 *Intraoperative management*: At surgery, following confirmation of the histologic diagnosis, a screening biopsy of the contralateral breast is done in most patients. (See Chap. 36.) Ordinarily, further surgery is not planned for the contralateral breast unless a clinically obvious contralateral cancer is present, or the patient has requested that everything possible be done at the first procedure.

For patients with lobular carcinoma in situ or noninfiltrating intraductal carcinoma, a total mastectomy with low axillary dissection is done, preserving both the pectoralis major and minor muscles. For patients with small infiltrating cancers and clinically negative axillary nodes, a Patey-type modified radical mastectomy is performed, consisting of total mastectomy and complete axillary dissection with excision of the pectoralis minor muscle. For patients with large or locally advanced breast cancers, or extensive clinical involvement of the axillary lymph nodes, a standard radical mastectomy is performed. In all patients with central or inner quadrant breast cancers, a screening biopsy of the internal mammary nodes (most commonly in the second interspace) is added to the above operative procedures. At present, extended radical mastectomy is performed in very few patients, primarily those with very large inner quadrant breast cancers and clinically positive axillary lymph nodes, in whom the risk of internal mammary nodal metastases may be as high as 60 percent; much more frequently in this group of patients a radical mastectomy is performed with screening biopsy of the internal mammary nodes and postoperative radiotherapy given to patients with proven internal mammary nodal metastases.

In a very small number of patients with early infiltrating carcinomas and all the favorable criteria noted above, we have performed wide local excision, axillary dissection, and radiotherapy. We do not feel that this approach should be recommended with absolute confidence until further documentation of long-term survival, patterns of local failure, and the late sequelae of radical radiotherapy are available, although in the few patients willing to accept these uncertainties, we have agreed to a breast-conserving approach.

3 *Postoperative follow-up*: Postoperative radiotherapy is given to a small number of patients, either those with biopsy-proven internal mammary nodal metastases or patients with locally advanced breast carcinomas in whom the risk of local recurrence is felt to be high. Adjuvant chemotherapy is recommended for many axillary node-positive patients, as well as a small number of node-negative patients felt to be at increased risk because of such histologic factors as lymphatic permeation by the primary carcinoma. All patients are examined in the office every 3 months for the first 2 years, and every 6 months thereafter. Mammography of the contralateral breast is performed about every 2 years, and chest x-rays, blood chemistries, and radioisotope scans are done selectively, primarily in patients with suspicious physical findings, symptoms, or a very high-risk primary tumor. Lifelong follow-up is maintained for all patients.

Immediate breast reconstruction is performed only in patients undergoing a prophylactic mastectomy. For patients with small infiltrating cancers and pathologically negative axillary nodes, reconstruction may be performed as early as 4 to 6 months postoperatively. For patients requiring postoperative radiotherapy and/or chemotherapy, in whom the risk of local relapse is much higher, breast reconstruction is ordinarily delayed 6 to 12 months beyond the completion of all postoperative adjuvant therapy.

REFERENCES

1. Fisher B: Laboratory and clinical research in breast cancer—a personal adventure: The David A. Karnofsky Memorial Lecture. *Cancer Res* 40:3863, 1980.
2. Veronesi U, Sacozzi R, Del Vecchio M, et al: Comparing radical mastectomy with quadrantectomy, axillary dissection and radiotherapy in patients with small cancers of the breast. *N Engl J Med* 305:6, 1981.
3. Cody HS, Bretsky SS, Urban JA: The continuing importance of adequate surgery for operable breast cancer: Significant salvage of node-positive patients without adjuvant chemotherapy. *CA* 32:242, 1982.

4. Maddox WA, Carpenter JT, Laws HL, et al: A randomized prospective trial of radical (Halsted) mastectomy versus modified radical mastectomy in 311 breast cancer patients. *Ann Surg* 198:207, 1983.
5. Durkin K, Haagensen CD: An improved technique for the study of lymph nodes in surgical specimens. *Ann Surg* 191:419, 1980.
6. Cody HS, Egeli RA, Urban JA: Rotter's node metastases: Therapeutic and prognostic considerations in early breast carcinoma. *Ann Surg* 199:266, 1984.
7. Urban JA, Baker HW: Radical mastectomy with en bloc resection of the internal mammary lymph node chain. *Cancer* 5:992, 1952.
8. Urban JA: Management of operable breast cancer: The surgeon's view. *Cancer* 42:2066, 1978.
9. Lacour J, Bucalossi P, Caceres E, et al: Radical mastectomy versus radical mastectomy plus internal mammary dissection: Five year results of an international comparative study. *Cancer* 37:206, 1976.
10. Veronesi U, Valagussa P: Inefficacy of internal mammary node dissection in breast cancer surgery. *Cancer* 47:170, 1981.
11. Haagensen CD: The choice of treatment for operable carcinoma of the breast. *Surgery* 76:685, 1974.
12. Osborne MP: Controversies in the management of primary breast cancer—surgical analysis. *Cancer Invest* 1:259, 1983.
13. Calle R, Pilleron JP, Schlinger P, et al: Conservative management of operable breast cancer: 10 year experience at the Foundation Curie. *Cancer* 42:1968, 1977.
14. Amalric R, Santamaria R, Robert F, et al: Radiation therapy with or without primary limited surgery for operable breast cancer: A twenty year experience at the Marseilles Cancer Institute. *Cancer* 49:30, 1982.
15. Harris JR, Connoly DL, Schmitt SJ, et al: Clinical-pathologic study of early breast cancer treated by primary radiation therapy. *J Clin Oncol* 1:184, 1983.
16. Atkins H, Hayward JL, Klugman DJ: Treatment of early breast cancer: A report after 10 years of a clinical trial. *Br Med J* 2:423, 1972.
17. Hayward JL: The surgeon's role in primary breast cancer. *Breast Cancer Res Treat* 1:27, 1981.
18. Harris JR, Recht A, Amalric R, et al: Time course and prognosis of local recurrence following primary radiation therapy for early breast cancer. *J Clin Oncol* 2:37, 1984.
19. Schain W, Edwards BK, Gorell RC, et al: Psychosocial and physical outcome of primary breast cancer therapy: Mastectomy vs. excisional biopsy and irradiation. *Breast Cancer Res Treat* 3:377, 1983.

21

Extended Radical Mastectomy

Katherine Yue-Yuin Li, M.D., M.S.
Zhen-Zhou Shen, M.D.

INTRODUCTION

Since Halsted in 1894 introduced the en bloc resection of primary breast cancer and the axillary lymph node chain, the operation was accepted as the standard cancer operation. In 1949, Handley and Thackray, from their biopsy of the internal mammary lymph nodes, pointed out that the internal mammary lymph nodes were also an important area of metastases from breast cancer. From 1954 to 1955,[1] we biopsied the second intercostal space during Halsted radical mastectomy (RM) consecutively in 119 patients and found the internal mammary lymph node metastasis to be involved in 19 percent (Table 21-1). Furthermore, breast cancer from all quadrants of the breast could metastasize to the internal mammary lymph nodes and some to the internal mammary lymph nodes only. In 1957 Turner-Warwick,[2] using isotopic tracing, proved that breast cancer could metastasize to both the axillary and internal mammary lymph nodes, irrespective of the site of the primary lesion; the axillary lymph nodes received 75 percent of the lymph flow and the internal mammary lymph nodes the remainder.

Our criteria of inoperability are supraclavicular lymph node metastases, edema of the ipsilateral arm, inflammatory breast cancer, and satellite nodules. We started with the Halsted radical mastectomy in 1952. Beginning in 1955 we began to use the en bloc intrapleural extended radical mastectomy in nine cases but changed to the en bloc extrapleural radical mastectomy, irrespective of the site of the primary lesion.

COMPARISON OF RADICAL MASTECTOMY AND EXTENDED RADICAL MASTECTOMY

From 1952 to 1978, we have performed 1831 cases of operable breast cancer with radical

The current TNM system of classification is used throughout.

Table 21-1 Biopsy of Internal Mammary Lymph Nodes in 119 Consecutive Radical Mastectomies

Site of Primary lesion*	Lateral	Medial	Central	Retro areolar	Entire breast
Total no. of cases	62	28	13	6	10
Internal mammary only (+)	0	0	2	1	0
Axillary only (+)	28	8	4	3	4
Axillary and internal mammary (+)	9	7	2	0	2
Axillary and internal mammary (−)	25	13	5	2	4

*Axillary lymph node (+) 67/119 cases, 56%.
Internal mammary lymph node (+) 23/119 cases, 19%.

Table 21-2 Age of 1831 Breast Cancer Patients

	<29	30-39	40-49	50-59	60-69	70-
Halsted RM	9	94	185	233	186	33
Extended RM	29	217	465	303	76	1
Total	38	311	650	536	262	34

Table 21-3 Staging of 1831 Cases of Breast Cancer

	Stage I	Stage II	Stage III	Unclassified
Halsted RM	32	259	397	52
Extended RM	77	479	374	161
Total	109 (5.9%)	738 (40.3%)	771 (42.1%)	213 (11.6%)

surgery. Among them, 740 cases were treated with Halsted radical mastectomy and 1091 cases with extended radical mastectomy. The ages of these 1831 cases are shown in Table 21-2, with the largest number of patients in the 40-to-59-age group. The staging of these two groups is given in Table 21-3, showing that over 80 percent of our patients were in stages II and III, with only 6 percent in stage I. This is very different from the breast cancer detected in Tianjin in 1977 from mass screening of 290,000 women.[3] There were 64 cases of breast cancer and among them 78 percent were stages I and II. This is also different from the BCDDP*[4] carried out in the United States from 1973 to 1978, where 4445 cancers were detected and 32.4 percent were in situ cancer or minimal breast cancer.

Pathological examination of the operative specimen from the 740 cases of Halsted

*Breast Cancer Detection Demonstration Project

Table 21-4 Site of Primary Lesion and Lymph Node Metastases (Halsted)

Site of primary lesion	Cases	Axillary (−)	Axillary (+), (%)
Lateral	359	160	199 (55.4)
Central	223	92	131 (58.7)
Medial	143	72	71 (47.6)
Unknown	15	7	8 (53.3)
Total	740	331 (44.7%)	409 (55.3)

Table 21-5 Site of Primary Lesion and Lymph Node Metastases (Extended Radical Mastectomy)

Site of primary lesion	Cases	Axillary (−)	Axillary (+), %	Internal mammary (+), %
Lateral	534	254	280 (52.4)	69 (12.9)
Central	227	108	119 (52.4)	51 (22.5)
Medial	287	156	131 (45.7)	63 (22.0)
Unknown	43	20	23 (53.5)	10 (23.3)
Total	1091	538	553 (50.7)	193 (17.7)

mastectomy showed the axillary metastatic rate to be 55.3 percent (Table 21-4). Of the 1091 cases of extended radical mastectomy, the axillary lymph node metastasis was 50.7 percent and the internal mammary lymph node metastasis, 17.8 percent (Table 21-5). Table 21-6 showed that even with the primary breast lesion situated laterally, there was 12.9 percent internal mammary lymph node metastasis. Analysis of the lymph node metastatic rate in the 534 laterally situated breast cancers shows that even in stage I, there was 2.7 percent internal mammary lymph node metastasis, rising to 23.8 percent in stage III. These results substantiate Turner-Warwick's observation that breast cancer could metastasize to both the axillary and internal mammary chain, irrespective of the site of the primary lesion.

There was no operative mortality. Postoperative complications of the two types of radical mastectomy are shown in Table 21-7. There was

Table 21-6 Lymph Node Metastases in 534 Cases with Lateral Breast Lesion

Stage	Cases	Axillary (−)	Axillary (+)	IM (+), (%)
I	37	29	8	1 (2.7)
II	249	143	106	20 (8.0)
III	189	45	144	45 (23.8)
Unclassified	59	37	22	3 (5.9)
Total	534	254	280	69 (12.9)

Table 21-7 Postoperative Complications

	Radical mastectomy, 740 cases	Extended radical mastectomy, 1091 cases
Pneumonia	1	7
Atelectasis	2	9
Pleural effusion		20
Necrosis of cartilage	2	4
Hemorrhage in wound		4
Infection of pleura		3
Pneumomediastinum		1
Cerebral edema	1	
Coronary infarction	1	
Slight paralysis of upper extremity	1	1
Total	8 (1.8%)	49 (4.5%)

Table 21-8 First Site of Failure after Operation

	No. of cases	Local	Local + distant	Distant metastasis	Uncertain
Halsted RM	740	70 (9.0%)	21 (2.8%)	174 (23.5%)	72 (9.7%)
Extended RM	1091	36 (3.3%)	26 (2.4%)	235 (21.5%)	54 (4.5%)

a higher percentage of postoperative complications after the extended radical mastectomy, 4.5 percent versus 1.8 percent after Halsted radical mastectomy.

Postoperatively, we compared the first site of recurrence in patients treated with Halsted radical mastectomy and the extended radical mastectomy. Recurrences were grouped as local recurrence only, local recurrence with distant metastasis, and distant metastasis only. Patients treated by the extended radical mastectomy showed a lower local recurrence rate than those treated by the Halsted radical mastectomy, 3.3 percent and 9 percent respectively. "Distant metastasis only" and "local recurrence with distant metastasis" were similar after both types of operation (Table 21-8).

The *survival rates* of the different stages of breast cancer treated by the two different methods are shown in Table 21-9. Comparison of the survival rates from the two types of radical mastectomy in stage I showed no statistical difference. However, the survival rates were significantly higher in stages II and III patients treated with the extended radical mastectomy.

Extending the Halsted radical mastectomy to include the internal mammary chain obviates the necessity of postoperative irradiation to the internal mammary chain when the axillary lymph nodes proved to be positive, thereby shortening the treatment time as well as decreasing medical expense. Table 21-10 shows the reported survival rates from using different methods in treating patients with positive internal mammary lymph nodes.[5–7] Surgery gave better results than a passive attitude or irradiation. (See Chap. 23 for alternate viewpoints.) Table 21-11 shows the survival rate after the extended radical mastectomy for patients with

Table 21-9 Comparison of Survival Rates of the Two Types of Radical Mastectomy

Stage	Type of Mastectomy	Cases	Survival rate (%) 10-year		20-year	
I	Halsted	32	74.4	$p > .05$	74.4	$p > .05$
	extended	77	88.2		82.5	
II	Halsted	259	50.6	$p < .01$	35.1	$p < .01$
	extended	479	69.3		63.3	
III	Halsted	397	25.3	$p < .01$	23.5	$p < .01$
	extended	374	41.3		37.3	
Unclassified	Halsted	52	46.7	$p > .05$	39.4	$p < .05$
	extended	161	72.4		72.4	

Table 21-10 Different Methods in Treating IM (+) Patients

Author	Cases	Method of treatment	Survival rate (%) 5-year	10-year
Donegan	113	Biopsy IM* when (+) no treatment	24	4
Handley	400	Biopsy IM when (+) 3000–3500 rads		
		Overall	36	16
		IM (+) only	37	35
		Axillary (+) IM (+)	33	12
Urban	455	En bloc excision of IM (intrapleural)		
		Overall	54	36
		IM (+) only	65	56
		Axillary (+) IM (+)	50	29
Cancer Hospital of S.F.M.C.	1091	En bloc excision of IM (extrapleural)		
		Overall	45.8	30.9
		IM (+) only	72.6	59.9
		Axillary (+) IM (+)	35.5	21.7

*IM = Internal mammary lymph nodes.

metastases to either the axillary or internal mammary lymph nodes to be similar.

In 1960,[8] when we analyzed the failures after curative surgery in 414 operable breast cancers, two-thirds of the failures were outside the operative field while only one-third were local recurrences (Table 21-12). Similarly, Table 21-8 shows that extending the scope of radical mastectomy decreased local recurrence.

OPERATIVE PROCEDURE: THE EXTRAPLEURAL EXTENDED RADICAL MASTECTOMY

We employed the original Halsted incision, after dissecting the breast with the axillary

Table 21-11 Prognosis in Relation to Site of Lymph Node Metastases (1091 Extended Radical Mastectomies)

Site of lymph node metastases	No. of cases	Survival rate (%) 10-Year	20-Year
Axillary (−) IM* (−)	505	83.4	76.4
Axillary (+) IM (−)	393	46.0	43.6
		NS†	NS
Axillary (−) IM (+)	33	59.9	54.3
Axillary (+) IM (+)	160	21.7	14.2

*IM = Internal mammary lymph nodes.
†NS = Not significant.

content, the pectoralis major was left attached to the sternal end and the operative specimen turned over the sternum. The internal mammary vessels were identified, ligated, and severed in the first intercostal space. Turning to the fourth intercostal space, the fourth costochondral junction was cut; lifting the cut end helped to identify the internal mammary vessels in this interspace. These were identified, ligated, and severed. From below upward, the pleura was pushed away from the thoracic cage with the transversus thoracic muscle, which is thickest in the fourth interspace and disappears in the first interspace. Pushing this muscle with the pleura helped to prevent perforating the pleura. After the pleura had been pushed away, the third and second ribs were cut at the costochondral junction. Their medial ends were dislocated from the sternum and severed. When the sternal ends of the pectoralis major were severed, the specimen was removed en bloc. If the pleura was perforated, placing a suction under the wound during suturing helped to remove any air in the thorax and there was no need for a chest drain. Using an electric knife for dissection, the loss of blood was practically nil.

Table 21-12 First Site of Recurrence after Surgery in 414 Breast Carcinomas*

Site of recurrence	No. of cases
Distant metastases (lung, liver, bone)	60
Skin flap	45
Supraclavicular lymph node	33
Internal mammary lymph node	11
Opposite breast and axilla	9

*Failure within treated area, 56 cases; failure outside treated area, 102 cases.

CONCLUSION

From our experience, we have come to the following conclusions:

1 Our data demonstrate a high incidence of metastases to internal mammary lymph nodes from all quadrants of the breast.

2 Improved survival rates are obtained by their surgical removal.

3 We believe that it is best that these nodes be treated surgically rather than relegate the control of internal mammary lymph node metastases to radiation or chemotherapy.

REFERENCES

1. Li YY et al: Metastasis to the internal mammary lymph node in cancer of the breast. *Chin J Surg* 5(6):441, 1957.
2. Turner-Warwick RT: Lymphatics of the breast. *Br J Surg* 46:574, 1957.
3. Li YY et al: Individualize the treatment of breast

cancer patient. *Tianjin Med J Suppl, J Oncol* 10(4):200, 1983.
4. Baker LH: Breast Cancer Detection Demonstration Project: Five-year Summary Report. *CA* 32(4):194, 1982.
5. Donegan WL: The influence of untreated internal mammary metastasis upon the course of mammary cancer. *Cancer* 39:533, 1977.
6. Handley RS: The conservative radical mastectomy of Patey: 10 yr. results of 425 patients. *Breast* 2:16, 1976.
7. Urban JA: Management of operable breast cancer. *Cancer* 42(4):2066, 1978.
8. Li YY et al: The treatment of 414 cases of breast cancer. *Chin J Surg* 8(5):420, 1960.

EDITORIAL ADDENDUM

The following table presents data from reported series of ERM, some of which show statistically significant improvement over that obtained from RM, while others do not show any difference. The series reported by Meier et al. where surgery was performed by one surgeon shows the most dramatic difference. This table was from Meier P, Ferguson D, Karrison T: A controlled trial of extended radical mastectomy. *Cancer* 55: 881, 1985.*

						Survival		
Reference	**% en bloc**	**Control**	**Randomized**	**Follow-up (years)**	**Group**	**No.**	**%**	***p***
Lacour *et al.*	61	RM	Yes	5	All RM	746	69	NS
					All ERM	697	72	
					Med N + $T_{1,2}$ RM	192	52	0.01
					Med N + $T_{1,2}$ ERM		71	
					Lat N-$T_{1,2}$ RM	239	87	0.05
					Lat N-$T_{1,2}$ ERM		78	
Lacour *et al.* †	61	RM	Yes	10	All RM	750	53	NS
					All RM	703	56	
Veronesi *et al.* ‡	100	RM	Yes	5	Med N + $T_{1,2}$ RM	57	58	NS
					Med N + $T_{1,2}$ ERM	63	52	
				10	All RM	374	61	NS
					All ERM	342	57	
Koszarowski §	100	RM	No	15	Med RM	270	36	NS
					Med ERM	103	39	
Kaae *et al.*	0	Simple irradiation	Yes	5	All simple	160	61	Not reported
					All ERM	146	64	
				10	All simple	199	44	Not reported
					All ERM	183	48	
Urban	100	RM	No	10	Lat RM	329	54	Not reported
					Med ERM	178	62	
Cacares	0	RM	No	10	All RM	113	44	NS
					All ERM	129	42	
Sugarbaker	0	RM	No	5	All RM	88	57	Not reported
					All ERM	158	70	
Meier *et al.*	112	RM	Yes	5	All RM	56	72	0.09
					All ERM	56	86	

*Published with permission of the author and publisher. References can be obtained from the original article.
† Same patients as above; medial tumors not separately analyzed at 10 years.
‡ These patients also in the study of Lacour *et al.*
§ Patients in the study of Lacour *et al.* were also analyzed.
RM: radical mastectomy; ERM: extended radical mastectomy; Med: medial; Lat: lateral; NS: not significant.

22

Intravascular Irradiation of the Internal Mammary Lymph Nodes

Irving M. Ariel, M.D.

INTRODUCTION

A technique has been described whereby radioactive sources are placed into the internal mammary artery at the time that a mastectomy is performed in order to irradiate a cylinder of tissue 6 cm in diameter. This area of tissue would then encompass the internal mammary lymph nodes (Fig. 22-1); 87 percent are within 1 cm and 97 percent are within 1.5 cm. The technique was originally described by Brasfield and Henschke but they never did present the end results of their treatment.[2–4] The technique has been used to treat 50 patients with breast cancer. This presentation details the results of such treatment.[1]

The current system of TNM classification is used throughout.

PATIENTS TREATED

Fifty patients on whom a radical mastectomy had been performed were candidates for the intravascular irradiation (Table 22-1). Those patients were chosen who had metastases to the axillary lymph nodes, proved by frozen section biopsy of the axillary nodes at the time of operation, regardless of the site of the primary cancer in the breast (i.e., whether located medially, centrally, or in a lateral position). These patients were in the fourth and fifth decades of life; the average age was 44 years and varied from 30 years to 67 years. Twenty-one were premenopausal and 29 were postmenopausal. Each patient suffered from infiltrating adenocarcinoma and was classified in the stage III category. Intraductal or lobular carcinoma in situ were not included as they were treated by a more conservative approach.

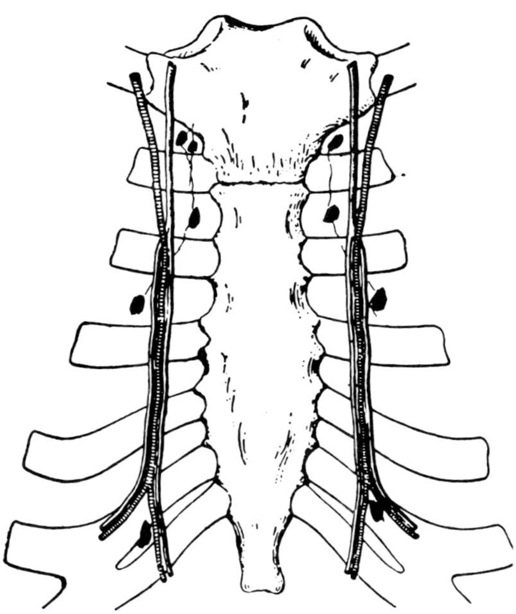

Figure 22-1 This shows the relationship of the internal mammary lymph nodes.

These patients were treated between 1955 and 1975.

TECHNIQUE OF IRRADIATING INTERNAL MAMMARY LYMPH NODES BY RADIOACTIVE ISOTOPES

At the conclusion of the radical mastectomy, a small transverse parasternal incision is made in the first or second intercostal space. The internal mammary artery and vein are found immediately beneath the intercostal muscles approximately 1 cm lateral to the edge of the sternum. The artery usually measures 2 to 5 mm in diameter, placed lateral to the vein, which is of slightly larger caliber. At times, a vein may be found on either side of the artery; a 0.1-cm-to-1.0-cm fat pad and one or two small lymph nodes separate the vessels from the pleura. The transverse thoracis which separates the pleura from the chest wall is thickened in the inferior location (fourth interspace) and disappears in the first interspace. The artery and vein mobilization is easily performed by the extrapleural approach, but, if necessary, the pleura may be transgressed (Fig. 22-2).

The internal mammary artery is ligated with no. 3-0 silk as high as possible. A second loop ligature is loosely placed at the lower portion of the interspace for traction and for anchoring the catheter in place. Next, a small slit is made in the artery between the ligatures, and a no. 21 gauge nylon catheter with a heat-fused tip is inserted for a distance of 15 cm, which is usually at the level of the xiphoid process. The lower silk ligature is tied around the vessel containing the catheter to prevent back bleeding and to stabilize the catheter. The intercostal muscles are not sutured in an effort to prevent the formation of mediastinal hematoma if bleeding should occur after the catheter is removed. Bleeding did not occur in any of our patients.

If desired, a similar technique is used for catheterizing the contralateral internal mammary artery. The pectoralis major muscle must be incised as a preliminary step. The mastectomy wound is closed and a dressing is applied. A closed suction drain is used. No chest drain is necessary unless the pleura has been incised.

When the patient returns to her room, a radioactive source (^{60}Co wire) is inserted into the entire length of the nylon tube in the internal mammary artery. The catheter containing the radioactive wire is removed when the desired calculated dosc is reached.

Radiologic Factors

Cobalt decays with a half-life of 5.25 years by beta emission accompanied by two gamma rays in cascade. The beta particles have a maximum energy of 0.3 MeV, while the two photons have energy of 1.17 and 1.33 MeV. For practical purposes, irradiations are considered monoenergic.

Most of our experience has been with the use of radioactive cobalt. The strength of the ^{60}Co source will determine the number of hours

Table 22-1 Patients Treated by Internal Mammary Lymph Node Irradiation (Stage III)

		No. of patients alive and well in 10 years	Percent of patients, %
Number of patients	50	—	—
Patients lost to follow-up	5	—	—
Patients with metastases to the internal mammary chain of lymph nodes + positive axillary lymph nodes	16	6	37
Patients without evidence of metastases to the internal mammary chain of lymph nodes + positive axillary lymph nodes	29	17	59

necessary to produce the given dose by usual calculations.[2]

Iridium-192 has been used on a few patients not included in this report.[8] Its availability makes it a useful isotope. Iridium-192 has a half-life of 74.5 days. Its maximum beta energy is 670 kV. The beta particles are readily absorbed in tissue. Its gamma spectrum, with 11 lines from 136 to 613 kV, is complex, but 94 percent of all the gamma energy is emitted by the four lines 296, 308, 316, and 468 kV. The effective energy of the ^{192}Ir gamma spectrum is about 340 kV, and the half value in lead is 2.3 mm. As with the ^{60}Co, the duration period that the iridium wire will stay in position will be calculated by the strength of the iridium inserted and the dose necessary to produce 7000 to 9000 rads. The no. 27 gauge ^{60}Co wire is 20 cm in length; however, the proximal 5 cm is inactive. This protects the skin from excessive irradiation near the point of exit. A cobalt wire of 15 mg radium equivalent will deliver 9000 rads to a 1-cm cylinder of tissue in 7 days. The half-life of ^{60}Co is 5.2 years, which will allow treatment for over 250 patients for each wire.

Of the 100 patients treated by Brasfield and Henschke, 30 had implants to each internal mammary artery.[2] Follow-up studies have indicated that 9000 rads delivered to the parasternal nodes is safe.

Complications

Complications were minimal. One patient developed painful osteochondritis of two ribs which was difficult to control, One patient developed a staphylococcal infection at the site of introduction of the polyethylene tube containing the cobalt wire. Five patients developed pneumothorax due to the fact that the pleura was transgressed during the procedure.

Results

Fifty patients have been treated from 1955 to 1975. Five were lost to follow-up and hence are not available for evaluation. Of the remaining 45 patients, 16 had metastases to the internal mammary lymph nodes as determined by a biopsy performed in the second interspace. It was our impression that if metastases occurred in the first and second interspaces, it indicated that metastases had occurred throughout the

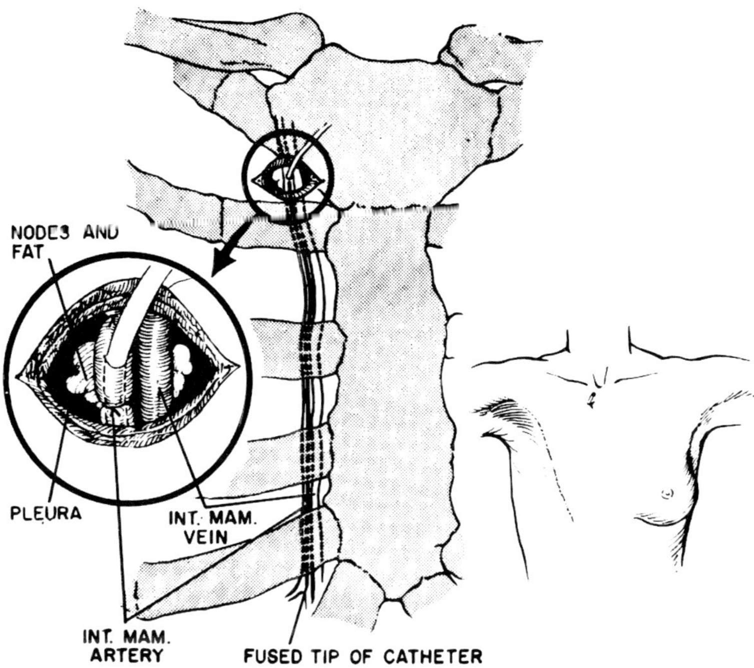

Figure 22-2 A method of catheterizing the internal mammary artery.

internal mammary chain. If no metastases were encountered in these interspaces, the patient was considered as being free of evidence of metastases of the internal mammary nodes for this presentation.

Of the 16 patients with evidence of metastases to the internal mammary lymph nodes, 6 have survived the 10-year period (37 percent). Of 29 patients who did not present evidence of metastases to the lymph nodes (according to our criteria) but were nevertheless treated; 17 have survived the 10-year period (59 percent). Li and Shen found that 132 patients had metastases to only one intercostal space, and 35, 53, 36, and 8 patients had metastases to the first, second, third, and fourth intercostal spaces, respectively.[10,11] In addition, 56 patients had metastases to two intercostal spaces, and 17 had metastases to three or more intercostal spaces. Thus, our criteria are not all-inclusive.

In one patient, a partial dissection of the lymph node was performed, and the lymph node was found to contain cancer. This patient was treated with ^{192}Ir therapy by the technique as described here. One year later the remainder of the node was excised but did not contain any residual carcinoma. This speaks well for the effects of the irradiation described. (This patient is not included in this evaluation.)

All patients who died did so due to generalized metastases. One woman who had positive metastases to her internal mammary chain of lymph nodes developed clinical evidence of metastasis to her brain 16 years after treatment and died soon after. The remainder developed generalized metastases from 1 to 10 years after treatment; 70 percent developed metastases within 3 years. None of the treated patients developed any signs of local recurrence.

DISCUSSION

Since attention was directed to the internal mammary lymph nodes being invaded by metastases from primary breast cancer many years ago, numerous studies have been performed to evaluate the incidence and methods of treating these metastases.[5,6,9,12] Handley in 1927 described the presence of metastases and advised the application of radium tubes for their control.[7] Li and colleagues in 1957 demonstrated that the internal mammary chain was a primary drainage site from the breast and focused attention to the need for its treatment.[11]

The incidence of 32 percent of patients with axillary metastases who will also harbor metastases to the internal mammary chain is noteworthy. Urban noted them positive for metastases in 35.4 percent of patients with medial tumors, whereas Li et al. found them positive in 19 percent of 1242 patients subjected to radical mastectomy.[10] The difference of her findings from those of Urban was that in her series the primary cancer was located in all parts of the breast and not limited to the medial quadrant. In our small series, we did not notice any correlation between the site of the primary cancer and the incidence of metastases to the internal mammary chain.

The two major treatment modalities for the internal mammary lymph nodes have been to expand the radical mastectomy to the extended radical mastectomy and external radiation therapy. Urban obtained a 35 percent alive-and-well value for 17 patients whose axillary and internal mammary nodes contained metastases and 60 percent alive-and-well value at 10 years for those patients whose axillae were positive but whose internal mammary nodes were negative following extended radical mastectomy.

Li and Shen observed a 22 percent survival of patients who had both chains involved with cancer, and a 46 percent 10-year survival for those with negative internal mammary lymph nodes but positive axillary lymph nodes following extended radical mastectomy. (See Chaps. 21 and 23.)

Results from external radiation therapy for proved metastases to the internal mammary lymph nodes are mostly conjectural, inasmuch as the radiation therapist seldom, if ever, examines the nodes. Handley, who administered 3000 to 3500 rads to the internal mammary nodes proved positive by biopsy, reported a 12 percent 10-year survival for 400 patients.[7]

Complications from external radiation are not insignificant and include radiation pneumonitis, mediastinal fibrosis, and others. Modern techniques of irradiation limit these complications.

The method described herein of brachytherapy of the internal chain is a novel manner of irradiating the nodes with results akin to those obtained by their extirpation, with no danger and minimal complication, to date. The procedure adds about 15 min to the operating time and, since the blank catheter is inserted at the time of operation, there is no radiation hazard to the operating room personnel. Radiation precautions, however, are necessary for all personnel after the radiation source has been inserted.

Our results of a limited number of patients treated by intravascular irradiation is comparable to that of other treatment methods. Our 10-year results of patients with biopsy-proved metastases to the internal mammary lymph nodes yielded a 37 percent survival, and the results of those with nodes proved negative by biopsy (which may have, nevertheless, contained metastases) yielded a 10-year survival of 59 percent.

The series is small but, inasmuch as these patients received no other treatment than the radical mastectomy and the intravascular irradiation, encouraging.

CONCLUSION

We have described a technique for irradiating the internal mammary lymph nodes which is atraumatic, effective, and has minimal complications. The 10-year survival of 37 percent for the 16 patients with proved metastases to the internal mammary lymph nodes and of 59 percent for those considered not to have metastases to those lymph nodes is encouraging. (The value is very conservative inasmuch as a biopsy of the second interspace was the determining feature for the presence or absence of metastases.) Each of the patients had proved metastases to the axillary lymph nodes.

In conclusion, metastasis to the internal mammary lymph nodes is not an ill-omened situation, as believed by Haagensen and others.[6]

REFERENCES

1. Ariel IM: Intravascular irradiation of the internal mammary lymph nodes. *Breast, Diseases of the Breast.* in press.
2. Brasfield RD, Henschke UK: Internal mammary irradiation implants, in Ariel IM (ed): *Progress in Clinical Cancer,* vol. 1. New York, Grune & Stratton, 1965, p. 450.
3. Brasfield RD, Henschke UK: Intravascular irradiation of the internal mammary lymph nodes in breast cancer. *Am J Roent Genol* 85(5):849, 1961.
4. Brasfield RD, Henschke UK: Intravascular irradiation of the internal mammary nodes in dogs. Personal Communication.
5. Caceres E: Radical mastectomy with resection of the internal mammary chain. *Acta Unio Int Contra Cancerum* 15:1061, 1959.
6. Haagensen CD: The choice of treatments for operable carcinoma of the breast. *Surgery* 76:685, 1974.
7. Handley RS: Parasternal invasion of the thorax in breast cancer and its suppression by the use of Radium tubes as an operative precaution. *Surg Gynecol Obstet* 45:721, 1927.
8. Henschke UK: Treatment of cancer with small sources of radioactive iridium, in Pack GT, Ariel IM (eds.): *Treatment of Cancer and Allied Diseases,* vol. 1, *Principles of Treatment.* New York, Paul Hoeber & Co., 1958.
9. Koszarowski T: Rational approach to the efficiency of internal mammary lymph node dissection in breast cancer cure. *Breast, Diseases of the Breast* 2(11):44, 1976.
10. Li KYY, Shen ZF: An analysis of 1242 cases of extended radical mastectomy. *Breast, Diseases of the Breast* 10(2):10, 1984.
11. Li KYY, et al: Biopsy of internal mammary lymph nodes during radical mastectomy and its significance in 119 cases. *Chin Surg J* 5:441, 1957.
12. Margottini M: Arguments in favor of super radical operations for carcinoma of the breast. *Acta Unio Int Contra Cancerum* 15:1037, 1959.
13. Urban JA: Clinical experience with excision of internal mammary lymph node chain in primary operable breast cancer. *Acta Unio Int Contra Cancerum* 15:1179, 1959.

23

The Role of Postoperative Radiotherapy in Breast Cancer

Maurice Tubiana, M.D.
Danielle Sarrazin, M.D.

INTRODUCTION

Postoperative radiotherapy (RT) has two aims: first, to decrease the incidence of local-regional recurrences through the control of residual subclinical disease, and second, to improve survival if metastatic dissemination can originate from local residual deposits, in particular those located in regional lymph nodes.

Postoperative RT may be carried out either after a mastectomy, simple or radical, or after a lumpectomy. For over half a century, postoperative RT has been widely used as a prophylactic measure following surgical treatment; however, its indications and even its usefulness remain highly controversial. Unfortunately, both supporters and opponents of postoperative RT do not make a sufficient effort to identify those subsets of patients in whom RT is effective and beneficial, and those in whom it might be useless or even detrimental. Moreover, most discussions concerning pre- or postoperative RT overlook the significance of the technique, the dose employed, the anatomical areas irradiated.

In this chapter, we shall discuss (1) radiation doses required to control residual disease; (2) effects of postoperative RT on local-regional recurrence, and the subsets of patients in whom it is indicated; (3) effects of postoperative RT on survival, and the identification of those subsets of patients in whom long-term survival is improved by postoperative RT; and (4) the side effects of RT both with and without chemotherapy (CT).

DOSE-EFFECT RELATIONSHIPS

Baclesse[4,5] pioneered the use of RT in the treatment of breast cancer and demonstrated that radiation alone can achieve long-term cures of breast cancer even when the primary tumor is

---

The current TNM system of classification is used throughout.

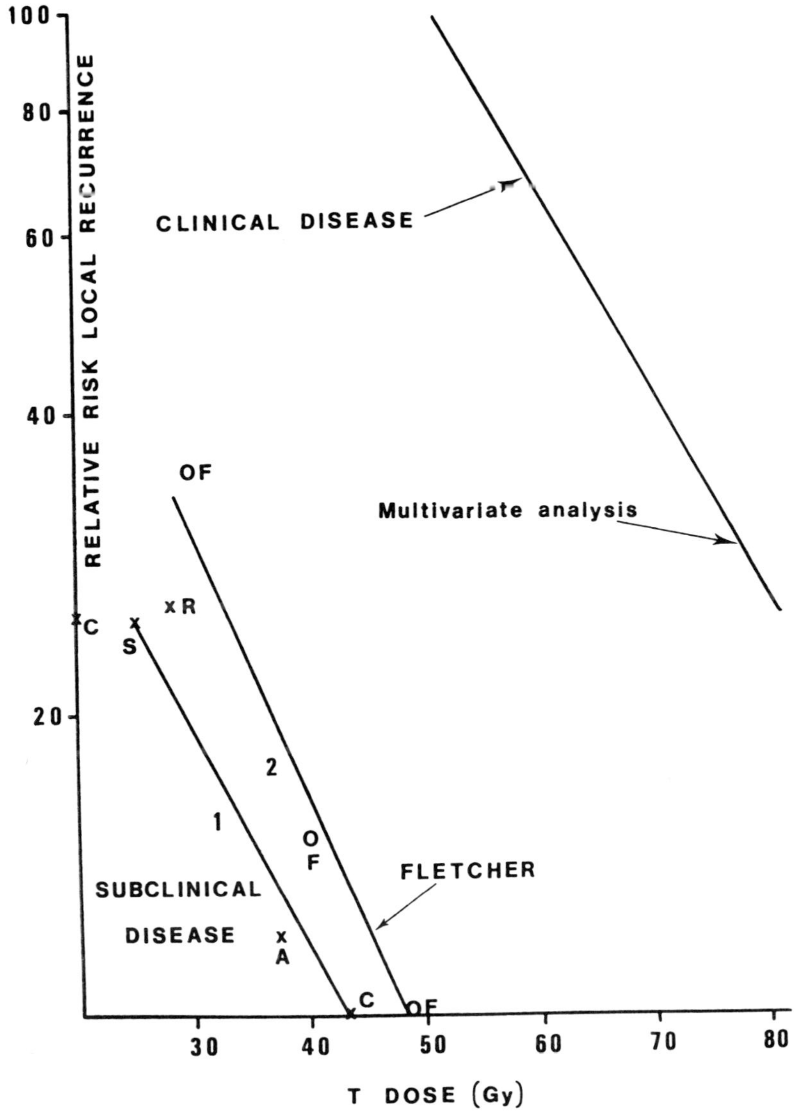

Figure 23-1 Relationship between tumor dose and probability of local recurrence. On the right are results of external radiotherapy of breast tumors treated by radiotherapy alone (multivariate analysis taking into account tumor size, skin involvement, and axillary and supraclavicular involvement). On the left are two sets of data concerning treatment of occult breast disease. A much smaller dose is sufficient to obtain a high rate of local control. Villejuif + P.M.H. (*Data from Arriagada et al.*[2])

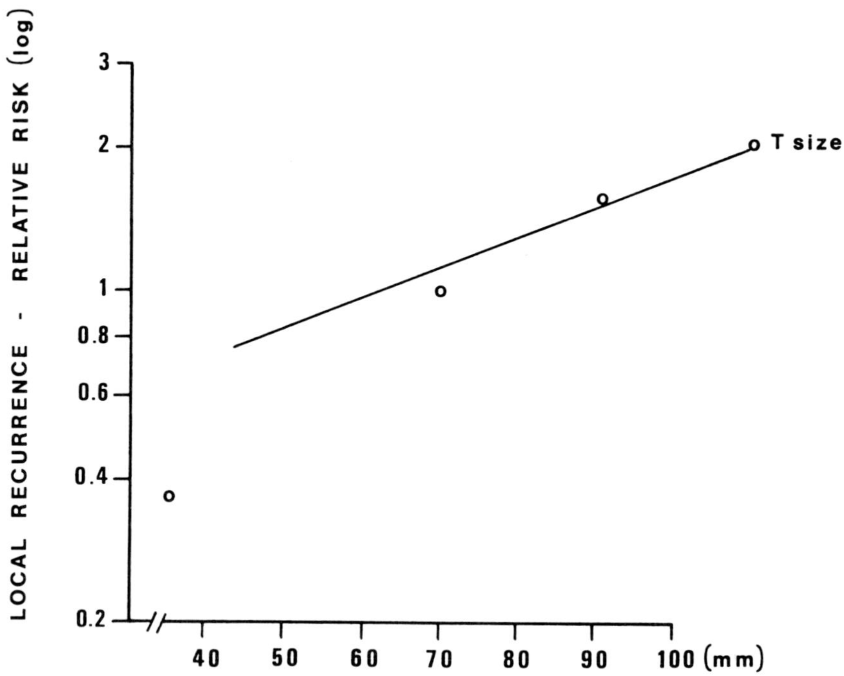

Figure 23-2 Relationship between tumor size and probability of local recurrence after treatment of breast tumor by radiotherapy alone (multivariate analysis taking into account tumor dose, skin involvement, and axillary and supraclavicular involvement). (*Arriagada et al.*[2])

bulky; however, he also showed that very high doses of approximately 8000 to 9000 rads are required to achieve local control. Such high doses induce significant sequelae. This is why the indications for RT alone are limited. The relationship between tumor dose and the probability of local relapse has been studied by different groups and the data are depicted in Fig. 23-1. A dose increase of 1500 rads decreases the relative risk of local recurrence twofold. Moreover, for a given dose the risk increases with tumor size (Fig. 23-2) but the influence of size is smaller than that of dose; a doubling of the tumor volume requires only an additional dose of a few hundred rads.

It has been shown by several authorities, in particular Fletcher,[17] that much smaller doses are sufficient to control residual occult deposits (Fig. 23-1). We have previously reviewed the experimental and clinical bases of the influence of tumor size on the relationship between dose and tumor control.[48] Briefly, subclinical disease corresponds to neoplastic masses of less than 5 to 6 mm in diameter. The number of clonogenic cells is therefore from 50 to 1000 times smaller than in primary breast tumors. This is consistent with clinical observations showing that the dose necessary to control the largest occult residual neoplastic mass is about two-thirds of that necessary to control large primary breast tumors.

Forty-five hundred to 5000 rads are sufficient to secure local control in virtually all patients, whereas after lower doses the incidence of local recurrence is appreciable. For example, Helle et al.[20] have recently reported the results of a prospective study showing a significantly higher rate of local-regional recurrence

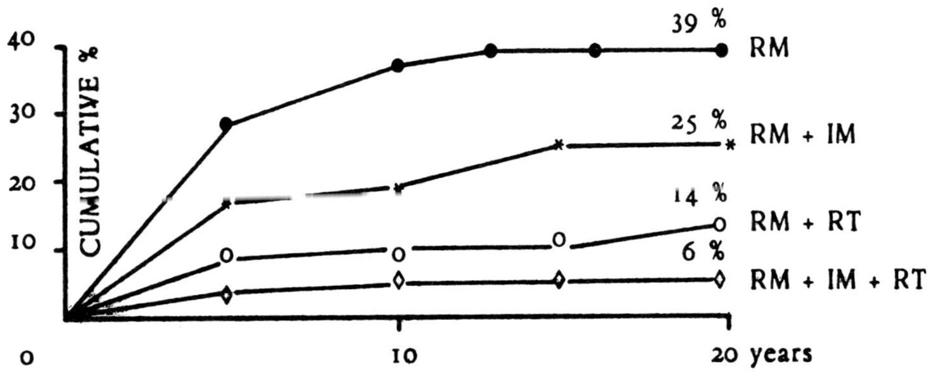

Figure 23-3 Cumulative incidence of local-regional failures in four groups of patients with breast tumors treated at Villejuif by radical mastectomy (RM), radical mastectomy and internal mammary chain dissection (RM + IM), radical mastectomy and postoperative radiotherapy of the regional lymphatic areas and the chest wall (RM + RT), radical mastectomy and internal mammary chain dissection plus postoperative radiotherapy (RM + IT + RT). (*From Sarrazin et al.,*[42,43] *and unpublished data from Arriagada et al.*)

following doses of 2000 rads than after 4000 or 5000 rads (47 percent versus 27 percent, and 24 percent in high-risk patients). After conservative treatment of breast cancer, Clarke et al.[9] have recently shown that there is significant correlation between dose expressed in terms of nominal single dose (NSD) and probability of local relapse. As the breast dose was 4500 rads in all patients, variations in the NSD value were related to variations in treatment duration.

INFLUENCE OF RADIOTHERAPY ON THE INCIDENCE OF LOCAL-REGIONAL RECURRENCE

Local-regional recurrence is defined as recurrence of the disease either within the operative scar and the chest wall, or in the regional lymph node areas. Following surgery alone, the incidence of local-regional recurrence varies widely (from 3 to 80 percent) with the characteristics of the treated patients and the type of surgical procedure. As discussed above, adequate doses of postoperative RT do decrease local-regional recurrences, particularly those in the supraclavicular fossa and the chest wall. This has been amply demonstrated by several controlled and noncontrolled studies.[13,14,16,17,22,42,43,57] For example, Fig. 23-3 shows our own data. The differences are significant and they demonstrate that the rate of local-regional recurrence is influenced by both the extent of the surgical procedure and the administration of postoperative RT. Despite the consistency of all available data on this point (Table 23-1), several questions remain under discussion.

Which subsets of patients require postoperative RT? Obviously, RT is not required for those patients in whom the incidence of local-regional recurrence is very low without postoperative RT.

For example, following radical or modified mastectomy, the incidence of local recurrence is low in patients with T_1 or T_2 tumors without axillary lymph node involvement.[13,22] It is not surprising that, for those patients, controlled trials have not revealed differences between irradiated and nonirradiated patients.[22,23] The histologic grade has also an important impact. For example, in the British cooperative trial,[12] the risk of local recurrence is low in grade 1 tumors and is not decreased in irradiated

Table 23-1 Prevention of Local-Regional Recurrences by Postoperative RT in Breast Cancers

	No RT (%)	Postoperative RT (%)	Reference
All local-regional recurrence			
Villejuif (at 20 years)			
Radical mastectomy	39	14 $p < .01$	Sarrazin et al.[42,43]
Extended mastectomy	25	6 $p < .01$	and unpublished Updating*
Norv. RA Inst. trial (at 5 years)			
Stage I	6.5	2.9 NS	
Stage II	25	9.5 $p < .01$	Høst[22,23]
Stockholm trial (at 10 years)			
Radical mastectomy	32	10 $p < .001$	Wallgren et al.[57,58]
British cancer campaign trial (at 10 years)			
Simple mastectomy without axillary dissection			
Clinically negative nodes	18.8	7.7 $p = .06$	
Clinically positive nodes	78	41 $p < .001$	Elston et al.[12]

**Source*: Unpublished data of M. Lê, R. Arriagada, D. Sarrazin, et al.

patients, whereas it is much higher in patients with grades 2 or 3. Furthermore, within grades 2 and 3 the risk tends to increase with increasing tumor size. At Villejuif, it has been shown that in patients treated by mastectomy without RT, the incidence of local-regional recurrence is higher in patients with tumors located in the inner quadrants than in tumors of the outer quadrants (at 15 years, 48 percent and 33 percent, respectively). This difference is not observed in patients having received postoperative RT or having undergone an internal mammary chain dissection.[42]

Since all the prognostic factors are interrelated, a multivariate analysis is necessary to identify the significant ones. Table 23-2 shows the results recently obtained in Villejuif using a Cox's model analysis on 1508 patients treated between 1954 and 1972 without adjuvant chemotherapy. The size of the breast tumor has only a small and nonsignificant influence. It is only in very small tumors (diameter approximately 1 cm) that the incidence of local recurrence is lower than in larger tumors. This is at variance from what is observed for distant metastases. For these, we have found that their incidence is significantly correlated with the size of the primary tumor.[25] On the other hand, two factors have an independent marked influence: the number of involved axillary nodes, and the histologic grade. Table 23-3 shows that in all subsets of patients, RT reduces by about half the incidence of local-regional recurrence. Dissection of the internal mammary chain is also effective in all subsets of patients (Tables 23-2 and 23-3); however, the differences are only marginally significant (Table 23-2). When the location of the tumors is taken into account, internal mammary chain dissection does not decrease the incidence of local-regional recurrence for tumors of the outer quadrants (33 percent and 28 percent, respectively) whereas it reduces markedly their incidence for tumors of the inner quadrants (48 percent and 22 percent, respectively, $p = .02$); however, the number of patients in each subset is small. In patients having received postoperative RT, internal mammary chain dissection does not exert any influence on the incidence of local-regional recurrence.

Some authors question the usefulness of postoperative RT when adjuvant CT is used. This is a point that we shall discuss below. It is

Table 23-2 Multivariate Study (Cox's Model) of the Factors Influencing Probability of Local-Regional Recurrence (1500 patients)

	Number of patients with the variable	Relative risk	*p* Value (trend)
Number of involved axillary nodes			
N-	543		
$1 \leq N \leq 3$	550	1.69	
$4 \leq N \leq 10$	283	2.80	10^{-6}
$N \geq 11$	132	5.41	
Histologic grade			
1	314	1	
2	722	1.66	10^{-4}
3	472	2.46	
Type of treatment			
Without RT	734	1	10^{-4}
With postoperative RT	774	0.44	
Without internal mammary chain dissection	791	1	0.08
With internal mammary chain dissection	717	0.76	

Source: Unpublished data of R. Arriagada, M. Lê, D. Sarrazin, et al.

sufficient here to say that in most studies the incidence of local recurrence is higher in patients who did not undergo postoperative RT, whether or not they have received adjuvant CT. For example, in a recent controlled clinical trial comparing segmental mastectomy with or without irradiation among patients with positive nodes, 98 percent of women treated with radiation and 64 percent of those receiving no radiation remained tumor-free at 5 years ($p < .001$), although both groups received chemotherapy.[15a]

Which areas should be irradiated? This depends on the type of surgery which has been performed. *After a mastectomy* (simple or radical), irradiation of the axilla is usually not performed in patients without lymph node involvement.[17,21,39] Recent data obtained in Villejuif suggest that after a careful, complete axillary dissection, irradiation of this lymphatic area may not be necessary, even when these nodes are involved.[44] When the axillary lymph nodes are involved, irradiation of the supraclavicular fossa and of the internal mammary chain should be performed since recurrence in these regions is not infrequent and surgical dissection of these areas is a procedure both mutilating and ineffective.[17,39] For tumors located in the inner quadrants, there is a probability of internal mammary chain involvement even if the axillary nodes are not involved[26,28]; hence,

Table 23-3 Histologic Grade. Relative Risk of Local-Regional Recurrence in Each Subset of Patients

	1				2				3			
	No RT		RT		No RT		RT		No RT		RT	
	No IMD*	IMD	No IMD	IMD	No IMD	IMD	No IMD	IMD	No IMD	IMD	No IMD	IMD
N–	1	0.74	0.45	0.33	1.65	1.22	.74	.55	2.46	1.82	1.11	0.82
1 ≤ N ≤ 3	1.65	1.22	0.74	0.55	2.72	2.01	1.22	.90	4.06	3.00	1.82	1.35
4 ≤ N ≤ 10	2.72	2.01	1.22	0.90	4.48	3.32	2.01	1.19	6.69	4.95	3.00	2.23
N ≥ 11	5.47	4.06	2.46	1.82	9.03	6.69	4.06	3.00	13.46	9.97	6.05	4.48

*IMD = Internal mammary chain dissection.
Source: Villejuif study. Unpublished data of R. Arriagada, M. Lê, D. Sarrazin, et al.

this region should be irradiated for all inner tumors.

The usefulness of chest wall irradiation is debated. For example, in the Manchester[33] and Oslo[22,23] studies, only the regional lymph nodes were irradiated and the incidence of chest wall recurrence was low. Since irradiation of the chest wall might impair later reconstructive surgery of the breast following a Patey's mastectomy, the target volume might be limited to only the supraclavicular and internal mammary lymph nodes. However, chest wall irradiation is indicated when there is an extensive axillary involvement, a multiple breast involvement, or skin or muscle infiltration.[17,59]

After a lumpectomy, it is generally agreed that the remainder of the breast must be irradiated.[7,8,19,35,37,41,44,54] Peters[34] has shown that in carefully chosen breast tumors it may be possible to avoid breast irradiation. However, in practice, not irradiating the breast after lumpectomy is exceptional. A recent paper[15a] has reported the results of a controlled clinical trial comparing segmental mastectomy with or without irradiation. The results clearly show that the incidence of breast recurrence is much lower in the irradiated breast. A total of 92 percent of women treated by irradiation remained free of breast tumors at 5 years as compared with 72 percent of those receiving no radiation ($p < .001$). (See also Chap. 18.)

In tumors less than 3 cm in diameter, following irradiation of 4500 to 5000 rads plus 1500 to 2000 rads boost, the incidence of local recurrence at 5 years is lower than 5 percent.[41,44] A multivariate analysis of Villejuif's data[9] shows that, besides the dose to the tumor bed, the prognostic indicator which has the main impact on the probability of relapse in the breast is histologic grade. There is also a trend toward an increased incidence of recurrence when the delay between biopsy and irradiation is longer than 6 weeks; this is in accordance with what has been observed in head and neck tumors,[56] and is consistent with experimental and clinical studies demonstrating the role of tumor repopulation.[51]

EFFECT OF IRRADIATION ON SURVIVAL

General Considerations

Besides avoidance of local recurrence, postoperative RT may decrease the incidence of distant metastases if local residual neoplastic tissue can act as a nidus for further hematologic or lymphatic dissemination. However, this point is highly controversial. It has even been claimed that irradiation may increase the probability of metastases by lowering immunological defenses and thereby increasing the probability that a small colony of neoplastic cells may develop into an overt metastasis.[45] It is true that, after a course of RT, there is a decrease in the number of T lymphocytes, but there is neither an increase in the severity of infectious disease nor any clinical or experimental evidence for an enhanced growth of micrometastases.[49] In fact, the statistical and biological data which were alleged to favor this hypothesis have been shown to be highly questionable, and considerable criticism has been expressed, both from a statistical and a biological point of view.[1,6,31,49]

Concerning the impact of local control on the incidence of metastases, it must be remembered that in most cases metastatic dissemination has occurred prior to initial treatment.[51] Some authors have claimed that local recurrences do not metastasize. In most studies, any improvement in local-regional control produced by postoperative RT has not been associated with any improvement in overall survival. However, some data suggest that distant metastases can originate from involved lymph nodes. For example, in the Guy's Hospital trial,[3] patients were randomized between radical mastectomy versus lumpectomy plus irradiation (2500 to 2700 rads in 10 days) at a dose which was insufficient to control all axillary disease. Among stage II patients with clinically positive lymph nodes, the frequency of axillary failures and of distant metastases was significantly higher in the group treated without axillary dissection.

This strongly suggests that lymph node metastases can be important foci for distant spread and is in accordance with the so-called multistep dissemination process.[55] Nevertheless, this model of cascade spread of blood-borne metastases is challenged by other data. In particular, in the NSABP study,[15] the group of clinically negative lymph node patients was randomized between simple mastectomy alone followed by subsequent removal of axillary nodes if they became positive, or by total mastectomy followed by regional irradiation. No difference was found in the incidence of distant metastases or survival up to the sixth year after initial treatment, although the incidence of local failure was 8.5 percent higher in the group treated without postoperative radiotherapy and axillary dissection. Moreover, Fisher et al.[15] calculated that approximately 40 percent of those patients treated by total mastectomy alone had a positive axillary lymph node unremoved and untreated. Thus, they concluded that a positive axillary lymph node is not a pivotal factor in the sequence of events leading to distant disease.

Although these data are extremely valuable, they are not conclusive. The follow-up is relatively short, the growth rate of tumors in clinically node-negative patients with breast cancer is relatively slow,[51,52] and it would be expected that most of the local recurrences and remote metastases will become clinically detectable only after relatively long periods.[51,52] From this point of view, it is noteworthy that only a small proportion of the expected 40 percent of axillary failures have been detected during the first 6 years. Also, if the patients have been carefully followed up, the positive nodes may have been detected at a time when their size was relatively small (approximately 1 to 2 g); it is known that, in patients with breast cancer without clinically involved lymph nodes, most disseminations occur when the size of the primary tumor is much larger than 1 to 2 g.[25]

These data do show that, among patients in whom distant dissemination has not occurred from the primary tumor at the time of initial treatment, only a relatively small proportion have regional occult disease present after surgery. Moreover, of these deposits, only a small proportion will have a chance to disseminate before becoming detectable. Thus, a comparison of the whole population of irradiated and nonirradiated patients has limited significance and an effort should be made to identify those subsets of patients in whom RT might be useful. It is well known that the natural history of breast cancer is influenced by prognostic factors such as the size of the primary tumor, number of metastasis-bearing axillary lymph nodes, and histologic grade.[10,11,42,52]

Any debate on the value of postoperative radiotherapy for breast cancer must take into account these characteristics as well as the location of the primary tumor (in the inner or outer quadrants), which affects the lymphatic drainage of that tumor. Obviously, postoperative radiotherapy is not equally effective for all patients. Pooling all of them might interfere with the identification of the subgroup(s) in which radiotherapy is worthwhile.

Another potential pitfall is the variation in quality of the RT technique. We have seen that, in order to prevent local recurrence, a sufficient dose should be delivered, of the order of 4000 to 5000 rads, in 4 to 5 weeks.[2,9] In studies in which irradiation was carried out with 200 kV RT, the doses were generally insufficient. Unfortunately, the dose was also insufficient or heterogeneous in some studies performed later with high-energy radiation.[22,46] Moreover, the target volumes have to be properly delineated. Progress has been accomplished in this respect. For example, in the last few years, the internal mammary lymph nodes have been more precisely located through the use of lymphoscintigraphy.[38] It has been shown that, although the average lateral displacement from the midsternal line is 2.5 cm, the actual distances range from 0 to 5.3 cm. Similarly, the depth from the skin ranges from 0.7 to 5 cm. With many formerly standard techniques, such as the opposed tangential chest wall fields, an appreciable proportion of patients had some of their internal mammary lymph nodes underdosed because they were located at the margin or out of the field.[46]

Another advance is the use of computer dosimetry, which allows the study of dose distribution, not only in the plane located at the level of the center of the target volume, but also in other parallel planes. It has been found that the dose distribution in some of these planes was inadequate. For example, in some patients, due to changes in the contours of the thorax, the internal mammary nodes located a few centimeters above the center of the field were grossly underdosed. Currently, we carry out a CT scan at three different levels and determine dose distribution in these planes.

Analysis of the Data

We shall now briefly review the available data and discuss whether some tentative conclusions can be reached despite their inconsistencies.

The first controlled trial was that of Paterson et al.,[33] which compared patients with operable breast cancer treated with or without postoperative radiotherapy of lymph node areas. Although immediate radiotherapy reduced the incidence of local recurrence, it did not improve survival; however, the criticism has been made that in this rather old study the crucial lymphatics of the internal mammary chain and the medial supraclavicular fossa received an uncertain dosage.

In two other trials the surgical technique was not the same in the two groups. The Copenhagen study[24] was initiated in 1951 and compared extended radical mastectomy (with internal mammary chain and supraclavicular fossa dissection) with simple mastectomy and irradiation. At 10 years the survival was identical in the two groups of patients. The Edinburgh trial, initiated in 1964, compared radical mastectomy (RM) with simple mastectomy plus postoperative RT of the axilla, supraclavicular fossa, and the internal mammary chain. The results were updated in 1980.[29] Follow-up data for the first 12 years show that survival in the RM group is significantly better ($p < .05$), particularly in stage I patients. Overall, there was a significantly prolonged survival after detection of recurrence in the RM group ($p < .05$), which was most marked when local recurrence and distant metastases coincided ($p < .01$). However, it should be pointed out that the RT technique which was used in this study is not that which would be used currently.

The international multicenter trial supported by the British Cancer Research Campaign[12] compared in 2268 patients from 1970 to 1975 (T_1 or T_2, N_0 or N_1, M_0 patients of less than 70 years of age) simple mastectomy followed by RT with simple mastectomy alone, without axillary dissection. With a 5-year follow-up, the incidence of local recurrence was significantly higher in the group treated by simple mastectomy alone, in particular in patients with positive axillary nodes (77.8 percent versus 41 percent rate of local-regional recurrence in patients without or with postoperative RT, respectively). In patients with negative nodes, the difference was much smaller and of only marginal statistical significance (18.8 percent versus 7.7 percent, $p = .06$). However, up to 10 years, metastasis-free survival and overall survival rates were identical in the two therapeutic groups, both for stages I and II patients.

The Manchester breast study[30] also compared simple mastectomy versus simple mastectomy followed by RT in patients treated from 1970 to 1975. The local-regional recurrence rate was higher in the group treated without RT but there was no difference in survival. However, the value of RT was greater for medial tumors and when the diameter of the primary tumor was larger than 2 cm.

Several National Surgical Adjuvant Breast Project (NSABP) trials have assessed the value of postoperative RT.[13–15] In the trial which started in 1961, premenopausal patients were all treated by radical mastectomy followed by postoperative RT (parasternal, axillary, and supraclavicular), placebo, or simple drug chemotherapy (TSPA). Regional recurrences were less frequent in the group treated by RT than in the two others, but there was no difference in survival rates or disease status. In the B-04 trial conducted between 1971 and 1974, patients with clinically positive or clinically negative axillary lymph nodes were randomized between three groups: radical mastectomy, simple mastectomy (without axillary dissection) followed by postoperative RT, and simple mastectomy alone followed by a watch policy. A comparison of the three groups showed that the addition of RT failed to reduce the probability of distant metastasis or of death. A program of radiation monitoring was carried out and it has been possible to assess protocol compliance regarding dose of radiation administered and to correlate any variation of radiation dosage with treatment outcome. Within the range of variation observed, there was no influence of the quantity of radiation administered.[14] This result is surprising and difficult to explain.

In summary, in all the trials analyzed above, postoperative RT did not improve the survival rate or decrease the incidence of distant metastases. There are three possible interpretations of this observation:

1 Postoperative RT is ineffective because local-regional recurrences do not serve as a source of further dissemination.

2 Postoperative RT is beneficial for only a small subset of patients and is ineffective in other patients or even detrimental in some subgroups of patients.

3 The RT technique was inadequate in these studies and any conclusion is not warranted.

Before discussing these possibilities, we shall concentrate on four recent sets of data which may provide answers to these questions.

In 1977 Høst and Brennhovd[22] reported the results of a controlled randomized trial which compared radical mastectomy with or without postoperative RT in 1090 patients. During the first years of the trial patients were irradiated with 200 kV x-rays, but in the period 1968 to 1972 telecobalt therapy was used. This allowed an increase in dose and a more uniform dose distribution within the target volumes. No effect of irradiation was demonstrated in stage I patients regarding survival, local recurrences, or metastases. In stage II, 200 kV irradiation reduced the incidence of local recurrences and local metastases but did not affect survival; cobalt therapy caused a similar reduction in local regional relapses but in addition increased survival significantly. This was due to a significantly lower number of patients with coincident regional and distant metastases, whereas the incidence of other types of metastases was the same in control and irradiated patients.[22]

A comparison of the two irradiation techniques helps to interpret this observation. Patients treated by kilovoltage x-rays had an adequate dose to the chest wall, the supraclavicular area, and the axilla, whereas the dose to the internal mammary nodes was low. With telecobalt the dose to the internal mammary chain was higher. The possible role of irradiation of the parasternal lymph nodes is substantiated by the fact that survival was not increased for tumors of the outer quadrants, whereas it was improved for medial quadrant tumors. Similarly, survival was not influenced by radiotherapy for patients without axillary lymph node involvement, whereas it was influenced in patients with four or more axillary lymph node metastases, that is, in patients with a high probability of parasternal lymph node involvement.[23]

The data were recently updated (Høst, 1984—personal communication). In the whole group of patients treated by ^{60}Co, the survival at 8.5 years is higher than in patients treated by surgery alone but the difference is not statistically significant (67 percent versus 55 percent). However, if patients are subgrouped into those with lateral tumors or those with central or medial tumors, there is no significant difference for patients with lateral tumors, whereas the difference is marginally significant for patients with mediocentral tumors (5-year survival rates: 80 percent versus 62 percent; 10-year survival rates: 58 percent versus 42 percent, log-rank $p = .08$). However, the numbers of patients are small.

Another important trial is that of the Radiumhemmet at Stockholm. Wallgren et al.[57,58] reported the results of a randomized trial comparing in 900 patients radical mastectomy alone with either preoperative or postoperative adjuvant radiotherapy. The target volume for irradiation included the breast or the chest wall postoperatively, and the axillary and supraclavicular lymph node regions. The dose in all regions was 4500 rads in 5 weeks. Preoperatively, the breast and the internal mammary node chain were encompassed within the same volume and treated by two tangential ^{60}Co fields. Postoperatively, the same volume was treated by a 10- to 15-MeV electron beam, and two techniques of treatment were used successively. During the first 2 years of the study, both the homolateral and the contralateral internal mammary lymph node chains were included; subsequently, only the homolateral internal mammary region was included.[46] For patients treated only to the homolateral region, the sharper falloff of the dose, especially at the margins and corners of the electron beam field compared to the tangential ^{60}Co fields, may have resulted in some underdosage of the internal mammary nodes. This was not the case in the other patients.[46]

Preoperative and postoperative radiotherapy increased the disease-free survival rate significantly and to the same extent. The lower disease-free survival rate in those treated by surgery alone is mainly but not entirely explained by the much higher frequency of local and regional recurrences. The first local or regional recurrence in these patients could often be treated by surgery and/or radiotherapy, but even if this first recurrence was disregarded, those treated with surgery alone had significantly lower disease-free survival.

The irradiated patients had a slightly lower frequency of distant metastases compared to those treated by surgery alone. The distribution of distant metastases in various sites did not seem to have been influenced by the mode of treatment.

Ten years after initial treatment, the survival of irradiated patients is higher than that of patients treated by surgery only, but the difference is not statistically significant. However, in the subgroup of patients with tumors located in the medial quadrants of the breast, survival is higher in patients treated by RT (survival rates at 10 years: 72 percent versus 63 percent). Comparisons of incidence of distant metastases and of mortality rates between patients treated preoperatively or postoperatively and, among patients treated postoperatively, between those treated with the wide versus those treated with the limited electron field technique suggest that RT was of benefit to patients treated with the wide field technique to the internal mammary chain and not to patients treated with the limited field. In these patients, radiation was delivered with a less adequate dose distribution.[46,58]

Thus the data tend to support the idea that irradiation could be ineffective or even deleterious when the treatment technique of the internal mammary chain is inadequate.

In a retrospective but informative study, Fletcher[16,17] compared the 10-year survival rates for patients treated with radical mastectomy alone, radical mastectomy followed by postoperative peripheral lymphatic irradiation or 4000 rads of preoperative irradiation followed by radical mastectomy. For those patients with histologically positive axillary lymph nodes, the 5-year survival rate is significantly higher for patients having received postoperative irradiation. The improvement of survival is striking for patients with four or more positive axillary lymph nodes. This comparison is instructive because the patients treated by surgery only were essentially patients with tumors of the outer quadrants, whereas the patients treated by postoperative radiotherapy were essentially patients with tumors of the medial quadrants whose prognosis is normally poorer,[17] probably due to the frequent involvement of the internal mammary chain.

Villejuif Studies

The results of what we shall call now the Villejuif studies may help to interpret these three sets of data. In 1963, an international group initiated a cooperative study with Villejuif acting as the coordinating center. The aim of this trial was to find out whether the theoretical advantages of internal mammary dissection were borne out by an increase in the survival rate; 1580 cases of breast cancer were included and the 5-year results were published by Lacour et al.[26] Briefly, it was shown that an extended mastectomy (EM) improved results in only one small subgroup: patients with medial quadrant T_1 or T_2 tumors with histologically positive axillary lymph nodes. This subset represented only 13 percent of the total group of patients. Therefore, it was not surprising that overall survival was not affected by the outcome of these patients. In this subgroup, 31 percent of the patients had their internal mammary lymph nodes involved. This incidence was much higher than in other $T_1 + T_2$ subgroups. Incidentally, it should be noted that, for tumors of the outer quadrants without axillary involvement, the survival rate was significantly lower in the extended mastectomy series. This suggests that removal of noninvolved lymph nodes may be detrimental.

The 10-year results were recently published[27] and the overall comparison did not demonstrate an increased survival in the group treated with internal mammary dissection. However, there were major differences between cooperative centers in the number of axillary nodes examined and therefore in the relative proportion of node-negative and node-positive patients and in the prognostic value of axillary involvement. Hence, it was of interest to study the results of each center separately. From 1963 to 1967, 243 patients had been included at Villejuif as part of this international trial. All patients have now been followed for at least 15 years. The difference in survival between extended mastectomy or radical mastectomy varies with the site of the breast tumor (medial or lateral) and the lymph node involvement. A multivariate analysis showed that, for patients with positive axillary nodes and medial tumors, the relative risk of death is 2.1 times higher in patients treated by radical mastectomy without internal mammary dissection than in patients treated by extended mastectomy (15-year survival rate: 28 percent and 53 percent, $p = .01$).[28]

Conversely, internal mammary dissection appears to be detrimental in patients with negative axillary nodes and lateral tumors (15-year survival rate: 83 percent and 58 percent, respectively, in patients without or with internal mammary dissection). Both differences are significant.[28] These data help to understand how, when pooling together node-negative and node-positive patients, the deleterious effect of internal mammary dissection in node-negative patients with lateral tumors might cancel out the beneficial effect observed in node-positive patients with inner or central tumors.

Thus, despite the relatively small number of cases, these surgical data strongly suggest that treatment of the internal mammary chain is beneficial for the small subset of patients with central or medial tumors and positive axillary nodes, whereas it is unnecessary in patients with other patterns of presentation who represent the vast majority. This conclusion is confirmed by the results obtained after postoperative RT of the internal mammary chain. In this study,[42,43,53] the patients included in the internal mammary chain surgical trial were used as controls.

During this period, some patients with breast cancer were not included in the trial for various reasons, e.g., those whose home was too far from Villejuif to allow regular intervals of follow-up, and patients related to a physician. These patients were treated according to the previous Villejuif protocol in which postoperative radiotherapy was systematically performed in patients in whom involvement of the axillary or internal mammary lymph nodes had been found. In those patients, the course of postoperative radiotherapy delivered 4500 rads to the axilla, internal mammary chain, supraclavicular fossa, and chest wall.

Thus, we can compare four groups of patients with metastasis-bearing axillary lymph nodes treated at Villejuif:

Group 1 Group 1 consisted of 73 patients included in the internal mammary chain trial but randomized to the group treated by radical mastectomy (without internal mammary chain dissection). These patients did not receive postoperative radiotherapy. In 36, the tumor was located in the inner quadrants.

Group 2 Group 2 consisted of 78 patients included in the trial and randomized to the group treated by extended mastectomy (radical mastectomy plus internal mammary chain dissection). No postoperative radiotherapy was performed. In 34 patients, the tumor was located in the inner quadrants.

Group 3 This group consisted of 87 patients not included in the trial and treated in Villejuif from 1958 to 1967. The surgical procedure was the same as that in group 1, i.e., radical mastectomy, but surgery was followed by postoperative radiotherapy. In 35 patients, the tumor was located in the inner quadrants.

Group 4 This group consisted of 182 patients not included in the trial and treated as in group 2 by extended mastectomy but followed by postoperative radiotherapy. In 122 patients, the tumor was located in the inner quadrants.

Adjuvant chemotherapy was not used in any of these patients. In the four groups of patients, radiotherapeutic castration was performed in premenopausal patients.

All patients treated during this period at Villejuif were included in this comparison if they were staged as having TNM T_0, T_1, T_2, T_3 (only when the largest tumor diameter was less than 7 cm) without tumor adherence to the chest wall and without definite invasion of the skin, classified as having N_0 or N_1 but with histologically positive lymph nodes, classified as having no detectable distant metastasis at diagnosis, and aged less than 70 years.

For each of the patients included in the four groups, the following information was available:

the UICC TNM stage, the quadrant in which the primary tumor was located, number of metastasis-bearing axillary lymph nodes, and number of noninvolved axillary lymph nodes. It was statistically verified that these groups did not differ with regard to the size of the primary tumor, histologic type of cancer, and histologic grade. We did not use a matching process because this statistical procedure would have considerably reduced the number of patients compared; however, adjustments were carried out for age and the number of metastasis-bearing lymph nodes, which were found to be significant prognostic factors in this series.

The mean follow-up of the patients is 15 years. Log-rank tests were used to assess the statistical significance of the differences observed. Survival and relapse-free survival were calculated by the actuarial method. When the groups are considered irrespective of the location of the tumor, no difference is observed for overall or relapse-free survival.

When the tumor location is taken into account, no difference is observed for patients with tumors of the outer quadrants; however, for patients with tumors of the inner quadrants, the overall or relapse-free survival is significantly lower for the group treated by radical mastectomy alone than for the three other groups in which the internal mammary chain had been treated either by surgical dissection or radiotherapy. The difference remains significant after adjustment for age and number of metastasis-bearing lymph nodes (log-rank test, $p < .05$).

Furthermore, the cumulative incidence of distant metastases is similar for tumors of the outer quadrants in the four therapeutic groups, whereas for tumors of the inner quadrants the cumulative incidence is significantly higher in the groups treated by radical mastectomy alone than in the three other groups (Figs. 23-4 and 23-5). *All these data strongly suggest that similar results are obtained by treatment of the internal mammary chain, either by radiotherapy or surgery. They also suggest that the main contribution of postoperative radiotherapy is the irradiation of the internal mammary chain, as we have previously pointed out.*[53] It should be emphasized that we did not observe any increase in the incidence of pleural or pulmonary metastases in patients with tumors of the inner quadrants treated by radical mastectomy without postoperative radiotherapy or internal mammary chain dissection.[42,43]

In summary, all these data seem to indicate that the internal mammary chain is a crucial area for tumors of the inner quadrants. The analysis of these four recent studies strongly suggests that these lymph nodes, when involved, are a likely nidus for further distant dissemination.

Since the proportion of patients with mediocentral tumors with axillary involvement is small, it is not surprising that when global comparisons are made, this beneficial effect is overlooked. Even among patients with tumors of the inner quadrants and axillary involvement, radiotherapy can decrease the occurrence of distant metastases only in patients with internal mammary chain involvement and without occult distant metastases at diagnosis; this subset of patients is probably very small. This is presumably why, even among patients with tumors of the inner quadrants, the differences are only marginally significant. However, the consistency of the four studies gives credence to this interpretation. Specially designed, controlled trials would be useful for providing unequivocal answers to this question.

Meanwhile, what are the therapeutic implications of these observations? Both surgical dissection and external radiotherapy give satisfactory results. Irradiation of the internal mammary chain is a nonmutilating procedure and improvements in the technique of irradiation have been made during the past decade. Similarly, surgical techniques also have improved; it is now possible to perform a dissection of the internal mammary chain by a nonmutilating

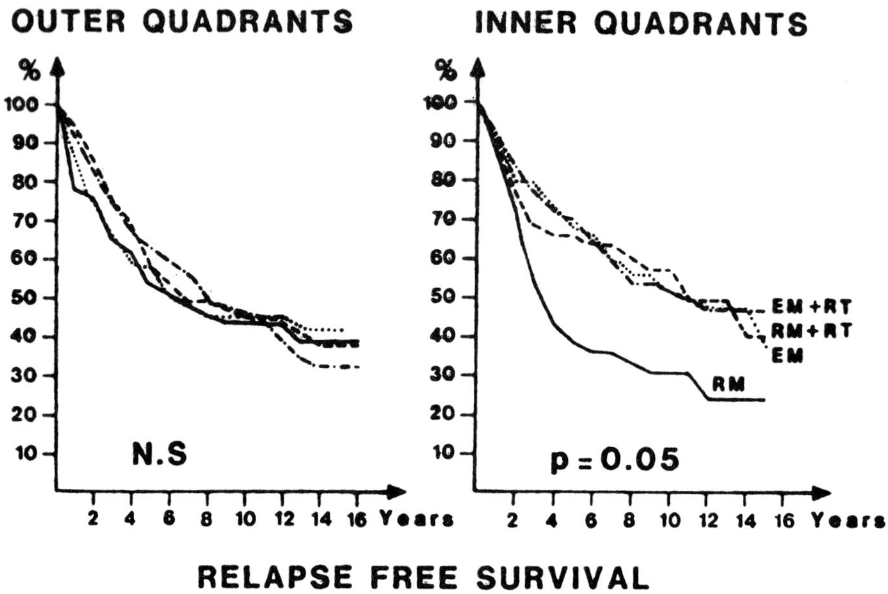

Figure 23-4 Relapse-free survival (RFS) in patients with breast tumors of the outer or inner quadrants treated by radical mastectomy (RM), radical mastectomy and internal mammary chain dissection (RM + IM), radical mastectomy and postoperative radiotherapy (RM + RT), radical mastectomy + internal mammary chain dissection + postoperative radiotherapy (RM + IM + RT). No difference is observed between the four groups in tumors of the outer quadrants. For tumors of the inner quadrants, the RFS is significantly lower in patients treated by radical mastectomy alone. RM,—; EM,....; RM + RT, ----; EM + RT, —. —.. (*Villejuif studies.*[42,43])

procedure. The great pectoral muscle can be conserved and reinserted after completion of the dissection.

In patients without internal mammary involvement, radiotherapy does not influence survival. In patients with tumors of the outer quadrants or in patients with mediocentral tumors without axillary involvement, the probability of internal mammary involvement is small. However, an isolated involvement of the internal mammary chain has been found in about 30 percent of patients without axillary lymph node involvement for T_2 tumors located in the inner quadrant. Thus, radiotherapy of the internal mammary chain and of the supraclavicular fossa may be considered for all T_2 tumors of the inner quadrants. For tumors of the outer quadrants, postoperative radiotherapy decreases the incidence of local and regional recurrences but does not improve the survival rate.

SIDE EFFECTS

Several studies have analyzed the immediate and late side effects of radiation therapy of the breast. The type and severity of complications are related to the total radiation dose, the dose per fraction, and the radiation technique.

With a proper technique, the dose of 4500 rads which is used in postoperative RT and conservative breast treatment is well tolerated. The incidence of complications is low.[17,21,39,40] The acute skin reaction following irradiation is moderate. Some patients experience esophagitis in the middle of the treatment, but medication is seldom necessary.

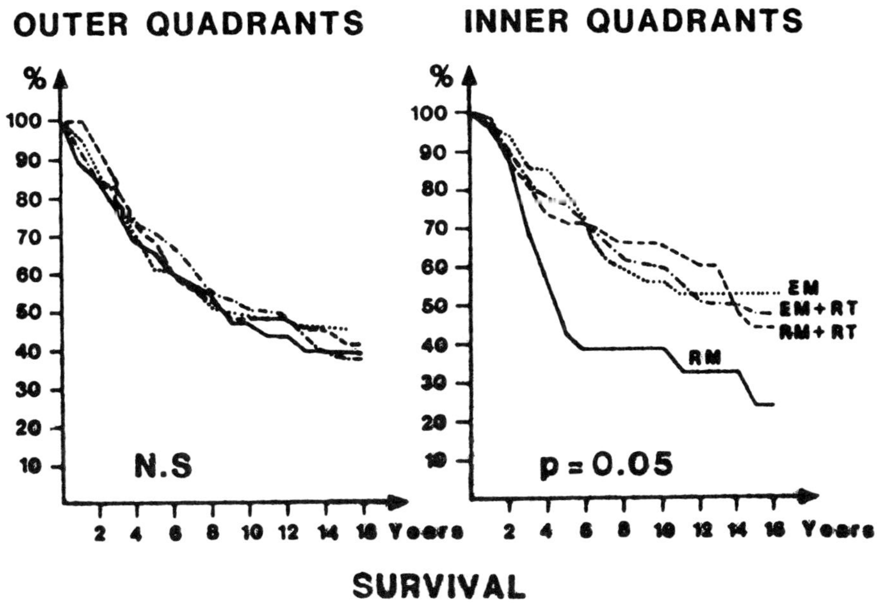

Figure 23-5 Overall survival in patients with breast tumors. See legend of Fig. 23-4. RM, —; EM, ...; RM + RT, ----; EM + RT, —. —.. (*Villejuif studies.*[42,43])

Late effects are more important to consider. *Mild skin telangiectasia* may occur, especially when patients have been treated with less than five sessions per week.

Arm edema is infrequent when 5000-rad tumor doses are delivered to an undissected axilla. Its incidence is higher in patients who were treated by both modalities.[3,37] In Villejuif, in patients receiving less than 6500 rads to the axilla, its incidence was 17 percent.[36] A comparison was carried out in Stockholm between the patients of the controlled trial treated by modified radical mastectomy with or without radiation therapy. In both groups, the volume of the affected arm was significantly greater than that of the control arm; it was at least 10 percent greater in 17 percent of the patients treated with radiotherapy versus 10 percent of those treated by surgery only. Generally, although the patients were not incapacitated, the mobility of the arm was significantly greater for the group not receiving RT; there was no significant difference in the gripping force between the two groups of patients.[47] Physical exercise instruction should begin during irradiation and be pursued throughout the course of treatment and follow-up.[17]

Brachial plexopathy is a rare but severe complication which occurs 2 to 5 years after treatment. At Villejuif, it was observed in 1.5 percent of patients who had received 5000 rads to the axilla during postoperative RT.[36] In patients whose axilla had been treated by RT alone, no plexopathy was observed for doses lower than 6000 rads. Two factors appear to increase the occurrence of this complication: a dose per fraction equal to or higher than 300 rads, and inadequate dose distribution within the axilla.[36]

Radiation-induced fractures of ribs are observed in approximately 7 percent of the patients receiving chest wall irradiation at a dose of 5000 rads.[17,40]

Radiation pneumonitis is probably the main side effect following postoperative RT.[18,32,40] Asymptomatic radiation fibrosis detected by systematic chest x-ray is observed in 50 percent[40] to 80 percent[23] of the irradiated patients. A small streak of fibrosis in the paramediastinal area may result in secondary emphysema of the nonirradiated part of the lung. However, symptomatic pneumonitis with cough and shortness of breath is observed in only a few percent of patients (3 percent in Villejuif); its frequency varies with the treatment technique, i.e., the volume of lung irradiated and the dose.[17,40]

Pectoral fibrosis and *skin necrosis* are very seldom observed following postoperative RT at 5000 rads.

In conclusion, minor side effects are frequent, but the incidence of serious late effects is low and the treatment is generally well tolerated. However, a small increment in dose (500 to 1000 rads) is sufficient to increase markedly the frequency and the severity of major complications and sequelae.

When radiotherapy and chemotherapy are combined, the incidence of complications depends upon both the total dose of radiation and/or drugs, the type of drug, and the chronology of delivery. Association of Adriamycin and mediastinal irradiation is particularly toxic when the time interval between the two agents is short. Severe cardiac complications have been reported.[50]

Sequential administration is preferred to concomitant administration since the additive toxic effect is decreased when the delay is longer than 1 week.[50] However, sequential treatments have the disadvantage of delaying administration of one of the two modalities. As adjuvant chemotherapy seems to control only very small neoplastic cell aggregates in breast cancers, a 2-month delay in its employment might be detrimental. We have seen above that a delay in the initiation of postoperative radiotherapy also reduces its effectiveness. This is why several authors feel that postoperative RT is inadvisable since it alters both the schedule and dosage of CT. Therefore, in the subsets of patients in whom both postoperative RT and adjuvant CT are indicated, it might be better to use alternating schedules in which both modalities are given without undue delays and toxic effects are limited.[50] The precise indications for combined treatments (postoperative RT and adjuvant CT) are not yet clear. The second Radiumhemmet breast trial in Stockholm compared postoperative RT versus adjuvant CT. Preliminary results suggest that in premenopausal patients CT gives better results, while the reverse is true for postmenopausal patients (Wallgren, personal communication, 1984). Thus, in premenopausal patients with tumors of the mediocentral quadrants, combined treatment might be indicated. It would be of interest to conduct a clinical trial investigating this therapeutic strategy.

REFERENCES

1. Alexander P: The bogey of the immuno-suppressive action of local radiotherapy. *Int J Radiat Oncol Biol Phys* 1:369, 1976.
2. Arriagada R, Mouriesse H, Sarrazin D, Clark RM, Deboer G: Radiotherapy alone in breast cancer. Analysis of tumor parameters, tumor dose and local control. *Int J Radiat Oncol Biol Phys* 11:1751, 1985.
3. Atkins H, Hayward JL, Klugman DJ, et al: Treatment of early breast cancer: A report after ten years of a clinical trial. *Br Med J* 2:423, 1972.
4. Baclesse F, Ennuyer A, Cheguillaume J: Est-on autorisé à pratiquer une tumorectomie simple suivie de radiothérapie en cas de tumeurs mammaires? *J Radiol Electrol Med Nucl* 41:137, 1960.
5. Baclesse F: Five-year results in 431 breast cancers treated solely by roentgen rays: *Ann Surg* 161:103, 1965.
6. Brady L, Fletcher GH, Levitt S: Cancer of the breast. The role of radiation therapy after mastectomy. *Cancer* 39:2868, 1977.
7. Bruce J: Operable cancer of the breast. A controlled clinical trial. *Cancer* 28:1443, 1971.

8. Calle R, Pilleron JP, Schlienger P, Vilcoq JR: Conservative management of operable breast cancer. The ten-year experience of the Fondation Curie. *Cancer* 42:2045, 1978.
9. Clarke DH, Lê MG, Sarrazin D, Lacombe MJ, Fontaine F, Travagli JP, May-Levin F, Contesso G, Arriagada R: Analysis of local-regional relapses in patients with early breast cancers treated by excision and radiotherapy: Experience of the Institut Gustave-Roussy. *Int J Radiat Oncol Biol Phys* 11:137, 1985.
10. Contesso G, Rouesse J, Mouriesse H, Sarrazin D, Genin J: Prognostic factors in breast cancers. (Submitted for publication.)
11. Contesso G, Rouesse J, Petit JY, Mouriesse H: Les facteurs anatomo-pathologiques du pronostic du cancer du sein. Bull Cancer (Paris) 64:523, 1977.
12. Elston CW, Gresham GA, Rao GS, Zebro T, Haybittle JL, Houghton J, Kearnay G: The cancer research campaign trial for early breast cancer. *Br J Cancer* 45:655, 1982.
13. Fisher B, Slack N, Cavanauch P, Gardner RB, Raudin R, and cooperating investigators: Postoperative radiotherapy in the treatment of breast cancer. Results of the NSABP Clinical Trial. *Ann Surg* 172:711, 1970.
14. Fisher B, Montague E, Redmond C, Deutsch M, Brown GR, Zauber A, Hanson WF, Wong A: Findings from NSABP protocol no. B-04: Comparison of radical mastectomy with alternative treatment for primary breast cancer. Radiation compliance and its relations to treatment outcome. *Cancer* 46:1, 1980.
15. Fisher B, Wolmark N, Redmond C, Deutsch M, Fisher E, and participating NSABP investigators: Findings from NSABP protocol no. B-04: Comparison of radical mastectomy with alternative treatments. II—The clinical and biologic significance of medial central breast cancer. *Cancer* 48:1863, 1981.
15a. Fisher B, Bauer M, Margolese R, et al: Five-year results of a randomized clinical trial comparing total mastectomy and segmental mastectomy with or without radiation in the treatment of breast cancer. *N Engl J Med* 312:665, 1985.
16. Fletcher GH, Montague ED: Does adequate irradiation of the internal mammary chain and supraclavicular nodes improve survival rates? *Int J Radiat Oncol Biol Phys* 4:481, 1978.
17. Fletcher GB: *Textbook of Radiotherapy*, 3d ed. Philadelphia, Lea & Febiger, 1980.
18. Hagen S, Kolbenstvedt A: Radiologic pulmonary changes following ^{60}Co treatment of mammary carcinoma. *Acta Radiol Ther Phys Biol* 11:386, 1972.
19. Hayward J: The conservative treatment of early breast cancer. *Cancer* 33:593, 1974.
20. Helle PA, Treurmet-Donker AD, Van Putten WLJ: Effect of post-operative radiotherapy on local and regional recurrence rate and survival in mammary carcinoma. An intercomparison of three different radiotherapy schedules. Proc. Third Meeting European Society Therapeutic Radiology and Oncology, Jerusalem, September 1984, p. 185.
21. Hery M, Sarrazin D: Valeur de la radiothérapie postopératoire systématique dans le cancer du sein opérable d'emblée. *Bull Cancer* 60:15, 1973.
22. Høst H, Brennhovd IO: The effect of postoperative radiotherapy in breast cancer. *Int J Radiat Oncol Biol Phys* 2:1061, 1977.
23. Høst H: Adjuvant radiation therapy in diagnosis and treatment of breast cancer. *International Clinical Forum*. Lewinson EF, Montague ACW (eds.). Baltimore, Williams & Wilkins, 1981, p. 201.
24. Kaae S, Johansen H: Simple mastectomy plus postoperative irradiation by the method of McWhirter for mammary carcinoma. *Ann Surg* 170:895, 1969.
25. Koscielny S, Tubiana M, Lê MG, Valleron AJ, Mouriesse H, Contesso G, Sarrazin D: Breast cancer: Relationship between the size of the primary tumour and the probability of metastatic dissemination. *Br J Cancer* 49:709, 1984.
26. Lacour J, Bucalossi P, Caceres E, et al: Radical mastectomy versus radical mastectomy plus internal mammary dissection: Five-year results of an international cooperative study. *Cancer* 37:206, 1976.
27. Lacour J, Lê M, Caceres E, Koszarowski T, Veronesi U, Hill C: Radical mastectomy versus radical mastectomy plus internal mammary dissection. Ten-year results of an International Cooperative Trial in breast cancer. *Cancer* 51:1941, 1983.

28. Lacour J, Lê M, Hill C, Kramar A, Contesso G, Sarrazin D: Is it useful to treat internal mammary nodes in operable breast cancer? (Submitted for publication.)
29. Langlands AO, Prescott JR, Hamilton T: A clinical trial in the management of operable cancer of the breast. *Br J Surg* 67:170, 1980.
30. Lythgoe JP, Leck I, Swindell R: Manchester regional breast study. Preliminary results. *Lancet* 1:744, 1978.
31. Montague ED, Fletcher GH: Is irradiation outdated in the primary treatment of nondisseminated breast cancer? in Dubois JB, Serrou B, Rosenfeld C (eds): *Immunopharmacologic Effects of Radiation Therapy*. New York, Raven Press, 1981.
32. Oppedal A, Kolbenstvedt A: Pulmonary contraction following ^{60}Co irradiation of mammary carcinoma. *Acta Radiol Ther Phys Biol* 15:329, 1976.
33. Paterson R, Russel MH: Clinical trials in malignant disease. Part III—breast cancer: Evaluation of post-operative radiotherapy. *Clin Radiol* 10:175, 1959.
34. Peters, MV: Wedge resection with or without radiation in early breast cancer. *Int J Radiat Oncol Biol Phys* 2:1151, 1977.
35. Pierquin P, Owen R, Maylin C, Otmezguine Y, Raynal M, Mueller W, Hannoun S: Radical radiation therapy of breast cancer. *Int J Radiat Oncol Biol Phys* 6:17, 1980.
36. Rawlings G, Arriagada R, Fontaine F, Bouhnik H, Mouriesse H, Sarrazin D: Plexite brachiale post-radiothérapique. *Bull Cancer (Paris)* 70:77, 1983.
37. Rissanen P: A comparison of conservative and radical surgery combined with radiotherapy in the treatment of stage I carcinoma of the breast. *Br J Radiol* 42:423, 1969.
38. Rose CM, Kaplan WD, Marck A: Lymphoscintigraphy of the internal mammary lymph nodes. *Int J Radiat Oncol Biol Phys* 2 (suppl. 2):102, 1977.
39. Sarrazin D, Hery H, Lê M: Rôle de l'irradiation post-opératoire systématique dans les cancers du sein opérables d'emblée, comportant un envahissement ganglionnaire. Etude de 209 observations. *Bull Cancer (Paris)* 60:31, 1973.
40. Sarrazin D, Fontaine F, Mouriesse H: Les complications de la radiothérapie des cancers du sein. *J Electr Radiol* 11:805, 1975.
41. Sarrazin D, Tubiana M, Lê M, Fontaine F, Arriagada R: Conservative treatment of minimal breast cancer, in Mouridsen HT, Palshof T (eds): *Breast Cancer: Experimental and Clinical Aspects*. Oxford, Pergamon Press, 1980, p. 251.
42. Sarrazin D, Lê M, Mouriesse H, Contesso G, Fontaine F, Arriagada R, Tubiana M: Radiotherapeutic studies on breast cancer at Villejuif. *The Cancer Bulletin (Houston)* 34:242, 1982.
43. Sarrazin D, Lê M, Lacour J, Tubiana M: Die post-operative strahlentherapie beim mammarkarzinom. Die Erkrankungen der Weiblichen Brustrdruse. Stuttgart, Georg Thieme Verlag, 1982, p. 196.
44. Sarrazin D, Lê M, Rouesse J, Contesso G, Petit JY, Lacour J, Viguier J, Hill C: Conservative treatment versus mastectomy in breast cancer tumors with macroscopic diameter of 20 mm or less. The experience of the Institut Gustave-Roussy. *Cancer* 53:1209, 1984.
45. Stjernsward J: Decreased survival related to irradiation post-operatively in early operable breast cancer. *Lancet* 2:1285, 1974.
46. Strender LE, Wallgren A, Arndt J, Arner O, Bergstrom J, Blomstedt B, Granberg PO, Nilsson B, Raf L, Silfversward C: Adjuvant radiotherapy in operable breast cancer: Correlation between dose in internal mammary nodes and prognosis. *Int J Radiat Oncol Biol Phys* 7:1319, 1981.
47. Swedborg I, Wallgren A: The effect of pre and postmastectomy radiotherapy on the degree of edema, shoulder-joint mobility and gripping force. *Cancer* 47:877, 1981.
48. Tubiana M: Post-surgical radiotherapy. Rationale and methods. *Recent Results Cancer Res* 67:107, 1979.
49. Tubiana M: Does post-operative radiotherapy facilitate metastatic dissemination?, in Dubois JB, Serrou B, Rosenfeld C (eds): *Immunopharmacologic Effects of Radiation Therapy*. New York, Raven Press, 1981, p. 399.
50. Tubiana M, Arriagada R, Cosset JM: Sequencing of drugs and radiations. The integrated alternating regimen. *Cancer* 55:2131, 1985.
51. Tubiana M: Cell kinetics and radiation oncology. *Int J Radiat Oncol Biol Phys* 8:1471, 1982.
52. Tubiana M, Pejovic MH, Chavaudra N, Contesso G, Malaise EP: The long-term prognostic

significance of the thymidine labelling index in breast cancer. *Int J Cancer* 33:441, 1984.

53. Tubiana M, Sarrazin D: A reappraisal of radiotherapy in the treatment of operable breast cancer: The new light on the internal mammary chain role, in Mouridsen HT, Palshof T (eds): *Breast Cancer: Experimental and Clinical Aspects*. Oxford, Pergamon Press, 1980, p. 243.
54. Veronesi U, Saccozzi R, Del Vecchio M, Banfi A, Clemente C, De Lena M, Gallus G, Greco M, Luini A, Marubini E, Muscolino G, Rilke F, Salvadori B, Zecchini A, Zucali R: Comparing radical mastectomy with quadrantectomy, axillary dissection, and radiotherapy in patients with small cancers of the breast. *N Engl J Med* 305:6, 1981.
55. Viadana E, Bross ID, Pickren JW: Cascade spread of blood-borne metastases in solid and non solid cancers of humans, in Weiss L, Gilbert HA (eds): *Pulmonary Metastasis*. Boston, G. K. Hall & Co., 1978.
56. Vikram B, Strong EW, Shah JP, Spiro R: Failure in the neck following multimodality treatment for advanced head and neck cancer. *Head Neck Surg* 6:724, 1984.
57. Wallgren A, Arner O, Bergstrom J, Blomstedt B, Granberg PO, Karnstrom L, Raf L, Silfversward C: The value of preoperative radiotherapy in operable mammary carcinoma. *Int J Radiat Oncol Biol Phys* 6:287, 1980.
58. Wallgren AA, Strender LE, Arner O, Bergstrom J, Blomstedt B, Granberg PO, Nilsson B, Raf L, Silfversward C: Pre- or post-operative radiotherapy in primary breast cancer, in Lewisson EF, Montague ACW (eds): *Diagnosis and Treatment of Breast Cancer. International Clinical Forum*. Baltimore, Williams & Wilkins, 1981, p. 209.
59. Weichselbaum RR, Marck A: The role of postoperative irradiation in carcinoma of the breast. *Cancer* 37:2682, 1976.

24

The Incidence and Significance of Local Recurrence

William H. Goodson III, M.D.

INTRODUCTION

Partial mastectomy has been proposed as an alternative to mastectomy for early breast cancer. Advocates of breast-preserving techniques assert, first, that mastectomy is excessive treatment for theoretically possible local recurrence. Second, they argue that local recurrence after a breast-preserving procedure does not have the same grave implications as local recurrence after mastectomy (i.e., it does not adversely affect survival, and it may in fact be a *local* problem). In most instances, those who advocate breast-preserving techniques have replaced total mastectomy with total breast irradiation.

The justification for either mastectomy or total breast irradiation is possible growth of either residual tumor or a separate focus of cancer in the same breast. These other foci of cancer are said to be "multicentric" and occur in at least 30 percent of mastectomy specimens after excision of the primary tumor. It is assumed that these foci of cancer will grow if not "treated."

The concern that multicentric or residual cancer will grow has led to two schools of thought concerning treatment. The traditional approach has been that this risk is high enough that all breast tissue should be removed. More recently, there has been interest in preserving the normal mound of breast tissue and destroying the epithelial tissue of the breast with ionizing radiation.

The risk that multicentric cancer will regrow has probably been overestimated for early tumors. Without any treatment multicentric cancer grows less often than anticipated,[31] and although radiation therapy retards growth it does not permanently reduce growth potential.

The staging system used varies and the specific meaning of the stage is indicated each time.

Breast Cancer Is Multicentric

After excision of a primary breast cancer, 21 to 31 percent of women have another focus of cancer in another quadrant of the breast,[22,25,31] 25 to 30 percent of women have cancer involving the nipple,[22,37] and 10.6 percent of patients had additional cancer in the same quadrant.[31] Characteristics of the primary tumor determine the probability of multicentric disease. Multicentric *invasive* cancer is more frequently associated with *larger cancers*. According to Lesser et al.[25] T_1 tumors had only 7 percent multicentric invasive cancer, while primary tumors over 4 cm in diameter were associated with 30 percent invasive multicentric cancers. The smaller tumors, however, were associated with a higher incidence of multicentric *noninvasive* cancers, 21 percent, in their series. Multicentric cancers were encountered more frequently when the primary cancer was infiltrating lobular carcinoma or infiltrating ductal carcinoma with a lobular carcinoma in situ component than when it was infiltrating ductal carcinoma alone. Morgenstern et al.,[31] found a higher average incidence (22 percent) of invasive multicentric cancer, but a lower incidence (10.8 percent) of in situ multicentric cancer.

Nipple invasion is more frequent when the primary tumor is under the areola. Lagios et al.[23] found that 34 percent of tumors within 2.5 cm of the nipple (a location which includes most tumors which extend underneath the areola) had nipple involvement. If the primary tumor was 2.6 cm or further from the base of the nipple (not subareolar), only 14 percent of patients had nipple invasion. The cancer in the nipple was evenly divided between invasive and in situ, although invasive cancer in the nipple was more common when the primary tumor extended beneath the areola.

If all multicentric or residual tumors grew, they would represent a continued threat to the patient. In this context, local control rates or their inverse expression, local recurrence rates, indicate the relative effectiveness of different forms of primary treatment of breast cancer.

THE NATURAL HISTORY OF UNTREATED MULTICENTRIC OR RESIDUAL BREAST CANCER

For small, early breast cancers there is a 15 to 20 percent probability that residual or multicentric cancer will grow. This constitutes a smaller threat than commonly predicted on the basis of pathologic studies of multicentricity. The observed rate is lower for two reasons: First, most of the studies of breast preservation with or without radiation therapy are limited to T_1 or small T_2 cancers. For these patients the risk of multicentric invasive cancer is only 7 percent,[25] not the average 30 percent for tumors of all sizes and stages. Second, it appears that not all lesions that are identified in an average series of pathology specimens have the potential to grow. The evidence for this is indirect, but as will be discussed below, most local recurrences are in fact failures of elimination of the original cancer, and only a small portion of local recurrences are actually new cancers. Only these new cancers can be attributed to multicentricity. The other local recurrences are failures of the original treatment.

Crile et al.[9,10] report 173 stage I and II patients followed for 8 to 23 years. All had had excision of the primary tumor alone, and only 13 percent had radiation therapy for those with clinically positive lymph nodes. They define local recurrence as regrowth of tumor at the original site and found it in 12 percent of their patients. In addition, they had six new tumors in other parts of the ipsilateral breast (3.4 percent). The latter 3.4 percent represents the risk of a second multicentric cancer, while the 12 percent represents the risks of treatment failure of the primary cancer. Therefore, for purposes of comparison this is a 15.4 percent rate. Eighty percent of their recurrences had been identified by the fifth year. With longer follow-up, they have similar local recurrence rates and they now project 15-year survival rates comparable to modified radical and simple mastectomy. The majority of the partial mastectomy patients did not have radiation therapy.[45]

Poisson et al.[36] treated 76 stage I patients with quadrantectomy and axillary dissection. Thirteen (17.1 percent) developed local recurrences. These patients have been followed 8 to 14 years, with a median follow-up beyond 10 years. Most recurrences were identified within the first 5 years. Of note is the 85.5 percent crude 10-year survival—this is excellent for any series of stage I patients and is not adversely affected by the local recurrences.

Clark et al.[8] report 154 stage I and II patients treated by excision alone. Many of their patients had short follow-up, but they present data as cumulative recurrences by years after treatment. They had 26 percent local recurrences by 6 years, but no additional local recurrences after the sixth year. Greening and Gowing[18] reported six local recurrences in 32 stage I patients followed 5 to 9 years after quadrantectomy and axillary dissection (19 percent local recurrence rate). Freeman et al.[14] had five local recurrences (11 percent) in 44 palpable and nonpalpable T_1 cancers for which the patients had been followed for 4 to 9 years. Both of these reports include patients with short follow-up, but since the first three reports cited above found almost all local recurrences by 6 years, latter rates are unlikely to change in a major way. *Based on these series one can estimate that the 10-year local recurrence rate for stage I cancer treated by partial mastectomy alone will be 15 to 20 percent and that the majority of local recurrences will be apparent within 5 years of treatment.*

MASTECTOMY TO REDUCE LOCAL RECURRENCE

The traditional approach of total mastectomy is the most successful way to reduce local recurrence of breast cancer. The risk of local recurrence for an individual patient varies with the size of the primary tumor and whether the cancer has spread to lymph nodes at the time of initial treatment. Histologic evaluation of excised nodes is the reliable way to evaluate nodal status, but many published series have used clinical evaluation alone. Since any group of patients called stage I on clinical evaluation will invariably include patients who are actually stage II (and therefore have a higher risk of local recurrence), patients who are staged clinically tend to have higher local recurrence rates.

For clinical stage I cancer of the breast (using the UICC or Revised American Joint Commission criteria) local recurrences range from zero to 4.4 percent.[39,24] In an alternative system, the Columbia Clinical Classification proposed by Haagensen, there is a 6.7 percent local recurrence in 402 "stage A" patients with clinically negative axillary lymph nodes[19] (this series includes patients with larger and therefore less favorable tumors and patients with positive nodes). In the 279 patients with histologically negative nodes presented by Haagensen there was a 3.2 percent local recurrence rate. These patients all had histologically negative nodes, but the group does include patients with larger primary tumors and therefore an increased risk of local recurrence. In another series with histologically negative nodes, Valagussa et al.[42] observed an 8 percent rate after treatment of T_1 and T_2 tumors. Again, they did not subdivide results by primary tumor size, and this is actually a rate for stage I patients and those who would usually be classified as stage II on the basis of a size T_2 tumor.

After mastectomy, most local recurrences are identified within 5 years of treatment. In a group of 704 consecutive patients with stages I, II, and III disease, Donegan et al.[13] observed 146 local recurrences. The local recurrence rate was 17.5 percent at 5 years and 20.2 percent at 10 years, so that 86.6 percent of their local recurrences were seen within 5 years of initial treatment. Haagensen[19] reported 54 chest wall and parasternal recurrences in stages A and B cases. Forty-two (70 percent) were identified in the first 5 years postoperatively. Identification of most local recurrences within 5 years is consistent in all series treated with surgery alone. This time course cannot be extrapolated to patients who have received radiation therapy.[16,27] Long-term follow-up is needed to establish true 10-year local recurrence rates after radiation therapy.[21]

EXCISION AND RADIATION THERAPY FOR LOCAL CONTROL OF EARLY BREAST CANCER

When excision of breast cancer is followed by radiation therapy, the early local recurrence rate is lower than after excision alone and similar to long-term rates reported after mastectomy. It is important to emphasize the word "early," since most reports of radiation therapy for breast cancer are based on early results.[17] The early difference between the rate predicted on the basis of multicentricity and the observed local recurrence rates has been interpreted as a success of radiation therapy. Long-term results, however, reveal that the rate of local recurrence continues to rise. When the long-term local recurrence rates are compared to local recurrence after excision alone, the data suggest that radiation does not cause a true reduction, but rather a delay in recognition of local treatment failure. For example, when a T_1 lesion has radiation therapy after excision about half the local recurrences are identified more than 5 years after primary treatment.[21]

Calle and Pilleron,[5] at the Curie Institute in Paris, report a 10-year follow-up of 89 patients with T_1 and small T_2 (up to 3 cm) tumors treated with excision and 5000 rads to the breast, plus 1000 rads boost to the tumor bed. There were 17 local recurrences (19 percent). Eleven of these were identified before 5 years and six between 5 and 10 years later. Thus, 35 percent of their local recurrences were identified after 5 years. Further data from the Curie Institute is presented by Vilcoq et al.,[44] with 14 biopsy-proven local recurrences in 240 patients followed for 3 years and 15 biopsy-proven local recurrences in 181 patients followed for more than 5 years. This gives progressive 3-, 5-, and 10-year local recurrence rates of 5.8, 8.2, and 19 percent, respectively, from the same institution.

Amalric et al.[1] report a 20-year experience from the Marseilles Cancer Institute, treating with 6000 rads over 6 weeks, plus a minimum of 1500-rads boost to the tumor area. One hundred fifty-one clinical stage I patients were followed for 5 years. Of 126 alive without evidence of disease, 113 had had their breasts preserved. Thus, 13 patients (8.6 percent) had had salvage mastectomy by 5 years. These authors had 60 patients followed 10 years. Of 41 alive without evidence of disease, 33 had had their breasts preserved. Thus, 8 had presumed local recurrences, a 10-year rate of 13 percent. In an addendum they cite a 10.5 percent local recurrence rate, but do not identify the type of patients in this group, and thus the exact 10-year rate in this study is unclear from this single paper. This uncertainty was resolved by Kurtz et al.,[21] who published data from the same institution, with a 10-year local recurrence rate of 13.5 percent for T_1 tumors. Particularly important is their observation that, among patients with the smaller T_1 tumors, 53 percent of the local recurrences were identified after 5 years.

Clark et al.[8] report 5- and 10-year local recurrence rates in two groups of patients treated with 4000 rads over 3 weeks. Those who received radiation to the breast only had 5- and 10-year local recurrence rates of 7.6 and 16.3 percent. Those who received radiation to the breast plus axilla had 5- and 10-year local recurrence rates of 12.3 and 21.5 percent. In both groups more than half the local recurrences were identified after 5 years.

Osborne et al.[33] reported a 20-year experience at the Royal Marsden Hospital, using 4500 rads to the entire breast and a 1000-rads boost to the primary tumor site. In a group of 115 clinical stage I patients, 5- and 10-year local recurrence rates were 18 and 26 percent, respectively. Again, 30 percent of these were identified after 5 years.

Recht et al.[46] claim, in their abstract, a 5-year local recurrence rate of 4 percent for clinical stage I patients and a 6-percent local recurrence rate at 10 years. They have, however, used the term "local recurrence" only if the recurrence was within the area of the iridium implant. Recurrences at the margins of the implant are called "marginal misses" and add another 4 percent at 10 years. Cancers recurring elsewhere in the breast are classified separately and total 8 percent at 10 years. Other authors usually combine these three classifications under the heading of local recurrence, and therefore this paper should be interpreted as showing a 16-percent local recurrence at 10 years for stage I cancer of the breast.

Other reports of lower local recurrence rates are for patients followed for shorter periods of follow-up. Pierquin et al.[35] reported two local recurrences in 40 patients (4.5 percent) treated with a minimum tumor dose of 7000 rads, but this was only a 5-year follow-up.

Montague et al.[30] had 162 patients with six local recurrences. However, 113 of these patients had been followed less than 5 years and 71 less than 3; i.e., 44 percent of the whole series had been followed less than 3 years. Since a significant number of recurrences are identified between the fifth and tenth years after treatment, a rate based on a large number of patients followed for a short time is unreliable. Unfortunately, the same method of reporting has been used many times.[2,7,26,32,34] (See also Chap. 18.)

Based on the publications cited one can estimate that local excision of a primary tumor and 4500 rads to the breast, followed by a boost to the tumor bed, will give a local recurrence rate of 13 to 26 percent. One-third to one-half of these local recurrences will become apparent more than 5 years after primary treatment. Thus, breast preservation with or without radiation therapy is associated with a higher local recurrence rate than after mastectomy. It has been asserted, however, that local recurrence after breast preservation is different from local recurrence after mastectomy.

THE CONSEQUENCES OF LOCAL RECURRENCE OF BREAST CANCER

Local Recurrence after Radical Mastectomy

The implication of local recurrence depends upon what method was used for the primary treatment of the breast. Local recurrence after radical mastectomy has grim implications, as shown by a high association with distant metastases and early mortality. Eleven of 13 local recurrences reviewed by Dao et al.,[11] occurred simultaneously with distant metastases. In the 146 local recurrences reported by Donegan et al.[13] the 1-year survival from the time of local recurrence was only 54.3 percent and the 5-year survival only 3.9 percent. Marshall et al.[29] reported a 57 percent 2-year survival among 57 patients. The high mortality was predictable, since 53 developed distant metastases and 29 already had distant metastases before or at the same as the local recurrence. Since the local recurrences and the distant disease occur nearly simultaneously, it is unlikely that either is the cause of the other. It is more likely that the occurrence of both at the same time reflects the aggressive nature of the primary cancer.

Local Recurrence after Partial Mastectomy

Local recurrence is more frequent when the breast is preserved, but reports of local recurrence after less-than-mastectomy treatment are less dismal. Clark et al.[8] report 55 percent 5-year survival from local recurrence after partial mastectomy and radiation. The 10-year survival was 33 percent. If recurrence was in the breast alone, 10-year survival was 77 percent, and survival in this group was virtually indistinguishable from patients who did not have local recurrence. Amalric et al.[1] reported a 69 percent 10-year crude survival, even with secondary surgery for local recurrence. Osborne et al.[33] found less satisfactory results, but theirs were still better than recurrence after mastectomy. They reported a 50 percent 5-year survival for 22 patients who had locally recurrent breast cancer (without metastases) after excision and radiotherapy.

The striking differences in the implications of local recurrence after mastectomy compared to breast-preservation techniques show they are different processes. Local recurrence after removal of all breast tissue implies a tumor of increased aggressiveness that had perhaps already invaded skin before the mastectomy or was seeded from lymphatics cut at surgery. In contrast, local recurrence after breast preservation includes such cases, but also includes patients with a locally extensive or multicentric tumor that was incompletely eradicated by the initial treatment. These latter recurrences constitute the increase in local recurrence seen with breast preservation compared with mastectomy.

The main question is whether these additional local recurrences can seed tumor cells and cause disseminated disease in the same manner we associate with primary cancer. However, since cancer takes 5 to 8 years to grow from a few cells (such as an early metastasis) to a 1-cm tumor, it will be many years after local recurrence before secondary metastases can be ruled out.

If it is found that local recurrences from breast preservation can seed secondary metastases, breast preservation with or without radiation therapy will carry an increased mortality. If, on the other hand, it is found that recurrence after breast preservation is not associated with an increased risk of metastases, then any possible difference in local recurrence with or without radiation will be insignificant. Thus, the decision whether to use radiation after partial resection of the breast will probably have less importance than the decision whether to do a mastectomy or a breast-preserving procedure.

RISK VERSUS BENEFITS OF RADIATION THERAPY AFTER LOCAL EXCISION OF EARLY BREAST CANCER

Since 10-year local recurrence rates after excision and radiation therapy are similar to those after quadrantectomy alone, one must evaluate whether all women who have a breast-preserving procedure should undergo radiation. With both methods, local recurrence rates are higher than after mastectomy (Table 24-1). The major difference is that *5-year local* recurrences are less when radiation therapy is used. This delayed recognition of local recurrence after radiotherapy is shown in all the studies reviewed and contrasts sharply to the earlier recognition of local treatment failure after either mastectomy or quadrantectomy without radiation.

It might be argued that the delay in local recurrence is emotionally beneficial. A woman has a longer "disease-free" interval before being confronted with treatment failure. However, this time is not actually disease-free, and it could be argued conversely that it would be beneficial to recognize treatment failure as soon as possible. This would allow earlier use of adjuvant therapy or salvage mastectomy. Radiation therapy also increases the dollar cost of treatment and the time commitment before a woman can consider her primary treatment complete.

In addition, radiation therapy may have long-term hidden risks. Published dosimetry for radiotherapy universally considers only the dose to the target breast. There are few data on the dose to the contralateral breast, but studies detect exposure of 150 to 300 rads.[4] This is largely scattered through the chest and cannot

Table 24-1 Local Recurrence Rates after Treatment of Early Breast Cancer (T_1, N_0 or N_{1A}, M_0, by UICC Staging)

	Years' follow-up	Number of patients	Number of local recurrences	Local recurrences, %
With clinical evaluation of axillary nodes				
Excision with radiation				
Curie Institute (6000 rads)	10	89	17	19[a,5]
Marseilles Cancer Institute (7500 rads)	10	60	8	13[1]
	10–21	139	19	13.3[21]
McGill University (1264 ret)	6–10	15	3	20[13]
Creteil, France (7000 rads)	5	43	2	4.5[35]
Royal Marsden Hospital (5000 rads)	10	115	30	26[33]
Excision without radiation				
Cleveland Clinic	9–23	173	27	15.4[b,9,10]
McGill University	6–10	32	5	16[14]
Mastectomy				
Columbia Presbyterian	10	608	39	7[c,19]
New York Medical College	10	446	20	4[c,24]
Memorial/Sloan Kettering	10	66	0	0[39]
With histologic evaluation of nodes in most patients				
Excision with radiation				
McGill University (1562 ret)	4–5	12	2	16[14]
Excision without radiation				
Royal Marsden Hospital	5–9	32	6	19[18]
McGill University	4–5	12	1	8[14]
St. Luc's, Montreal	8–14	76	13	17[d,36]
Mastectomy				
Columbia Presbyterian	10	418	7	2[19]
Milan Tumor Institute	10	335	27	8[c,e,42]

[a] Includes some 2–3-cm tumors, data not further classified.
[b] Includes 32% clinically stage II patients.
[c] Includes 2–5-cm tumors, data not further classified.
[d] Wide local excision of the malignant lesions, including easily a quarter to a third of the breast parenchyma around it, with resection margins proven clear of all invasion at the time of operation.
[e] Includes supraclavicular recurrences, data not further classified.

be eliminated by routine shielding. As shown by several studies,[3,28] this dose is carcinogenic in human breast tissue, but there is a 15- to 20-year lag time between radiation and recognition of induced tumors. Women with advanced cancer are unlikely to live this long; however, women with T_1, N_0 tumors do live 20 years. For these women the possibility of radiation-induced cancer is a relevant issue. It will be many years before this possibility will be adequately evaluated clinically, but there is evidence that therapeutic radiation given to the breast area can cause cancer of adjacent tissues.[15]

FACTORS ASSOCIATED WITH LOCAL RECURRENCE OF BREAST CANCER

Factors associated with local recurrence of breast cancer are very similar no matter what the initial treatment. They include positive nodes, residual tumor, extensive in situ

Table 24-2 Factors Predisposing to Local Recurrence

Primary treatment		
Mastectomy	**Excision and radiotherapy**	**Quadrantectomy**
(+) Nodes	(+) Nodes	(+) Nodes
(?) Narrow skin margins	(+) Resection margins	(+) Resection margins
In situ CA (lobular)	In situ CA (intraductal)	In situ CA (intraductal)
High grade primary tumor	High mitotic rate	
	Undifferentiated nuclei	

carcinoma, and aggressive undifferentiated cancer (Table 24-2).

Deck and Kern,[12] in a study of 68 local recurrences after mastectomy, found a significantly higher rate of local recurrence in patients with *infiltrating lobular carcinoma* (29 percent) than in those with *infiltrating ductal carcinoma* (5.7 percent). Only 3.6 percent of patients with negative axillary lymph nodes had local recurrence, compared to 11.2 percent of those with positive lymph nodes. They found no relationship between the margin of skin excised and local recurrence, although Donegan, et al.[13] found a higher incidence of local recurrence if there was less than a 3-cm skin margin. Donegan also found that local recurrence was more frequent (18.2 to 23.4 percent) with high-grade tumors than low-grade tumors (zero to 11.1 percent).

After segmental resection without radiation therapy, Lagios et al.[23] found that 36 percent of patients had recurrences *if nodes were positive*, but 17.6 percent had recurrences if nodes were negative. If there was residual disease at the resection margin, 71 percent had recurrences, but only 13 percent did if the margins were free of tumor. (In their study they included tumors up to 5 cm in diameter, which contributes to their high overall local recurrence rate.) When the recurrent cancer was invasive the histology was similar to the primary tumor. Intraductal carcinoma was present at the resection margins in their cases with local recurrence. A high incidence of positive nodes or very large tumors probably explains the high recurrence rates reported by other authors.[35]

When radiation is added to excision, local recurrence rate is influenced by the *pathology of the tumor*, the *extent of excision*, and the *status of axillary nodes*. Schnitt et al.[40] analyzed 12 local recurrences identified within the first 5 years of treatment. Local recurrence was more likely if over 25 percent of the primary tumor was intraductal, when there was extensive noninvasive carcinoma adjacent to the primary, when the nuclei were undifferentiated, or when there were two or more mitoses per high-power field. Local control was less (77 percent) in patients with positive nodes compared to those with negative nodes (92 percent), but this difference did not reach statistical significance, probably because of the small number in their series. Adequate excision was an extremely important factor. There was a 5-year local control probability of 64 percent in those who had an incisional biopsy, but a 92 percent probability of "cure" in patients who had an excisional biopsy. Similarly, Calle et al.[6] found that 59 percent of patients who did not have excision of the primary tumor required salvage surgery, the majority of which took place within $4\frac{1}{2}$ months of the completion of irradiation. In Schnitt's study the highest risk of local recurrence was in those women who had extensive intraductal carcinoma with poorly differentiated nuclei. Notably, a boost to over 6000 rads to the tumor bed did not significantly reduce the local recurrence rate in this group.

Age

Excision and radiation therapy is less successful in young patients. Vilcoq et al.[44] observed a 35 percent local recurrence rate in patients 21 to 30 years old when treated. They had a 7 percent rate in those who were 31 to 50, and no local recurrences in patients 51 or older at the time of treatment. This difference was highly significant ($p < .001$) by their own statistics.

The importance of adequate excision is further illustrated by the two most successful studies of breast preservation with radiation therapy: Both used quadrantectomy rather than lumpectomy. Romsdahl et al.[38] reported 8.1 percent local recurrences with limited excision and 2.8 percent in patients who had wide excision done primarily by them. They define wide excision as taking all the breast tissue "from the areola to the edge of the breast" in the affected quadrant. Veronesi et al.[43] also used quadrantectomy (although some authors have cited this report as an example of lumpectomy and radiation therapy). In an update after a minimum of 8 years' follow-up, there are only 14 recurrences of cancer in the 352 breasts treated with quadrant resection and radiation therapy. This is a rate of 4 percent at 8 years, suggesting that the quadrantectomy which they use may approach the results obtained with mastectomy.[47]

Other than the work of Pierquin,[35] these are the only studies of less-than-mastectomy combined with radiation that show a low local recurrence rate. The dramatic drop in the local recurrence rate associated with an extensive surgical procedure suggests that it is the latter, rather than radiation therapy, which produces better local control. This is reinforced by Clark's observation[8] that only three of the local recurrences he saw were in areas other than the site of the primary tumor and Criles' observation that he had 12 percent recurrence of the primary cancer and only 3.4 percent new cancer in the same breast. These studies emphasize that inadequate treatment of the original cancer constitutes the main risk for treatment failure.

SELECTION OF PATIENTS FOR QUADRANTECTOMY WITHOUT RADIATION THERAPY

It is not clear that irradiation should be used routinely after breast-preserving surgery for cancer. We are forced to confront a risk-benefit analysis in which the benefits are not permanent and the risks may be higher than initially contemplated. For this reason we must reassess the information and advice we give women with early breast cancer. For every woman with breast cancer, selection of treatment is based on her understanding of treatment results. Each patient should be informed not only of the existence of alternative treatments, but also of the known differences in results. Although there are many preliminary studies of breast preservation procedures, *modified radical mastectomy remains the standard, and women should be so informed.* If, however, a decision is made to use a breast-preserving treatment it seems appropriate that some women be treated with quadrantectomy alone. As with all reported studies of less-than-mastectomy treatment, these participants should be carefully selected.

There are several factors which are consistently associated with local recurrence, no matter what treatment is used (Table 24-2). These should be considered exclusions from quadrantectomy alone. (The similarity of factors leading to local failure and the fact that the same factors are associated with an increased probability of disseminated disease support those who feel that local treatment is a minor factor in patient outcome.) Positive lymph nodes are strongly associated with local failure, as well as with systemic treatment failure. This is logical, since if a cancer is located in one part of the breast and tumor has spread to lymphatic tissue outside the breast, some tumor nests would be in the lymphatics between the primary tumor and the node-bearing region. If these tumor nests are untreated they would be expected to grow. Therefore, patients with positive lymph nodes should be excluded from treatment with quadrantectomy alone.

Incomplete excision of the tumor or positive resection margins are associated with treatment failure. Again, residual tumors would be expected to grow and patients with positive margins should be advised to have more than excision alone.

Analysis of treatment failure with[40] or without[23] radiation therapy shows a strong association with an extensive intraductal component of the primary. Similarly, an extensive lobular in situ component is associated with local recurrence in mastectomy patients.[12] Until further information is available to determine if there is a difference between recurrence associated with a lobular in situ or intraductal component, patients with extensive in situ carcinoma of either kind should be excluded. Probably, those with undifferentiated nuclei and high mitotic rates should also be excluded.

Quadrantectomy alone should not be offered to women with 2-cm or larger tumors because of the higher incidence of invasive multicentric cancers.[2] Initially, it is probably appropriate to limit this treatment to women with tumors 1 cm or less in size.

CONCLUSION

Once a decision has been made to use breast-preserving treatment for early breast cancer, it seems appropriate to treat selected patients with quadrantectomy alone, that is, without radiation therapy. The 5-year local recurrence rate is lower when radiation is used, but 10-year rates are similar. Balanced against the lower 5-year rate is the possible long-term carcinogenic effect of radiation therapy on the opposite breast or other tissue. This is a major consideration for women with small, early breast cancers who are likely to survive the 20-year lag time for radiation-induced cancer to develop. Excluded from treatment with quadrantectomy alone should be women with any one of the following: positive nodes, tumor at the resection margins, undifferentiated carcinoma, extensive in situ component, or a primary tumor larger than 2 cm (or possibly 1 cm). At present, modified radical mastectomy is the standard treatment.

REFERENCES

1. Amalric R, Santamaria F, Robert F, et al: Radiation therapy with or without primary limited surgery for operable breast cancer: A 20-year experience at the Marseilles Cancer Institute. *Cancer* 49:30, 1982.
2. Balawajder I, Antich PP, Boland J: The management of breast carcinoma by primary radiotherapy at Mount Sinai Hospital from 1962–1979. *Cancer* 49:1587, 1982.
3. Baral E, Larsson L-E, Matisson B: Breast cancer following irradiation of the breast. *Cancer* 40:2905, 1977.
4. Bloomer WD: Late sequelae of radiation therapy, in Harris J, et al. (eds): *Conservative Management of Breast Cancer*, Philadelphia, Lippincott, 1983, p. 273.
5. Calle R, Pilleron JP: Radiation therapy, with and without lumpectomy, for operable breast cancer: Ten-year results. *Breast* 5:2, 1979.
6. Calle R, Pilleron JP, Schlienger P, et al: Conservative management of operable breast cancer. Ten years' experience at the Foundation Curie. *Cancer* 42:2045, 1978.
7. Chu AM, Cope O, Russo R, et al: Treatment of early stage breast cancer by limited surgery and radical irradiation. *Int J Radiat Oncol Biol Phys 6:25, 1980.*
8. Clark RM, Wilkinson RH, Mahoney LJ, et al: Breast cancer: A 21-year experience with conservative surgery and radiation. *Int J Radiat Oncol Biol Phys* 8:967, 1982.
9. Crile G Jr: The incidence of local recurrence of carcinoma of the breast. *Surg Gynecol Obstet* 156:497, 1983.

10. Crile G Jr, Cooperman A, Esselstyn, CB Jr : Results of partial mastectomy in 173 patients followed for from five to ten years. *Surg Gynecol Obstet* 150:563, 1980.
11. Dao TL, Nemoto T: The clinical significance of skin recurrence after radical mastectomy in women with cancer of the breast. *Surg Gynecol Obstet* 117:447, 1963.
12. Deck KB, Kern WH: Local recurrence of breast cancer. *Arch Surg* 111:323, 1976.
13. Donegan WL, Perez-Mesa CM, Watson FR: A biostatistical study of locally recurrent breast carcinoma. *Surg Gynecol Obstet* March 1966, p. 529.
14. Freeman CR, Belliveau NJ, Kim TH, et al: Limited surgery with or without radiotherapy for early breast carcinoma. *J Can Assoc Radiol* 32:125, 1981.
15. Goffman T, McKeen E, Curtis R, Schein P: Esophageal carcinoma following irradiation for breast cancer. *Cancer* 52:1808, 1983.
16. Goodson WH, III: The next big question in the treatment of carcinoma of the breast. *Surg Gynecol Obstet* 156:795, 1983.
17. Goodson WH III: Radiotherapy (letter). *N Engl J Med* 310:1055, 1984.
18. Greening WP, Gowing NFC: Treatment of breast cancer by quadrantic excision with axillary dissection. *J R Soc Med* 72:710, 1979.
19. Haagensen CD: Figures 34.6 and 34.12, *Diseases of the Breast.* Philadelphia, London, Toronto, W. B. Saunders Co., 1971, pp. 707, 714.
20. Harris J, Recht A, Amalric R, et al: Time course and prognosis of local recurrence following primary radiation therapy for early breast cancer. *J Clin Oncol* 2:37, 1984.
21. Kurtz JM, Spitalier J-M, Amalric R: Late breast cancer recurrence after lumpectomy and irradiation. *Int J Radiat Oncol Biol Phys* 9:1191, 1983.
22. Lagios MD, Gates EAS, Wesdahl PR, et al: Guide to the frequency of nipple involvement in breast cancer. A study of 149 consecutive mastectomies using a serial subgross and correlated radiographic technique. *Am J Surg* 138:135, 1979.
23. Lagios MD, Richards VE, Rose MR, et al: Segmental mastectomy without radiotherapy. Short term followup. *Cancer* 52:2173, 1983.
24. Leis Jr, HP: Modified radical mastectomy: Definition and role in breast cancer surgery. *Int Surg* 65:211, 1980.
25. Lesser ML, Rosen PP, Kinne DW: Multicentricity and bilaterality in invasive breast carcinoma. *Surgery* 91: 234, 1982.
26. Levene MB, Harris JR, Hellman S: Treatment of carcinoma of the breast by radiation therapy. *Cancer* 39:284, 1977.
27. Loeffler J, Recht A, Harris J: Letter, *N Engl J Med* 310:1056, 1984.
28. McGregor D, Land C, Choi K, et al: Breast cancer incidence in atom bomb survivors, Hiroshima and Nagasaki. *J Nat Cancer Inst* 59:799, 1977.
29. Marshall KA, Redfern A, Cady B: Local recurrence of carcinoma of the breast. *Surg Gynecol Obstet* 139: 406, 1974.
30. Montague ED, Gutierrez AE, Barker JL, et al: Conservation surgery and irradiation for the treatment of favorable breast cancer. *Cancer* 43:1058, 1979.
31. Morgenstern L, Kaufman PA, Friedman NB: The case against tylectomy for carcinoma of the breast. *Am J Surg* 130: 251, 1975.
32. Nobler MP, Venet L: Twelve years' experience with irradiation as the primary treatment for breast cancer. *Int J Radiat Oncol Biol Phys* 7:33, 1981.
33. Osborne MP, Ormiston N, Harmer CL, et al: Breast conservation in the treatment of early breast cancer. A 20-year follow-up. *Cancer* 53:349, 1984.
34. Peters MV: Wedge resection with or without radiation in early breast cancer. *Int J Radiat Oncol Biol Phys* 2:1151, 1977.
35. Pierquin B, Owen R, Maylin C, et al: Radical radiation therapy of breast cancer, *Int J Radiat Oncol Biol Phys* 6:17, 1980.
36. Poisson R, Legault-Poisson S, Mercier J-P, et al: Étude pilote sur le traitement individualisé et non-mutilant des cancers du sein. (Expérience personnelle de Saint-Luc de 1970-1976), L'Union Medical du Canada 113:494, 1984.
37. Quinn RH, Barlow JF: Involvement of the nipple and areola by carcinoma of the breast. *Arch Surg* 116:1139, 1981.
38. Romsdahl MM, Montague ED, Ames FC, et al: Conservation surgery and irradiation as treatment for early breast cancer. *Arch Surg* 118:521, 1983.
39. Schottenfeld D, Nash AG, Robbins GF, et al: Ten-year results of the treatment of primary operable breast carcinoma. A summary of 304 patients evaluated by the TNM system. *Cancer* 38:1001, 1976.

40. Schnitt SJ, Connolly JL, Harris JR, et al: Pathologic predictors of early local recurrence in stage I and II breast cancer treated by primary radiation therapy. *Cancer* 53:1049, 1984.
41. Tagart REB: Partial mastectomy for breast cancer. *Br Med J*, November 1978, p. 1268.
42. Valagussa P, Bonadonna G, Veronesi U: Patterns of relapse and survival following radical mastectomy. *Cancer* 41:1170, 1978.
43. Veronesi U, Saccozzi R, del Vecchio M, et al: Comparing radical mastectomy with quadrantectomy, axillary dissection and radiotherapy in patients with small cancers of the breast. *N Engl J Med* 305:6, 1981.
44. Vilcoq JR, Calle R, Stacey P, et al: The outcome of treatment by tumorectomy and radiotherapy of patients with operable breast cancer. *Int J Radiat Oncol Biol Phys* 7:1327, 1981.
45. Hermann RE, Esselstyn CB Jr, Crile G Jr, et al. Results of conservative operations for breast cancer. *Arch Surg* 120:746, 1985.
46. Recht A, Silver, Schnitt S, et al. Breast relapse following primary radiation therapy for early breast cancer. I. Classification, frequency and salvage. *Int J Radiat Oncol Biol Phys* 11:1271, 1985.
47. Veronesi U, Zucali R, del Vecchio M. Conservative treatment of breast cancer with the QU.A.RT. technique. *World J Surg* 9:676, 1985.

25

Neoadjuvant (Preoperative) Chemotherapy

J. Ragaz, M.D.
A. Coldman, Ph.D.
F. Salinas, D.V.M.
A. Worth, M.D.
M. Manji, M.D.
J. Goldie, M.D.

INTRODUCTION

Adjuvant therapy for cancer has developed as a result of extensive experimental data documenting the clear superiority of early over late treatment.[79,80] To improve cure in the absence of new, more potent agents, attention has focused on the optimal scheduling of the administration of available drugs. Neoadjuvant (preoperative) therapy is an example of this approach.

Neoadjuvant therapy, introduced by Frei several years ago,[28] is defined as treatment

1 given at the earliest possible time in the tumor's natural history;
2 given before the definitive local-regional treatment; and
3 consisting of the most effective treatment regimens.

TUMOR BIOLOGY

As a tumor grows, several biological events occur simultaneously. The speed of proliferation of individual cells decreases with time; the exponential rate of growth in the initial period is replaced by exponential growth retardation as expressed by a gompertzian function.[83,89,90] Establishment of micrometastases occurs in most patients before the clinical diagnosis is made.

Along with the expansion of tumor cell burden (TCB) and the formation of micrometastases, malignant clones, exhibiting unstable genotypes, mutate toward resistance.[33] The appearance of the first resistant mutant cell eliminates the chance of a cure. Computer simulation results confirmed by experimental data

The current TNM system of classification is used throughout.

indicate that the transition toward incurability is rapid, particularly in tumors with a high mutation rate. Therefore, even minor delays in beginning chemotherapy may convert a curable condition into one which can only be palliated.

Present concepts in the biology of metastases[11,21–24,36] indicate that the tumor burden consists of heterogeneous populations of cells with different metastatic potentials, and only the most viable metastases, forming the most aggressive subclones, survive and repopulate the host. In their latest work, Clifone and Fidler[11] suggest that the high metastatic potential of the subclones of aggressive cells is associated with increased genetic instability. This, in turn, may be a primary cause of their more aggressive behavior. Although these phenomena probably vary greatly between individual patients, it is to be expected that all individuals with high-risk lesions are at a certain risk for perioperative dissemination of the disease, albeit to different degrees. Hence, preoperative reduction of tumor cell burden seems a desired strategy to be tested in the clinical setting.

KINETICS

Animal Studies

In theory, any noncurative reduction of TCB may shift the proliferation rate of the remaining cells from the flat to the steep portion of the gompertzian curve, resulting in acceleration of the division rate in the remaining local and systemic metastases.

The evidence in experimental systems for the enhancement of formation of metastases by surgery is now quite convincing. As early as the turn of the century, Clunet[12] documented an increased incidence of systemic metastases in a mouse model after resection of the primary tumor. In 1913 Tyzzer,[96] summarizing Clunet's experiments, discussed the concept of athrepsia, i.e., competition for overall nutrition in the tumor system, as a principal explanation for this phenomenon. The early experiments indicated that perisurgical tumor manipulation, combined with noncurative cytoreduction, may play an important part in subsequent evolution of the disease. In the next several decades, experiments documenting a remaining tumor increased proliferation rate after noncurative surgery were reported by Gorelik,[35] De Wyss,[17] Simpson-Herren et al.,[84] Fisher et al.,[25] and others.

Human Studies

The enhancement of dormant metastases by noncurative therapeutic intervention, observed in animals, has not been documented adequately in human tumors. Nevertheless, similar phenomena, perhaps at a different magnitude, are also expected to take place in the clinical setting. Delarue[15] summarized the incidence of increased local and systemic perisurgical spread of malignant cells in patients undergoing surgical treatment for newly diagnosed cancer. Perisurgical vascular spread was documented by an increase of circulating cancer cells in the bloodstream. Other workers confirmed these observations, reporting the presence of circulating cancer cells for 7 to 9 days after surgery with the yield of circulating cells varying with the tumor stage and type of tumor.

Although several workers found no clear association between circulating cancer cells and subsequent survival, Roberts et al.[77] reported that patients exhibiting circulating tumor cells during surgery had a 5-year survival frequency only half that of those with no such cells. Similarly, Watne et al. in 1960[97] reported improved 18-month survival in patients without circulating cancer cells, and Drye et al.[18] reported recurrences only in patients with circulating cancer cells. This suggests, therefore, that although the majority of circulating cells fail to establish metastases,[21] a certain proportion of these cells may enhance established metastases with adverse effects on survival. The role of host

Table 25-1 Effects of Surgery on the Effector Mechanisms of Immune Response

Surgical procedure or perioperative condition	Immunological consequence	Reference
Prostatic carcinoma (*n* = 15) following cryosurgery or transurethral resection	Depression of PHA-stimulated lymphocytes	Ablin et al.[1]
General surgery (*n* = 135); anesthetic agents: thiobarbiturate and *d*-tubocurarine	Inhibition of diapedesis, reduction of phagocytosis and lymphocyte/neutrophil ratio	Francisci et al.[27]
Total hip replacement surgery (*n* = 8)	Transient increase of NK cell activity, followed by postoperative decline	Tonnessen et al.[95]
Effects of surgery and anesthesia on patients with (*n* = 20) or without (*n* = 34) malignant tumors	Decreased postsurgical cell-mediated response	Micheels et al.[60]
Removal of primary malignant melanoma (*n* = 47)	Cell-mediated cytotoxicity reduced at day 1, 50% restored at day 6; number of macrophages or ability to produce IFN unchanged	Moller-Larsen et al.[62]
Splenectomy in Hodgkin's (*n* = 5) and non-Hodgkin's disease (*n* = 26) patients	Decreased responses to primary immunization	Sullivan et al.[92]
Cholecystectomy in guinea pigs	Impaired memory function and delayed hypersensitivity in early postsurgical period	Cooper et al.[14]
Cancer patients (*n* = 250) with no systemic spread	Invalid correlations between primary response to DNCB and prognosis after anesthesia or surgery	Tarpley et al.[94]
Murine anesthesia induced by thiopental	Increase in pulmonary metastasis following immunosuppression	Lundy[55]
Local anesthetic effects of tertiary amines in PBC from healthy donors	Inhibition of NK cell activity by lidocaine and procaine	Takagi et al.[93]

Abbreviations: PHA, phytohemagglutinin; NK, natural killer; DNCB, dinitrochlorobenzene; IFN, interferon.

immunity (see Table 25-1) in the survival of circulating malignant cells, although suspected to be important, has not been fully clarified. It also remains to be shown whether preoperative chemotherapy in these cases has a beneficial effect.

QUANTITATIVE ASPECTS OF PREOPERATIVE CHEMOTHERAPY

As a result of gompertzian growth relationships, major differences in doubling time (DT) between macro- and micrometastases are expected.[82,89] Recent estimates of DT, as obtained from calculations of the first recurrence after mastectomy, have shown, as in animal models, a significantly shorter doubling time in microscopic breast cancer than in established measurable disease. Furthermore, if the post-mastectomy DT of micrometastases is expected to decrease and may vary anywhere from 10 to 60 days, delaying the initiation of adjuvant chemotherapy by 25 or 50 days after mastectomy will mean that the clinician will have to deal with a TCB two or three times that which is present at diagnosis.

The following series of calculations attempt to express quantitatively several biological phenomena relevant to the timing of adjuvant chemotherapy. It is assumed that the growth curve is exponential, as is DT. For the quantitative expression of the log fractional cell kill of the chemotherapy treatments *KsN*, the formula of Lloyd and Skipper[86] is used:

$$K_sN = K_s \times N - \left[\frac{\log 2}{\mathrm{DT}}(N-1) \times I\right] \quad (25\text{-}1)$$

where K_sN = overall log cell kill for the duration of treatment
K_s = log cell kill per course of treatment
N = number of courses
I = interval between courses

Let the average cell kill per course of treatment [e.g., cyclophosphamide, methotrexate, fluorouracil (CMF) regimen] be estimated as 0.5 log (a reasonable estimate, judging from the responses of metastatic breast cancer with measurable disease), the number of treatments N = 9, the interval I between the treatment courses be 21 days, and DT = 40 days. Following formula 25-1, the net cell kill will be approximately 3 logs. In other words, cure will be possible if, in the absence of resistant mutants, less than 10^3 cells are present at the time of starting the chemotherapy treatment. As the minimum number of cells needed to establish a clinical diagnosis is 10^9 (i.e., a size of 1 cm^3) and a large proportion of patients presenting with newly diagnosed breast cancer harbor more than 10^4 stem cells (micrometastases) outside the primary tumor, the majority of cases treated by the adjuvant treatments where the average cell kill is 0.5 logs per course of treatment, will be incurable with the presently available regimens.

A more effective drug combination, where the cell kill per treatment (K_s) is increased to 1.5 logs, may be simulated. The net cell kill over a 6-month course of therapy in this instance will be 11 logs. In other words, with the treatment achieving a cell kill of 1.5 logs per treatment, all patients with no resistant cells harboring up to 10^{11} tumor cells could be cured.

In order to obtain a higher cell kill, new agents and treatment combinations will have to be developed. In their absence, the lowest possible TCB should be secured at the time of starting adjuvant treatment. Maximal chance for an approach such as this will be achieved with the neoadjuvant (preoperative) setting.

Assuming the presence of micrometastases, what kind of difference in systemic TCB can be expected with preoperative chemotherapy timed 7 days before mastectomy, as opposed to 28 days later? Taking the DT of micrometastases to be 40 days and using the formula for the tumor cell burden (TCB) (excluding the primary) as

$$TCB = N_o \times 2^{t/DT} \quad (25\text{-}2)$$

where N_o is the number of systemic tumor cells at diagnosis, excluding the primary, N is the number of cells on the day of instituting adjuvant chemotherapy, and t is the time between surgery and the first cycle of chemotherapy. If $N_o = 5 \times 10^4$ (estimated by Skipper[85]), the systemic TCB 7 days prior to mastectomy is 4.3×10^4 cells, whereas the TCB 28 days after surgery is 8.1×10^4 cells. When, in addition to a 35-day delay in starting chemotherapy, a decrease in the DT of micrometastases due to the probable acceleration of the growth rate in connection with surgery[17,25,84] is taken into account, an even greater increase of the tumor volume will be seen in the short interval of 35 days. For tumors with simulated decreases (lasting for 28 days) of the postsurgical DT of 30, 20, and 10 days, the TCB on day 28 after surgery was calculated to be 9.5×10^4, 1.3×10^5, and 3.5×10^5 cells, respectively. It should be remembered that during the short delay of 5 weeks, in addition to a net quantitative increase in TCB, the malignant cells exhibiting unstable genotype may undergo a qualitative change, namely a transition to a state of resistance,[33] further reducing the chance of a cure.

CONVENTIONAL ADJUVANT CHEMOTHERAPY: REVIEW OF WORK ON DELAYS

Human studies, in contrast to animal experiments, have not fully clarified the question of timing of adjuvant chemotherapy. It is believed by many investigators that because of the relatively long doubling time generally seen in established breast cancer, delays of weeks or days may be of secondary importance. In view of the new data on acquired resistance and kinetic phenomena accompanying surgery and the appreciation of a significantly shorter DT of micrometastases,[82] the approach toward optimal timing of adjuvant therapy has to be reassessed. There are several clinical studies documenting benefits of an early start,[43,66,91] but others disagree.[8,31] In a study of Nissen-Meyer and coworkers,[66,67] a significant long-term survival advantage of treated patients was seen in 10 participating institutions where chemotherapy was started on day 1 after surgery, whereas there was no such difference in one hospital where therapy was delayed by 2 to 4 weeks.

A similar conclusion was reached at the University of Arizona, where adjuvant chemotherapy was used with doxorubicin (Adriamycin) and cyclophosphamide.[43] Patients treated with a chemotherapy delay of more than 4 weeks had a significantly lower relapse-free survival than those treated earlier. Sulkes et al.[91] showed that the actuarial disease-free survival in patients who started the CMF adjuvant chemotherapy after more than a 3-month interval was significantly lower than in patients who started the therapy within the first 90 days of surgery. In contrast, Glucksberg et al.[31] reported no difference in the rates of treatment failure in patients given a CMF vincristine, prednisone regimen at less than 14 days, 14 to 28 days, and 29 to 42 days. Similarly, negative results on the impact of timing the start of fluorouracil, Adriamycin, cyclophosphamide (FAC) chemotherapy regimen were reported by Buzdar et al.,[8] although their recent update showed that in patients with more than four positive axillary lymph nodes, the outcome was improved in those who were given FAC chemotherapy in the first 4 weeks.

Several other studies point to the adverse effects of delaying institution of adjuvant chemotherapy in connection with postoperative radiotherapy preceding chemotherapy.[40] Interpretation of these studies, however, is complicated by other factors, such as bone marrow suppression interfering with the ability of patients to receive maximum-intensity chemotherapy,[91] or immune suppression due to radiotherapy adversely affecting survival.[30] On the other hand, adverse effects of radiotherapy in combination with chemotherapy were not found by some investigators.[54] In summarizing the effects of delay in starting adjuvant chemotherapy, the following conclusions can be made:

1 Most animal data and some clinical data indicate that the optimal time for starting adjuvant chemotherapy is as soon as possible after the diagnosis of breast cancer is obtained.

2 In view of recent data on resistance and postsurgical kinetics of the remaining tumor, the immediate period after diagnosis and surgery may

be the critical one; afterwards, the extent of delaying conventional adjuvant chemotherapy may be less important.

PREOPERATIVE CHEMOTHERAPY IN LOCALLY ADVANCED INOPERABLE BREAST CANCER

The recent introduction on a large scale of chemotherapy before radiation or surgery for locally advanced inoperable breast cancer (LAIBC) began the era of neoadjuvant therapy for breast cancer. Papaioannou pioneered preoperative chemotherapy for solid tumors in humans,[69,70] and has concluded that preoperative chemotherapy of locally advanced breast cancer using a relatively aggressive Adriamycin-containing regimen is safe.

Morris et al.[63,64] discussed the results of a CMF regimen given preoperatively for two to four cycles to a small group of patients with LAIBC. Mastectomy was subsequently done in all patients without any serious postoperative complications and without need for a skin graft. Of importance was a 74 percent objective response rate of the measurable disease in the primary tumor prior to the mastectomy. The reduction of the local regional tumor raises a very intriguing suggestion that such a response could provide an in vivo test of responsiveness to preoperative chemotherapy. Schick et al.[81] reported a group of patients with LAIBC treated preoperatively with CMF or cyclophosphamide, Adriamycin, fluorouracil (CAF) regimens and concluded that the treatment is not only safe, but that it enables more effective surgery to be done with curative intent. Also, the lower the primary tumor cell burden at the time of surgery, the safer is the procedure. Recent data from the U.S. National Cancer Institute[88] showed encouraging results using a novel synchronized hormone chemotherapy and radiotherapy regimen using conjugated estrogen (Premarin), tamoxifen, cyclophosphamide, Adriamycin, methotrexate, and fluorouracil, with a greater than 60 percent histological complete remission rate after such preoperative treatment. The value of postoperative chemotherapy, in addition to possibly increasing long-term survival, stems from its potential for permitting use of different therapeutic strategies according to the response to preoperative treatment, as seen from the clinical and pathological assessment of the primary tumor. In summary, recent reviews of the management of patients with inoperable breast cancer indicate benefits of early systemic treatment, preceding local-regional therapy. The adoption of preoperative chemotherapy for operable patients with stages I to III breast cancer would be a logical extension of this observation.

PREOPERATIVE CHEMOTHERAPY IN STAGES I AND II BREAST CANCER

Since 1980, Jacquillat et al.[42] have conducted a nonrandomized study of neoadjuvant chemotherapy for stages T_1 to T_4, N_0, N_1, M_0 breast cancer. Preliminary results showed that in 87 percent of patients a reduction of more than 50 percent in the size of the primary tumor by preoperative chemotherapy was documented before the local-regional treatment had begun; 4-year disease-free survival frequency was 81 percent. Furthermore, a higher recurrence rate (20 percent) was seen in 56 patients whose initial tumor regression in response to preoperative chemotherapy was < 75 percent, compared to a recurrence rate of 8 percent in 87 patients whose initial tumor regression was $>$ 75 percent. In this preliminary analysis, therefore, a correlation between the in vivo sensitivity to the preoperative chemotherapy and outcome was found. Caution is advised, however, as the primary tumor, although a marker of sensitivity to preoperative chemotherapy, is likely to remain a source of resistant cells. These may continue expanding and disseminating throughout the duration of response, as such a response probably represents a reduction of the population of sensitive clones only. Accordingly, an early removal of primary tumor soon after the first cycles of preoperative chemotherapy and radiotherapy, regardless of the magnitude of response, would be the optimum strategy.

At the Vancouver Cancer Institute, work on preoperative adjuvant chemotherapy for stages I and II breast cancer patients started in 1981.[84–86] During the project's first phase, 43 patients were treated in a pilot study with one course of preoperative CMF chemotherapy (Table 25-2). During the second phase, initiated in 1983, a randomized trial of preoperative vs. postoperative adjuvant chemotherapy was started (Table 25-3). Presently, 101 premenopausal patients with stages I and II breast cancer have been randomized.

Randomization is performed by the referring surgeons. Patients allocated to the preoperative arm will receive the first cycle of the CMF chemotherapy regimen intravenously (IV) as soon as possible after the randomization; the definitive surgery (partial or modified radical mastectomy) follows. Hence, only one course of preoperative chemotherapy is given and the timing of surgery is not altered. High-risk patients (those with positive axillary nodes, vascular invasion, or lymphangitic spread) from both treatment arms continue postoperative chemotherapy for 6 months; low-risk patients will have no further treatment. The results of the pilot study[85] led to the conclusions:

1 One course of preoperative chemotherapy given a median of 7 days before mastectomy is safe.

2 Reduction of the median delay between the day of diagnosis and the first day of adjuvant chemotherapy to 2 (range 0 to 11) days is a substantial reduction compared with the conventional postoperative chemotherapy (range 28 to 60 days).

3 Survival of patients receiving preoperative chemotherapy has not been adversely affected by such treatment.

An additional aspect of this work includes the introduction of fine-needle aspiration (FNA) as a primary diagnostic method for breast cancer.[73,75] Recent reviews have shown that, in the hands of experienced cytologists, the diagnostic errors of FNA, in particular, instances of false-positive diagnosis, can be kept at a

Table 25-2 Protocol of the CCABC Pilot Study for Preoperative Chemotherapy with CMF for Newly Diagnosed Patients with Breast Cancer

Time (days)	Pretreatment	1	4–7	8	21
Biopsy and diagnosis (including estrogen receptors)	x				
Investigations:	x				
CBC	x			x	
LFTs	x				
CEA, sialic acid	x				
Chest x-ray	x				
Bilateral mammograms	x				
Bone scan	x				
Surgery + (modified radical, simple, or partial mastectomy)			x		
Cyclophosphamide, 600 mg/m^2 IV		x			x
MTX, 40 mg/m^2 IV		x			x
5-FU, 600 mg/m^2 IV		x			x

Abbreviations: CBC, complete blood count; MTX, methotrexate; 5-FU, fluorouracil.

Table 25-3 Outline of the CCABC Randomized Study of Preoperative versus Postoperative Adjuvant Chemotherapy for Premenopausal Patients with Newly Diagnosed Breast Cancer

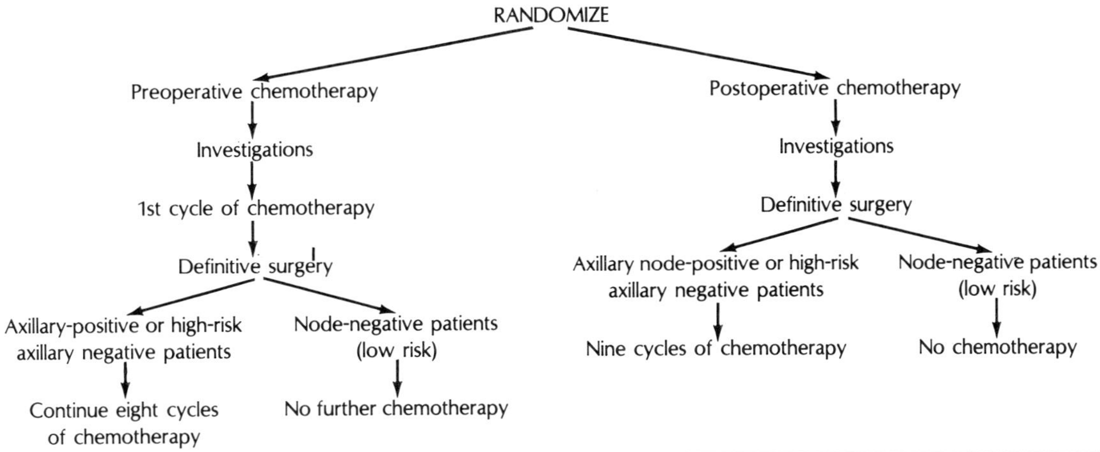

minimum.[26,46,49,76,78,98] It is anticipated that FNA will induce less tissue trauma than the conventionally performed open biopsy. Adverse kinetic changes in connection with cytoreduction and immunosuppression (Table 25-1) are also expected to occur to a lesser degree.

CHEMOTHERAPY: NEOADJUVANT REGIMENS

Experimental and clinical data indicate several consistent features of the optimal treatment regimens (Fig. 25-1). These are

Dose-intensity relations
Selection of appropriate agents and their combination
Timing of administration
Routes and schedules of administration

All four are important and interdependent.

Dose Intensity

Most of the available experimental data on dose-intensity of postoperative adjuvant chemotherapy indicate a superiority of intensive regimens.[80,87] In human adjuvant studies however, the question of dose intensity is more controversial. Hryniuk and Bush,[41] in a detailed review of more than 35 published studies, documented a clear association between the intensity of the delivered dose and the response as well as the median survival of patients with advanced stage IV breast carcinoma. Their most recent update (presented at the NIH Consensus Development Conference on Adjuvant Chemotherapy and Endocrine Therapy for Breast Cancer, Washington, 1985) documenting the same conclusion, included a retrospective review of adjuvant studies. Bonadonna and Valagussa's data[4] indicate that patients receiving more than 85 percent of the calculated dose did significantly better than those patients receiving less than 65 percent. Relevant to this type of analysis is a study by Lee[53] which showed that among the 58 patients who received six or more cycles of CMF adjuvant chemotherapy, only 21 percent were able to receive more than 85 percent of the calculated dose because of neutropenia and gastrointestinal toxicity, noted particularly in postmenopausal patients. Therefore, the practical realities may result in a situation wherein the large proportion of patients may be unable or unwilling to receive the calculated dose of the medications,

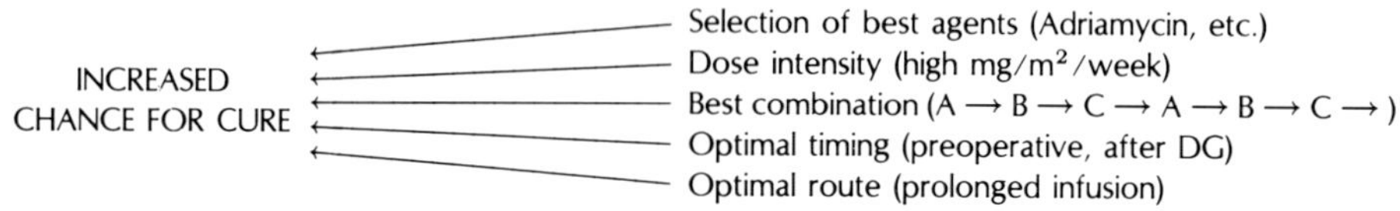

Figure 25-1 Outline of features of neoadjuvant regimens. Note that the best combination includes, in addition to the selection of most active agents, early alternations of effective regimens.

despite the scientific awareness of its importance. Thus, a careful and continuous assessment of cost versus benefit of treatment intensity is required.

Selection of Agents

Until recently there was not much evidence indicating a superiority of individual chemotherapy agents within combination regimens used in adjuvant therapy of breast cancer. Lately, however, along with the concept of dose intensity, the role of selection of the most active agents in combination has been emphasized. Misset et al.[61] randomly distributed 329 patients between the CMF and AVCF (Adriamycin, vincristine, cyclophosphamide, fluorouracil) arms. Overall, the 5-year disease-free survival was significantly better with AVCF (65.5 percent) as opposed to CMF (57 percent); ($p = 0.015$). This difference was most pronounced in the high-risk premenopausal patients with more than three positive nodes (70 percent vs. 43 percent; $p = 0.01$).

The University of Arizona's natural history data base in 1981 reviewed and analyzed 1971 cases receiving postoperative adjuvant chemotherapy with L-phenylalanine mustard (L-PAM); CMF; CMF with vincristine and prednisone; Adriamycin–cyclophosphamide; or FAC BCG.[44] The highest disease-free survival curves were seen with the regimen of FAC as given at the M.D. Anderson Hospital[7] with documented overall superiority over other adjuvant regimens ($p = 0.01$). The most consistent differences between FAC and other combinations are the higher dose intensity, the use of Adriamycin, and longer duration of the treatment.

There are, however, several studies which dispute the need for high-intensity treatment in an adjuvant setting.[2,10] The cost/benefit analysis of all regimens must remain a high priority in overall reviews of long-term results of adjuvant therapies. If the high-intensity regimens lead to a significant increase in cures, then the cost, including side effects and even a low mortality rate, will be more acceptable. Analysis of long-term results of controlled studies of dose intensity regimens has to be completed before a final conclusion can be made. Testing of high-intensity regimens, along with the question of chemotherapy timing, remains the most exciting aspect of clinical research on malignancies.

Combination of Regimens

Combining active agents is a well-recognized method for increasing the therapeutic efficacy of chemotherapy. The main objective of such an approach is to increase the number of cells within the heterogeneous population which are sensitive to the individual drugs in the combination regimen. All known active drugs, however, cannot be given in combination simultaneously in adequate dosage; individual regimens may be given in sequence, though, either switching at the nadir or alternating at each cycle.[34] Sequential alteration has been found mathematically to minimize the likelihood that multiply resistant subtypes will emerge during the period of active therapy. However, this conclusion rests on assumptions regarding the equal efficacy of the drugs or combinations which are to be alternated.

Several clinical studies suggest superiority of such an approach. The results with Hodgkin's disease,[5] where MOPP [mechlorethamine (nitrogen mustard), vincristine, procarbazine, prednisone] combination alternates with ABVD (Adriamycin, bleomycin, vinblastine, dactinomycin), show better outcome than a sequential combination where MOPP is followed later by ABVD. More frequent alternations of individual agents or regimens, matching closely the concepts of the computer simulations,[34] resulted in development, at the Vancouver Cancer Institute, of novel combinations for treatment of Hodgkin's disease (MOPP-ABV hybrid),[47] non-Hodgkin's lymphoma (MACOP-B),[13,48] stage IV breast cancer (CMF with Adriamycin),[72] and oat cell lung cancer.[65] Preliminary analysis of some of these indicates encouraging results.[47,48]

Scheduling

Metabolic and kinetic types of resistance are recognizable causes of treatment failure (Fig. 25-2). Taking the generation time of most malignant tumors to be more than 48 h and the duration of S phase more than 8 h, only one-sixth of the tumor population will be in S phase when exposed to the chemotherapeutic agents administered as an IV bolus. Previous investigators have worked out concepts of intensity of treatment delivered over time, indicating that it is not only the dose but also the duration of intensity of treatment which improves the therapeutic ratio.[16,39] There are also experimental data pointing to the superiority of continuous exposure to drugs (infusions) compared with short IV injections, particularly with cell cycle–specific agents.

1. Genetic → Enzymes, Transport, DNA repair
2. Kinetic
3. Metabolic
4. Toxicity to host

Figure 25-2 Commonly recognized types of resistance to chemotherapy treatments.

Improved technical aspects of continuous maintenance of indwelling catheters, as well as increasing availability of portable infusion pumps, may convert the concept of long-term infusion chemotherapy into a reality. Japanese workers reported on preoperative continuous intraarterial infusion with fluorouracil and mitomycin in inoperable breast cancer,[29,50] and Hellman et al.[37] and MacKenzie-Pratt et al.[57] reported encouraging results of regional arterial perfusion in the preoperative setting for locally advanced breast cancer.

SELECTION OF HIGH-RISK PATIENTS: NEOADJUVANT STAGING

With the introduction of preoperative chemotherapy, a more effective presurgical treatment may possibly sterilize the micro- or macroscopic tumor foci in the lymph glands, hence altering the conventional staging. In these instances, information gathered at the time of initial staging, before the first course of preoperative chemotherapy and before definitive surgery, would be used to identify high-risk and low-risk patients. This information would subsequently determine the intensity and duration of neoadjuvant therapy. The proposed prechemotherapy staging criteria are outlined in Fig. 25-3.

Estrogen Receptors

Recent evidence indicates that not only the level of estrogen receptors (ER) may predict response to hormonal treatments, but also that their presence correlates with survival. Workers at the

1. Tumor size
2. Tumor pathology
3. Differentiation, LI, grade
4. ER
5. DNA + ploidy flow cytometry
6. Mammograms–history
7. Internal mammary lymphoscintigram

Figure 25-3 Prognostic factors used for assessment of high- versus low-risk patients–neoadjuvant staging.

Vancouver Cancer Institute[32] have shown in 583 patients that cases with positive axillary lymph nodes but high estrogen receptor content had a better survival rate than those with negative axillary lymph glands but negative estrogen receptors. Therefore, the data suggest that ER as assessed at diagnosis may be an independent prognostic factor.

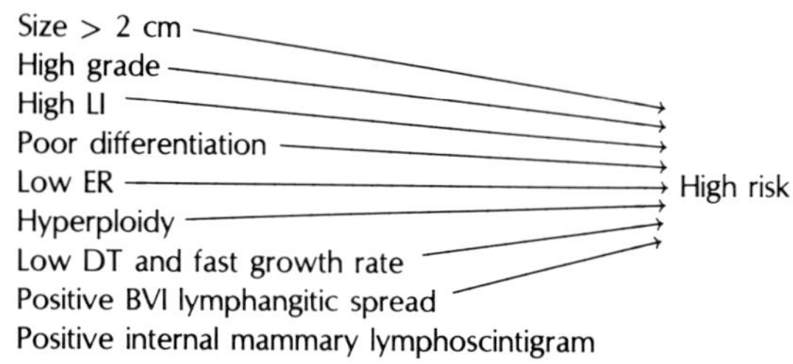

Figure 25-4 Definition of high-risk patients with breast carcinoma at the time of diagnosis—neoadjuvant staging.

Mammogram, History, and Labeling Index

Heuser et al.[38] analyzed case histories of 10,120 women receiving mammograms, in which calculations of DT of the newly diagnosed malignant tumors had been made. The authors concluded that the fast-growing tumors: (1) had a significantly closer association with positive axillary lymph nodes; (2) exhibited no mammographically detectable calcification; (3) were discovered in patients of younger age; (4) were associated with higher yield of lymphangitic vessel invasion, higher mitotic index, larger tumor size, and poor cellular differentiation; and (5) resulted in a lower 5-year survival rate in comparison to slowly growing tumors.

Similar data were published by Boyd et al.,[6] analyzing the significance of tumor growth rate as assessed by the duration of symptoms leading to diagnosis. Comparison of several prognostic factors showed the growth rate to be as good a predictor of relative death rate as was lymph node status, clinical stage, or Bloom's tumor grade. In multivariate analysis, the growth rate was shown to be independent of nodal status, clinical stage, or tumor grade ($p = .0002$).

Further evidence for useful information obtained from the labeling index (LI) and doubling time of primary tumors at the time of diagnosis has come from other workers,[51,56,90] suggesting that, independent of nodal status, a group of higher-risk patients can be identified before surgery or chemotherapy (Fig. 25-4).

Internal Mammary Node Lymphoscintigram

Up to 25 to 30 percent of patients with negative axillary lymph nodes at diagnosis will have a tumor recurrence in a 10-year follow-up. The state of the internal mammary lymph glands as determined by lymphoscintigraphy can effectively predict survival. Recent data suggest that patients with negative axillary but positive internal mammary lymph glands are at a similar risk of recurrence to those with positive axillary lymph nodes.[20,58] Therefore, information from internal mammary and/or axillary scintigrams, obtained after initial diagnosis but before therapy, can help to assess the stage of the disease without the need for information on axillary lymph node status.

Flow Cytometry

Recent reviews have shown that DNA measurements by flow cytometry from FNA at diagnosis[3,52,68] correlate well with survival and with other parameters affecting prognosis. Furthermore, DNA determination by flow cytometry permits assessment of histological grade, ER status,[68] and percent of cells in S phase,[56] enhancing the value of this technique for selecting high- and low-risk patients. Durand and Olive[19] found a good correlation between the cell kill and the mean cellular Adriamycin fluorescence as determined by flow cytometry, representing effects of Adriamycin on DNA synthesis. Since FNA allows repeated sampling of the accessible tumors, it can be used both at the time of primary diagnosis (for cytology and ER determination) and subsequently at relapse. With the help of flow cytometry, it thus may permit continuous assessment of cell cycles during treatment, antedating the measurable clinical response. Thus, kinetic differences induced by treatment modalities can be assessed, allowing more precise changes of treatment strategies.

CONCLUSION

Neoadjuvant chemotherapy represents a further escalation in the quest to offer curative treatment to more patients. The assurance of the lowest possible systemic TCB at the time of definitive local-regional treatment by preoperative chemotherapy is the main rationale for neoadjuvant treatment. Such therapy, according to theoretical and experimental evidence, may not only maximally decrease the chance of development of resistance but may also minimize the adverse kinetic effects of noncurative surgery and extensive tissue trauma. Adoption of high-intensity chemotherapy schedules administered by the optimal routes is another component of the neoadjuvant approach.

With the help of more sophisticated diagnostic techniques, selection of high- versus low-risk patients may become more accurate. Thus, early intensive preoperative systemic chemotherapy can be given to a better-selected subpopulation of patients, while low-risk patients may benefit from a less-aggressive approach. Also, with the introduction of effective preoperative chemotherapy, a more uniform adoption of conservative surgery with the possible elimination of radical mastectomy and extensive axillary explorations is a realistic possibility.

The increasing use of fine needle aspiration (FNA) may substantially reduce the need for incisional open biopsies. In addition to the assessment of histology, the FNA may provide information on ER status, flow cytometry assessment, and in vivo sensitivity of the tumor to the initially introduced chemotherapy courses.

Therefore, the timing of the first cycle of chemotherapy before the local-regional treatment, though the main element, is not the only aspect of the concept of neoadjuvant therapy.

Neoadjuvant chemotherapy may result in profound practical changes in the management of breast cancer. Therefore, before it can be introduced on a large scale, a thorough reassessment of all its aspects must be done. Well-organized future studies and organization of an effective mechanism of cooperation of academic centers with practitioners are essential parts of the neoadjuvant approach. It is likely that if practical reality allows the adoption of all the concepts discussed in this report a fundamental improvement in the outcome of breast cancer may be expected.

REFERENCES

1. Ablin RJ, Bruns GR, Guinan PD, et al: Alteration in host responsiveness in patients with prostatic cancer following cryosurgery or transurethral resection. *Am Surg* 43:144, 1977.
2. Ahmann DL, O'Fallon JR, Scanlon PW, et al: A preliminary assessment of factors associated with recurrent disease in a surgical adjuvant clinical trial for patients with breast cancer with special emphasis on the aggressiveness of therapy. *Am J Clin Oncol* 5:371, 1982.
3. Auer G, Tribukait B: Comparative single cell and flow DNA analysis in aspiration biopsies from breast carcinoma. *Acta Pathol Microbiol Scand* 88A:355, 1980.
4. Bonadonna G, Valagussa P: Dose response effect of adjuvant chemotherapy in breast cancer. *N Engl J Med* 304:10, 1981.
5. Bonadonna G, Viviani S, Bonfante V, et al: Alternating chemotherapy with MOPP/ABVD in Hodgkin's disease: Updated results. *Proc Am Soc Clin Oncol* 3:C-994, 254, 1984.
6. Boyd NF, Meakin JW, Hayward JL, et al: Clinical estimation of the growth rate of breast cancer. *Cancer* 48:1037, 1981.
7. Buzdar A, Blumenschein G, Gutterman J, et al: Adjuvant therapy with 5-fluorouracil, Adriamycin, cyclophosphamide and BCG for stage II or III breast cancer, in Jones SE, Salmon SE (eds): *Adjuvant Therapy of Cancer II.* New York, Grune & Stratton, 1979, pp 277.

8. Buzdar AU, Smith TL, Powell KC, et al: Effect of timing of initiation of adjuvant chemotherapy on disease free survival in breast cancer. *Breast Cancer Res Treat* 2:163, 1982.
9. Buzdar AU: Personal Communications.
10. Chlebowski RT, Weiner JM, Luce J, et al: Significance of relapse after adjuvant treatment with combination chemotherapy or 5-fluorouracil alone in high risk breast cancer: A western cancer study group project. *Cancer Res* 41:4399, 1981.
11. Clifone MA, Fidler IJ: Increasing metastatic potential is associated with increasing genetic instability of clones isolated from murine neoplasms. *Proc Natl Acad Sci USA* 78:6949, 1981.
12. Clunet J: *Recherches Experimentales sur les Tumeurs Malignes*. Paris, France, Steinhil G, 1910.
13. Connors JM, Klimo P: MACOP-B: Treatment of advanced diffuse large cell lymphoma (DLL) with an innovative 12 week intensive program. *Proc Am Soc Clin Oncol* 3:C9-29,238, 1984.
14. Cooper AJ, Irvine JM, Turnbull AR: Depression of immunological responses due to surgery. *Immunology* 27:393, 1974.
15. Delarue NC: The free cancer cell. *Can Med Assoc J* 82:1175, 1960.
16. DeVita VT Jr: Principles of chemotherapy, in DeVita VT Jr, Helman S, Rosenberg SA (eds): *Cancer: Principles and Practice of Oncology*. Philadelphia, Lippincott, 1982, pp 132.
17. De Wyss WD: Studies correlating the growth rate of a tumor and its metastases and providing evidence for tumor related systemic growth retarding factors. *Cancer Res* 32:374, 1972.
18. Drye JC, Rumage WT Jr, Anderson D: Prognostic importance of circulating cancer cells after curative surgery: A long time follow up study. *Ann Surg* 155:733, 1962.
19. Durand RE, Olive PL: Flow cytometry studies of intracellular Adriamycin in single cells in vitro. *Cancer Res* 41:3489, 1981.
20. Ege GN: Internal mammary lymphoscintigraphy: A rational adjunct to the staging and management of breast carcinoma. *Clin Radiol* 29:453, 1978.
21. Fidler IJ: Recent concepts of cancer metastasis and their implications for therapy. *Cancer Treat Rep* 68:193, 1984.
22. Fidler IJ, Hart IR: Biological diversity in metastatic neoplasms: Origins and implications. *Science* 217:998, 1982.
23. Fidler IJ, Poste G: Macrophage mediated destruction of malignant tumor cells and new strategies for the therapy of metastatic disease. *Springer Semin Immunopathol* 5:161, 1982.
24. Fidler IJ, Zeidman I: Enhancement of experimental metastasis by x-ray: A possible mechanism. *J Med* 3:172, 1972.
25. Fisher B, Gunduz N, Saffer EA: Influence of the interval between primary tumor removal and chemotherapy on kinetics and growth of metastases. *Cancer Res* 43:1488, 1983.
26. Frable WJ: Fine needle aspiration biopsy: A review. *Hum Pathol* 14:9, 1983.
27. Francisci de G, Giacomo M, Scrascia E, et al: Aspects of the immunological involvement in general anesthesia: Transvascular diapedesis, circulatory leukocytes and phagocytosis. *Adv Exp Med Biol* 73 (Part A):462, 1976.
28. Frei E III, Cancellos GP: Dose: A critical factor in cancer chemotherapy. *Am J Med* 69:585, 1980.
29. Fujimori M, Sakauchi G, Izuo M, et al: Studies on regional perfusion and intra-arterial infusion for cancer chemotherapy. *Surgery* 55:630, 1964.
30. Glick J, Donoff B, Haller D, et al: Integration of full dose adjuvant chemotherapy with definitive radiotherapy for primary breast cancer, in Salmon SE, Jones SE (eds): *Adjuvant Therapy of Cancer*. New York, Grune & Stratton, 1984, p 291.
31. Glucksberg H, Rivkin SE, Rasmussen S, et al: Combination chemotherapy (DMFVP) versus L-phenylalanine mustard (L-PAM) for operable breast cancer with positive axillary nodes. *Cancer* 50:423, 1982.
32. Godolphin W, Elwood JM, Spinelli JJ: Estrogen receptor quantitation and staging as complementary prognostic indicators in breast cancer: A study of 583 patients. *Int J Cancer* 28:677, 1981.
33. Goldie JH, Coldman AJ: A mathematical model for relating the drug sensitivity of tumors to their spontaneous mutation rate. *Cancer Treat Rep* 63:1727, 1979.
34. Goldie JH, Coldman AJ, Gudauskas GA: Rationale for the use of alternating non-cross-resistant chemotherapy. *Cancer Treat Rep* 66:439, 1982.
35. Gorelik E, Segal S, Feldman M: Growth of a local tumor exerts a specific inhibitory effect on progression of lung metastases. *Int J Cancer* 21:617, 1978.

36. Hanna H, Fidler IJ: Role of natural killer cells in the destruction of circulating tumor emboli. *JNCI* 65:801, 1980.
37. Hellman P, Bennett B: Intra-arterial cytotoxic therapy and x-ray therapy for cancer of the breast. *Br J Surg* 55:419, 1968.
38. Heuser L, Spratt JS, Polk HC Jr: Growth rates of primary breast cancers. *Cancer* 43:1888, 1979.
39. Hill BT: Biochemical and cell kinetic aspects of drug resistance, in Bruchovsky N, Goldie JH (eds): *Drug and Hormone Resistance in Neoplasia*, Boca Raton, Fla., CRC Press, 1982, vol 1, p 21.
40. Holland JR, Glidwell O: Adverse effect of radiotherapy on adjuvant chemotherapy for carcinoma of the breast. *Surg Gynecol Obstet* 150:817, 1980.
41. Hryniuk W, Bush H: The importance of dose intensity in chemotherapy of metastatic breast cancer. *J Clin Oncol*: 1984.
42. Jacquillat CI, Weil M, Auclerc G, et al: Neoadjuvant chemotherapy in the conservative management of breast cancers,: Study of 143 patients, in Ragaz J, Band PR, Goldie JH (eds): *Recent Results in Cancer Research*. New York, Springer-Verlag, 1986, vol 103, p 113.
43. Jones SE, Brooks RR, Takasugi BJ, et al: Current results of the University of Arizona adjuvant breast cancer trials (1974–1984), in Senn HJ (ed): *Recent Results in Cancer Research*. New York, Springer-Verlag, 1985, vol 96, p 133.
44. Jones SE, Moon T, Bonadonna G, et al: The use of a natural history data base (NHDB) to compare selected adjuvant trials for women with operable stage II (node positive) breast cancer, in Salmon SE, Jones SE (eds): *Adjuvant Therapy of Cancer IV*. New York, Grune & Stratton, 1984, p 235.
45. Karpas CM, Madden RE: Tumor cells and megakaryocytes in the blood: Their detection and importance, in Ariel IM (ed): *Progress in Clinical Cancer*. New York, Grune & Stratton, 1970, vol 4, p 62.
46. Kern WH: Diagnosis of breast cancer by fine needle aspiration smears. *JAMA* 241: 1979.
47. Klimo P, Connors JM: MOPP/ABV (hybrid) in treatment of advanced or recurrent Hodgkin's disease (initial experience). *Proc Am Soc Clin Oncol* 2:C-813,208, 1983.
48. Klimo P, Connors JM: MACOP-B chemotherapy for the treatment of diffuse large cell lymphoma. *Ann Intern Med* 102:396, 1985.
49. Kline RS: Masquerades of malignancy: A review of 4,241 aspirates from the breast. *Acta Cytol* 24:263, 1981.
50. Koyama H, Wada T, Takahashi Y, et al: Intra-arterial infusion chemotherapy as a preoperative treatment for locally advanced breast cancer. *Cancer* 36:1603, 1975.
51. Kusama S, Spratt JS, Donegan WL, et al: The gross rates of growth of human mammary carcinoma. *Cancer* 30:594, 1972.
52. Kute TE, Muss HB, Anderson D, et al: Relationship of steroid receptor, cell kinetics and clinical status in patients with breast cancer. *Cancer Res* 41:3524, 1981.
53. Lee YT: Adjuvant chemotherapy (CMF) for breast carcinoma. Patients' compliance and total dose achieved. *Am J Clin Oncol* 6:25, 1983.
54. Lippman M, Lichter A, Danforth D, et al: The influence of primary breast cancer treatment—mastectomy (M) or excisional biopsy plus radiation (E + RT)—on the ability to deliver adjuvant chemotherapy, in Salmon SE, Jones SE (eds): *Adjuvant Therapy of Cancer IV*. New York, Grune & Stratton, 1984, 301.
55. Lundy J: Anesthesia and surgery: A double-edged sword for the cancer patient. *J Surg Oncol* 14:61, 1980.
56. MacDivitt RW, Stone KR, Craig RB, et al: A proposed classification of breast cancer based on kinetic information. *Cancer* 57:269, 1986.
57. MacKenzie-Pratt RM, Betteridge TJ, Dixon P: Regional arterial cytotoxic perfusion combined with radical operation in breast cancer. *Br J Surg* 50:833, 1963.
58. Manji MF: Internal mammary lymphoscintigraphy in breast carcinoma: Possible significance in relation to current treatment. *J Can Assoc Radiol* 33:10, 1982.
59. Meyer JS, Bauer WC: In vitro determination of tritiated thymidine labeling index (LI). *Cancer* 36:1374, 1975.
60. Micheels JM, Degiovanni G, Cayet AM: Effect of surgery and anesthesia on cell mediated immunity. *Acta Anaesthesiol Belg* 30(suppl):33, 1979.
61. Misset JL, De Vassal F, Jasmis C, et al: 5 Year results of the French adjuvant trial for breast cancer comparing CMF to a combination of Adriamycin, vincristine, cyclophosphamide and 5-fluorouracil, in Salmon SE, Jones SE (eds): *Adjuvant Therapy*

of Cancer IV. New York, Grune & Stratton, 1984, p 243.

62. Moller-Larsen F, Moller-Larson A, Haahr S: The influence of general anesthesia and surgery on cell-mediated cytotoxicity and interferon production. *J Clin Lab Immunol* 12:69, 1983.
63. Morris DM: Inoperable stage III carcinoma of the breast. *South Med J* 76:615, 1983.
64. Morris DM, Aisner J, Elias EG, et al: Mastectomy as an adjunct to combination chemotherapy. *Arch Surg* 113:282, 1978.
65. Murray N, Hadzic E, Shah A, et al: Alternating chemotherapy and thoracic radiotherapy with concurrent cisplatin for limited stage small carcinoma of the lung (SCCL). *Proc Am Soc Clin Oncol* 3:C-835,214, 1984.
66. Nissen-Meyer R: One short chemotherapy course in primary breast cancer: 12 year follow up in series 1 of the Scandinavian adjuvant chemotherapy study group, in Jones SE, Salmon SE (eds): *Adjuvant Therapy of Cancer II*. New York, Grune & Stratton, 1979, p 207.
67. Nissen-Meyer R, Kjellgren K, Malmio K, et al: Surgical adjuvant chemotherapy: Results with one short course with cyclophosphamide after mastectomy for breast cancer. *Cancer* 41:2088, 1978.
68. Olszewski W, Darzynkiewicz Z, Rosen PP, et al: Flow cytometry of breast carcinoma: Relation of DNA ploidy level to histology and estrogen receptor. *Cancer* 48:980, 1981.
69. Papaioannou AN: Chemotherapy before mastectomy may be a more effective therapeutic sequence than its reverse in primary operable breast cancer. *Eur J Cancer* 1 (suppl):255, 1980.
70. Papaioannou AN: Perspective in cancer research: Preoperative chemotherapy for operable solid tumours. *Eur J Cancer* 17:263, 1981.
71. Papaioannou AN, Lissaios B, Vasilaros S, et al: Pre- and postoperative chemoendocrine treatment with or without postoperative radiotherapy for locally advanced breast cancer. *Cancer* 51:1284, 1983.
72. Plenderleith IH: Personal Communication.
73. Ragaz J, Baird R, Goldie J, et al: Neoadjuvant-preoperative (preop) adjuvant chemotherapy (CT) for breast cancer—new approach for the management of breast cancer. *Proc Am Soc Clin Oncol* 2:C-434, 111, 1983.
74. Ragaz J, Baird R, Goldie J, Rebbeck P, et al: Neoadjuvant (preoperative) chemotherapy for breast cancer, in Salmon SE, Jones SE (eds): *Adjuvant Therapy of Cancer IV*. New York, Grune & Stratton, 1984, p 425.
75. Ragaz J, Baird R, Rebbeck P, et al: Neoadjuvant (preoperative) chemotherapy for breast cancer. *Cancer* 56:1241, 1985.
76. Rimsten A, Stenkvist B, Johanson H, et al: The diagnostic accuracy of palpation and fine-needle biopsy and an evaluation of their combined use in the diagnosis of breast lesions: Report on a prospective study in 1244 women with symptoms. *Ann Surg* 182:1, 1975.
77. Roberts S, Jonasson O, Long L, et al: Clinical significance of cancer cells in the circulating blood: Two to five year survival. *Ann Surg* 154:362, 1961.
78. Rosen R, Hajdu SI, Robins G: Diagnosis of carcinoma of the breast by aspiration biopsy. *Surg Gynecol Obstet* 134:837, 1972.
79. Schabel FM Jr: Concepts for systemic treatment of micrometastases. *Cancer* 35:15, 1975.
80. Schabel FM Jr, Simpson-Herren L: Some variables in experimental tumor systems which complicate interpretation of data from in vivo kinetic and pharmacologic studies with anticancer drugs. *Antibiot Chemother* 23:113, 1978.
81. Schick P, Goodstein J, Moor J, et al: Preoperative chemotherapy followed by mastectomy for locally advanced breast cancer. *J Surg Oncol* 22:278, 1983.
82. Shackney WE, McCormack GW, Cuchural GJ Jr: Growth rate patterns of solid tumors and their relation to responsiveness to therapy. *Ann Intern Med* 89:107, 1978.
83. Simpson-Herren L, Corbett TH, Griswold DP: The cell population kinetics and response to a S-phase specific agent of three transplantable colon tumor lines. *Cell Tissue Kinet* 13:613, 1980.
84. Simpson-Herren L, Sanford AH, Holmquist JP: Effects of surgery on the cell kinetics of residual tumor. *Cancer Treat Rep* 60:1749, 1976.
85. Skipper HE: Repopulation rates of breast cancer cells after mastectomy (judged from break points in remission-duration curve). Southern Research Institute, 1979, booklet 12, p 63.
86. Skipper HE: Additional thoughts on the model of Goldie and Coldman. Southern Research Institute, 1980, booklet 10, p 19.

87. Skipper HE: Influence of dose intensity of C and A and S in CAF-containing regimens and the response of an experimental neoplasm (mammary adenocarcinoma 16/C) in advanced breast cancer in women. Southern Research Institute, 1985, booklet 7, p 27
88. Sorace RA, Bagley CS, Lichter AS, et al: The management of non-metastatic locally advanced breast cancer using primary induction chemotherapy with hormonal synchronization followed by radiation with or without debulking surgery. *World J Surg* 9:775, 1985.
89. Steel GG: *Growth Kinetics of Tumors.* Oxford, Clarendon, 1977, p 20.
90. Straus MJ, Moran RE: The cell cycle kinetics of human breast cancer. *Cancer* 46:2634, 1980.
91. Sulkes A, Brufman G, Rizel S, et al: The effect of postoperative radiotherapy on the feasibility of optimal dose adjuvant CMF chemotherapy in stage II breast carcinoma. *Int J Radiat Oncol Biol Phys* 9:17, 1983.
92. Sullivan JL, Ochs HD, Schiffman G, et al: Immune response after splenectomy. *Lancet* 1:178, 1978.
93. Takagi S, Kitagawa S, Oshimi K, et al: Effect of local anesthetics on human natural killer cell activity. *Clin Exp Immunol* 53:477, 1983.
94. Tarpley JL, Twomey PL, Catalona WJ, et al: Suppression of cellular immunity by anesthesia and operation. *J Surg Res* 22:195, 1977.
95. Tonnessen E, Mickley H, Grunnet N: Natural killer cell activity during premedication, anesthesia and surgery. *Acta Anaesthesiol Scand* 27:238, 1983.
96. Tyzzer EE: Factors in the production and growth of tumor metastases. *J Med Res* 28:309, 1913.
97. Watne AL, Sandberg AA, Moore GE: Prognostic implications of tumor cells in the blood. *Am Assoc Cancer Res Proc* 3:160, 1960.
98. Zajicek J: *Aspiration Biopsy Cytology, Part 1: Cytology of Supradiaphragmatic Organs.* New York, S. Krager, 1974.

26

Adjuvant Chemotherapy of Breast Cancer

Merrill S. Kies, M.D.

INTRODUCTION

Significant changes have taken place over the last 15 years in the treatment of "early" stage, infiltrating ductal and lobular breast cancer. Stages I and II tumors, which are generally considered resectable, are defined clinically as less than 5 cm in size, not fixed to the chest wall, and not associated with palpable fixed axillary adenopathy. Once the standard of therapy, the radical mastectomy is no longer routinely performed in most cancer centers. Procedures such as total mastectomy with an axillary lymph node dissection, a technique which preserves the chest wall musculature and only rarely results in long-term arm edema or swelling, is now the more common surgical approach.[1] The axillary sampling ranges from removal of only a few lymph nodes to a meticulous "clean-out" of the axilla, and provides important prognostic information, since the number of lymph nodes with demonstrable involvement by tumor correlates directly with risk of later recurrence. For some breast cancer patients, an alternative approach to primary treatment is local tumor excision with radiation therapy to the remaining breast tissue and draining regional lymph nodes.[2] Preliminary results indicate that, in terms of survival, this breast-saving approach is equivalent to surgery.

Certainly for best therapeutic and cosmetic results, an understanding of the wishes of the patient and cooperation between the surgeon and radiation oncologist are necessary. Size of the tumor and breast, the presence or absence of multicentric tumors, bilateral breast cancers, and axillary node status all must be considered before treatment strategy is determined.

Another recent change from traditional practice is that a two-step procedure is now generally advocated.[1] First, a diagnostic biopsy is obtained and studied so that definitive therapeutic planning, with the patient participating, can be carried out in a deliberate manner. This avoids the old practice of performing a biopsy with the patient under anesthesia, then proceeding directly to mastectomy if the frozen section shows breast cancer upon pathologic examination.

The observation that more than 50 percent of breast cancer patients are at risk of disease recurrence, irrespective of the choice of initial therapy, argues that despite the efforts of public education and increased use of mammography to detect smaller primary cancers, the disease is frequently systemic at the time of diagnosis. Risk of recurrence has been found to be highest in women with demonstrable metastases to axillary nodes, when the primary tumor is found to have low or no estrogen receptor-binding activity, and with larger primary tumor size.[3] This has led to the application of so-called surgical adjuvant therapy with chemotherapy or hormone manipulation in patients at high risk of having disseminated microscopic disease undetectable by routine clinical and radiographic techniques. Initial clinical trials were designed to determine whether or not the elective use of systemic cytotoxic therapy given to women at high risk of tumor recurrence following surgery would produce increased survival comparing treated patients to prospectively randomized control groups receiving standard surgical and radiation therapy alone. On a scientific level, the hypothesis that micrometastases with higher proliferative indices would be quite sensitive to available cytotoxic drugs is being examined.

SURGICAL ADJUVANT CHEMOTHERAPY

Studies by Fisher et al.[4] and Bonadonna et al.[5] have offered strong evidence that node-positive patients who receive chemotherapy after mastectomy have prolonged recurrence-free survival, compared to patients treated with mastectomy alone. In the United States, the National Surgical Adjuvant Breast Project (NSABP)[4] randomized patients to receive or not receive L-phenylalanine mustard (L-PAM) orally for 5 days every 6 weeks for 2 years. The results of this study were favorable for premenopausal patients. Disease-free survival was statistically significantly greater for treated patients, particularly those less than 39 years of age. In Milan,[5] cyclophosphamide, methotrexate, and 5-fluorouracil (CMF) were given in monthly cycles for 1 year. The updated Milan data, listed in Table 26-1, show the disease-free and overall survival advantages in treated premenopausal

Table 26-1 Disease-Free Survival at 6 Years for Patients Treated with CMF in Milan Trial

	Disease Free (%)		
N	Mastectomy only (179)	Mastectomy CMF (207)	*p*
All patients	43.8	55.7	.001
Nodes 1–3	45.6	65.1	.001
Nodes ≥ 4	31.8	35.7	.27
Postmenopausal	44.9	50.5	.35
Premenopausal	42.7	59.8	.001
Nodes 1–3	48.6	73.7	.005
Nodes ≥ 4	26.8	41.4	.05
Survival			
All patients	64.5	73.9	.12
Premenopausal	62.5	77.6	.02

Table 26-2 Prospective Adjuvant Chemotherapy Trials Including a Control Group of Patients Given Surgery and/or Radiation without Adjuvant Systemic Treatment in Stage II Breast Cancer

Group	No. patients	Adjuvant therapy tested	Findings
NSABP[6]	370	L-PAM	Improved RFS and OS in premenopause; 1–3 nodes
Bonadonna[7]	386	CMF	Improved RFS and OS in premenopause
Senn[8]	118	LMF + BCG	Improved RFS in postmenopause; no OS difference
Wheeler[9]	227	CVFM	Improved RFS in postmenopause; no OS difference
Rubens[10]	312	L-PAM	No difference
Morrison[11]	512	AVCMF	Improved RFS in premenopause; no OS difference
Smith[12]	322	CMF, CMF + RT	Improved RFS in premenopause and postmenopause after RT + CMF and CMF vs postoperative RT alone; improved OS after RT + CMF vs RT alone

NSABP = National Surgical Adjuvant Breast Project; RFS = relapse-free survival; L-PAM = L-phenylalanine mustard; M = methotrexate; L = Leukeran; A = Adriamycin; OS = overall survival; C = cyclophosphamide; F = 5-fluorouracil; V = vincristine; RT = postoperative radiation.

Source: After Bonadonna and Valagussa.[7]

women. Recent follow-up at 9 years shows an overall survival advantage for treated premenopausal women (66 percent) versus controls (43 percent) with $p = .02$. There remains a lack of statistically significant differences in survival for treated and control postmenopausal patients. These data suggest that early observed differences in relapse-free survival do not necessarily precede differences an overall survival. Bonadonna and coworkers have also examined the quality and intensity of therapy given to study patients *after* relapse and find no evidence that ultimate survival differences could be explained on that basis.

Results of these and other prospective studies (Table 26-2) indicate that relapse-free and survival advantages have been most convincingly demonstrated in premenopausal patients with one to three positive axillary nodes, while those with four or more nodes positive at diagnosis may primarily benefit from extended relapse-free survival. Results in postmenopausal women have been mixed and the value of adjuvant cytotoxic therapy in this larger group remains unclear. Interestingly, the risk of local-regional recurrence in the chemotherapy treatment arms has appeared to be reduced in comparisons with patients treated only by mastectomy, suggesting that the routine use of radiation for this purpose is probably not warranted.

These well-designed prospective trials helped establish the potential value of adjuvant chemotherapy, although a number of important questions remain and are the subject of clinical studies currently being carried out in Europe and North America: (1) Is adjuvant therapy appropriate for postmenopausal women? (2) What is the optimal drug regimen, dose, and timing with respect to surgery or radiation? (3) Should hormones be used or added to cytotoxic programs?

(4) Does adjuvant chemotherapy result in a higher percentage of ultimate cures, or does it only delay recurrence? (5) Are there significant long-term, chemotherapy-related side effects?

Other studies comparing single-agent therapy with multiple drug programs have shown improved relapse-free survival for combination chemotherapy regimens in pre- and postmenopausal patients.[6,13] The NSABP tested L-PAM versus L-PAM and 5-fluorouracil (PF) in 741 patients with the result that pre- and postmenopausal women with four or more positive nodes had improved disease-free survival. The Southwest Oncology Group (SWOG) contrasted L-PAM with CMF, vincristine, and prednisone (CMFVP), and again demonstrated improved relapse-free survival in the pre- and postmenopausal patients given combination chemotherapy. In view of the prospectively randomized trials with no treatment control arms mentioned earlier, these results suggest some contradictions.

Treatment Intensity

A recent retrospective analysis of the Milan experience[14] showed that a subgroup of the treated postmenopausal patients given a higher percentage of the planned drug dosages actually did better than the untreated controls. One study, of advanced disease, prospectively randomized patients to one of two relatively intensive multidrug regimens or low-dose Leukeran, methotrexate, 5-FU, and prednisone with a resultant lower response rate (32 percent versus 50+ percent) and shortened survival in the milder treatment arm.[15] Another study[16] of high- versus low dose 5-FU, Adriamycin, and Cytoxan failed to show a significant response duration or survival difference. At present, while there has been no convincing demonstration of a reliable dose-response or dose-survival effect relationship in breast cancer, it is theorized that major cytoreduction depends on maintenance of high drug dose levels and that frivolous dose reductions should be avoided, especially in the adjuvant setting. Steep dose-response effects have been demonstrated in experimental systems for most cytotoxic agents and are likely to be operative in human breast cancer.

At Milan, investigators theorized that maximal cell kill was likely to occur within 3 to 6 months from treatment start, and a second trial matching 6 versus 12 months of CMF was performed[17] with no differences in either disease-free or total survival evident in premenopausal patients at 7 years follow-up. The question of optimal duration of chemotherapy is obviously not yet resolved; however, it is likely to depend on drug selection, dose, and the patient population to be treated. Thus, a number of trials are under way examining this issue, and current recommendations are that 12 months of therapy remain the standard for comparison, at least for CMF or modifications.

The Milan group[7] has also recently reported the sequential administration of initial adjuvant therapy consisting of six cycles of CMFP followed by four cycles of Adriamycin and vincristine (AV). The design of the study called for treatment delays but maximal dosage administration in the face of myelosuppression to minimize the risk of compromising treatment results by injudicious dose reductions. In an early analysis, 5-year disease-free survival (76 percent) and overall survival (87 percent) compared favorably with earlier results in control postmenopausal patients (50 percent and 73 percent, respectively), but further follow-up is needed.

Influence of Menopausal Status

Other issues also need clarification. There is a lack of consistency of the criteria for classification to pre- or postmenopausal status. In the SWOG trial there were no apparent differences in results according to age. Stratification before randomization to L-PAM or CMFVP was by menopausal status and extent of nodal involvement. In 356 evaluable patients with a median follow-up time of 5 years, relapse-free survival was virtually identical for premenopausal (CMFVP, 68 percent; L-PAM, 51 percent) versus postmenopausal (CMFVP, 71 percent; L-PAM, 56 percent), stratified for treatment assignment. A similar lack of differences in relapse-free survival has been evident in the experience at the M. D. Anderson Hospital,[18] while other studies bearing on this issue show mixed results, making interpretation hazardous. It is fair to say that the postmenopause benefits of adjuvant chemotherapy are not clear and that the use of adjuvant chemotherapy in this setting should be reserved for controlled clinical investigations.

Table 26-3 Some Selected Trials of Adjuvant Tamoxifen with or without Cytotoxic Therapy In Stage II Breast Cancer

Group	Study design
NSABP[19]	PF vs PFT
ECOG[20]	CMF vs CMFP vs CMFPT[I]
	CTR vs CMFP vs CMFPT*
Rose[21]	CTR vs T*

NSABP = National Surgical Adjuvant Breast Project; ECOG = Eastern Cooperative Oncology Group; PF = L-PAM + F; CTR = control; I = premenopausal patients; * = postmenopausal patients.

Adjuvant Combined Hormone–Chemotherapy

The addition of hormones to surgical adjuvant chemotherapy and the use of hormone manipulation alone as adjuvant therapy are being studied. Earlier reports of adjuvant oophorectomy or oophorectomy with prednisone demonstrated little or no advantage for the treated subgroups, but over the last few years interest in this approach to adjuvant therapy has reawakened because of the availability of hormone receptor determinations to identify patients more likely to benefit from hormone therapy, and the development of tamoxifen (T), a relatively safe and well-tolerated oral antiestrogen. Table 26-3 presents selected trials designed to assess the effect of tamoxifen alone or with chemotherapy as an adjuvant maneuver. Results have been mixed, follow-up is early, and details regarding postrelapse salvage therapy are not available, making it necessary to delay definitive conclusions regarding the overall contribution of endocrine adjuvant therapy. At this time, there are no convincing data showing that survival is prolonged after adjuvant treatment with hormonal manipulation.

In 1977, the Eastern Cooperative Oncology Group (ECOG) initiated two surgical adjuvant chemotherapy studies for pre- and postmenopausal patients, after mastectomy, who had at least one involved axillary lymph node.[20] Patients were stratified according to the degree of nodal involvement and estrogen receptor status. Premenopausal patients were randomized to receive chemotherapy with CMF alone, the same regimen with the addition of prednisone (P), or the four-drug chemotherapy combination plus tamoxifen (T). Postmenopausal patients were similarly stratified and randomized either to a no-treatment control or 12 cycles of CMFP or CMFP and tamoxifen.

At a median follow-up time exceeding 4 years, there were no statistically significant differences in outcome with respect to disease-free or overall survival measured from time of diagnosis. In premenopausal women there were no major differences in outcome among subgroups. In postmenopausal patients, relapse-free survival was superior in treated patients contrasted with the control arm in the subgroup of patients with estrogen receptor-negative tumors. As expected, patients who were estrogen receptor (ER) positive at diagnosis and who had one to three lymph nodes involved did significantly better than ER-negative patients and patients with four or more nodes involved, respectively. Thus, a preliminary analysis of these two ECOG studies failed to show evidence that the addition of tamoxifen has resulted in a substantial benefit for either pre- or postmenopausal women. Again, it is not clear that the cytotoxic surgical adjuvant therapy increases survival in postmenopausal patients. Note, however, that the median time to relapse is approximately $2\frac{1}{2}$ years, and since median follow-up in those studies is only slightly in excess of that figure, it is far too early to draw firm conclusions.

The ECOG is currently enrolling patients into the two studies outlined in Table 26-4. Premenopausal patients will receive 12 cycles of CMFT or CMFPT and Halotestin. In the latter group, while the tamoxifen and Halotestin are continued, the CMF will be alternated with thiotepa, Velban, and Adriamycin for 12 months. At the end of 1 year, patients will be randomized to discontinue all treatment, or to tamoxifen for an additional 4 years. This arduous study will evaluate the treatment efficacy of drug-resistant tumor cell clones. Also, it will examine the potential benefit of prolonged tamoxifen therapy. Postmenopausal patients will be entered on EST4181, which also tests the value of long-term tamoxifen after cytotoxic chemotherapy. Additionally, in one treatment arm all therapy will be discontinued after only four cycles, in order to determine more precisely the optimal duration of chemotherapy.

CURRENT STATUS

We are coming to recognize that tumor cell heterogeneity may underlie problems we face in eradicating undetected micrometastases. Over time, neoplastic cells spontaneously and probably randomly mutate with the consequent emergence of drug resistance. It is estimated that resistant subclones of tumor cells become

Table 26-4 Current Eastern Cooperative Oncology Group Adjuvant Breast Cancer Trials for Stage II Patients after Mastectomy

Stratify		Step one		Step two
EST 5181—Premenopausal adjuvant therapy trial				
Degree of nodal involvement	R	CMFPT	R	Observation
(histological)	A	for 12	A	
1–3 positive	N	cycles	N	Continue T
4–10 positive	D		D	to total of
> 10 positive	O		O	5 years
	M		M	
	I	CMF (P) TH	I	Observation
Estrogen receptor result	Z	alternating	Z	
Positive	E	with	E	Continue T
Negative		T^{S}AV TH		to total
		for 12 cycles		of 5 years
EST 4181—Postmenopausal adjuvant therapy trial				
Degree of nodal involvement		R		
(histological)		A		CMFPT for 12 cycles +
1–3 positive		N		continuous TAM to
4–10 positive		D		a total of 5 years
> 10 positive		O		
		M		CMFPT for 12 cycles
		I		+ observation
		Z		
Estrogen receptor result		E		CMFPT for 4 cycles
Positive				+ observation
Negative				

T^{S} = Thiotepa; A = Adriamycin; V = vinblastine; T = tamoxifen; H = Halotestin.

clinically evident as tumor recurrences after variable periods of time, despite cytoreductive therapy, and that to improve upon current results strategies will require the addition of new cross-resistant drug combinations as proposed in the Milan and ECOG studies mentioned previously. There may also be considerable heterogeneity with respect to hormone receptor-binding protein concentration, perhaps in part accounting for the typical mixed or partial responses observed after hormone manipulation and for unpredictable effects on tumor cell kinetics that may affect tumor responsiveness to cytotoxic chemotherapy. One preliminary report[19] has already suggested the potential deleterious effects of adding tamoxifen to adjuvant cytotoxic chemotherapy in some subgroups of high-risk women.

Our understanding of prognostic factors has become muddled given the biologic heterogeneity of breast cancer. In turn, caution must be exercised in interpreting complex clinical trials of numerous drug and hormone combinations given by different institutions from around the world. The extent of histologic axillary node involvement and the absence of estrogen receptors correlate with risk of relapse and ultimate survival. Other factors such as tumor grade, progesterone receptor content, primary tumor size and histology, age, and myriad other clinicopathologic factors may influence the clinical course and response to therapy, making further study of potential prognostic indicators necessary. Comparison of treatments either within a trial or between two case series from separate centers requires careful balance of patient groups based on the accurate identification of reliable prognostic indicators to avoid mistaken interpretation of results.

With the achievement of improved survival in high-risk premenopausal women after mastectomy, pressure to treat node-positive postmenopausal women, heavy demands from patients and society at large to develop improved adjuvant treatment programs, and a steady supply of patients, it is clear that thousands more women will be treated in the future with cytotoxic therapy, with or without hormone adjuncts. In fact, the early success of adjuvant therapy in node-positive premenopausal women has prompted the widespread application of adjuvant cytotoxic treatment to groups of patients at high risk of eventual tumor relapse (e.g., the node negative–estrogen receptor negative patient) but for whom scientific evidence of therapeutic benefit has not yet been demonstrated. Paradoxically, a significant minority of these patients would not have relapsed without the adjuvant treatment and thus will have been exposed to the potential hazards of drug treatment without realizing any benefit.

Nonetheless, the much larger number of high-risk women requiring systemic adjuvant therapy for metastatic microscopic disease will prompt continuation of adjuvant treatment programs until diagnostic methods are sufficiently sensitive to identify microscopic metastases. Thus, there is a pressing need to consider the potential hazards, as well as the benefits, of adjuvant treatment. lThis chapter will now turn to toxic effects of adjuvant chemotherapy in women, most of whom have been treated following mastectomy. Toxicities are considered according to whether host effects appear to be immediate and temporary, or represent long-term, more permanent changes in organ function.

IMMEDIATE COMPLICATIONS

The most commonly used drugs over the last 10 years for surgical adjuvant chemotherapy have been L-PAM, cyclophosphamide (Cytoxan, C), methotrexate (M), 5-fluorouracil (F), doxorubicin (Adriamycin, A), vincristine (V), and prednisone (P). These drugs have most often been used in three- or four-drug combinations and are well known to be associated with many short-term ill effects such as nausea, alopecia, mucositis, dermatitis, hemorrhagic cystitis, constipation, conjunctivitis, peripheral neuropathy, and others that are now generally predictable. As would be expected, nausea, vomiting, and malaise are much more common in patients receiving combination therapy such as CMF or CMFVP,[5,6,13] than after single-agent treatment with L-PAM.[3,4] The psychological aspects of treatment-related nausea should be emphasized as anticipatory nausea and vomiting may occur in about 25 percent of patients severely affected. Noticeable alopecia occurs in about 60 percent of patients receiving cyclophosphamide-based combinations, virtually all patients receiving doxorubicin, and only a few treated with L-PAM alone.

Similarly, observations of patients receiving combined chemotherapy–hormone adjuvant therapy have revealed immediate toxic side effects as expected on the basis of the broad general past experience with hormonal therapy utilizing estrogens, Halotestin, tamoxifen, or castration. Ongoing follow-up of the Case Western (low-dose CMF ± tamoxifen) and NSABP (L-PAM + F ± tamoxifen), as well as the ECOG projects mentioned earlier, will provide additional information with respect to this question.

We should consider in more detail such life-threatening side effects as infection occurring during periods of leukopenia, congestive heart failure associated with doxorubicin, and problems peculiar to the patient undergoing adjuvant chemotherapy for breast cancer: coagulation disturbances, endocrine disturbances and early menopause, psychologic considerations, and problems associated with pregnancy.

Serious Infections

Although bone marrow suppression is the dose-limiting side effect in a majority of patients overall, probably occurring in 75 percent, severe leukopenia (less than 500/mm^3) and/or thrombocytopenia (less than 50,000/mm^3) are much less common, perhaps affecting fewer than 10 percent of patients. There is much variation from center to center with respect to what level of white cell and platelet nadir is acceptable, and reporting of hematologic toxicity has not been uniform. Most treatment protocols have dose modification plans to avoid repeated episodes of life-threatening bone marrow suppression. Because drug dose may be an important factor with respect to treatment efficacy,[14] as well as toxicity, we can expect to see more clinical trials designed to address the issue of treatment intensity as it relates to long-term disease-free survival.

With current drug programs, the incidence of prolonged serious myelosuppression is surprisingly low and the incidence of marrow toxicity has not been observed to be very different in young versus older women.[14,22] Furthermore, the reported rate of treatment-related deaths due to infection occurring during periods of profound leukopenia is less than 0.5 percent of patients treated. See Table 26-5 for a summary of reported drug-related fatalities in some series.

Future studies are likely to test cytotoxic agents given in combination and in high doses for relatively short periods of time, 3 to 6 months. This approach is patterned after successful drug treatment programs for other advanced malignancies such as Hodgkin's disease[27] and testicular cancer.[28] Highly intensive radiation and chemotherapy treatment

Table 26-5 Lethal Infectious Complications

Group	Regimen	Drug deaths
NSABP[4,23]	L-PAM	0
	LFCM	2/300
OSAKO[23]	LMF + BCG	2/118
Milan[5,18]	CMF 12	0/243
CALGB[24]	CMF/CMFVP	2/499
MDA[25]	FAC + BCG	0/222
Arizona[26]	AC	0
SWOG[13]	L-PAM	0/777
	CMFVP	0/187

Source: Modified after Senn.[23]

regimens with successful bone marrow reconstitution after autologous bone marrow transplant in breast cancer patients are also now reported,[29,30] further reflecting the widespread interest in aggressive treatment regimens.

We can conclude that the heretofore reported incidence of lethal infectious complications appears to be less than 0.5 percent of patients treated, a figure considered acceptable in most major centers. As the intensity of drug treatment is increased, however, this risk could change drastically.

Toxicity Associated with Radiation

An important practical concern relates to the combined use of radiation and chemotherapy as components of the multimodal therapy of primary breast cancer. Any injury to bone marrow may lead to enhanced myelotoxicity with subsequent compromise of drug doses, especially in breast cancer programs consisting largely of middle-aged to older women who may have preexistent depletion of marrow stem cell reserves simply related to aging, other unassociated marrow problems, or undetected marrow infiltration by breast cancer. Nonetheless, this potentially serious problem has faded for the patient following mastectomy because of recognition that postoperative radiation does not produce a salutary effect on survival despite reduction in local-regional tumor relapse rates.

A question of emerging significance relates to patients receiving radiation as primary therapy and adjuvant chemotherapy. Myelosuppression is a function of radiation portal size, necessitating dose reduction of CMF of about 25 percent during periods of concomitant treatment. Programs consisting of sequential radiation followed by chemotherapy are expected to be well tolerated from the standpoint of toxicity but delays of 4 to 8 weeks before starting systemic therapy may be hazardous. Most therapeutic trials to date have primarily included women after mastectomy, with the result that few data are available addressing this issue.

Certainly, concurrent radiation–Adriamycin chemotherapy may result in a marked enhancement of cutaneous and pulmonary reaction and may lead to a compromise of the efficacy of radiation as well as chemotherapy. These concerns will need to be addressed cautiously as increased numbers of women turn to radiation as the definitive local treatment. Lippman et al.[31] have studied node-positive stages I and II patients randomized to total mastectomy versus excisional biopsy followed by radiation. All patients received chemotherapy with Adriamycin and Cytoxan, with the first cycle given 1 to 2 weeks following mastectomy or preceding radiation. They observed that aggressive chemotherapy could be administered to patients concurrently receiving radiation to breast and draining regional nodes but that drug dose reductions were necessary because of depressed granulocyte counts in 50 percent more patients treated with radiation than with mastectomy. Effects of these dose reductions on ultimate outcome are not yet known. For larger radiation volumes, concurrent CMF regimens and radiation may require changes in drug dose or scheduling in 25 percent of patients.[32]

Miscellaneous Problems

Miscellaneous potential problems include hepatotoxicity, especially in view of prolonged methotrexate exposure. The Milan group[33] found no evidence of liver damage in their patients who had been treated with adjuvant CMF. Neither has cardiomyopathy, a potential consequence of doxorubicin therapy, been observed in either the Milan[34] or Arizona[26] experience. Congestive heart failure has been reported in three of 222 patients treated at the M. D. Anderson Hospital with FAC to a total cumulative doxorubicin dosage of 300 mg/m^2. Current recommendations[34] are to avoid cumulative doxorubicin levels greater than 280 to 300 mg/m^2.

Interestingly, many patients have been observed to gain weight on therapy. This occurs on programs consisting of cytotoxic therapy, with or without hormonal adjuncts. The basis for this problem in general is not well understood and is probably multifactorial, occurring as a consequence of hormone treatment with resulting salt and water retention, endocrine changes, and secondary depression. As well, increased oral intake, a result of a conscious effort by many patients to sustain optimal general health and immune function may be a factor.

Coagulation Abnormalities

Coagulation abnormalities have long been associated with cancer, in particular with widely disseminated adenocarcinomas. And although consumptive coagulopathy is not a commonly recognized consequence of adjuvant chemotherapy, subclinical coagulation abnormalities manifested by slight shortening of the activated partial thromboplastin time (aPTT), borderline to slightly elevated fibrin split products (FSP), and dropping fibrinogen levels may identify the patient at increased risk of thrombosis or disseminated intravascular hemorrhage following chemotherapy.[35] Lipton et al.[36] have reported seven breast cancer patients who developed deep venous thrombosis or nonfatal pulmonary embolization within 6 months of the start of tamoxifen therapy. Two of these patients had no clinical evidence of metastatic disease, one was receiving concomitant therapy with CMF and aminoglutethimide, the others no other treatments. Of special note is the recent observation that 17 of 817 eligible patients on the NSABP protocol B-12, comparing PFT with or without Adriamycin in axillary node-positive patients with positive estrogen or progesterone receptors, had possible embolic or phlebitic events. Two cases of cerebral thrombosis, two cases of arterial embolization, and 13 cases of suspected or confirmed deep vein thrombosis were described. Overall, reports of disordered coagulation in patients on adjuvant chemotherapy are too infrequent to warrant special precaution over that normally observed in the cancer patient on treatment. But the potential for this complication should be recognized, especially for patients with a prior history of deep vein thrombosis, pulmonary embolus, or cerebral vascular accident.

Endocrine Consequences

Considerable attention has been given to the endocrine consequences of adjuvant chemotherapy, particularly in premenopausal women. Although a number of older studies[37–39] failed to show a significant benefit from postoperative hormonal treatments, many investigators have questioned the mechanism by which cytotoxic therapy appears to effect improved disease-free survival predominately in premenopausal patients and have suggested that favorable effects of adjuvant chemotherapy may largely result from "medical oophorectomy."[40] There are strong arguments against this position. Fisher et al.[41] note that the most striking benefits in the prospective studies of the NSABP have occurred in women less than 39 years of age, while women in the 40 to 49 year age range were far more likely to have a clinical menopause during or following adjuvant treatment. Bonadonna, too, has been unable to correlate drug-induced amenorrhea with improved disease-free survival, though there was a trend toward lower recurrence rates for patients with drug-induced amenorrhea compared to those with continuing normal menses.[34]

Nonetheless, cytotoxic drugs are well known to affect endocrine function, and amenorrhea secondary to primary ovarian failure in premenopausal patients is well documented.[42–44] Dnistrian and colleagues[42] performed serial measurements of estrogens, androgens, pituitary gonadotropins, and prolactin in an attempt to monitor the endocrine effects of CMF adjuvant chemotherapy in pre- and postmenopausal patients. As expected, ovarian suppression was observed to occur and persist in premenopausal patients aged 40 or older, most often within 2 to 4 months from treatment start; younger women required much larger cumulative doses before ovarian dysfunction was evident. No decrement in pituitary and adrenal function was found. Hormonal levels appeared unaffected in postmenopausal patients, suggesting that any observed benefit of adjuvant chemotherapy in those patients is not a result of endocrine changes.

In Milan,[7] amenorrhea induced by alkylating agents was also observed to be age-related. In an experience with 549 menstruating women, of those 40 years of age or younger, the incidence of amenorrhea was 54 percent, reversible in 23 percent. Of patients older than 40, the incidence was 96 percent, reversible in 4 percent. There were no obvious differences according to whether 6 or 12 months of CMF was given. Thus, it appears that adjuvant therapy hastens the onset of ovarian failure in older premenopausal women and is generally permanent in this group, but may be reversible in younger patients.[45] The contribution of ovarian suppression to observed survival benefit of adjuvant treatment in premenopausal patients remains conjectural.

Psychologic Effects

Most centers are aware of the negative psychologic impact that many women experience as they endure inconvenient and toxic treatment programs with or without having metastatic disease. Unfortunately, few sophisticated efforts have been made to more precisely define the psychologic effects of participating in adjuvant chemotherapy programs, or even to record psychologic responses that occur following drug therapy. Major problems may be encountered with respect to changes in self-esteem, sexuality, family, and at work. Although adjuvant chemotherapy may not appear threatening to the "well-adjusted" individual, physical changes such as alopecia, frequent inconvenient physician visits, nausea and vomiting following therapy, secondary endocrine changes, alteration of self-image after mastectomy, and the omnipresent reminder of possible treatment failure in the clinic setting—the cachectic patient with advanced disease—may be of great concern to any patient. Very practical issues such as loss of employment, loss of physical attractiveness, threat of divorce, and decreased energy levels are common problems that the physician frequently ignores.

Thoughtful consideration of a patient's problems with sex and sexual adequacy is especially necessary for the patient undergoing adjuvant chemotherapy treatments because, by definition, the majority of these women should be functioning at normal or near normal performance status and in general have an expected survival of many years. Cytotoxic therapy may result in diminished estrogen production, loss of fertility, lessened libido, dyspareunia with loss of normal vaginal lubrication, and diminished feelings of self-worth. Psychotherapy, support groups, and continuing interest and counsel from concerned physicians and nurses are needed to minimize the potential negative impact of both cancer chemotherapy and the setting in which it is given. A corollary of this is the need for medical and nursing personnel to recognize that intensive chemotherapy may have substantial physical and psychological effects which are best recognized and minimized by open discussion. Review of major adjuvant chemotherapy trials[4,5,13,23–25] fails to reveal meaningful toxicity data regarding the psychologic consequences of adjuvant chemotherapy largely because of inherent difficulties in quantitating behavioral and emotional responses after mastectomy and medical therapy.

Pregnancy

Special problems arise for young women who become pregnant and either may benefit from chemotherapy after mastectomy or who may become pregnant while on adjuvant chemotherapy. As it is well documented that many if not all chemotherapy agents may be teratogenic if the fetus is exposed during the first trimester of pregnancy, most authorities would consider therapeutic abortion for patients less than 20 weeks pregnant. Of course, such decisions must be made only after careful consideration of available medical information, the indications for cytotoxic or hormonal therapy, and the religious and personal feelings of the patient.

There are now multiple reports of patients becoming pregnant while receiving combination chemotherapy.[46–48] A recent review[49] of the effects of receiving chemotherapy during the first trimester suggests that the incidence of fetal malformations is probably in excess of 10 percent, a fivefold increase. It remains uncertain as to whether or not fetal exposure during the second and third trimesters results in teratogenicity. Risk of developing a malignancy in later life after fetal exposure to chemotherapeutic agents is not known.

LATE EFFECTS

Second Malignancies

Acute myelocytic leukemia has become a widely recognized complication of chemotherapy and combined modality treatment programs for hematologic malignancies and solid tumors.[50–52] Alkylating agents, alone, when given with other chemotherapeutic agents, or when combined with radiation, have been implicated as an important etiologic factor. Frequently, a period of blood cytopenia associated with bone marrow hypocellularity precedes the overt development of fulminant acute leukemia which then is generally considered to carry an ominous prognosis. The extent of cytogenetic abnormalities may be increased in comparison to patients without previous exposure to chemotherapy. This has been interpreted by some[53] to be a reflection of the leukemogenic actions of chemotherapy-induced DNA damage. Concern over possible chemotherapy-related malignancies in women receiving adjuvant chemotherapy is especially acute because the value of chemotherapy in the majority of the patients treated, postmenopausal patients, remains unproven, and because 5 to 20 percent of patients receiving treatment could be expected to be disease-free at 10 years follow-up after mastectomy or primary therapy with radiation alone.

Acute leukemia has been reported after adjuvant chemotherapy by several groups. Rosner et al.[54] have described the occurrence of leukemia in 27 breast cancer patients, four of whom had received adjuvant chemotherapy (three are known to have been treated with thiotepa). He reviewed an additional 67 cases and found that the mean interval from the diagnosis of breast cancer to the occurrence of leukemia was 6.9 years. In a startling report, Lerner[55] described the development of acute myelogenous leukemia in three of 13 women treated with adjuvant chlorambucil for 4 or more years after mastectomy. Ershler[56] reported the association of breast cancer and acute leukemia in 11 patients, and also reviewed the literature. It was not reported how many in the Ershler series had had adjuvant chemotherapy.

Nowell et al.[53] performed cytogenetic studies in 20 breast cancer patients, including three who had developed acute myelocytic leukemia 2 to 30 months after completing adjuvant chemotherapy with Cytoxan-based drug combinations. Abnormalities were found in two of the three leukemia patients but none of the others. All three patients had received L-PAM following surgery. In all, significant myelosuppression was observed during or after therapy and each patient had a period of leukopenia preceding the development of overt leukemia at 25, 31, and 39 months from diagnosis.

Most recently, Fisher et al [57] reviewed the NSABP experience with 8483 patients and found that leukemia or myeloproliferative disorders were side effects of both postoperative radiation (5 of 646 patients) and adjuvant chemotherapy (34 of 5299 patients) consisting of L-phenylalanine mustard-containing regimens at

10 years. Moreover, leukemia was observed in 3 of 2068 patients treated by operation alone, indicating that leukemia is not a common element in the natural history of breast cancer.

The question of how frequent multiple primary cancers are in patients with breast cancer is now a subject of international study.[58] In the United States, women with breast cancer have a three- to fivefold increase in risk for cancer of the opposite breast and probably an increased risk of ovarian, endometrial, and colon cancer. "Cancer families" have been recognized in which hereditary neoplasms occur, consistent with autosomal dominant inheritance patterns, accounting for as many as 5 percent of breast cancers, with or without other associated adenocarcinomas. Albain and Ultmann[59] reported a case of ileocecal diffuse histiocytic lymphoma occurring in a patient with metastatic breast cancer who had received large doses of cyclophosphamide.

Careful analysis of the Milan experience,[34] with follow-up ranging from 5 to 8 years, fails to show an increased incidence of second neoplasms in the chemotherapy-treated population (1.1 percent) compared to the control patients (1.7 percent). In a report with longer follow-up, Kardinal and Donegan reported no difference in incidence of second cancers.[60]

In summary, there are reports of chronic bone marrow injury and induction of myeloproliferative disease and acute leukemia in patients treated with adjuvant chemotherapy for breast cancer, although the risk is low. The Fisher report [57] provides compelling data that hematologic disorders are side effects of radiation and adjuvant chemotherapy. Efforts to identify patient subgroups responding favorably to such treatment should be continued so that only those expected to benefit from adjuvant therapy will be exposed to the risk. Current attempts to reduce treatment duration (e.g., CMF for six cycles, CA for three cycles) while intensifying the chemotherapy should tend to reduce the risk of induction of secondary neoplasms.

Response to Secondary Therapy

Despite implementation of early systemic treatments for high-risk patients after mastectomy, a significant number of these women do subsequently develop recurrent disease and will require reinstitution of systemic treatment. There are few studies which focus on these patients, and response and survival data after resumption of hormone or cytotoxic treatments. Buzdar et al.[61] did report that of 58 evaluable patients, all previously treated with doxorubicin-based combination chemotherapy, 33 (57 percent) achieved partial or complete tumor response to a variety of hormonal and cytotoxic treatments with median survival from relapse of 15 months for the entire group and 25.7 months for responding patients. Some responding patients were treated with the same drugs (FAC) given during the adjuvant treatment period with no clear correlation between response upon retreatment and time from completion of adjuvant therapy until tumor relapse. Bitran et al.[62] also reported responses to secondary therapy after relapse following adjuvant treatments in 6 of 21 patients. More data are needed with respect to this potential problem and should emerge from follow-up studies of the major adjuvant chemotherapy trials, but to date there are no data which indicate a serious compromise in tumor responsiveness to standard treatment after relapse following adjuvant chemotherapy.

CONCLUSION

We can conclude that surgical adjuvant chemotherapy studies will continue to require close surveillance, as large numbers of patients have now been treated 5 or more years ago and are probably entering a period of heightened risk for the development of secondary malignancies. To date, observed acute and late toxic effects from chemotherapy have been largely predictable and tolerable. We have witnessed improved survival after adjuvant treatments in premenopausal women, but serious questions remain regarding drug selection, treatment intensity and duration, use of hormones, and long-term complications of therapy. Participation in well-designed clinical trials directed toward this end should provide some answers and is necessary for continued progress.

REFERENCES

1. Moxley JH III, Allegra JC, Henney J, Muggia F: Treatment of primary breast cancer: Summary of the National Institutes of Health Consensus Development Conference. *JAMA* 244:797, 1980.
2. Bluming A: Treatment of primary breast cancer without mastectomy: Review of the literature. *Am J Med* 72:820, 1982.
3. Carter SK: Surgery plus adjuvant chemotherapy: A review of therapeutic implications. I. Breast cancer. *Cancer Chemother Pharmacol* 4:147, 1980.
4. Fisher B, Carbone P, Economou SG, other NSABP investigators: L-Phenylalanine mustard (L-PAM) in the management of primary breast cancer: A report of early findings. *N Engl J Med* 292:117, 1975.
5. Bonadonna G, Brusamolino E, Valagussa P, Rossi A, Brugnatelli L, Brambilla C, De Lena M, Tancini G, Bajetta E, Musumeci R, Veronesi U: Combination chemotherapy as an adjuvant treatment in operable breast cancer. *N Engl J Med* 294:405, 1976.
6. Fisher B, Redmond C, Fisher ER, other NSABP investigators: A summary of findings from NSABP trials of adjuvant therapy, in Jones SE, Salmon SE (eds): *Therapy of Cancer IV*. Orlando, FL, Grune & Stratton, 1984, p. 185.
7. Bonadonna G, Valagussa P: Adjuvant systemic therapy for resectable breast cancer. *J Clin Oncol* 3:259, 1985.
8. Senn HJ, Jung WF: Swiss adjuvant trials with LMF(+BCG) in N− and N+ breast cancer patients, in Jones SE, Salmon SE (eds): *Adjuvant Therapy of Cancer IV*. Orlando, FL, Grune & Stratton, 1984, p. 261.
9. Wheeler TK: Full drug combination chemotherapy following surgery in breast cancer, in Jones SE, Salmon SE (eds): *Adjuvant Therapy of Cancer II*. Orlando, FL, Grune & Stratton, 1979, p. 269.
10. Rubens RD, Hayward JL, Knight RK et al: Controlled trial of adjuvant chemotherapy with melphalan for breast cancer. *Lancet* I:839, 1983.
11. Morrison JM, Howell A, Grieve RJ, Monypenny IJ, Kelly KA, Marson A, Waterhouse JA: The West Midlands trial of adjuvant chemotherapy for axillary node positive breast cancer: A controlled clinical trial, in Jones SE, Salmon SE (eds): *Adjuvant Therapy of Cancer IV*. Orlando, FL, Grune & Stratton, 1984, p. 253.
12. Smith DC, Crawford D, Dykes EH, Calman KC, Russell AR, McArdle CS: Adjuvant radiotherapy/chemotherapy in breast cancer, in Jones SE, Salmon SE (eds): *Adjuvant Therapy of Cancer IV*. Orlando, FL, Grune & Stratton, 1984, p. 283.
13. Glucksberg H, Rivkin SE, Rasmussen S, Tranum B, Gad-El-Mawla N, Costanzi J, Hoogstraten B, Athens J, Maloney T, McCracken J, Vaughn C: Combination chemotherapy (CMFVP) versus L-phenylalanine mustard (L-PAM) for operable breast cancer with positive axillary nodes: A Southwest Oncology Group Study. *Cancer* 50:423, 1982.
14. Bonadonna G, Valagussa P: Dose-response effect of adjuvant chemotherapy in breast cancer. *N Engl J Med* 304:10, 1981.
15. Cavalli F, Pedrazzini A, Martz G, et al: Randomized trial of three different regimens of combination chemotherapy in patients receiving simultaneously a hormonal treatment for advanced breast cancer. *Eur J Cancer Clin Oncol* 19:1615, 1983.
16. Malik R, Blumenshein GR, Legha SS, Hortobagyi GN, Buzdar A, Yap HY, Hill S, Bodey GP: A randomized trial of high-dose 5-fluorouracil (F), doxorubicin (A) and cyclophosphamide (C) vs. conventional FAC regimen in metastatic breast cancer. *Proc Am Soc Clin Oncol* 1:79, 1982.
17. Tancini G, Bonadonna G, Valagussa P, Marchini S, Veronesi U: Adjuvant CMF in breast cancer: Comparative 5-year results of 12 versus 6 cycles. *J Clin Oncol* 1:2, 1983.
18. Buzdar AU, Smith TL, Blumenschein GR, Hortobagyi GN, Marcus CE, Hersh EM, Martin RG, Gehan EA, Freireich EJ: Breast cancer adjuvant therapy trials of M. D. Anderson Hospital: Results of two studies, in Jones SE, Salmon SE (eds): *Adjuvant Therapy of Cancer IV*. Orlando, FL, Grune & Stratton, 1984, p. 217.
19. Fisher B, Redmond C, Brown A et al: Influence of tumor estrogen and progesterone receptor levels

in the response to tamoxifen and chemotherapy in primary breast cancer. *J Clin Oncol* 1:227, 1983.

20. Tormey DC, Taylor SG IV, Kalish LA, Olson JE, Grage T, Gray R: Adjuvant systemic therapy in premenopausal (CMF, CMFP, CMFPT) and postmenopausal (observation, CMFP, CMFPT) women with node positive breast cancer, in Jones SE, Salmon SE (eds): *Adjuvant Therapy of Cancer IV*. Orlando, FL, Grune & Stratton, 1984, p. 359.
21. Rose C, Thorpe SM, Mouridsen HT et al: Antiestrogen treatment of postmenopausal women with primary high risk breast cancer: 36 months of life table analysis and steroid hormone receptor status. *Breast Cancer Res Treat* 3:77, 1983.
22. Glass A, Wieand HS, Fisher B, other NSABP investigators: Acute toxicity during adjuvant chemotherapy for breast cancer: The NSABP experience from 1717 patients receiving single and multiple agents. *Cancer Treat Rep* 65:363, 1981.
23. Senn HJ: Current status and indications for adjuvant therapy in breast cancer. *Cancer Chemother Pharmacol* 8:139, 1982.
24. Tormey DC, Weinberg VE, Holland JF, other participating CALGB investigators: A randomized trial of five and three drug chemotherapy and chemoimmunotherapy in women with operable node positive breast cancer. *J Clin Oncol* 1:138, 1983.
25. Buzdar AU, Blumenschein GR, Gutterman JU, Toshimo CK, Hortobagyi GN, Smith TL, Campos LI, Wheeler WL, Hersh EM, Freireich EJ, Gehan EA: Postoperative adjuvant chemotherapy with fluorouracil, doxorubicin, cyclophosphamide, and BCG vaccine: A follow up report. *JAMA* 242:1509, 1979.
26. Allen J, Brooks R, Jones SE, Chase E, Heusinkveld RS, Giordano GF, Ketchel SJ, Jackson RA, Davis S, Moon T, Salmon SE: Adjuvant treatment for stage II (node positive) breast cancer with Adriamycin-cyclophosphamide (AC) ± radiotherapy (XRT), in Salmon SE, Jones SE (eds): *Adjuvant Therapy of Cancer III*. New York, Grune & Stratton, 1981, p. 453.
27. Devita JT Jr, Simon RN, Hubbard SM, Young RC, Berard CW, Moxley JH, Frei E III, Carbone PP, Canellos GP: Curability of advanced Hodgkin's disease: Long term follow-up of MOPP-treated patients at the National Cancer Institute. *Ann Intern Med* 92:587, 1980.
28. Einhorn LH, Donohue J: *Cis*-diaminedichloroplatinum, vinblastine, and bleomycin combination chemotherapy in disseminated testicular cancer. *Ann Intern Med* 87:293, 1977.
29. Kies MS, Vriesendorp HM, Gordon LI, Kucuk O, Rosen ST, Fey TA, McDonough C, Prachand S: Autologous bone marrow transplantation in patients with cancer. *Exp Hematol* 11(suppl 5):128, 1983.
30. Gale RP, Cline MJ: Autologous bone marrow transplantation in patients with cancer. *Exp Hematol* 7(suppl 5):351, 1979.
31. Lippman ME, Lichter AS, Danforth D, Ellenberg S, d'Angelo T, Gorrell C: The influence of primary breast cancer treatment—mastectomy or excisional biopsy plus radiation—on the ability to deliver adjuvant chemotherapy, in Jones SE, Salmon SE (eds): *Adjuvant Therapy of Cancer IV*. Orlando, FL, Grune & Stratton, 1984, p. 301.
32. Levine JF, Coleman CN, Cox RS, et al: The effect of post-operative and primary radiation on delivered dose of adjuvant cyclophosphamide, methotrexate, and 5-fluorouracil (CMF) chemotherapy in breast cancer. *Cancer* 53:237, 1984.
33. Bajetta E, Buzzoni R, Giardini R, Bonadonna G: Liver assessment in women receiving adjuvant CMF chemotherapy. *Tumori* 67:27, 1981.
34. Bonadonna G, Valagussa P: Chemotherapy of breast cancer: Current views and results. *Int J Radiat Oncol Biol Phys* 9:279, 1983.
35. Kies MS, Kwaan HC: Thromboembolism in cancer patients, in Kwaan HC, Bowie EJW (eds): *Thrombosis*. Philadelphia, W. B. Saunders Co., 1982.
36. Lipton A, Harvey HA, Hamilton RW: Venous thrombosis as a side effect of tamoxifen treatment. *Cancer Treat Rep* 68:887, 1984.
37. Nissen-Meyer R: The role of prophylactic castration in the therapy of human mammary cancer. *Eur J Cancer* 3:395, 1967.
38. Ravdin RG, Lewison EF, Slack NH, Gardner B, State D, Fisher B: Results of a clinical trial concerning the worth of prophylactic oophorectomy for breast carcinoma. *Surg Gynecol Obstet* 131:1055, 1970.
39. Cole MP: Suppression of ovarian function in primary breast cancer, in Forrest APM, Kunkler PB (eds): *Prognostic Factors in Breast Cancer*. Edinburgh, Livingston, 1968, p. 145.

40. Pourquier H: The results of adjuvant chemotherapy are predominately caused by the hormonal changes such therapy induces. In favor, in Van-Scoy-Mosher MB (ed): *Medical Oncology. Controversies in Cancer Treatment.* Boston, G. K. Hall & Co., 1981, p. 83.
41. Fisher B, Redmond C, Wolmark N, Wieand HS: Disease-free survival at intervals during and following completion of adjuvant chemotherapy: The NSABP experience from three breast cancer protocols. *Cancer* 48:1273, 1981.
42. Dnistrian AM, Schwartz MK, Fracchia AA, Kaufman RJ, Hakes TB, Currie VE: Endocrine consequences of CMF adjuvant therapy in premenopausal and postmenopausal breast cancer patients. *Cancer* 51:803, 1983.
43. Recchione C, Rossi A: Hormonal study in patients developing amenorrhea during adjuvant chemotherapy for breast cancer. *Tumori* 65:93, 1979.
44. Rose DP, Davis TE: Ovarian function in patients receiving adjuvant chemotherapy for breast cancer. *Lancet* 1:1174, 1977.
45. Samaan NA, DeAsis DN, Blumenschein GR, Buzdar AU: Pituitary-ovarian function in breast cancer patients on adjuvant chemoimmunotherapy. *Cancer* 41:2084, 1978.
46. Garrett MJ: Teratogenic effects of combination chemotherapy. *Ann Intern Med* 80:667, 1974.
47. Thomas PRM, Peckham MJ: The investigation and management of Hodgkin's disease in the pregnant patient. *Cancer* 38:1443, 1976.
48. Sweet DL, Kinzie J: Consequences of radiotherapy and antineoplastic therapy for the fetus. *J Reprod Med* 17:241, 1976.
49. Schapira DV, Chudley AE: Successful pregnancy following continuous treatment with combination chemotherapy before conception and throughout pregnancy. *Cancer* 54:800, 1984.
50. Casciato DA, Scott JL: Acute leukemia following prolonged cytotoxic agent therapy. *Medicine* 58:32, 1979.
51. Rosner F: Acute leukemia as a delayed consequence of cancer chemotherapy. *Cancer* 37:1033, 1976.
52. Reimer RR, Hoover R, Fraumani JF, Young R: Acute leukemia after alkylating-agent therapy of ovarian cancer. *N Engl J Med* 297:177, 1977.
53. Nowell P, Glick JH, Bucolo A, Finan J, Creech R: Cytogenetic studies of bone marrow in breast cancer patients after adjuvant chemotherapy. *Cancer* 48:667, 1981.
54. Rosner F, Carey RW, Zarrabi MH: Breast cancer and acute leukemia: Report of 24 cases and review of the literature. *Am J Hemat* 4:151, 1978.
55. Lerner HJ: Acute myelogenous leukemia in patients receiving chlorambucil as long-term adjuvant chemotherapy for stage II breast cancer. *Cancer Treat Rep* 62:1135, 1978.
56. Ershler WB, Robbins HI, Davis HL, Hafez G, Meisner LF, Dahlberg S, Arndt C: Emergence of acute non-lymphocytic leukemia in breast cancer patients. *Am J Med Sci* 284:23, 1982.
57. Fisher B, Rockette H, Fisher ER, Wickerham L, Redmond C, Brown A: Leukemia in breast cancer patients following adjuvant chemotherapy or postoperative radiation: The NSABP experience. *J Clin Oncol* 3:1640, 1985.
58. Harris CC, Suemasu K: Multiple primary neoplasms (meeting report). *Cancer Res* 43:5629, 1983.
59. Albain KS, Ultmann JE: Aggressive large cell lymphoma of the ileum after long-term cyclophosphamide therapy for breast carcinoma. *Am J Med* 75:882, 1983.
60. Kardinal CG, Donegan WL: Second cancers after prolonged adjuvant Thiotepa for operable carcinoma of the breast. *Cancer* 45:2042, 1980.
61. Buzdar AU, Legha SS, Hortobagyi GN, Yap H, Wiseman CL, Distefano A, Schell FC, Barnes BC, Compos LT, Blumenschein GR: Management of breast cancer patients failing adjuvant chemotherapy with Adriamycin-containing regimens. *Cancer* 47:2798, 1981.
62. Bitran JD, Desser RK, Shapiro CM, Michel A, Kozloff MF, Billings AA, Recent W: Response to secondary therapy in patients with adenocarcinoma of the breast previously treated with adjuvant chemotherapy. *Cancer* 51:381, 1983.

Part Six

Treatment of Advanced Breast Cancer

27

Surgical Treatment of Advanced Breast Cancer

Richard E. Wilson, M.D.

INTRODUCTION

For purposes of definition and ease of presentation, the surgical treatment of advanced breast cancer can be divided into the management of four categories of disease:

1 Primary breast cancer—stage III
2 Primary breast cancer—stage IV
3 Recurrent breast cancer which is still local or regional in nature
4 Recurrent breast cancer which presents with distant metastases

Each of these forms of advanced breast cancer has a different prognosis, and different treatment options are available to the surgeon for them. Obviously, a thorough evaluation of the patient is essential to define the exact stage in each category. While it is realized that noninvasive staging is fraught with inaccuracies, the use of bone scan, liver scan, liver function tests, CEA determination, and newer imaging modalities such as CT scan and magnetic resonance will all serve to delineate the full extent of the potentially or proven systemic breast cancer in each of these groups of patients. This is particularly true for the first and third categories, those with either stage III primary cancer of the breast or those with local-regional recurrent cancer.

In part, the treatment of patients with recurrence depends upon the treatment initially used for any given patient.[1] For example, if prior radiation was used to manage the primary breast lesion, local-regional recurrence within the breast can no longer be managed with further radiation therapy. On the other hand, recurrence in the chest wall after mastectomy may best be treated by radiation, not further surgery.

Surgical therapy in these four categories of patients with advanced breast cancer must be integrated with other modalities of treatment. Selection of a surgical approach should be based upon a comparison of its advantages and disadvantages with other forms of therapy. In patients with proven metastatic disease, the choice of a surgical procedure for therapy must be weighed for its risks and benefits. Prevention of pain and minimization of disability should be the primary goals of therapy in all forms of advanced breast cancer. There is abundant evidence that patients who achieve a response to therapy for metastatic breast cancer do live longer and valuable palliation can frequently be obtained.[2] The problem lies in selecting the proper approach and sequence of therapies for any given patient.

For each of the four categories of advanced disease, surgical considerations will be discussed in greatest detail, with appropriate reference to the role of other forms of treatment—either jointly or alternatively. The indications for surgical therapy will be presented in comparison with other treatment options.

The disease status in patients with advanced breast cancer, be it regional or distant, may be extremely variable—patient for patient—and it is difficult to categorize women for any one form of treatment. Rather, the physician treating such patients must be aware of all the alternatives and select the most appropriate therapy or set of therapies for each patient with her particular set of circumstances. Nonetheless, surgical therapy has a great deal to offer some breast cancer patients with advanced stage disease.

PRIMARY CANCER—STAGE III

Considering stage III breast cancer, a division into two subtypes of disease is necessary (Table 27-1). Stage IIIA consists of those women with T_3 disease which is either N_0, N_{1a} or N_{1b}. Women with this type of disease, while definitely at greater risk for local and distant recurrence, should still be placed in the group considered to have operable breast cancer. That means that the treatment of choice remains modified radical mastectomy. The surgeon should be alert to identify pectoral muscle extension in these patients, and to extend the resection to include involved contiguous structures, if found. These lesions are too large to consider partial mastectomy and radiation therapy, since the degree of cosmesis will be inadequate and the risk for recurrence high. As stated in the classification, these women may have uninvolved lymph nodes in the axilla or they may be clinically and/or microscopically involved. Because of the higher risk for both local and distant metastases, adjuvant radiation therapy and chemotherapy should be considered in a more routine manner for these women. The radiation is to reduce regional recurrence that is associated with larger lesions, while the chemotherapy would be considered the best method of altering the incidence of systemic micrometastases. Treatment of the primary lesion by radiation alone or by radiation and chemotherapy—without mastectomy—is much less likely to achieve good local control, which is so essential for adequate treatment of this lesion. Patients with T_3 lesions have an opportunity for 5-year survival in the range of 50 percent and, therefore, should be candidates for aggressive treatment.

Table 27-1 Stage III Breast Cancer

IIIA: T_3, N_0 or N_1	Tumor size only—still operable
IIIB: Either T_4 or N_2, N_3	Locally or regionally inoperable

Patients with stage IIIB disease are those who have either T_4 lesions or N_2 or N_3 nodal disease. This group of patients includes those with inflammatory cancer and locally advanced, inoperable malignancy. They may be inoperable either because of the involvement of the skin of the breast itself, or the fixation and extent of disease within the draining lymph nodes. The initial determinate of subsequent therapy for these women should be the *response to aggressive chemotherapy*. This would usually mean an Adriamycin-containing treatment plan generally given in at least three courses. Evidence of response to chemotherapy places the patient into a category where more aggressive local control is justified. This could be with either radiation alone, or surgical mastectomy followed by radiation. In general, our experience has been that radiation alone is not as likely to produce subsequent control of the local cancer in these patients as is a total mastectomy followed by radiation. This, then, is the most ideal form of therapy for these stage IIIB patients. The chemotherapy initiates local control and demonstrates the sensitivity of micrometastases. Continued local control with surgery and radiation may be followed by systemic chemotherapy with the same program of treatment as was shown to be successful when measurable tumor was in place (Table 27-2).

For those women who fail to respond to chemotherapy, there is no justification for mastectomy. They are doomed to extensive chest wall recurrence even with radiation following surgery, and any attempt at mastectomy, even a "toilet mastectomy," (resection of bulk cancer without concern for margins) is unwise. The only form of toilet mastectomy that is justified is that used in the chemotherapy-sensitive patient mentioned above, who would receive radiation therapy after this total mastectomy (Fig. 27-1). Total mastectomy alone in the chemotherapy-insensitive patient is ill-advised, because the life span of these patients is too short and radiation therapy will usually provide adequate palliation and not run the risk of rapid chest wall recurrence with its serious side effects. Cancer *en cuirasse* has always been recognized as a terrible consequence of inappropriate toilet mastectomy

Table 27-2 Indications for Mastectomy in Stage IIIB Disease

1. If excellent local response to systemic therapy (tamoxifen or chemotherapy)
2. As part of a plan for regional radiotherapy
3. For symptomatic local disease despite systemic treatment and radiation

Ulcerated Breast Cancers

1. Biopsy—ER status
2. Stage for systemic disease
3. ER+ → Antiestrogen
   → ± Radiotherapy, ± Mastectomy
   → ± Chemotherapy
4. ER− → Chemotherapy
   → ± Radiotherapy, ± Mastectomy
5. Mastectomy rarely indicated

Figure 27-1 A stepwise approach to the management of ulcerated breast cancers. Determination of the estrogen receptor status is of paramount importance. Patients whose tumors are estrogen receptor-positive are best treated with antiestrogen, and the addition of other modalities such as radiation therapy, chemotherapy, and surgery must be made on an individual basis. For estrogen receptor-negative tumors, chemotherapy is the treatment of choice to be followed by radiation and/or mastectomy as indicated. Only if all therapy fails to produce local tumor control and healing of the ulcer should mastectomy be contemplated.

and therefore this procedure should be avoided when the risk of rapid chest wall recurrence is likely.

This proposal for combination chemotherapy, surgery, and radiation is similar to that described by Hortobagyi et al. in 1983.[3] In their program of therapy for 52 women, patients with complete responses ($n = 8$) and those with no responses ($n = 9$) were to receive radiation but no mastectomy. Those women with partial responses to chemotherapy ($n = 35$) were selected to have mastectomy. A total of 34 patients in this series had mastectomy with a 21 percent incidence of local recurrence. For patients receiving chemotherapy and mastectomies, 2/7 had recurrence; 4/18 patients with chemotherapy and radiation therapy had recurrence; while 5/27 patients treated with all three modes recurred. Hortobagyi et al. utilized a program of 2 years of treatment. Of course, treatment compliance was a serious problem, as it would be with any such group. However, at 16 months, 40 percent of the women remained disease-free.

Balawajder et al. in 1983[4] analyzed their experience with 108 patients treated for advanced stage III disease. About 25 percent of these patients were stage T_3, N_0, or N_1.

For patients treated with all three modalities of therapy, there was a local control rate of 88 percent. Mastectomy with radiation gave a local control rate of 55 percent. Radiation and chemotherapy had a local control rate of 54 percent, and radiation alone only controlled 38 percent of the patients. There was no difference in survival seen in all four subsets, and the authors did point out that the possible increases in radiation dosage would have been equivalent to performing a mastectomy. Obviously, these types of studies need further evaluation and further experience. Mastectomy must be considered as a method of achieving local control in conjunction with other forms of treatment, rather than as the sole therapy.

For both types of stage III disease, evaluation and identification of the estrogen and progesterone receptor status of the cancer are essential. These patients are at high risk for early recurrence, either locally or distantly, and the use of antihormone therapy or some other type of hormone alteration may be contemplated if proper sensitivity is demonstrated. Whether or not "adjuvant" therapy with an antihormone such as tamoxifen would be indicated is a point for further consideration. Unquestionably, should hormone sensitivity of the primary tumor be identified, management of subsequent metastatic disease would be best handled with hormone alteration, particularly if chemotherapy has already been used in the primary therapy, as would be necessary for stage IIIB disease.

It should be emphasized that, whenever possible, every biopsy of recurrent breast cancer should be tested for persistence of estrogen receptor sensitivity. The potential for tumor heterogeneity and the possibility that the initial clones of cancer will have altered their growth characteristics when they metastasize makes documentation of hormone sensitivity necessary prior to treatment decisions for metastases. While this is not always possible, documentation of hormone status should be attempted whenever tissue is accessible.

PRIMARY CANCER—STAGE IV

Patients who present with an untreated primary cancer and distant metastases are an unusual group of women. They often have a long history of a progressively growing breast mass before seeking medical attention for a metastatic lesion. Sometimes the primary lesion is not even detectable at the time that metastases are identified. Of all patients with metastatic disease, they are the most likely to have tumor sensitivity to hormonal manipulation. In fact, their therapy is truly dependent on the estrogen receptor status of the tumor and the localization of their metastases. As stated above in "Primary Cancer—Stage III," every attempt should be made to obtain tissue for estrogen and progesterone receptor assays in these women. Since the primary tumor is always present on the chest wall, such a sampling can usually be performed under local anesthesia. About a 1-cm^3 portion of tumor is required; it is important to obtain frozen sections on the tissue both to be certain that the diagnosis is correct and that the breast carcinoma tissue is actually sent for the assay.

If the patient is shown to have a tumor which is estrogen receptor-positive, then administration of the antiestrogen, tamoxifen, is the treatment of choice. This substance is so free of side effects and has such a good chance of producing a long-term remission that there is definitely no better therapy to be considered. There is an occasional temporary "flare" of symptoms due to the agonistic estrogen action of tamoxifen. If the patient is premenopausal, it is not defined as yet as to whether or not oophorectomy should be performed in conjunction with the antiestrogen therapy. One approach that this author has used is to perform oophorectomy on women who are strongly estrogen receptor-positive and who are premenopausal with metastatic disease and untreated primary cancers. When the estrogen receptor is minimally elevated, antiestrogen is used to ascertain if there is a chance for response. It is well documented that the degree of estrogen receptor present in the tumor can be quantitated with the response to tamoxifen.[5] For postmenopausal patients, antiestrogen therapy is far better than any ablative approach to hormone alteration. For patients who are estrogen receptor-positive and who have a satisfactory response to tamoxifen, relapse of metastatic disease, even if it cannot be biopsy-proven as being estrogen receptor-positive, should be considered for therapy with either adrenalectomy or aminoglutethimide.[6]

It is rarely necessary to perform a mastectomy in these patients with stage IV disease who are responsive to hormone treatment. In our experience, as reported in the past, the use of ablative therapy with or without chemotherapy usually resulted in control of symptoms from the untreated breast cancer.[7,8] In most cases, the breast cancer shrank and was under excellent control with systemic management. In some patients, the previously biopsied intramammary breast cancer had responded so completely that it was no longer apparent when the patient finally came to autopsy. Again, noninvasive techniques such as radiation therapy would be much more appropriate in patients with systemic disease under treatment with hormonal therapy whose local disease relapses and becomes symptomatic. The reason for this approach is the high risk of rapid chest wall recurrence after removal of a fungating breast cancer. Obviously, decisions for or against surgical resection must be made on an individual basis.

For patients whose cancers are estrogen receptor-negative, there is only one course of action: systemic chemotherapy. In general, it is possible to achieve an initial remission of disease with systemic chemotherapy in these patients, but, unfortunately, persistence of response after chemotherapy has been discontinued is usually short-lived. When the disease reactivates, local control may be more difficult. Once again, radiation would be the most likely consideration, since subsequent courses of chemotherapy have less likelihood of affecting the systemic disease. An unnecessary operative procedure—even a mastectomy—would be inappropriate.

For those patients presenting with malignant pleural effusions, either with estrogen receptor-positive or -negative disease, the surgeon should consider the valuable role of pleurodesis. Initial response to therapy may eliminate the need for this procedure, but if there is persistent pleural effusion and symptomatic dyspnea, placement of a chest tube to evacuate the fluid, followed by tetracycline sclerosis of the pleura, will achieve a fine palliative result. It should be considered not only in this group of stage IV patients, but also in those with recurrent disease after initial primary treatment.

RECURRENT BREAST CANCER—LOCAL-REGIONAL DISEASE

Experience with local recurrence after radical mastectomy has been dismal. With rare exceptions, every patient with local recurrence eventually dies of metastatic disease. While the time to death may be longer for patients with local recurrence than those with systemic[9] metastases, the inevitable outcome still is to be predicted. Palliation can be achieved with proper therapy but there is no evidence that the poor end results have been altered by palliative forms of treatment. While specific characteristics of the primary cancer such as size of tumor, number of involved lymph nodes, and estrogen receptor status may be correlated with the risk of recurrence, other factors such as the width of the skin margins, the location of the tumor within the breast, and the type of histologic definition of the tumor do not appear to serve as prognostic factors for recurrence.[10] On the other hand, with local-regional recurrence after mastectomy, three factors have been defined by Bedwinek et al. as being valuable prognostic indicators of better survival.[11] The number of recurrences, the size of the largest recurrence and the disease-free interval from primary treatment all influenced outcome. Five-year survival figures were 45 percent for single metastases versus 22 percent for multiple lesions; for patients with up to a 1-cm recurrent lesion, 51 percent lived 5 years while only 18 to 23 percent of patients with larger lesions did so; if the disease-free interval was greater than 24 months, 56 percent survived 5 years, while only 17 percent of patients with disease-free intervals less than 24 months lived 5 years.

Gilliland et al. found that stage I patients lived a mean of 7.2 years after recurrence, while stage III patients survived only an average of 2.5 years.[12] Therefore, the extent of the primary disease may affect the outcome should recurrence take place. Bedwinek and his colleagues, on the other hand, did not identify the original stage of the disease, the number of histologically positive lymph nodes, the menopausal status, or the location of local recurrence as prognostic factors for survival after local-regional recurrence.[11]

An area of great interest is the question as to whether or not patients with local-regional recurrence after having had partial mastectomy and radiation have a different prognosis than those who have local-regional recurrence after modified or Halsted mastectomy. The data available at this time indicate that there is a difference in these groups of patients and that some women with local-regional recurrence after partial mastectomy and radiation have a real opportunity for salvage by subsequent mastectomy. Hayward's data from the Guy's Hospital trial first pointed this out.[13] In that series, there was more than twice the recurrence for stage I and stage II cancer patients at 5 and 10 years, who had been treated with partial mastectomy and radiation as compared with Halsted mastectomy. Yet, after "salvage mastectomy" there was no statistical difference in survival for the two groups in either stage. For patients with stage I disease, the site of recurrence was in the axilla in 22 percent, and in the breast in 5 percent. For the stage II patients with wide excision, 26 percent had axillary recurrence, 22 percent skin recurrence, and 10 percent "in-breast" recurrence. The authors drew no conclusions as to whether patients with in-breast recurrences had a different outcome than those with other local-regional recurrences. Clark et al., however, identified better survival for patients who had in-breast recurrence compared to those with recurrence in the axilla alone, the axilla and the breast, or in other local sites.[14] In their series, patients with in-breast recurrence had no difference in survival from those patients who never recurred at all. However, in many patients, as in the review by Harris et al.,[15] local-regional recurrence in women primarily treated with partial mastectomy and radiation does appear to alter the ultimate survival. In their report, which encompasses the treatment of primary cancer by partial mastectomy and radiation at the Princess Margaret Hospital in Toronto, the Marseilles Cancer Center, and the Institute Curie in Paris, 50 percent of the patients remained free of distant disease at 10 years who had a salvage mastectomy, while for the entire series the 15-year actuarial distant disease-free rate was 71 percent. It would be inappropriate at this time to believe that salvage after partial mastectomy and radiation can be as successful as original mastectomy, or that patients who recur can survive as well as those who do not. This statement is supported by the recent report of Osborne et al.[16] These authors demonstrated that, at the Royal Marsden Hospital, 20-year survival statistics after partial mastectomy and radiation showed that the *initial stage of the disease* had a great deal to do with salvageability, should recurrence take place. There was a 42 percent 5-year survival with salvage mastectomy for patients who did not have positive nodes initially. On the other hand, patients with clinically positive nodes were not able to be salvaged when recurrence took place within the radiated breast. Also, there was a somewhat different pattern of local recurrence in these patient populations. For patients with earlier-stage disease and clinically negative lymph nodes there was a progressive increase of local recurrence over 20-year follow-up. On the other hand, for those with positive lymph nodes and more advanced local disease, recurrence took place most frequently within the first 5 years, and there was not a great increase in the incidence of recurrence through the next 15-year period. Thus, it is safe to state that, as we are more careful in our staging, we will most certainly define populations of patients best suited to one form of primary treatment or the other.

The major variables in the treatment of women with local-regional recurrence after radical or modified radical mastectomy are (1) whether previous radiation has been given, (2) whether previous chemotherapy has been administered, and (3) the estrogen receptor status of the metastatic disease. If possible, excision of the recurrent tumor on the chest wall should be carried out. Extensive surgical resection may be required to achieve this, even to the use of full chest wall excision with pedicle flaps. Shah and Urban reported a 43 percent 5-year survival when such radical excisions were performed,[17] and it is well accepted that local control achieves the best possible palliation. If radiation therapy has not been previously given, total field radiation should be used following excisional biopsy. Bedwinek et al. demonstrated that less radiotherapy was required if total excision could be achieved.[18] Total excision, however, is not a substitute for radiation therapy. Those patients without residual tumor required about 5000 rads, whereas those with tumor present on the chest wall after biopsy required 5500 to 6500 rads for local control. The use of antiestrogen therapy with or without chemotherapy, if the tumor is hormone-positive, is probably worthwhile. Cocconi et al. have reported response rates when tamoxifen was added to cyclophosphamide, methotrexate and 5-fluorouracil therapy in a randomized trial for postmenopausal patients who have had measurable recurrent disease on the chest wall.[19] Unquestionably, the initial chemotherapeutic attack on the recurrent disease is the most important and should be the most intensive. Once a patient has recurred following systemic chemotherapy, the chance of a subsequent chemotherapy response is quite restricted.

For patients with recurrence after partial mastectomy, total mastectomy is essential for in-breast recurrence. If axillary dissection had not been previously performed, it should be included. Chemotherapy is probably best added for positive lymph node disease, but this is by no means certain. Likewise, the use of antiestrogen medication is optional. Until we have a better understanding of whether treatment at this phase is capable of achieving cure or just palliation, the extent of therapy with systemic modalities is a matter of controversy. The primary role is to achieve local-regional control, and this is performed with surgery and/or radiation. Supraclavicular lymph node metastases, likewise, can best be treated with radiation therapy, although these are more to be considered as systemic metastases. In the presence of estrogen sensitivity of the tumor, they might well be treated with antiestrogen medication.

Women who have had partial mastectomy without radiation must be considered at risk for either axillary recurrence or in-breast recurrence. It would probably be best to perform total mastectomy and axillary dissection for either type of recurrence in this patient population, but in some circumstances axillary radiation and radiation to the breast might suffice for axillary recurrence once it was certain there was no additional in-breast active cancer. It is unwise to radiate the breast which has a local recurrence without removal of this recurrent disease. Control rate will be inadequate if this is done. If the patient refuses mastectomy and has not had radiation therapy, then removal of residual in-breast disease is a possible option with radiation therapy to follow.

The management of local-regional recurrence is certain to be modified as greater experience with recurrence after partial mastectomy and radiation is seen. The surgeon must remain alert to identify recurrence at its earliest time and to treat it as though the primary cancer is still curable. There is sufficient evidence to justify aggressive follow-up of patients who have partial mastectomy and radiation with mammograms, physical examination, and biopsy when necessary. Patients selecting this option of primary therapy should be informed about the need for such thorough and careful follow-up and should be encouraged to carry out self-examination on a monthly basis as well. The breast and overlying skin will always have some degree of thickening after this form of therapy, so that sequential evaluation is essential to defining any new disease.

Recurrent Disease with Distant Metastases

Prognosis for patients with distant metastases is related to the disease-free interval and the distribution of their metastases. Certain general patterns of metastatic disease can be seen with specific sites predominating but not exclusively involved. These are (1) skeletal, (2) soft-tissue, and (3) visceral.

Skeletal Metastases

Skeletal metastases are generally in the spine, proximal long bones, skull, and pelvis. Frequently, these tumors are estrogen receptor-positive and may be associated with long disease-free intervals. It is for these patients that endocrine ablative surgical procedures had the most to offer in the past. The definition of the estrogen receptor status and its clinical application, along with determination of progesterone receptors, has helped to define more accurately a population of patients with metastatic breast cancer who will have a high response rate to hormone manipulation.[20]

It is critical that surgeons be concerned about skeletal metastases in these patients from the standpoint of fracture prevention or fixation. For non-weight-bearing sites, such as the ribs, clavicle, humerus, and iliac crest, radiation can be used to prevent fractures and speed callus formation in bones already fractured. Internal fixation may be required for some displaced fractures of the humerus. Fractures in weight-bearing portions of the pelvis can easily be controlled with radiation, as well. Imminent fractures of the femur should have prophylactic nailing performed. Frank femoral fractures may require resection of the head of the femur and a Moore type of prosthesis or full joint replacement if standard hip nailing is impossible. Radiation should be added to internal fixation. The use of methylmethacrylate glue may also aid in fracture stabilization. The ability of patients to reambulate is important palliation and should not be overlooked.

One extremely dangerous area of bone metastases is that which involves the spine. Insidious spinal cord injury can result from involvement of the body or pedicle of the cervical, thoracic, or lumbar spine. Fractures of the bone, with or without tumor growth into the spinal canal, can produce rapidly progressive spinal cord damage. Weakness of the legs, rectal or bladder incontinence, and sensory signs such as paresthesia or numbness of the extremities should be recognized as warning signs of impending irreversible cord compression. Prompt myelography or CT examination of the spine and neurosurgical consultation to determine whether decompression is required are essential. Even with decompression, radiation therapy is generally used. The reversal of this type of complication can provide acceptable palliation for the patient for many months.

A decade ago, only ablative procedures such as oophorectomy, adrenalectomy, and hypophysectomy, or high-dose estrogen therapy, were available approaches for patients presumed to have hormonally sensitive tumors. Results of therapy were good and ablative hormone procedures were widely performed. The availability of antiestrogen therapy has dramatically altered the standards of care for these patients. Tamoxifen, the commonly available agent for antiestrogen therapy, competes at the cytoplasmic estrogen receptor site in the tumor cell with estrogen for receptor activation. Its greatest benefit is its virtual absence of side effects and its reversibility when discontinued. For premenopausal females, as stated above, there are no clear data to indicate whether oophorectomy should be included with antiestrogen treatment or not. It is well known that tamoxifen therapy does not cause cessation of menstrual cycles, and, in fact, circulating estrogen levels can rise in these women. One has the option of initiating tamoxifen therapy first, proceeding with oophorectomy first, or combining both as initial therapy. As stated before, my preference has been to start with tamoxifen first when the estrogen receptor level was only minimally elevated, or when patients have complications of their disease that make operative procedures less appropriate. For patients with higher estrogen receptor levels, the probability of response is greater and an operative procedure such as oophorectomy is most justified. In the patients who respond to tamoxifen, relapse should be treated by oophorectomy if the patient was premenopausal at the outset.

For postmenopausal patients, antiestrogen therapy is clearly the initial treatment of choice, especially if metastases can be demonstrated to be estrogen receptor-positive. It is well recognized that because of tumor cell heterogeneity not all metastases follow the same hormonal pattern as the primary lesion. With the virtual absence of side effects from tamoxifen, however, patients whose primary lesions were estrogen receptor-positive should receive antiestrogen treatment when they have metastases. The response to tamoxifen by metastases may be particularly useful in defining whether the tumor cell populations are still estrogen receptor-positive. If response occurs with tamoxifen therapy, no other treatment need be contemplated, but when relapse occurs, other hormonal alterations should be considered. Surgical adrenalectomy, so frequently used in the past, can still provide excellent responses in some of these patients. Likewise, aminoglutethimide, as mentioned earlier, may also achieve successful remission. For patients with hormonally responsive tumors, continued therapy in the direction of hormonal alteration should be used rather than switching to chemotherapy.

Soft-Tissue Metastases

For patients with soft-tissue metastases (primarily the chest wall, lymph nodes in the supraclavicular region, or opposite axilla) rebiopsy for determination of estrogen receptor status is easiest and should be performed. If tumors are estrogen receptor-positive, the same treatment options exist as mentioned for skeletal disease. If the tumors are receptor-negative, then chemotherapy should be selected for management.

Visceral Metastases

Patients with visceral metastases—lung, liver, heart, or brain—are generally candidates for systemic chemotherapy. Brain metastases and pleural metastases represent two special areas. As discussed earlier, pleural metastases are best managed by sclerosis of the tumor cavity with tetracycline. Brain metastases should be treated with total brain irradiation (3000 rads) after dexamethasone has been initiated. The dexamethasone is given in a dose of 16 mg/day by mouth. We have seen that a good response to dexamethasone is usually associated with a salutory response to radiation. Occasionally, craniotomy for resection of "solitary" brain metastases is to be considered. This is rarely done, however, since solitary metastases are unusual and the response rate to radiation for brain metastases from breast cancer is sufficiently high as to make surgical resection of metastases unnecessary.

CONCLUSION

Treatment of patients in all of these categories of advanced breast cancer must be directed at achieving the best quality of life for the individual. Only patients with stage IIIA cancer have any reasonable chance for any long-term disease-free survival, or "cure." They should be treated aggressively in an attempt to achieve that objective. The other patients mentioned in this chapter require more selective and individual treatment to provide them with the best possible control of symptoms or potential symptoms. Surgeons should participate at all levels in the care of these patients. Often, simple surgical procedures added to other therapeutic approaches can contribute to the palliative benefit of these women. On the other hand, inappropriate or poorly planned surgical operations may have disastrous outcomes. Clinical judgment and experience are essential, in addition to consultation with one's colleagues.

REFERENCES

1. Wilson RE: Surgical management of locally advanced and recurrent breast cancer. *Cancer* 53:752, 1984.
2. Wilson RE, Piro AJ, Aliapoulios MA, Moore FD: Evaluation of adrenalectomy and hypophysectomy in the treatment of metastatic cancer of the breast. *Cancer* 24:1322, 1969.
3. Hortobagyi GN, Blumenschein GR, Spanos W, Montague ED, Buzdar AU, Yap HY, Schell F: Multimodal treatment of loco-regionally advanced breast cancer. *Cancer* 51:763, 1983.
4. Balawajder I, Antick PP, Boland J: An analysis of the role of radiotherapy alone and in combination with chemotherapy and surgery in the management of advanced breast carcinoma. *Cancer* 51:574, 1983.
5. Fisher B et al: Treatment of primary breast cancer with chemotherapy and tamoxifen. *N Engl J Med* 305:1, 1981.
6. Santen RJ et al: A randomized trial comparing surgical adrenalectomy with aminoglutethimide plus hydrocortisone in women with advanced breast cancer. *N Engl J Med* 305:545, 1981.
7. Moore FD, Van DeVanter SB, Boyden CM, Lokich J, Wilson RE: Adrenalectomy with chemotherapy in the treatment of advanced breast cancer: Objective and subjective response rates; duration and quality of life. *Surgery* 76:376, 1974.
8. Wilson RE, Donegan WL, Mettlin C, Natarajan N, Smart CR, Murphy GP: The 1982 national survey of carcinoma of the breast in the United States by the American College of Surgeons. *Surg Gynecol Obstet* 159:309, 1984.
9. Ferguson DJ, Meier P, Karrison T, Dawson PJ, Straus FH, Lowenstein FE: Staging of breast cancer and survival rates. An assessment based on 50 years of experience with radical mastectomy. *JAMA* 248:1337, 1982.
10. Donegan WL, Perez-Mesa CM, Watson FR: A biostatistical study of locally recurrent breast carcinoma. *Surg Gynecol Obstet* 122:529, 1966.
11. Bedwinek JM, Lee J, Fineberg B, Ocwieza MA: Prognostic indicators in patients with isolated local-regional recurrence of breast cancer. *Cancer* 47:2232, 1981.
12. Gilliland MD, Barton RM, Copeland, EM III: The implications of local recurrence of breast cancer as the first site of therapeutic failure. *Ann Surg* 197:284, 1983.
13. Hayward JL: Steroid excretion in early breast cancer. *Br J Surg* 51:224, 1964.
14. Clark RM, Wilkinson RH, Mahoney LJ, Reid JG, MacDonald WD: Breast cancer: A 21 year experience with conservative surgery and radiation. *Int J Radiat Oncol Biol Phys* 8:967, 1982.
15. Harris JR, Connolly JL, Schnitt SJ, Cohen RB, Hellman S: Clinical-pathologic study of early breast cancer treated by primary radiation therapy. *J Clin Oncol* 1(3):184, 1983.
16. Osborne MP, Ormiston N, Harmer CL, McKinna JA, Baker J, Greening WP: Breast conservation in the treatment of early breast cancer: A 20 year follow-up. *Cancer* 53(2):349, 1984.
17. Shah JP, Urban JA: Full thickness chest wall resection for recurrent breast cancer involving the bony chest wall. *Cancer* 35:567, 1975.

18. Bedwinek JM, Fineberg B, Lee L, Ocwieza M: Analysis of failures following local treatment of isolated local-regional recurrence of breast cancer. *Int J Radiat Oncol Biol Phys* 7:581, 1981.
19. Cocconi G, DeLisi V, Boni C, Mori P, Malacarne P, Amadori D, Giovanelli E: Chemotherapy versus combination of chemotherapy and endocrine therapy in advanced breast cancer: A prospective randomized study. *Cancer* 51:581, 1983.
20. McGuire WL, Carbone PP, Volmen EP: *Estrogen Receptors in Human Breast Cancer.* Philadelphia, Raven Press, 1975.

28

Hormone and Chemotherapy: Fundamental Clinical Concepts

Stephen K. Carter, M.D.

INTRODUCTION

The therapy of advanced breast cancer is currently a palliative mode of therapy. The goal of treatment is to alleviate symptoms and prolong survival with therapy which will not in itself diminish functional capability. Chemotherapy must be integrated into a sequential flow of palliative therapeutic options which include hormonal manipulations and radiation therapy. The choice of therapy depends upon critical variables such as the metastatic pattern, tempo of disease progression, hormonal receptor status, and performance status and response, or lack thereof, to previous therapeutic manipulations.

When a woman with breast cancer first presents with metastatic disease, a triage plan must be developed for the manifold therapeutic options, involving an analysis of the prognostic variables just mentioned. A decision tree for triage is given in Fig. 28-1. The physician must first determine the metastatic pattern and the tempo of disease. If either of these two variables precludes waiting 8 to 12 weeks for the potential benefits of hormonal therapy, then this option must be excluded, regardless of hormone receptor status or other factors. Examples of situations where this would be the case include patients with lymphangitic pulmonary metastases, hepatic metastases with liver function impairment, and pleural effusion.

If hormonal manipulation is not precluded by the metastatic pattern, it then becomes the prime choice for consideration. Whether hormonal therapy is used today depends upon the estrogen receptor (ER) status of the patient. If the ER status is negative then the probability of endocrine response is low and chemotherapy becomes the prime choice. If the ER status is unknown, then a pragmatic attempt at endocrine therapy is warranted since it is less toxic than chemotherapy. In the days before routine ER status determinations, empirical initial endocrine therapy was the standard approach

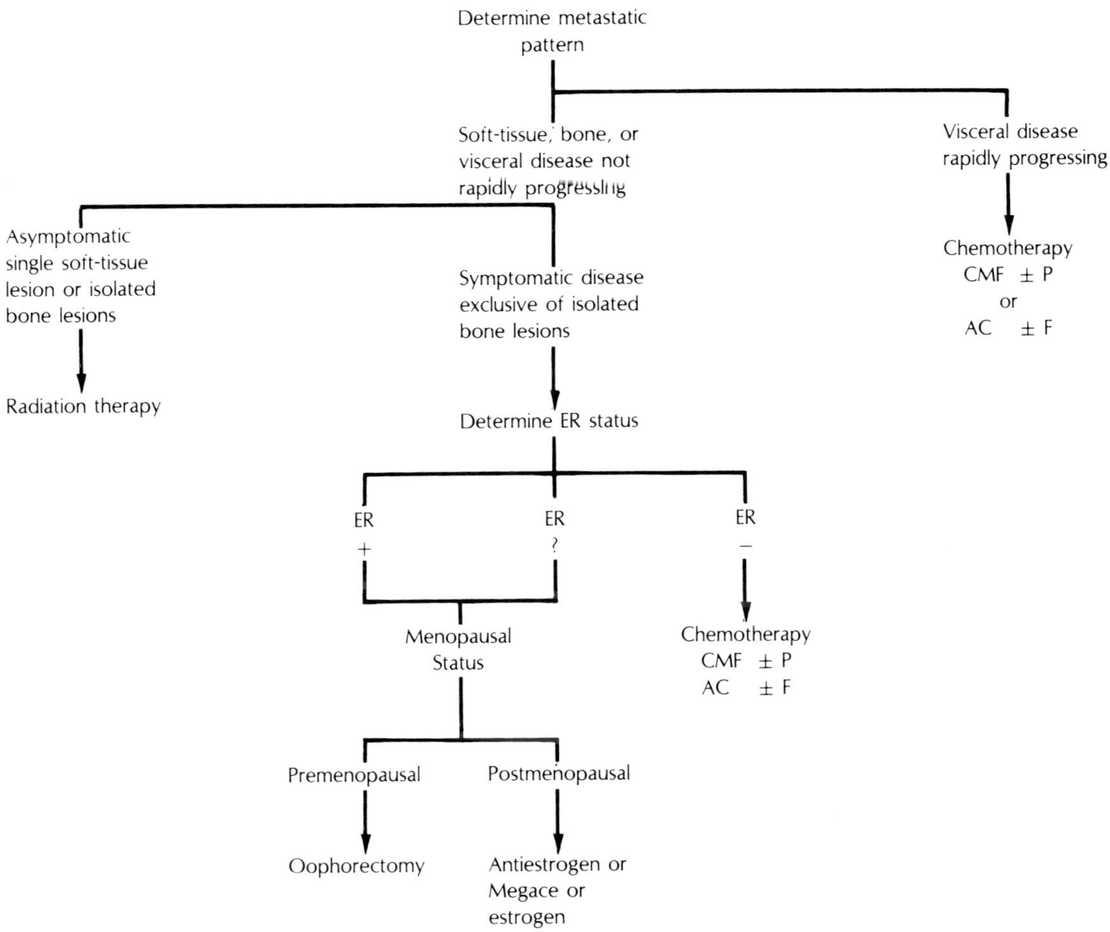

Figure 28-1 Advanced breast cancer triage for primary therapy.

with response, or lack thereof, serving as a poor man's ER status evalution.[1]

The ultimate value of a breast cancer therapy regimen involves evaluating the therapeutic index, both alone and within the total sequence of palliative regimens used. The efficacy end points include objective response rate, duration of response, time to treatment failure in all patients, and survival. The survival end point is a difficult one to utilize in a comparative fashion between different studies. The reason for this is that survival is usually calculated from the onset of therapy which, in advanced breast cancer, can be a very heterogeneous zero point. A chemotherapy regimen utilized as the initial cytotoxic palliative intent can be either the first, second, third, or even fourth overall therapeutic thrust within the palliative sequence of therapies. One example for first use of chemotherapy could be a woman with her first evidence of metastatic relapse being hepatic metastases with an elevated bilirubin. A second example would be a woman with her first evidence of metastatic relapse being skin or nodal but with a negative estrogen receptor assay. A third example could be a woman who had been previously treated with an oophorectomy, adrenalectomy, and then tamoxifen. It should be obvious that comparing median survival from onset of treatment among various small series, testing the same regimen, might be very difficult to interpret meaningfully. All clinical research experiences with individual regimens should be reported within the context of all therapies administered and survival given both from onset of treatment and from the clinical diagnosis of advanced disease.

ENDOCRINE THERAPY

Hormonal therapy has had a resurgence in the management of advanced breast cancer, due to three major factors: (1) the discovery of the estrogen-progesterone receptor assay, (2) the discovery of new, less-toxic hormonal therapies, and (3) the recognition that chemotherapy has plateaued at a much lower level of activity than had been anticipated a decade ago.

Retrospective analysis and empiric observation has determined that the ideal patient for endocrine therapy would have the following prognostic aspects independent of hormone receptor status: (1) a long disease-free interval, (2) disease primarily in soft tissue and bone, (3) prior hormone response, (4) late premenopausal or late postmenopausal status, and (5) have a limited number of metastatic sites.

With the advent of the estrogen receptor (ER) assay, this has become the predominant determinant for endocrine therapy response potential. The ER is a protein found in the cytoplasm of roughly two-thirds of all women with breast cancer. More recently, the progesterone receptor (PgR) has also become of investigative interest. Both these receptors are measured by an in vitro assay. In this assay a tumor cell homogenate is made and the supernatant is incubated with radiolabeled estrogen or progesterone. The assay can be interpreted in a qualitative way as either positive or negative at a particular cutoff level. The assay can also be analyzed in a quantitative manner focusing on the absolute level reported. This is deemed important since it appears that the higher the receptor level, the higher the response rate potential to endocrine therapy. The cumulative frequency distribution of standard receptors, as analyzed by McGuire and Clark, is shown in Table 28-1.[1]

In the past, the empiric response to appropriate endocrine therapy was about 30 percent. This involved treating all patients except those with aggressive visceral dominant disease.[2] McGuire and Clark[1] have demonstrated the predictability of ER and PgR for response to be in the range of 32 to 71 percent (Table 28-2). Their data would seem to indicate that the PgR is critically important since the ER+ or PgR− group had a response rate (32 percent) similar to what is reported for empirical endocrine treatment.

One of the difficulties with hormone receptors is the discordance which can exist in measurement. This discordance is of two types: The first involves simultaneous assays on two different specimens from the same patient, and the second involves sequential measurements on different specimens from the same patient over a period of time. Gross et al.[3] have recently

Table 28-1 Cumulative Frequency Distributions of Steroid Receptors

Hormone receptor level in cytosol protein (Fmol/mg)	Percent estrogen receptor $N = 7197$	Percent progesterone receptor $N = 5877$
<3	30	44
<5	35	52
<10	42	61
<20	50	69
<50	65	79
<100	76	86
<500	99	98
<1000	100	99

Source: Derived from McGuire and Clark.[1]

Table 28-2 Response to Hormonal Therapy in Advanced Breast Cancer Related to Estrogen and Progesterone Receptor Status[1]

Receptor status	Number of patients	CR + PR, percent
ER − / PgR −	171	9
ER − / PgR +	15	53
ER + / PgR −	189	32
ER + / PgR +	263	71

reviewed the PgR assay results from more than 5500 patients, focusing on 283 patients in whom multiple breast cancer specimens were analyzed. Multiple biopsy specimens from 109 patients were studied for the PgR assay results. In this group 15 patients (14 percent) had a major discordance in which the results were interpreted as PgR+ in one and PgR− in another. In addition, a further 20 patients (18 percent) had a "minor" discordance in which one specimen was read as PgR+ or PgR−. Taken together, this type of discordance exists in nearly a third of patients, which is sobering for therapeutic decision making.

Progesterone receptor content was studied in 174 sequential pairs of assays. A major discordance was observed in 9 percent of 106 patients whose initial biopsy was PgR− and in a striking 44 percent of patients whose initial biopsy was PgR+ (Table 28-3). A correlation with the ER assay was done where data permitted. If the initial PgR was positive and remained so at second biopsy, a positive ER of the same specimen remained positive in 91 percent of the cases. If an initial PgR+ assay was discordant, then there was an ER discordance of 47 percent. It therefore seems that the PgR assay selects a subset of patients whose ER, when evaluated as well, fluctuates in parallel with the PgR.

Discordance for simultaneous hormone receptor assays can be caused by inadequate sample size, lack of assay reproducibility, or tumor heterogeneity. The importance of tumor sample size is illustrated in the study by Hull et al.,[4] in which discordance in ER assay was found in 56 percent of samples less than 2 cm in size as against only 7 percent when the tumor sample size was larger than 2 cm. Additional causes of sequential discordance could be either the so-called "biological drift" or gradual loss of PgR over time, and/or changes in the endogenous hormonal milieu. Gross et al.[3] feel that these are less important than the impact of intervening endocrine therapy. In a multivariate

Table 28-3 Discordance and Concordance in Sequential Progesterone Receptor Assays

		Correlation with second sequential assay		
Initial progesterone receptor status	Number	Concordance	Minor discordance	Major discordance
+	55	27 (49%)	4 (7%)	24 (44%)
−	106	94 (89%)	3 (3%)	9 (8%)
±	3	0 (0%)	13 (100%)	0 (0%)

± = Progesterone receptor level between 5 and 10 Fmol/mg protein.
Source: Data of Gross, et al.[3]

Table 28-4 Objective Response to Combination Chemotherapy Correlated With Estrogen Receptor Status

Investigators	Chemotherapy regimens	Number treated and percent CR + PR	
		ER+	ER−
Lippman et al.[5]	Various	25 (12%)	45 (76%)
Kiang et al.[6]	Various	28 (86%)	36 (36%)
Jonat et al.[7]	Various	14 (43%)	28 (71%)
Marsland et al.[8]	CMF ± P	29 (78%)	15 (46%)
Chang et al.[9]	CMF	16 (88%)	17 (35%)
Rubens et al.[10]	CMF, AV	29 (59%)	15 (60%)
Bonadonna et al.[11]	CMF, AV	28 (50%)	16 (44%)

analysis this was the predominant independent factor observed.

A debate has also existed in the literature regarding the correlation of ER status and response to cytotoxic drugs. The data are variable and subject to the vagaries of retrospective analysis in a highly heterogeneous disease. A tabulation of seven series (Table 28-4) demonstrates no clear evidence for a correlation. Recent commentaries by Levine and Lippman[12] and Kiang[13] now emphasize the problems inherent in this type of analysis and they no longer diverge dramatically regarding interpretation.

Prednisone

Prednisone is a drug whose exact mechanism of action against breast cancer is still unknown. It may function as a cytolytic agent or as an endocrine-mediated agent. It may be mediated by the presence of glucocorticoid receptor, which is present in about half the breast cancer specimens. In the review by Siebert and Lippman,[14] the response to corticosteroids correlated strongly with presence of estrogen receptor. The response rate in ER-positive patients was 34 percent (28/83) while in ER-negative patients it was 2 percent (1/46). For this reason, prednisone-containing combination chemotherapy regimens may obfuscate the true relationship between ER and response to cytotoxic chemotherapy.

Surgical Ablative Procedures

Surgical ablative procedures used to be quite common in the management of advanced breast cancer. Remission rates with these procedures have generally ranged from 25 to 50 percent.[15] Whether oophorectomy, adrenalectomy, or hypophysectomy, these procedures are associated with an appreciable morbidity and a low, but significant, mortality.[15] These procedures are used less today as a result of the introduction into clinical practice of the antiestrogen, tamoxifen, and the adrenal blocking agent, aminoglutethimide. These agents appear to induce remissions as often as do surgical procedures, and they are associated with a lower morbidity and a negligible mortality.

The surgical procedure still used the most is oophorectomy, which remains for many the initial endocrine treatment of choice for premenopausal women. When performed for women whose tumors are not clearly estrogen receptor-poor or -negative, the response rate is in the range of 50 to 60 percent. In ER-negative women, benefit is seen in less than 10 percent. In postmenopausal women the initial endocrine therapy is now mainly with antiestrogens, although medroxyprogesterone acetate and diethylstilbestrol will give equivalent response rates. The use of second-line surgical ablative procedures is being replaced with aminoglutethimide and hydrocortisone to accomplish a "medical adrenalectomy."

Tamoxifen

Tamoxifen is at present the most widely used hormonal additive treatment for advanced breast cancer. It is a synthetic antiestrogen which appears to compete with estradiol for the cytoplasmic estrogen receptor and produces a receptor complex which is not able to interact properly with the genome specific for the receptor-estrogen complex.[16] The exact efficacy potential of tamoxifen is not a simple matter to elucidate. A wide range of response rates have been reported in trials involving patients with widely different mixes of prognostic variables. Depending upon the patient selection factors involved, response rates appear to fluctuate within a range of 15 to 55 percent.

The usual dose of tamoxifen ranges from 20 to 40 mg daily with the drug being given in two equally divided doses each day. There is no evidence from trials to date of a dose-response relationship. In one randomized trial, Ward[17] compared 10 mg twice daily with 20 mg twice daily in 68 patients and found response rates of 36 and 40 percent, respectively. Tormey et al.[18] found a similar lack of a dose-response effect using doses which ranged from 2 to 100 mg/m^2 twice daily. Rose et al.[19] studied 30 versus 90 mg daily of tamoxifen in a randomized trial involving 143 women. The response rates were 36 and 37 percent, respectively, with no differences in response duration and time to treatment failure.

Patterson et al.[20] collected information on 45 different studies totaling 2889 patients. The cumulative overall response rate was 34 percent (971/2889) with complete responses being uncommon. The response range in these studies was from 14 to 57 percent and can be explained by differences in the prognostic mixes of patients studied along with differences in response criteria and data reporting techniques. When patients with no prior systemic therapy were separated out, the cumulative response rate was 43 percent (176/407). In patients with prior chemotherapy it was similar at 41 percent (96/223). The lowest response rate was in nonresponders to prior endocrine therapy which was 21 percent (34/165). In prior endocrine therapy responses, it was 59 percent (119/201).

Margreiter and Weigele[21] have reported a study of 44 previously untreated premenopausal women with measurable or evaluable breast cancer treated with tamoxifen. Excluded were patients with hepatic or cerebral metastases. In 23, bone lesions were the predominant site, followed by 15 soft-tissue dominant, and 7 with lung or pleural disease. In 35, hormone receptors were known with 18 being positive and 17 being negative. Response was observed in 12/44 (27 percent) of the patients. Three of the 12 responses were complete. The median duration of response was 12.7 months. The greatest benefit was obtained in patients with soft-tissue dominant disease where 9/15 (60 percent) responded. On the other hand, only 1/7 (14 percent) with bone and 2/22 with visceral and bone dominant disease responded. Responses broken down by hormone receptor status were as follows: ER+ and PgR+, 7/10; ER+ and PgR−, 2/6; ER− and PgR+, 1/1; and ER− and PgR−, 0/18. It therefore appears that tamoxifen offers a viable alternative to oophorectomy in hormone receptor-positive women.

The randomized trials which have been performed comparing tamoxifen with either estrogens or androgens (Table 28-5) demonstrate roughly comparable response. The major benefit for tamoxifen in these studies appears to be diminished side effects.

Aminoglutethimide

Aminoglutethimide (AG) is a drug which can be used in place of an adrenalectomy. It was

Table 28-5 Randomized Clinical Trials of Tamoxifen versus Either Estrogens or Androgens

Investigators	Selection criteria	Treatment regimen	Number of evaluable patients	Percent CR + PR
Ingle et al[22] for North Central Cancer Treatment Group	Postmenopausal—no prior hormones, 31% had prior chemotherapy	1. Tamoxifen 20 mg daily	69	33
		2. DES 5 mg three times daily	74	41
Stewart et al.[23]	Postmenopausal—no prior hormones or chemotherapy	1. Tamoxifen 30 mg daily	29	31
		2. DES 5 mg three times daily	27	22
Beex et al.[24]	More than 2 years from last menstrual period—12% with prior hormones and 15% with prior chemotherapy	1. Tamoxifen 40 mg daily	30	33
		2. Ethinyl estradiol 3 mg daily	29	31
Westerberg[25]	Postmenopausal—no prior hormones or chemotherapy	1. Tamoxifen 40 mg daily	37	30
		2. Fluoxymesterone 10 mg twice daily	42	19

originally used as an anticonvulsant agent unsuccessfully. Aminoglutethimide was found to inhibit the synthesis of pregneninolone from cholesterol, resulting in a reduction in synthesis of steroid hormones, especially hydrocortisone, aldosterone, and sex steroid hormones, synthesized by various tissues, particularly the adrenal. Subsequently it was found that AG blocks the aromatase enzymes necessary for the conversion of androgens to estrogens and that in postmenopausal women this conversion is the main source of estrogens.

The initial trials of AG were undertaken as a medical alternative to adrenalectomy. Powles[26] has reported on 213 postmenopausal women treated with AG, with 190 being deemed evaluable (Table 28-6). His group observed 6 complete and 47 partial responses for an overall response rate of 28 percent. The breakdown by previous therapy is given in Table 28-7. Analysis by the site of metastases indicated good control of disease in bone (54 percent), soft tissue (47 percent), and lung (45 percent). Liver metastases generally responded poorly (22 percent). The median duration of response to AG was about 14 months. Toxicity included transient lethargy (33 percent) and nausea (15 percent), which were dose-limiting for some patients. A widespread macular rash (self-limiting) sometimes associated with fever appeared in 23 percent of patients about 10 days after the start of therapy. Overall, only 5 percent of patients had to cease medication because of toxicity.

Two trials comparing AG with tamoxifen are outlined in Table 28-8. Both trials demonstrate comparable response rates in the populations under study. Since tamoxifen has fewer side

Table 28-6 Aminoglutethimide in Postmenopausal Women

Total	213	
Early death (<4 weeks)	23	
Assessable for response	190	
CR	6	3%
PR	47	25%

Source: Data of Powles.[26]

Table 28-7 Aminoglutethimide Treatment of Advanced Breast Cancer

Previous therapy breakdown	Number of patients	Number response	Percent response
None	62	19	30
Previous systemic R_X	125	34	27
Previous artificial menopause	36	7	19
Previous chemotherapy	53	13	25
No previous endocrine R_X	75	22	29
Previous endocrine R_X	112	31	28
Previous response	26	10	38
No previous response	53	10	19
Unassessable response	33	11	33

Source: Data of Powles.[26]

effects it would appear the preferable drug to use first.

Progestational Agents

Progestational agents are now receiving increasing emphasis within the framework of a sequential therapeutic palliative strategy for women with advanced breast cancer. The agents most commonly used are megestrol acetate and medroxyprogesterone acetate. Megestrol acetate has been reported as achieving response rates of 29 percent in 160 women treated by Ansfield et al.,[29] and 40 percent in 102 women studied by Alexieva-Figusch et al.[30] Similar

Table 28-8 Randomized Clinical Trials of Tamoxifen versus Aminoglutethimide

Investigators	Selection criteria	Treatment regimen	Number of evaluable patients	Percent CR + PR
Smith et al.[27]	No menopausal status limitation with 9% being premenopausal, 26% with prior hormones and 38% with prior chemotherapy	1. Tamoxifen 10 mg twice daily	60	30
		2. AG 250 mg three times daily plus hydrocortisone 20 mg twice daily	57	30
Lipton et al.[28]	"Menopausal or castrate" with 41% having prior hormonal therapy	1. Tamoxifen 20 mg twice daily	39	38
		2. AG 250 mg twice daily for 2 weeks, then four times daily plus hydrocortisone 100 mg daily in divided doses for 2 weeks, then 40 mg daily in divided doses	36	36

response rates have been reported for medroxyprogesterone acetate by the Cooperative Breast Cancer Group[31] (25 percent in 24 women). Pannuti et al.[32] have reported somewhat higher response rates with high-dose medroxyprogesterone acetate, but follow-up studies have failed to demonstrate a meaningful dose-response relationship for this agent.

Several randomized trials have been performed comparing tamoxifen with medroxyprogesterone acetate (Table 28-9). In all these trials response rates have not significantly differed between the two approaches in the patient populations under study.

Megestrol acetate is an effective second-line hormonal therapy after tamoxifen response and progression. Ingle et al.[36] and Ross et al.[37] have reported response rates of 33 and 31 percent, respectively, in these populations.

CHEMOTHERAPY

The chemotherapy of breast cancer is almost exclusively combination chemotherapy involving combinations utilizing six drugs:

1 Cyclophosphamide (C)
2 Methotrexate (M)
3 5-Fluorouracil (F)
4 Vincristine (V)
5 Prednisone (P)
6 Adriamycin (A)

The single-agent activities of these drugs are in the range of 20 to 40 percent. These single-agent response rates are mainly derived from older studies in which the drugs were used prior to common acceptance of combination chemotherapy. The one exception is Adriamycin. Adriamycin is the only commonly used drug for breast cancer which has been tested, as a single agent, in comparison to combinations. In one study of the Southwest Oncology Group (SWOG), Adriamycin was compared to CMFVP administered either continuously or intermittently. In this study the overall response rate for the single agent was not significantly different from that observed with the combinations, although survival favored the continuous five-drug regimen.[38]

Combination chemotherapy was first demonstrated to give high response rates by Greenspan

Table 28-9 Randomized Clinical Trials of Tamoxifen versus Medroxyprogesterone Acetate

Investigators	Selection criteria	Treatment regimen	Number of evaluable patients	Percent CR + PR
Mattson[33]	Over age 50, 16% with prior hormone therapy and 95% with prior chemotherapy	1. Tamoxifen 10 mg three times daily	32	47
		2. MPA 1000 mg/IM daily × 30, then weekly	26	54
Pannuti et al.[34]	Over 1 year postmenopausal, no prior hormones, and 13% with prior chemotherapy	1. Tamoxifen 10 mg twice daily	26	27
		2. MPA 1000 mg orally twice daily for 30 days, then for 15 days a month	27	37
Beretta et al.[35]	Postmenopausal with 75% having "other antitumor treatments"	1. Tamoxifen 20 mg daily	39	28
		2. MPA 400–1200 mg/day orally	40	25

in the 1960s.[39,40] Greenspan's work was almost totally ignored by the rest of the breast cancer research community and no cooperative group ever attempted to confirm or reproduce his results. In 1969, Cooper[41] submitted an abstract to the American Association for Cancer Research (AACR) which reported on a five-drug regimen including cyclophosphamide, methotrexate, 5-fluorouracil, vincristine, and prednisone (CMFVP) administered in a continuous fashion. The abstract stated that in 60 patients treated, complete responses were observed in 90 percent. The abstract was short, even as abstracts go, and was never followed up by a full literature presentation of the data. It is one of the anomalies of cancer clinical research history that this slim abstract had a major impact on the research community while the two publications of Greenspan were totally ignored. Subsequent to Cooper's abstract, every National Cancer Institute-sponsored cooperative clinical trials group undertook trials utilizing CMFVP or modifications thereof. The following five combination regimens derived from the original abstract have received the greatest degree of study:

1 CMFVP (continuous)
2 CMFVP (intermittent)
3 CMFP
4 CMF
5 CFP

The results of the various studies can be summarized as follows: (1) No one has confirmed the 90 percent complete response rate originally reported by Cooper; (2) the complete response rate is in the range of 5 to 15 percent; (3) the overall response rate is in the 40 to 60 percent range; (4) there does not appear to be a major difference between any of these regimens, although randomized comparisons are not extensive; and (5) when compared to the single-agent components in randomized studies, the response rate is higher but the survival advantage is not great.

Adriamycin's discovery has had a significant impact in the design of advanced breast cancer drug studies. Adriamycin is generally considered to be the most active of the single agents. This statement is based primarily on its single-agent response rate of approximately 40 percent when used as firstline cytotoxic chemotherapy. Adriamycin has been extensively tested in combination with various components of the CM-FVP regimen. The most commonly used combinations are

1 CAFVP
2 CAF or FAC
3 AC
4 AV

One of the most common approaches has been to substitute Adriamycin for methotrexate in either the CMFVP or CMF regimens, with the CAF or FAC combination being the most widely investigated. These data can be summarized as follows: (1) Adriamycin-containing regimens seem to result in an increased partial response rate in the range of 10 to 20 percent; (2) there is no convincing evidence that FAC or CAF is superior to AC; and (3) survival from onset of treatment is somewhat longer with Adriamycin-containing regimens.

A representative experience with two commonly used regimens in advanced breast cancer has been reported by Smalley et al.[42] for the Southeastern Cancer Study Group (SECSG). They compared low-dose intermittent CMFVP with CAF in 362 patients entered on study between April 1, 1974 and July 1, 1977. In addition, 79 women with bone metastases only were treated with CAF in an unrandomized fashion. None of the patients had received prior chemotherapy. All the premenopausal women had been treated with an oophorectomy. A total of 265 of the 362 randomized individuals was evaluable for analyzing. The reasons for not being evaluable were incomplete data (9 percent), ineligible (11 percent), and protocol violations (7 percent).

Table 28-10 Comparison of CAF versus CMFVP Broken Down by Metastatic Pattern

	CAF				CMFVP			
Pattern	Number	Number CR	Number PR	Percent response	Number	Number CR	Number PR	Percent response
1 = Bone only metastases	50	0	8	16	--	--	--	--
2 = Subcutaneous metastases to anterior chest wall	32	11	15	81	29	2	13	52
3 = Pleural metastases with effusion and frequently large chest wall ulceration	17	2	4	35	14	2	2	29
4A = Nodular lung metastases	26	3	11	54	22	1	6	32
4B = Lymphangitic lung metastases	12	2	3	42	9	0	3	33
5 = Widespread disease	25	3	8	44	30	0	12	40
0 = Stage III–IV disease with no primary surgical or radiation treatment	23	2	10	52	26	2	9	42

The response rate was higher with CAF (55 percent) than with CMFVP (40 percent), $p = .01$. If all the ineligible patients plus protocol violations are added to the analysis, CAF achieved a response in 80/167 (48 percent) and CMFVP in 56/165 (34 percent). The complete response rate was 17 percent after CAF and only 5 percent after CMFVP. This difference is highly significant ($p = .005$). In the patients with bone disease, only five patients (10 percent) responded to CAF while 43 (86 percent) remained objectively stable. All those achieving stability had improvement in performance status and a decrease in pain.

When duration of response was examined, the two regimens gave similar results. The time to progression for all patients favored CAF. At the time of the paper, 80 percent of those treated with CMFVP had died, while with CAF 65 percent had died. The two survival curves are not statistically significantly different, although there is a trend favoring CAF. In terms of toxicity, CAF induced a greater degree of myelosuppression and more nausea and vomiting than CMFVP.

The response rates were correlated with metastatic pattern using a clinical staging system developed by this group (Table 28-10). Patients with a good risk pattern of metastases, i.e., those with nodular lung involvement, with local chest wall recurrence, and/or with bone-only metastases had substantially better palliation from chemotherapy than did their poor-risk counterparts. In this group CAF gave a higher response rate, more complete responses, a longer duration of disease control, and a trend toward improved survival. In poor-risk patients, the two regimens were relatively the same.

Cancer and Leukemia Group B (CALGB)[43] has reported on a large-scale, three-arm study involving five-drug chemotherapy. This study involved 396 patients, of whom 302 were deemed evaluable. The study involved patients with no prior chemotherapy and measurable or evaluable disease. One group was treated with CM-FVP administered continuously. A second group was treated with CMFVP intermittently, with 28-day cycles consisting of 14 days of treatment and 14 days of rest being utilized. The third regimen was identical to CMFVP administered continuously, except that Adriamycin was substituted for methotrexate (CAFVP).

The results are shown in Table 28-11. The response rates were identical for the two schedules of CMFVP, while the CAFVP regimen gave a significantly higher response rate, mostly due to more partial responses being observed. The time to first response was shortest with CMFVP administered continuously and longest with CAFVP. In terms of prognostic subsets, the CAFVP regimen was superior in patients having osseous dominant or visceral dominant disease, a natural menopause, a performance status of 1 to 3, no additive chemical hormonal therapy, a modified radical or radical mastectomy, or no prior radiotherapy.

The remission duration was best for CAFVP (median = 14 months) as compared to CMFVP administered continuously (median = 9 months) and CMFVP administered intermittently (median = 7 months). The differences between the two CMFVP regimens were not statistically significant. There was a distinct overall survival advantage with CAFVP compared to intermittent CMFVP, but not to continuous CMFVP. The major side effects were similar in each regimen.

A summary of some additional selected randomized trials is given in Tables 28-12 and 28-13. When looked at in totality, the differences in response rates and duration of response and survival are not dramatic. They indicate some slight advantage for adding prednisone to CMF and for substituting Adriamycin for methotrexate.

Unfortunately, complete response (CR) is not common in advanced breast cancer after cytotoxic chemotherapy. When it does occur, long-term disease-free survival is also uncommon so that it is not meaningful to speak about cure with the current armamentarium of drugs. Decker et al.,[57] in reviewing the Mayo Clinic experience in 438 patients, treated on a range of protocol studies, reported that CR was observed in only 49 (11 percent). Of interest was the fact that the highest CR rate was seen with a single agent (Adriamycin at 20 percent) as

Table 28-11 CALGB* Study of CMFVP versus CAFVP

Treatment regimen	Number of evaluable patients	Percent (%) CR	PR	CR + PR	Median time to first response (weeks)	Median duration remission (months)	Median time to treatment failure (months)	Median survival (months)
CMFVP-C	86	9	41	50	3.3	9.0	9.0	16.0
CMFVP-I	109	11	39	50	4.0	7.0	8.0	13.0
CAFVP	107	15	56	71	4.3	14.0	11.0	19.0

*CALGB = Cancer and Leukemia Group B.

Table 28-12 Selected Randomized Trials Comparing Regimens Derived from the Original CMFVP Combination

Group	Treatment regimen	Number of patients	Percent CR + PR	Median duration of response (months)	Median survival (months)
Swiss group[44]	1. CMFVP	91	49	8.0	16.0
	2. CMP	78	43	7.3	15.4
ECOG[45]	1. CMF	90	49	5.3	14.8
	2. CMFP	88	59	8.5	18.0
	3. AV	178	53	8.0	13.0
Fox Chase[46]	1. CMF	39	49	11.5	--
	2. CAMF	39	62	12.5	--
CALGB * [47]	1. CMF	96	34	7.0	14.0
	2. CAF	80	54	13.5	24.0
	3. CAFVP	77	57	10.0	16.0
Milan[48,49]	1. CMF → AV	57	61	12.0	22.0
	2. AV → CMF	57	59	11.0	23.0
ECOG† [50]	1. CMF	46	56	7.6	12.4
	2. CMFP	47	70	6.0	19.3
	3. CMF → AV	50	58	12.4	18.2

* CALGB = Cancer and Leukemia Group B.
† ECOG = Eastern Cancer and Oncology Group.

against the various combinations they studied. Of the 49 in CR only, one remained continuously disease-free at the time of the report. The M.D. Anderson Hospital group[58] reviewed their experience of 619 women treated with Adriamycin-containing combinations. Their experience was that 116 (19 percent) achieved CR. Of these, 49 remained in CR more than 2 years, while 28 had relapsed a median of 19 months after cessation of treatment.

Several approaches have been undertaken to attempt to improve the results with combinations derived from the six major drugs:

1 Chemotherapy plus immunotherapy
2 Chemotherapy plus endocrine therapy
3 Sequential use of non-cross-resistant combinations

To date, none of these has been demonstrated to be superior to standard approaches, although clinical investigations still continue, particularly with the chemohormonal therapy approach. Nonspecific stimulation of the immune system with materials such as BCG, *Corynebacterium parvum*, methanol extraction residue of BCG (MER), and levamisole have all been disappointing. Every prospectively randomized trial has failed to reveal any increase in response rate, response duration, or survival when immunotherapy is added to chemotherapy. Recently Samal et al.[59] have reported that levamisole appears to lower survival when added to CMFP chemotherapy in comparison to CMFP alone (Fig. 28-2).

COMBINATION HORMONE AND CHEMOTHERAPY

The combination of chemotherapy and endocrine therapy has been conceptually attractive for a long time. Since these two modalities work through presumably different mechanisms

Table 28-13 Selected Randomized Trials Comparing Adriamycin-Containing Regimens

Group	Treatment regimen	Number of patients	Percent CR + PR	Median duration of response (months)	Median survival (months)
SWOG[51]	1. AC	105	42	5.5	15.3
	2. ACF	103	43	8.3	15.3
	3. ACFM	105	49	8.8	16.3
SWOG[52]	1. ACe	140	44	7.3	22.3
	2. FAC	160	48	13.0	21.0
	3. A + CMFVP	148	49	9.3	19.0
Yale[53]	1. AC	26	50	10.0	--
	2. AC → MF	22	55	10.0	--
SECSG[54]	1. CAF	40	63	7.0	--
	2. CAF → Cameleon	80	42	12.0	--
Mayo Clinic[55]	1. A + PAM	27	52	12.0	24.0
	2. CFP	23	48	16.0	22.0
	3. CFP → A + PAM	23	83		
NCI[56]	1. CAF	46	63	16.5	--
	2. DAV → CMF	48	71		--

NCI = National Cancer Institute.
SECSG = Southeastern Cancer Study Group.
SWOG = Southwest Oncology Group.

of action and do not have overlapping toxicity patterns, it has been hoped that their combined effects would be at least additive and hopefully synergistic. The possibility also exists that the two different mechanisms would combine together in an antagonistic fashion. Since the treatment of advanced breast cancer is a sequence of hormones and drugs, any evaluation of a combined approach must include a comparison with the sequence of the drugs and endocrine therapies in question. The most critical end point for that evaluation would be survival from onset of therapy within the context of overall survival, utilizing first diagnosis of metastatic disease as the zero point. The early results of clinical trials tend to focus mainly on the response rate, which may not be the most important issue in terms of treatment recommendations to the practicing oncologist. An increased response rate with the combination, which does not translate into a survival advantage over the sequence of the two components, may have little practical value.

Some selected randomized trials are outlined in Table 28-14. These trials do not make a convincing case for the combined approach utilizing the end point of survival. The heterogeneity of advanced breast cancer and its treatment make interstudy comparisons very difficult. The potential combinations of drugs plus hormones regarding the choice of components, as well as schedules and sequences, are practically unlimited. Only a few possibilities have been empirically tested.

The difficulty of interpretation of these trials can be seen in a trial of the CALGB,[67] which has studied CAF in a protocol testing the value of adding tamoxifen in postmenopausal women. This study entered patients from January 1980 until August 1982 and involved only women with first recurrence. Patients who had completed adjuvant chemotherapy greater

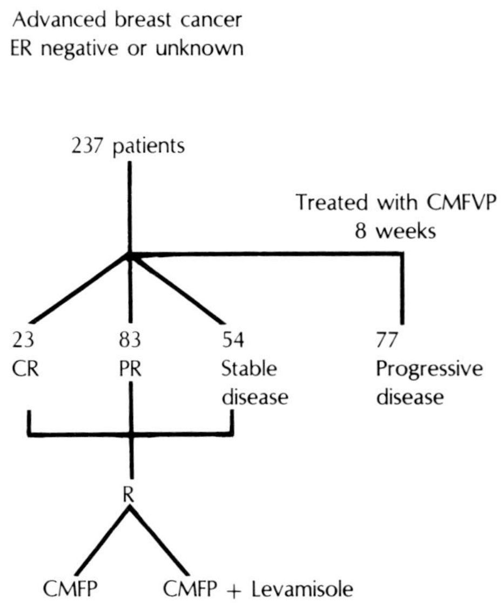

	CMFP	CMFP + Levamisole	
Median duration response (weeks)	29	18	$p = .04$
Median survival (weeks)	86	65	$p = .007$

Figure 28-2 The negative impact of chemoimmunotherapy maintenance with levamisole compared to chemotherapy alone.[59]

than 6 months prior to entry were eligible, provided it was their first documented recurrence. The patients were stratified by ER status, dominant site of metastatic disease, and by no prior therapy versus prior adjuvant chemotherapy.

A total of 246 patients were entered and 232 were evaluable for response. The overall response rate was 51 percent with CAF and 56 percent with CAF-T. The complete response rates were 15.5 percent and 14 percent, respectively. The projected median duration of response is 17.3 months with tamoxifen added and 14.6 months with chemotherapy alone. The response rate correlated with ER status is given in Table 28-15. No differences exist in the ER+ or ER− subgroups but in the ER unknown group, the response rate favors CMF-T, but appears due to an unexplainable lower response rate with CAF alone. The response rates were similar in women who had, and had not, required prior adjuvant chemotherapy (Table 28-16).

The concept of utilizing fixed sequences of non-cross-resistant combinations has been intuitively attractive to oncologists and has been empirically studied in breast cancer where it was felt enough active drugs existed to test the concept. In recent years, this approach has received additional hypothetical support by the mathematical models of Goldie and Coldman.[68] In breast cancer, the most frequently studied sequence has been CMF alternating with AV. The first to test this was the group of Bonadonna.[69] When all the data are evaluated,[70,71] there is no convincing evidence that this particular sequence meaningfully improves the therapeutic index over utilizing the two combinations in the usual sequential manner. The same is true for other sequences which have been tried (see Tables 28-12 and 28-13).

Table 28-14 Randomized Trials of Chemotherapy Plus Endocrine Therapy versus Chemotherapy Alone or Endocrine Therapy Alone

Group	Menopausal status	Treatment regimen	Number of patients	Percent CR + PR	Median duration of response (months)	Median survival (months)
EORTC[60]	Post	1. CMF	73	45	--	--
		2. CMF + T	77	70	--	--
SAKK[61]	Post	1. Chemotherapy + T	118	44	--	17.8
		2. T → Chemotherapy	113	40	--	25.6
Kiang et al.[62]	Post	1. DES	38	37	10	--
		2. DES + CF	48	67	10	--
Cocconi et al.[63]	Post	1. CMF	71	51	11.7	27.7
		2. CMF + T	62	74	12.7	19.5
Pellegrini[64] et al.	Post	1. VAC + MPA	88	49	>15	--
		2. VAC	89	47	15	--
SAKK[61]	Pre	1. 0 + Chemotherapy	42	57	--	22.5
		2. 0 → Chemotherapy	38	45	--	20.5
Mayo Clinic[65]	Pre	1. 0 + CFP	36	29	13.3	32.8
		2. 0 → CFP	36	25	4.3	22.0
CALGB[66]	Pre	1. 0 + CMFVP	53	72	17	26
		2. 0 + C	54	65	16	23
		3. 0 → CMFVP	38	18	5	30
Mayo Clinic[65]	Post	1. CMF → CMF + T	133	51	47 weeks	51 weeks
		2. CMF + T		74	111 weeks	78 weeks
CALGB[67]	Post	1. CAF	232	51	14.6	--
		2. CAF + T		56	17.3	--

CALGB = Cancer and Leukemia Group B.
EORTC = European Organization For Research and Treatment of Cancer.
SAKK = Swiss Chemotherapy Group.

CHEMOTHERAPY AND STAGE III BREAST CANCER

Despite the large number of women with breast cancer, the subset classified as having stage III disease is both the smallest and the most heterogeneous. Stage III disease can be a primary lesion larger than 5 cm with no involvement of axillary nodes ($T_3N_0M_0$). It can involve a primary lesion of any size with involvement of skin or chest wall. It can include those with inflammatory breast cancer. This encompasses a wide range of prognostic variables and potential for disease-free survival after local therapy.

The majority of patients with stage III disease ultimately develop metastatic disease despite the achievement of "local control." Because of this, chemotherapy has been integrated into the initial picture. This can involve several cycles of drugs given prior to radiotherapy and/or surgery as well as "adjuvant" type therapy given after local control procedures. The literature reports tend to be almost exclusively relatively small uncontrolled series because of the relatively low incidence of this subset. These small numbers, combined with the great heterogeneity within stage III, make these uncontrolled series difficult to evaluate in comparison

Table 28-15 CAF ± Tamoxifen in Advanced Breast Cancer: Response Rate Correlated with ER Status

	ER−				ER+				ER?			
Treatment regimen	No. Rx	No. CR	No. PR	Percent response	No. Rx	No. CR	No. PR	Percent response	No. Rx	No. CR	No. PR	Percent response
CAF - T	39	9	12	54	34	2	14	47	43	7	21	65
CAF	37	4	22	70	40	7	13	50	39	5	8	33

to each other. In addition, it is difficult to decide how they should be translated into everyday practice.

In any evaluation of a combined modality approach to stage III disease, it is important to conceptually separate the value of "local control" versus "systemic control." As Canellos[72] has recently pointed out, a review of literature in this area "leaves the reader with no definite conclusions as to the importance of local control." The morbidity of failure of local control is not easily discernible from the published papers, although the avoidance of this is the paramount goal of radiotherapeutic and surgical treatment. The potential for local failure is so different between $T_3N_0M_0$ versus $T_{1-2}N_3M_0$ disease that case selection becomes a dominant issue in the evaluation of therapeutic approaches.

Garewal et al.[73] have analyzed 130 patients with primary tumors larger than 5 cm derived from a natural history data bank, including patients from the University of Arizona, the Milan Cancer Institute, and the Royal Marsden Hospital. These 130 patients broke down into 112 with histologically involved axillary nodes and 18 without. Only two of the 18 patients without axillary involvement have relapsed so far, both with local-regional relapses at 11 and 22 months after surgery. This group ($T_3N_0M_0$) has a projected relapse-free survival superior to women with $T_{1-2}N{+}M_0$ disease in this analysis. Therefore, this small subset of stage III has an excellent prognosis and probably should not be included in trials of stage III patients.

The Milan Group[74,75] has been one of the pioneers in the use of chemotherapy as part of a combined modality attack against stage III disease. In their first study, they administered Adriamycin plus vincristine as initial treatment for women with T_{3b}–T_4 lesions. After four cycles of drug, they achieved a 70 percent response rate and then administered radiation therapy to achieve local control. Their three-year survival rate was 52 percent which was superior to their historical experience with x-ray alone. Their second study involved three cycles of the same regimen (Adriamycin plus vincristine) followed by a randomization to either x-ray or surgery. After local control therapy,

Table 28-16 CAF ± Tamoxifen: Response Rate Correlated with Prior Adjuvant Chemotherapy Treatment

	No Prior Adjuvant Chemotherapy				Prior Adjuvant Chemotherapy			
Treatment regimen	No. Rx	No. CR	No. PR	Percent response	No. Rx	No. CR	No. PR	Percent response
CAF - T	103	17	43	58	13	1	4	38
CAF	99	13	38	51	17	3	5	47

with either modality, seven further cycles of drug were administered. At last report, the two arms were similar with about 50 percent survival at 4 years. This study, of course, does not address the issue of what the drugs may be accomplishing.

At M.D. Anderson Hospital[76] the chemotherapy regimen used has been FAC plus the addition of BCG. They treated 52 women with $T_{3b}N_{2-3}$ lesions. They first gave three cycles of the chemoimmunotherapy. This was followed by either simple mastectomy or irradiation in a nonrandomized fashion. Subsequent to this, 2 years of chemotherapy was given with methotrexate substituting for Adriamycin when a critical total dose was reached. Their 5-year survival was 40 percent.

Summary

If the role of chemotherapy as part of a combined modality attack in stage III disease is ever to be properly determined, it will require collaborative multicenter trials which will bring in the large number of patients required to answer the critical questions within the framework of the heterogeneity of breast cancer in general, and of stage III disease in particular.

REFERENCES

1. McGuire WL, Clark GM: The prognostic role of progesterone receptors in human breast cancer. *Semin Oncol* 10:2, 1983.
2. Carter SK: Hormonal treatment of advanced breast cancer, in Carter SK, Glatstein E, Livingston RB (eds): *Principles of Cancer Treatment*. New York, McGraw-Hill, 1982, p. 342.
3. Gross GE, Clark GM, Chamness GC, McGuire WL: Multiple progesterone receptor assays in human breast cancer. *Cancer Res* 44:836, 1984.
4. Hull DF III, Clark GM, Osborne CK et al: Multiple estrogen receptor assays in human breast cancer. *Cancer Res* 43:413, 1983.
5. Lippman ME, Allegra JC, Thompson EB, Simon R, Barlock A, Green L, Huff KK, Do HMT, Aitken SC, Warren R: The relation between estrogen receptors and response rate to cytotoxic chemotherapy in metastatic breast cancer. *N Engl J Med* 298:1223, 1978.
6. Kiang DT, Frenning DH, Goldman AT, Ascensaŏ VF, Kennedy BJ: Estrogen receptors and responses to chemotherapy and hormonal therapy in advanced breast cancer. *N Engl J Med* 299:1330, 1978.
7. Jonat W, Maass H: Some comments on the necessity of receptor determination in human breast cancer. *Cancer Res* 38:4305, 1978.
8. Marsland TA, Rosenbaum C, Stollbach LL, Cohen JL: Estrogen receptors (ER) and chemotherapy (CT) in breast cancer. *Proc ASCO*, abstract 316, 1979, p. 367.
9. Chang JC, Hill GW, Wergorski G: Estrogen receptors and response to cyclophosphamide, methotrexate, and 5-fluorouracil (CMF) in advanced breast cancer. *Proc ASCO*, abstract 367, 1980, p. 411.
10. Rubens RD, King RJB: Oestrogen receptors and response to cytotoxic chemotherapy. *Proc ASCO*, abstract 52, 1979, p. 304.
11. Bonadonna G, DiFronzo G, Tancini G: Estrogen receptors (ER) and response to chemotherapy in advanced and early breast cancer. *Proc ASCO*, abstract 281, 1979, p. 359.
12. Levine RM, Lippman MF: Relationship between estrogen receptor proteins and response to chemotherapy in breast cancer, *Cancer Treat Rep* 68:573, 1984.
13. Kiang DT: Correlation between estrogen-receptor and response to chemotherapy in patients with breast cancer. *Center Treat Rep* 68:577, 1984.
14. Siebert K, Lippman ME: Hormone receptors in breast cancer. *Clin Oncol* 1:735, 1982.
15. Wells SA, Santen RJ: Ablative procedures in patients with metastatic breast cancer. *Cancer* 53:762, 1984.
16. Lippman M, Bolan G, Huff K: The effects of estrogens and antiestrogens on hormone responsive human breast cancer in long term tissue culture. *Cancer Res* 36:4595, 1976.
17. Ward HWC: Anti-oestrogen therapy for breast cancer: A trial of tamoxifen at low dose levels. *Br Med J* 1:13, 1983.
18. Tormey DC, Lippman ME, Edwards BK, Cas-

without fluoxymesterone in advanced breast cancer. *Ann Intern Med* 98:139, 1983.

19. Rose C, Theilade K, Boesen E et al: Treatment of advanced breast cancer with tamoxifen: Evaluation of the dose-response relationship at two dose levels. *Breast Cancer Res Treat* 2:395, 1982.
20. Patterson JS, Battershy LA, Edwards DG: Review of the clinical pharmacology and international experience with tamoxifen in advanced breast cancer. *Rev Endocrine Related Cancer* (suppl 9), 1982, p. 563.
21. Margreiter R, Weigele J: Tamoxifen (Nolvadex) for premenopausal patients with advanced breast cancer. *Breast Cancer Res Treat* 4:45, 1984.
22. Ingle JN, Ahmann DL, Green SJ et al: Randomized clinical trial of diethylstilbestrol versus tamoxifen in postmenopausal women with advanced breast cancer. *N Engl J Med* 304:16, 1981.
23. Stewart HJ, Forrest APM, Gunn JM et al: The tamoxifen trial: A double-blind comparison with stilboestrol in postmenopausal women with advanced breast cancer, in Mouridsen HT, Palshof T (eds): *Breast Cancer: Experimental and Clinical Aspects.* Oxford, Pergamon Press, 1980, p. 83.
24. Beex L, Pieters G, Smals A, Koenders A, Benraad T, Kloppenborg P: Tamoxifen versus ethinyl estradiol in the treatment of postmenopausal women with advanced breast cancer. *Cancer Treat Rep* 65:179, 1981.
25. Westerberg H: Tamoxifen and fluoxymesterone in advanced breast cancer. A controlled clinical trial. *Cancer Treat Rep* 64:117, 1980.
26. Powles TJ: The role of aromatase inhibitors in breast cancer. *Semin Oncol* 10:20, 1983.
27. Smith IE, Harris AL, Morgan M et al: Tamoxifen versus aminoglutethimide in advanced breast carcinoma: A randomized cross-over trial. *Br Med J* 283:1432, 1981.
28. Lipton A, Harvey HA, Santen RJ, et al: Randomized trial of aminoglutethimide versus tamoxifen in metastatic breast cancer. *Cancer Res* 42(suppl):3434s, 1982.
29. Ansfield FJ, Kallas GJ, Singson JP: Clinical results with megestrol acetate in patients with advanced carcinoma of the breast. *Surg Gynecol Obstet* 155:888, 1980.
30. Alexieva-Figusch J, Van Gilse AA, Hop WCJ et al: Progestin therapy in advanced breast cancer: Megestrol acetate, an evaluation of 160 treated cases. *Cancer* 46:2369, 1980.
31. Cooperative Breast Cancer Group: Results of studies by the Cooperative Breast Cancer Study Group 1961–1963. *Cancer Chemother Rep* 41(suppl):1, 1964.
32. Pannuti F, Martoni A, Lenaz GR et al: A possible new approach to the treatment of metastatic breast cancer: Massive doses of medroxyprogesterone acetate. *Cancer Treat Rep* 62:499, 1978.
33. Mattson W: A phase III trial of treatment with tamoxifen versus treatment with high-dose medroxyprogesterone acetate in advanced postmenopausal breast cancer, in Iacobelli S, DiMarco A (eds): *Role of Medroxyprogesterone in Endocrine-Related Tumors. Progress in Cancer Research and Therapy.* New York, Raven Press, 15:65, 1980.
34. Pannuti F, Martoni A, Fruet F, Burroni P, Canova N, Hall S: Oral high-dose medroxyprogesterone acetate versus tamoxifen in postmenopausal patients with advanced breast cancer, in Iacobelli S, Lippman ME, Robustelli Della Cuna G (eds): *The Role of Tamoxifen in Breast Cancer.* New York, Raven Press, 1982, p. 85.
35. Beretta G, Tabiadon D, Tedeschi L, Luporini G: Hormonotherapy of advanced breast cancer: Comparative evaluation of tamoxifen citrate versus medroxyprogesterone acetate, in Iacobelli S, Lippman ME, Robustelli Della Cuna G (eds): *The Role of Tamoxifen in Breast Cancer.* New York, Raven Press, 1982, p. 113.
36. Ingle JN, Ahmann DL, Green SJ: Randomized clinical trials of megestrol acetate versus tamoxifen in paramenopausal or castrated women with advanced breast cancer. *Am J Clin Oncol* 5:155, 1982.
37. Ross MB, Buzdar AV, Blumenschein GR: Treatment of advanced breast cancer with megestrol acetate after therapy with tamoxifen. *Cancer* 49:413, 1982.
38. Hoogstraaten B, George SL, Samal B et al: Combination chemotherapy and Adriamycin in patients with advanced breast cancer. *Cancer* 38:13, 1976.
39. Greenspan EM: Regression of metastatic hepatomegaly from mammary carcinoma. *NY State J Med* 64:2442, 1964.
40. Greenspan EM: Combination cytotoxic chemotherapy in advanced disseminated breast carcinoma. *J Mt Sinai Hosp* 33:1, 1966.

41. Cooper R: Combination chemotherapy in hormone resistant breast cancer. *Proc AACR* 10:15, 1969.
42. Smalley RV, Lefante J, Bartolucci A et al: A comparison of cyclophosphamide, Adriamycin, and 5-fluorouracil (CAF) and cyclophosphamide, methotrexate, 5-fluorouracil, vincristine and prednisone (CMFVP) in patients with advanced breast cancer. *Breast Cancer Res Treat* 3:209, 1983.
43. Tormey D, Weinberg VE, Leone LA et al: A comparison of intermittent vs. continuous and of Adriamycin vs. methotrexate 5-drug chemotherapy for advanced breast cancer. *Am J Clin Oncol* (CCT) 7:231, 1984.
44. Brunner KW, Sonntag RW, Martz G, Senn HJ, Obrecht P, Alberto P: A controlled study in the use of combined drug therapy for metastatic breast cancer. *Cancer* 36:1208, 1975.
45. Carbone PP, Bauer M, Band P, Tormey D: Chemotherapy of disseminated breast cancer: Current status and prospects. *Cancer* 39:2916, 1977.
46. Creech RH, Catalano RB, Harris DT, Engstrom PF, Grotzinger PJ: Low dose chemotherapy of metastatic breast cancer with cyclophosphamide, Adriamycin, methotrexate, 5-fluorouracil (CAMFP) versus sequential cyclophosphamide, methotrexate, 5-fluorouracil (CMF) and Adriamycin. *Cancer* 43:51, 1979.
47. Aisner J et al for CALGB: Chemoimmunotherapy for advanced breast cancer: A randomized comparison of 6 combinations (CMF, CAF vs. CAFVP) each with or without MER immunotherapy. A CALGB study (abstr. C-433). *Proc Am Soc Clin Oncol* 22:443, 1981.
48. Brambilla C, Valagussa P, Bonadonna G: Sequential combination chemotherapy in advanced breast cancer. *Cancer Chemother Pharmacol* 1:35, 1978.
49. Valagussa P, Brambilla C, Bonadonna G: Advanced breast cancer: Are the traditional stratification parameters still of value when patients are treated with combination chemotherapy? *Eur J Cancer* 15:565, 1977.
50. Tormey DC, Gelman R, Band P, Carbone P: Comparison of single to alternating combination therapy in metastatic breast cancer (abstr. 686). *Proc Am Assoc Cancer Res* 21:171, 1980.
51. Tranum B et al: Adriamycin in combination for the treatment of breast cancer: A Southwest Oncology Group Study. *Cancer* 41:2078, 1978.
52. Tranum B et al: Adriamycin combinations in advanced breast cancer. A Southwest Oncology Group Study. *Cancer* 49:835, 1982.
53. Kennealy GT et al: Combination chemotherapy for advanced breast cancer: Two regimens containing Adriamycin. *Cancer* 42:27, 1978.
54. Vogel CL, Lefante J, East D, Rogers B, Smalley R: Cyclophosphamide, Adriamycin and 5-fluorouracil (CAF) alternating with a cycle-active regimen in metastatic breast cancer: A randomized Southeastern Cancer Study Group Trial (abstr. C-417). *Am Soc Clin Oncol* 22:439, 1981.
55. Ahmann DL et al: Evaluation of a fixed alternating treatment in patients with advanced breast cancer. *Cancer Clin Trials* 1:219, 1978.
56. Tormey DC et al: A randomized comparison of two sequentially administered combination regimens to a single regimen in metastatic breast cancer. *Cancer Clin Trials* 2:247, 1979.
57. Decker DA, Ahmann RL, Bisel HF et al: Complete responders to chemotherapy in metastatic breast cancer. *JAMA* 242:2075, 1979.
58. Legha SS, Buzdar AV, Smith TL et al: Complete remissions in metastatic breast cancer treated with combination drug therapy. *Ann Intern Med* 91:847, 1979.
59. Samal BA, Foulkes MA, McDonald B: Levamisole probably shortens response and survival in CMFP-maintained advanced breast cancer patients. *Proc ASCO* 3:126, 1984.
60. Mouridsen HT, Palshof T, Engelsman E, Sylvester R: CMF versus CMF plus tamoxifen in advanced breast cancer in postmenopausal women. An EORTC trial, in Mouridsen HT, Palshof T (eds): *Breast Cancer. Experimental and Clinical Aspects.* Oxford, Pergamon Press, 1980, p. 119.
61. Cavalli F et al for the Swiss Group for Clinical Research (SAKK): Hormono-chemotherapy versus hormono-therapy followed by chemotherapy in the treatment of disseminated breast cancer, in Mouridsen HT, Palshof T (eds): *Breast Cancer. Experimental and Clinical Aspects.* Oxford, Pergamon Press, 1980, p. 119.
62. Kiang DT, Kennedy BJ: Chemoendocrine therapy of advanced breast cancer. *Breast Cancer Res Treat* 1:105, 1981.
63. Cocconi G, De Lisi V, Boni C, Mori M: CMF vs CMF plus tamoxifen (T) in postmenopausal metastatic breast cancer. A prospective randomized

study (abstr. C-287). *Proc Am Soc Clin Oncol* 1:75, 1982.

64. Pellegrini A et al: Vincristine, Adriamycin, cyclophosphamide (VAC) versus vincristine, Adriamycin, cyclophosphamide plus high dose medroxyprogesterone acetate (VAC + HD MPA): A randomized multinational clinical trial in metastatic breast cancer. *Proc XIII Intl Cancer Congress*, Seattle, 1982 (abstract 01629).
65. Ahmann DL, O'Connell MJ, Hahn RG, Bisel HF, Lee RA, Edmondson JH: An evaluation of early or delayed adjuvant chemotherapy in premenopausal patients with advanced breast cancer undergoing oophorectomy. *N Engl J Med* 297:356, 1977.
66. Falkson G, Falkson HC, Glidewell O, Weinberg V, Leone L, Holland JF: Improved remission rates and remission duration in young women with metastatic breast cancer following combined oophorectomy and chemotherapy. *Cancer* 43:2215, 1979.
67. Kardinal CG, Perry MC, Weinberg V et al: Chemoendocrine therapy vs. chemotherapy alone for advanced breast cancer in postmenopausal women. *Breast Cancer Res Treat* 3:365, 1983.
68. Goldie JH, Coldman AJ: A mathematical model for relating the drug sensitivity of tumors to their spontaneous mutation rate. *Cancer Treat Rep* 63:1727, 1979.
69. Brambilla C, Valagussa P, Bonadonna G: Sequential combination chemotherapy in advanced breast cancer. *Cancer Chemother Pharmacol* 1:35, 1978.
70. Ahmann DL, O'Fallen J, O'Connell MJ et al: Evaluation of a fixed alternating treatment in patients with advanced breast cancer. *Cancer Clin Trials* 1:219, 1978.
71. Tormey DC, Falkson G, Simon RM et al: A randomized comparison of two sequentially administered combination regimens to a single regimen in metastatic breast cancer. *Cancer Clin Trials* 2:247, 1979.
72. Canellos G: The treatment of locally advanced breast cancer. *J Clin Oncol* 2:149, 1984.
73. Garewal HS, Taksugi B, Jones G, et al: Is $T_3N_0M_0$ breast cancer with pathologically negative nodes truly stage III? *J Clin Oncol* 2:242, 1984.
74. DeLena M, Zucali R, Viganotti G, et al: Combined chemotherapy-radiotherapy approach in locally advanced (T_{3b}–T_4) breast cancer. *Cancer Chemother Pharmacol* 1:53, 1978.
75. DeLena M, Varini M, Zucali A, et al: Multimodal treatment for locally advanced breast cancer. *Cancer Clin Trials* 4:229, 1981.
76. Hortobagyi GN, Blumenschein GR, Spanos W, et al: Multimodal treatment of locoregionally advanced breast cancer. *Cancer* 51:763, 1983.

29

Hormone and Chemotherapy Selection of Specific Options

James N. Ingle, M.D.

INTRODUCTION

Hormone therapy plays an important role in the management of many women with metastatic breast cancer. These approaches have received high priority because of the generally lower morbidity compared with chemotherapy or surgical ablative procedures. Once metastatic, breast cancer is generally not curable. Even with aggressive chemotherapy programs, complete responses are seen in only about 10 to 20 percent of patients, and the vast majority of these patients eventually relapse and succumb to their cancer.[1] The general lack of curability of metastatic breast cancer with current treatment programs has stimulated much work in hormonal agents, combinations of hormonal agents, and the use of hormonal manipulations in combination with chemotherapy.

The reader must be aware of variability between studies in criteria for classification of patients (e.g., menopausal status) and in characteristics of patients studied especially as they relate to hormonal receptor status and prior therapy exposure.[2]

Commonly used additive hormonal agents are listed in Table 29-1. Those studied most intensively in the recent past include tamoxifen (an antiestrogen), aminoglutethimide (an aromatase inhibitor), and megestrol acetate and medroxyprogesterone acetate (progestins).

HORMONAL THERAPY IN POSTMENOPAUSAL WOMEN

Prior to the introduction of the newer hormonal agents (i.e., antiestrogens and aromatase inhibitors), estrogens and androgens were the agents most commonly used. The large nonrandomized study reported by the Committee on Research of the American Medical Association[3] found that estrogens produced a higher response rate in postmenopausal women

Table 29-1 Commonly Used Additive Hormonal Agents

Estrogens
Diethylstilbestrol (DES)
Ethinyl estradiol (EE_2)
Androgen
Fluoxymesterone
Progestins
Medroxyprogesterone acetate
Megestrol acetate
Antiestrogen
Tamoxifen
Corticosteroids
Variety of preparations
Aromatase inhibitor
Aminoglutethimide

than did androgens. This position was corroborated by several randomized trials (Table 29-2). Kennedy[4] found a higher response rate with diethylstilbestrol (DES) than with testosterone propionate. Kennedy and Brown[5] found that a combination of DES and testosterone propionate was not superior to DES alone, and again they found DES to be superior to testosterone. Ahmann et al.[6] found that the addition of a progestin to DES was not superior to DES alone. Thus, entering the decade of the 1970s, DES was generally considered to be the hormonal agent of choice for postmenopausal women with advanced breast cancer.

Comparative Trials of Estrogens or Androgens with Tamoxifen

Following phase II trials of tamoxifen, several comparative trials were performed comparing this agent with estrogens or androgens (Table 29-3). Two trials compared DES to tamoxifen in a prospective randomized fashion. Ingle et al.[7] and Stewart et al[8] both reported no statistically significant difference between the two agents, but less toxicity with tamoxifen. Tamoxifen was compared with ethinyl estradiol (EE_2) by Beex at al.[9] and they concluded that the two agents were equally effective but more side effects were found with the estrogenic agent. Tamoxifen was compared with fluoxymesterone by Westerberg,[10] and a higher response rate was found for patients treated with tamoxifen as well as a better survival for the patients treated with tamoxifen initially in this crossover trial.

On the basis of these four randomized trials, tamoxifen has generally been considered to be the preferred hormonal agent in postmenopausal women with advanced breast cancer.

Comparative Trials of Tamoxifen versus Aminoglutethimide

Two major trials have compared tamoxifen with aminoglutethimide (AG) (Table 29-4). Smith et al.[11] studied 117 women randomized between the two agents and found a 30 percent objective response rate for both agents and no significant difference in predicted median duration of response. Objective responses in osseous metastases, however, were seen more commonly in patients treated with AG (11 responses in 31 patients, 35 percent) than patients treated with tamoxifen (five responses in 29 patients, 17 percent). Toxicity was higher with AG in that seven (7 percent) of 97 patients receiving AG as initial or secondary crossover treatment required discontinuation of the drug. No patients treated with tamoxifen experienced toxicity requiring its discontinuation. It was concluded by these authors that both agents appeared to be equally effective.

Lipton et al.[12] found similar response rates for the two agents and, like Smith et al.,[11] found a higher response rate for AG in patients with osseous metastases but this difference was not statistically significant ($p = .10$). They also concluded that AG appears to be at least equivalent to tamoxifen in the management of postmenopausal women with advanced breast cancer, and suggested that site of involvement may be important in selection of therapy. It would appear, however, that in clinical practice the use of tamoxifen would be preferable to that of AG primarily because of the toxicity.

Table 29-2 Randomized Clinical Trials Involving Estrogens

Reference	Regimen (dose)	Number of evaluable patients	Response rate, % (CR + PR)	Comments
Kennedy[4]	Testosterone Propionate (100 mg IM three times per week) versus	59	10	Included patients castrated < 1 year and those 1 or more years after last menstrual period.
	Diethylstilbestrol (5 mg three times daily)	55	29	
Kennedy and Brown[5]	Testosterone Propionate (100 mg IM three times per week) versus	22	14	Included patients castrated < 1 year and those 1 or more years after last menstrual period. Study blinded.
	Diethylstilbestrol (5 mg three times daily) versus	22	45	
	Both	12	41	
Ahmann et al.[6]	Diethylstilbestrol (5 mg three times daily) versus	20	40	All patients > 5 years postmenopausal. No prior systemic therapy. Study blinded.
	Medrogestone (100 mg four times daily) versus	18	22	
	Both	19	37	

Comparative Trials of Tamoxifen versus Progestins

Because of phase II data showing efficacy of progestins, several trials have compared medroxyprogesterone acetate (MPA) and megestrol acetate to tamoxifen (Table 29-5). Mattsson et al.[13] compared high-dose IM MPA to tamoxifen and found relatively high response rates for both agents. Survival was reported to be approximately the same for the two regimens. They noted that MPA provided better subjective benefits than tamoxifen in terms of increased appetite, weight gain, and sense of well-being.

Pannuti et al.[14] compared high-dose MPA to tamoxifen and found a higher response rate for MPA, although this was not statistically significant. The objective remission duration was longer for patients treated with tamoxifen (15 months versus 5.5 months), but the median survivals were quite similar (tamoxifen, 14 months; MPA, 15 months). They also found that subjective benefit was observed more often in the MPA regimen.

Beretta et al.[15] examined oral MPA in a variety of doses against tamoxifen in their randomized trial. In addition to similar response rates, there appeared to be no significant difference in median response duration or survival.

Muss et al.[16] reported preliminary results of an ongoing randomized trial of tamoxifen versus megestrol acetate in women at least 5 years postmenopausal. At the time of their communication, 11 (29 percent) of 38 patients on megestrol acetate and seven (21 percent) of 34 patients on tamoxifen had achieved a response. Time to progression and survival were similar.

Ingle et al,[17] in a select group of women 1 to 5 years after the last menstrual period or

Table 29-3 Randomized Trials of Estrogens or Androgens versus Tamoxifen

Reference	Regimen (dose)	Number of evaluable patients	Response rate, % (CR + PR)	Comments
Ingle et al.[7]	Diethylstilbestrol (5 mg three times daily)	74	41	5 years or more from last menstrual period; no prior hormones; 31% had prior chemotherapy.
	versus			
	Tamoxifen (10 mg twice daily)	69	33	
Stewart et al.[8]	Diethylstilbestrol (5 mg three times daily)	27	22	More than 5 years from last menstrual period; no prior hormones or chemotherapy.
	versus			
	Tamoxifen (10 mg three times daily)	29	31	
Beex et al.[9]	Ethinyl estradiol (3 mg daily)	29	31	More than 2 years from last menstrual period; 12% had prior hormonal therapy; 15% had prior chemotherapy.
	versus			
	Tamoxifen (20 mg twice daily)	30	33	
Westerberg[10]	Fluoxymesterone (10 mg twice daily)	42	19	"Postmenopausal"; no prior hormones or chemotherapy.
	versus			
	Tamoxifen (20 mg twice daily)	37	30	

previously castrated, found no significant difference in response rates for the two agents, but a longer survival for those patients treated with megestrol acetate. They noted that this survival advantage was difficult to interpret given the results of analysis of response and time to treatment failure.

It is apparent that the precise role of progestins in management of women with advanced breast cancer needs further elucidation.

Comparative Trials of Tamoxifen Alone or Combined with Other Hormonal Agents

The concept of combination hormonal therapy has been evaluated in numerous clinical trials (Table 29-6). Tamoxifen alone or combined with DES was evaluated by Mouridsen et al,[18] and no superiority for the combination was identified. Tamoxifen alone was compared to tamoxifen plus prednisolone by Stewart et al.,[19] and a significantly higher response rate ($p <$ .01) and longer survival ($p < .025$; medians: 21 months versus 12 months) were found with the combination; however, further studies are needed to corroborate these findings because of the relatively low response rate observed with tamoxifen alone.

Tormey et al.[20] compared tamoxifen alone to tamoxifen plus fluoxymesterone. In this phase I and II trial the dosage level of tamoxifen varied from 2 to 100 mg/m^2 twice daily. The response rate for the combination was significantly better, as was the time to treatment failure. Survival for the two groups, however, was not significantly different. The superiority of this combination approach needs confirmation in a randomized trial utilizing a fixed dose of tamoxifen.

Mouridsen et al.[21] found no significant difference between tamoxifen alone or in combination

Table 29-4 Randomized Trials of Tamoxifen versus Aminoglutethimide

Reference	Regimen (dose)	Number of evaluable patients	Response rate, % (CR + PR)	Comments
Smith et al.[11]	Tamoxifen (10 mg twice daily)	60	30	Included premenopausal (9% patients), perimenopausal, postmenopausal patients; 26% had prior hormonal therapy; 38% had prior chemotherapy.
	versus			
	AG (250 mg three times daily for 2 weeks then four times daily) plus Hydrocortisone (20 mg twice daily)	57	30	
Lipton et al.[12]	Tamoxifen (20 mg twice daily)	39	38	"Menopausal or castrate"; 41% had prior hormonal therapy.
	versus			
	AG (250 mg twice daily for 2 weeks then four times daily) plus Hydrocortisone (100 mg daily in divided doses for 2 weeks then 40 mg daily in divided doses)	36	36	

AG = Aminoglutethimide.

with medroxyprogesterone acetate (MPA). It should be noted that the MPA dose utilized was low—100 mg per day orally.

Powles et al.[22] performed a large randomized trial of tamoxifen plus aminoglutethimide plus hydrocortisone plus danazol (TAD), or tamoxifen alone initially followed by the other two agents, in sequence if possible. Evaluable for response were 198 patients; objective responses were seen more often in the TAD patients (43 percent) than in those treated initially with tamoxifen alone (31 percent). Unfortunately, this high response rate did not translate into either a longer time to disease progression or survival.

Ingle et al.[23] presented preliminary results of an ongoing randomized trial of tamoxifen alone or combined with aminoglutethimide. Although the response rate was higher for the combination regimen, the data were too preliminary for any firm conclusions.

Garcia-Giralt et al.[24] randomized patients to tamoxifen alone or sequential tamoxifen for 15 days alternating with MPA for 15 days. The response rate was higher for the sequential approach, but not statistically significant. The duration of response favored the sequential approach (medians: 25 + months versus 9.5 months); but, unfortunately, no significant difference in terms of survival was noted.

Several studies of combination hormonal therapy involving tamoxifen have provided provocative data and, in view of the apparent advantage of adding prednisone or fluoxymesterone, further work is indicated in this area.

HORMONAL THERAPY ALONE OR COMBINED WITH CHEMOTHERAPY IN POSTMENOPAUSAL PATIENTS

Several studies have addressed the question of whether or not therapeutic gain can be achieved by the addition of chemotherapy to tamoxifen. Cavalli et al.[25] performed an excellent large randomized trial involving 297 evaluable postmenopausal patients with metastatic breast cancer who had not received prior systemic therapy. These patients were randomized to receive either tamoxifen alone (in which chemotherapy was started after 6 weeks unless an objective

Table 29-5 Randomized Trials of Tamoxifen versus Progestins

Reference	Regimen (dose)	Number of evaluable patients	Response rate, % (CR + PR)	Comments
Mattsson et al.[13]	Tamoxifen (10 mg three times daily) versus	33	52	Older than 50 years; 16% had prior hormonal therapy; 44% had prior chemotherapy.
	MPA (1000 mg intramuscularly every day for 30 days and then weekly)	30	70	
Pannuti et al.[14]	Tamoxifen (10 mg twice daily) versus	26	27	More than 1 year postmenopausal or castrated; only one patient had prior hormonal therapy; 13% had prior chemotherapy.
	MPA (1000 mg orally twice daily for 30 days then for 15 days a month)	27	37	
Beretta et al.[15]	Tamoxifen (20 mg daily) versus	39	28	"Postmenopausal"; "three-fourths" had "other antitumor treatments."
	MPA (400–1200 mg/day orally; median dose: 600 mg)	40	25	
Ingle et al.[17]	Tamoxifen (10 mg twice daily) versus	27	26	One to less than 5 years postmenopausal or castrated (51%); no prior additive hormonal therapy;
	MA (50 mg/m^2 three times daily)	28	14	

MPA = Medroxyprogesterone acetate; MA = megestrol acetate.

regression had occurred) or tamoxifen plus chemotherapy. The chemotherapy program utilized was determined by further randomization to one of three regimens considered "minimal, conventional, or maximal." The overall response rates were quite similar, being 33 percent in the group treated initially with tamoxifen alone and 40 percent in the group treated with concurrent chemohormonal therapy. Survival was somewhat better in the group treated with tamoxifen alone initially (median survival: 27.5 months versus 23.7 months) but there was no significant difference overall. These investigators identified 80 patients who were considered to have good prognostic factors from a clinical standpoint, and they found that survival was significantly better in those who received sequential treatments beginning with tamoxifen alone initially. They concluded that postmenopausal patients should probably be treated initially with a trial of hormonal therapy; chemotherapy should be used for patients in whom hormonal therapy fails.

Glick et al.[26] treated 89 postmenopausal patients with a 12-week induction program of tamoxifen alone. The estrogen receptor status was either positive or unknown. Following this induction period, patients without disease progression were randomized to either continue treatment with tamoxifen alone or to tamoxifen plus combination chemotherapy with cyclophosphamide, methotrexate, and 5-fluorouracil. There were no survival differences between the patients in the two treatment groups, and the authors concluded that the addition of chemotherapy offered no benefit to these patients.

Bezwoda et al.[27] examined a subset of patients known to be estrogen receptor-positive. These patients were randomized to either tamoxifen alone followed by chemotherapy (with cyclophosphamide, methotrexate, and 5-fluorouracil) at the time of disease progression or the use of both modalities initially. Response rates and survivals for the two groups were similar, thus no advantage was demonstrated for the addition of chemotherapy to the initial treatment regimen.

These three studies[25–27] utilizing tamoxifen would appear to provide a reasonable basis for the choice of hormonal therapy alone rather than chemohormonal therapy as initial treatment for postmenopausal women. The exception to this practice would be those patients who were clinically not candidates for a hormonal manipulation alone because of sites, extent, or tempo of disease progression, or because of known lack of hormonal receptors. Whether this statement is true for all hormonal agents is a matter of debate. Kiang and Kennedy[28] have recently reported that they found a survival benefit, with a *p* value approaching .05, from combined chemohormonal therapy in a subset of patients with "ER-rich tumors." In their study, 22 patients were randomized to DES plus cyclophosphamide plus 5-fluorouracil; 19 patients were randomized to DES initially followed by the two chemotherapeutic agents upon disease progression.

Although the numbers of patients involved in this trial are quite small, the results do point out that generalizations based on the tamoxifen data with regard to chemohormonal therapy may be incorrect. One would expect that future work in utilizing hormones to manipulate tumor cell kinetics, as will be discussed below, will lead to more effective combined chemohormonal therapy.

Sequencing of Hormonal Agents in Chemotherapy

The most provocative data at present relate to laboratory and clinical observations with respect to the use of sequencing for hormonal agents in breast cancer. Lippman et al.[29] noted that in MCF-7 human breast cancer cells physiologic concentrations of estradiol stimulate cell division, whereas tamoxifen is inhibitory. This inhibitory effect of tamoxifen was reversible by addition of estradiol. In one experiment they demonstrated that estradiol was able to "rescue" cells previously incubated with tamoxifen such that thymidine incorporation rose to levels higher than both control and estradiol-treated cells. Osborne[30] has outlined the hypothesis that the interaction between hormone and chemotherapy in a clinical setting may result in an adverse effect on cell kill. He and his group have shown that tamoxifen causes endocrine-responsive MCF-7 cells to accumulate in G_1 phase and that this transition delay is dose-dependent.[31,32] Because some cytotoxic agents have not been effective against cells in prolonged G_1 phase, this alteration in cell kinetics may decrease the effectiveness of chemotherapy.

Two investigators have taken the lead in examining the sequencing concept. Lippman et al.[33] randomized patients to either a four-drug chemotherapy program alone (cyclophosphamide and doxorubicin on day 1 and 5-fluorouracil and methotrexate 1 week later in a 21-day cycle), or this chemotherapy combined with tamoxifen (20 mg/m^2 on days 2 to 6) and Premarin (0.625 mg every 12 h for three doses beginning on day 7). Although the response rates were identical, they found that, among patients with a partial response, the times to progression and survival were significantly longer for patients who received the chemohormonal therapy approach. Allegra[34] examined this concept using a somewhat different treatment scheme and chemotherapy program. This approach involved 18-day cycles consisting of tamoxifen (10 mg) for 10 days, followed by Premarin (0.625 mg twice daily) for 4 days, followed by moderately high-dose methotrexate, then 5-fluorouracil and leucovorin rescue. In this phase II trial 32 patients were evaluable and the overall response rate was 69 percent. Of greatest note, however, is that 15 patients (47 percent) achieved a complete remission. The favorable characteristics of these patients were noted but the high proportion of complete responders would support further attention to this approach.

Much is yet to be learned regarding usefulness of hormonal agents for altering cell kinetics in breast cancers, and one can expect much additional work in this area. For example, Rosso et al.[35] showed that DES can recruit resting breast cancer cells even in the case of receptor-negative breast cancers. A lack of substantial improvements in efficacy with the empirical approaches previously noted indicates the need for carefully designed trials in this area, utilizing information obtained from these more basic studies.

Table 29-6 Randomized Trials of Tamoxifen Alone or Combined with Other Hormonal Agents

Reference	Regimen (dose)	Number of evaluable patients	Response rate, % (CR + PR)	Comments
Mouridsen et al.[18]	Tamoxifen (10 mg three times daily)	65	39	> 6 months after last menstrual period, > 3 months after surgical castration, > 6 months after radiation castration; no prior additive hormonal therapy; 40% had prior chemotherapy.
	vs			
	Tamoxifen (10 mg three times daily) plus Diethylstilbestrol (1 mg three times daily)	57	37	
Stewart et al.[8]	Tamoxifen (10 mg twice daily)	72	13	≥ 6 months since last menstrual period, ≥ 50 years if hysterectomy without oophorectomy; no prior endocrine therapy; 19% had prior chemotherapy.
	vs			
	Tamoxifen (10 mg twice daily) plus Prednisolone (5 mg twice daily)	73	36	
Tormey et al.[20]	Tamoxifen (2-100 mg/m^2 twice daily)	52	15	Included premenopausal (6% of patients), castrated, and naturally postmenopausal patients; 60% had prior hormonal therapy and 85% had prior chemotherapy.
	vs			
	Tamoxifen (2-100 mg/m^2 twice daily) plus Fluoxymesterone (7 mg/m^2 twice daily)	56	38	
Mouridsen et al.[21]	Tamoxifen (10 mg three times daily)	45	44	> 6 months after last menstrual period, > 3 months after surgical castration; 67% had prior chemotherapy; > 6 months after radiation castration.
	vs			
	Tamoxifen (10 mg three times daily) plus Medroxyprogesterone acetate (100 mg orally every day)	55	26	
Powles et al.[22]	Tamoxifen (10 mg twice daily)	57	33	More than 1 year postmenopausal; 8% had prior hormonal therapy; 10% had prior chemotherapy.
	vs			
	Tamoxifen (10 mg twice daily) plus Aminoglutethimide (250 mg three times daily) plus Hydrocortisone (20 mg twice daily) plus Danazol (100 mg three times daily)	50	50	

Table 29-6 Randomized Trials of Tamoxifen Alone or Combined with Other Hormonal Agents *(continued)*

Reference	Regimen (dose)	Number of evaluable patients	Response rate, % (CR + PR)	Comments
Ingle et al.[20]	Tamoxifen (10 mg twice daily)	27	26	More than 1 year postmenopausal or castrated; 18% had prior hormonal therapy; 38% had prior chemotherapy.
	vs			
	Tamoxifen (10 mg twice daily) plus Aminoglutethimide (125 mg four times daily for 2 weeks then 250 mg four times daily) plus Hydrocortisone (100 mg daily in divided doses for 2 weeks then 40 mg daily in divided doses)	28	39	
Garcia-Giralt et al.[24]	Tamoxifen (20 mg/m² daily)	44	48	No prior additive hormonal therapy.
	vs			
	Tamoxifen (20 mg/m² daily for 15 days) then medroxyprogesterone acetate (350 mg/m² orally for 15 days)	35	60	

HORMONAL THERAPY IN PREMENOPAUSAL WOMEN

At the present time, oophorectomy remains the standard hormonal treatment in premenopausal women with advanced breast cancer. Stoll's review[36] of major reports on surgical castration shows response rates ranging from 24.5 to 37 percent. McGuire et al.[37] found that 65 percent responded to castration in a pooled series of patients known to be estrogen receptor-positive.

Several additive hormonal agents have been utilized recently in premenopausal women with advanced breast cancer. Two larger studies dealing with the use of tamoxifen have demonstrated efficacy. Pritchard et al.[38] reported a phase II trial of tamoxifen (20 mg twice daily) and found that 13 (32 percent) of 42 evaluable patients achieved complete or partial response. Of the 13 patients who had disease progression without a response on tamoxifen, none responded to subsequent oophorectomy; whereas six of eight patients with complete or partial response or stability on tamoxifen did have a response to subsequent oophorectomy.

Hoogstraten et al.[39] utilized tamoxifen in a dose of 10 mg twice daily and found that 14 (37 percent) of 38 evaluable patients achieved an objective response. In their study, none of the 14 prior tamoxifen responders had a response to oophorectomy.

Tamoxifen has been shown to induce responses in premenopausal women with advanced breast cancer. It has not been established what its relative efficacy is compared with bilateral oophorectomy. Clearly, such a study needs to be done before tamoxifen can be considered a replacement for the surgical procedure in clinical practice.

Provocative data have recently been published by Harvey et al.,[40] in which they utilized a gonadotropin-releasing hormone analogue (Leuprolide) and found a 44 percent partial regression rate in 25 premenopausal patients. This class of drugs will certainly receive further attention.

A number of investigators have examined the concept of adding chemotherapy to oophorectomy in premenopausal patients (Table 29-7). Ahmann et al.[41] randomized patients to either oophorectomy alone with delayed CFP chemotherapy (cyclophosphamide, 5-fluorouracil, prednisone) given at time of disease progression, or the use of this chemotherapy beginning 3 weeks after oophorectomy. Time of progression was significantly longer for the group of patients receiving both modalities than for those undergoing oophorectomy alone. However, when one considers time of progression following both oophorectomy and chemotherapy, the progression curves for the two treatment approaches are nearly identical. In addition, a log-rank test of the equality of survival distributions showed no significant difference ($p = .91$). Thus, in this study there did not appear to be an advantage to the routine use of chemotherapy following oophorectomy.

Falkson et al.[42] reported improved response rates and response duration with the use of chemotherapy in addition to oophorectomy, but again there was no survival advantage. Rossof,[43] in a small series of premenopausal patients randomized to either oophorectomy alone or oophorectomy plus chemotherapy, also found no survival advantage for the addition of chemotherapy. Cavalli et al.[25] randomized 109 premenopausal patients to either oophorectomy alone followed by chemotherapy or both modalities together. The chemotherapy regimen employed was randomly allocated to one of three different regimens representing "minimal, conventional, or intensive program." The overall response rate was 46 percent in the concurrent group and 43 percent in the sequential treatment approach. Of note is that

Table 29-7 Trials Comparing Oophorectomy Alone or Combined with Chemotherapy (See Text)

Reference	Schema		Number of evaluable patients
Ahmann et al.[41]	Oophorectomy fail ——→	CFP	39
	versus		
	Oophorectomy plus CFP		37
Falkson et al.[42]	Oophorectomy plus VPCMF		54
	versus		
	Oophorectomy plus C		56
	versus		
	Oophorectomy If progression after response, or stable, or progression after 4 weeks, then VPCMF		38
Rossof et al.[43]	Oophorectomy No progression at 12 weeks →	CMF	20
		Observation	14
Cavalli et al.[25]	Oophorectomy plus chemotherapy*		55
	versus		
	Oophorectomy If no response at 6–8 weeks, then chemotherapy		54

* Randomization to one of three chemotherapy regimens (LMFP or LMP/FVP or LMFP/D).
C = Cyclophosphamide, F = 5-fluorouracil, P = prednisone, V = vincristine, M = methotrexate, L = chlorambucil, D = doxorubicin.

the overall survival was not significantly different between the two treatment approaches (i.e., median survivals of 25.3 months for the concurrently treated patients and 21.0 months for the sequential approach, $p = .29$).

Hormonal receptor data were not available in these studies and it is not clear if there are subsets in which a chemohormonal therapy approach might be advantageous. It is clear, however, that no survival advantage has been demonstrated in any of these studies for the addition of chemotherapy to an oophorectomy.

TRIALS COMPARING MAJOR ENDOCRINE ABLATION WITH TAMOXIFEN OR AMINOGLUTETHIMIDE

Major endocrine ablations have established efficacy in the management of metastatic breast cancer, and this topic has been recently reviewed[44]. Several trials have been performed comparing tamoxifen or aminoglutethimide (AG) in a randomized setting with a major endocrine ablation. Kiang et al.[45] performed a randomized trial with a crossover design in 26 patients comparing tamoxifen (20 mg twice daily) with a transsphenoidal hypophysectomy. There were no significant differences in response rates or durations of response between the two treatment regimens in the initial treatment phase. However, the authors concluded that the sequence of hypophysectomy followed by tamoxifen was preferable.

Nemoto et al.[46] performed a randomized trial with a crossover design comparing tamoxifen (10 mg twice daily) with a surgical adrenalectomy in 51 patients who were either postmenopausal or postoophorectomy. Although the response rates were somewhat higher in the adrenalectomy group (52 percent) than in the tamoxifen group (35 percent), this was not statistically significant. Also, the overall response rates (i.e., response to one or both treatment modalities) for the different sequences and the overall survival of the two groups were not significantly different.

Harvey et al.[47] randomized 35 patients to either a transsphenoidal hypophysectomy or AG. The response rates were 21 percent and 47 percent, respectively, and the authors concluded that AG offers an acceptable alternative to hypophysectomy in women with metastatic breast cancer.

Santen et al.[48] randomized 96 patients, 69 of whom were evaluable to either AG or surgical adrenalectomy. They found objective response rates in 53 and 45 percent respectively, and concluded that AG can be chosen as a treatment modality in place of a surgical adrenalectomy.

The relatively small sample sizes in these studies do impose limitations on conclusions which can be drawn. However, the results of these trials have provided a basis for emphasis on the use of additive hormonal approaches rather than major endocrine ablations.

CONCLUSION

Hormonal therapy is still the mainstay of systemic therapy for women with advanced breast cancer. At present, it would appear that hormonal manipulations alone are preferable for the initial treatment of most patients with metastatic breast cancer. The exception to this practice would be those patients who are clinically not candidates for hormonal therapy because of sites, extent, or tempo of disease, or because of known absence of hormonal receptors.

Whether the use of hormonal agents in combination will result in increased efficacy remains to be seen. Further work is clearly needed on the use of hormonal agents as manipulators of tumor-cell kinetics to improve the effectiveness of cytotoxic chemotherapy programs. The information obtained from the laboratory should be taken into account in the design of future-generation clinical trials. With such an approach, we may be optimistic about improving the efficacy of systemic therapy approaches for the treatment of women with advanced breast cancer.

REFERENCES

1. Decker DA, Ahmann DL, Bisel HF, Edmonson JH, Hahn RG, O'Fallon JR: Complete responders to chemotherapy in metastatic breast cancer. Characterization and analysis. *JAMA* 242:2075, 1979.
2. Ingle JN: Additive hormonal therapy in women with advanced breast cancer. *Cancer* 53:766, 1984.
3. Council on Drugs: Androgens and estrogens in the treatment of disseminated mammary carcinoma: Retrospective study of 944 patients. *JAMA* 172:1271, 1960.
4. Kennedy BJ: Diethylstilbestrol versus testosterone propionate therapy in advanced breast cancer. *Surg Gynecol Obstet* 120:1246, 1965.
5. Kennedy BJ, Brown JH: Combined estrogenic and androgenic hormone therapy in advanced breast cancer. *Cancer* 18:431, 1965.
6. Ahmann DL, Hahn RG, Bisel HF: Disseminated breast cancer: Evaluation of hormonal therapy utilizing stilbestrol and medrogestone (AY-62022) singly and in combination. *Cancer* 30:651, 1972.
7. Ingle JN et al: Randomized clinical trial of diethylstilbestrol versus tamoxifen in postmenopausal women with advanced breast cancer. *N Engl J Med* 304:16, 1981.
8. Stewart HJ et al: The tamoxifen trial: A double-blind comparison with stilboestrol in postmenopausal women with advanced breast cancer, in Mouridsen HT, Palshof T (eds): *Breast Cancer: Experimental and Clinical Aspects.* Oxford, Pergamon Press, 1980, p. 83.
9. Beex L, Pieters G, Smals A, Koenders A, Benraad T, Kloppenborg P: Tamoxifen versus ethinyl estradiol in the treatment of postmenopausal women with advanced breast cancer. *Cancer Treat Rep* 65:179, 1981.
10. Westerberg H: Tamoxifen and fluoxymesterone in advanced breast cancer: A controlled clinical trial. *Cancer Treat Rep* 64:117, 1980.
11. Smith IE et al: Tamoxifen versus aminoglutethimide in advanced breast carcinoma: A randomized cross-over trial. *Br Med J* 283:1432, 1981.
12. Lipton A et al: Randomized trial of aminoglutethimide versus tamoxifen in metastatic breast cancer. *Cancer Res* 42(suppl):3434s, 1982.
13. Mattsson W, Von Eyben F, Hallsten L, Tennvall L: A trial of tamoxifen versus high-dose medroxyprogesterone acetate in advanced postmenopausal breast cancer: A final report. *Excerpta Med Int Congr Ser* 611:276, 1982.
14. Pannuti F, Martoni A, Fruet F, Burroni P, Canova N, Hall S: Oral high-dose medroxyprogesterone acetate versus tamoxifen in postmenopausal patients with advanced breast cancer, in Iacobelli S, Lippman ME, Robustelli Della Cuna G (eds): *The Role of Tamoxifen in Breast Cancer.* New York, Raven Press, 1982, p. 85.
15. Beretta G, Tabiadon D, Tedeschi L, Luporini G: Hormonotherapy of advanced breast cancer: Comparative evaluation of tamoxifen citrate versus medroxyprogesterone acetate, in Iacobelli S, Lippman ME, Robustelli Della Cuna G (eds): *The Role of Tamoxifen in Breast Cancer.* New York, Raven Press, 1982, p. 113.
16. Muss HB et al: Megestrol acetate (M) versus tamoxifen in postmenopausal women with advanced breast cancer: A prospective randomized trial of the Piedmont Oncology Association (POA) (abstract). *Breast Cancer Res Treat* 3:323, 1983.
17. Ingle JN et al: Randomized clinical trial of megestrol acetate versus tamoxifen in paramenopausal or castrated women with advanced breast cancer. *Am J Clin Oncol* (CCT) 5:155, 1982.
18. Mouridsen HT et al: Therapeutic effect of tamoxifen versus combined tamoxifen and diethylstilboestrol in advanced breast cancer in postmenopausal women, in Mouridsen HT, Palshof T (eds): *Breast Cancer: Experimental and Clinical Aspects.* Oxford, Pergamon Press, 1980, p. 107.
19. Stewart JF et al: Contribution of prednisone to the primary endocrine treatment of advanced breast cancer. *Eur J Cancer Clin Oncol* 18:1307, 1982.
20. Tormey DC, Lippman ME, Edwards BK, Cassidy JG: Evaluation of tamoxifen doses with and without fluoxymesterone in advanced breast cancer. *Ann Intern Med* 98:139, 1983.
21. Mouridsen HT, Palshof T, Rose C: Therapeutic effect of tamoxifen alone versus tamoxifen in combination with gestagen and oestrogen in advanced breast cancer, in Henningsen B, Linder F, Steichele C (eds): *Endocrine Treatment Of Breast Cancer: A*

New Approach. Recent Results in Cancer Research. Berlin, Springer-Verlag, 71:169, 1980.

22. Powles TJ et al: Treatment of disseminated breast cancer with tamoxifen, aminoglutethimide, hydrocortisone, and danazol used in combination or sequentially, *Lancet* 1(8391):1369, 1984.
23. Ingle JN et al: Progress report on two clinical trials in women with advanced breast cancer. Trial 1: Tamoxifen versus tamoxifen plus aminoglutethimide. Trial II: Aminoglutethimide in patients with prior tamoxifen exposure. *Cancer Res* 42(suppl):3461s, 1982.
24. Garcia-Giralt E et al: Sequential administration of tamoxifen and medroxyprogesterone acetate in disseminated breast cancer (abstract). *Proc ASCO* 3:129, 1984.
25. Cavalli F et al: Concurrent or sequential use of cytotoxic chemotherapy and hormone treatment in advanced breast cancer: Report of the Swiss Group for Clinical Cancer Research. *Br Med J* 286:5, 1983.
26. Glick JH et al: Tamoxifen plus sequential CMF chemotherapy versus tamoxifen alone in postmenopausal patients with advanced breast cancer: A randomized trial. *Cancer* 45:735, 1980.
27. Bezwoda WR, Derman D, de Moor NG, Lange M, Levin J: Treatment of metastatic breast cancer in estrogen receptor positive patients: A randomized trial comparing tamoxifen alone versus tamoxifen plus CMF. *Cancer* 50:2747, 1982.
28. Kiang DT, Kennedy BJ: Survival data of chemoendocrine therapy in advanced breast cancer (abstract). *Proc ASCO* 3:119, 1984.
29. Lippman M, Bolan G, Huff K: The effects of estrogens and antiestrogens on hormone-responsive human breast cancer in long-term tissue culture. *Cancer Res* 36:4595, 1976.
30. Osborne CK: Combined chemo-hormonal therapy in breast cancer: A hypothesis. *Breast Cancer Res Treat* 1:121, 1981.
31. Osborne CK, Boldt DH, Clark GM, Trent JM: Effects of tamoxifen on human breast cancer cell cycle kinetics: Accumulation of cells in early G_1 phase. *Cancer Res* 43:3583, 1983.
32. Osborne CK, Boldt DH, Estrada P: Human breast cancer cell cycle synchronization by estrogen and antiestrogens in culture. *Cancer Res* 44:1433, 1984.
33. Lippman ME, Cassidy J, Wesley M, Young RC: A randomized attempt to increase the efficacy of cytotoxic chemotherapy in metastatic breast cancer by hormonal synchronization. *J Clin Oncol* 2:28, 1984.
34. Allegra JC: Methotrexate and 5-fluorouracil following tamoxifen and Premarin in advanced breast cancer. *Semin Oncol* 10(no.2, suppl. 2):23, 1983
35. Rosso R et al: Presurgical cytokinetic chemotherapy in locally advanced breast cancer (abstract). *Proc Int Conf Adjuvant Therapy Cancer.* Tucson, Arizona, March 21–24, 1984, p.85.
36. Stoll BA: Castration and oestrogen therapy, in Stoll BA (ed): *Endocrine Therapy in Malignant Disease.* London, W.E. Saunders, 139, 1972.
37. McGuire WL, Carbone PP, Sears ME, Escher GC: Estrogen receptors in human breast cancer: An overview, in McGuire WL, Carbone PP, Vollmer EP (eds): *Estrogen Receptors in Human Breast Cancer.* New York, Raven Press, 1975, p. 1.
38. Pritchard KI, Thomson DB, Myers RE, Sutherland DJA, Mobbs BG, Meakin JW: Tamoxifen therapy in premenopausal patients with metastatic breast cancer. *Cancer Treat Rep* 64:787, 1980.
39. Hoogstraten B et al: Tamoxifen and oophorectomy in the treatment of recurrent breast cancer. *Cancer Res* 42:4788, 1982.
40. Harvey HA, Lipton A, Max DT, Pearlman HG, Diaz-Perches R, de la Garza J: Effective medical castration produced by the GnRH analog leuprolide in metastatic breast cancer (abstract). *Proc ASCO* 3:111, 1984.
41. Ahmann DL et al: An evaluation of early or delayed adjuvant chemotherapy in premenopausal patients with advanced breast cancer undergoing oophorectomy: A later analysis. *Am J Clin Oncol* 5:355, 1982.
42. Falkson G et al: Improved remission rates and remission duration in young women with metastatic breast cancer following combined oophorectomy and chemotherapy. *Cancer* 43:2215, 1979.
43. Rossof AH, Gelman R, Creech RH: Randomized evaluation of combination chemotherapy vs observation alone following response or stabilization after oophorectomy for metastic breast cancer in premenopausal women. *Am J Clin Oncol* 5:253, 1982.
44. Badellino F, Canavese G, Margarino G: Endocrine surgery in breast cancer, in Leclerq G, Toma S, Paridaens R, Heuson JC (eds): *Clinical Interest of*

Steroid Hormone Receptors in Breast Cancer. Recent Results in Cancer Research. Berlin, Springer-Verlag, 91:222, 1984.

45. Kiang DT, Frenning DS, Vosika GJ, Kennedy BJ: Comparison of tamoxifen and hypophysectomy in breast cancer treatment. *Cancer* 45:1322, 1980.
46. Nemoto T, Patel J, Rosner D, Dao TL: Tamoxifen (Nolvadex) versus adrenalectomy in metastatic breast cancer. *Cancer* 53:1333, 1984.
47. Harvey HA, Santen RJ, Osterman J, Samojlik E, White DS, Lipton A: A comparative trial of transsphenoidal hypophysectomy and estrogen suppression with aminoglutethimide in advanced breast cancer. *Cancer* 43:2207, 1979.
48. Santen RJ et al: A randomized trial comparing surgical adrenalectomy with aminoglutethimide plus hydrocortisone in women with advanced breast cancer. *N Engl J Med* 305:545, 1981.

30

Radiation Treatment for Palliation of Metastatic Breast Cancer

Zelig A. Tochner, M.D.
Zvi Fuks, M.D.

INTRODUCTION

Despite major advances in the management of breast cancer and increases in survival time for individual patients, the mortality rate (27 per 100,000 females) has remained remarkably stable throughout the last 50 years.[2,23,28] Approximately 80 percent of all patients with carcinoma of the breast still succumb to the disease, regardless of the mode of therapy employed.[40] Studies involving large numbers of patients indicate that the most common causes of breast cancer-related death result from its metastatic dissemination.[40,47] Approximately 30 percent of patients initially present with widespread metastatic disease.[18] Furthermore, only 60 percent of patients presenting with disease still apparently localized are appropriate candidates for a curative attempt with radical or modified mastectomy,[11] and only approximately half these eventually remain relapse-free. Of patients treated with a curative intent and in whom a relapse does occur, one-third recur with chest wall and/or regional lymph node metastases, and two-thirds recur with distant metastases.[11,19,27] Although postoperative radiotherapy significantly reduces the rates of local and regional lymph node recurrences in Stage II cases, it does not affect the overall relapse rate, due to the high frequency of distant metastases.[11]

Of the patients who fail and develop distant spread, nearly 20 percent have evidence of multiorgan involvement at the time of first relapse.[54] Of those who present with single-organ dissemination nearly 50 percent have skeletal metastases, approximately one-third have either lung or pleural involvement,[19,27] and less than 5 percent present with metastases to the liver. Only in a minority of patients does the tumor remain confined to the site of initial relapse; in most cases other organs become progressively involved. While the tumor may subsequently spread to almost any organ, the central nervous system is a relatively frequent target for such metastatic dissemination, and either the brain or the leptomeninges are involved in approximately 30 percent of the patients who succumb to metastatic breast cancer.[60]

The prognosis of patients who develop metastatic dissemination is extremely poor, since metastatic carcinoma of the breast is essentially incurable. Since survival may not be prolonged by the treatment, the patient's quality of life represents the major consideration in treatment design. Furthermore, since treatment is palliative in nature, the treatment option which has a reasonable chance of achieving response with minimal side effects should be employed first. Hormonal manipulations and combination chemotherapy have recently become the most common therapeutic modalities for metastatic breast cancer, but for specific local metastatic problems, radiotherapy is still the modality of choice. Radiation has been most commonly used in the treatment of metastases to the bone and brain, but treatment of other sites has also been occasionally explored.

GENERAL THERAPEUTIC CONSIDERATIONS

The shape and distribution of radiation fields and the dose and fractionation schemes employed in the treatment of various cancers usually represent a compromise between the need to encompass with radiation the total tumor volume carried to tumoricidal dose levels, and the desire to avoid significant injury to the surrounding normal tissues. The tumoricidal dose levels for breast cancer have not been accurately defined. François Baclesse was one of the first to show that high doses of radiation result in long-term local control of primary inoperable breast tumors.[3,4] In a more recent study, Fletcher and Montague administered 6000 rads in 6 weeks and obtained local control in 72 percent of patients with inoperable breast cancer.[22] These authors also suggested that the tumoricidal dose level for subclinical microscopic amounts of breast cancer is 4500 to 5000 rads, whereas permanent eradication of gross disease requires doses exceeding 6000 rads.[21,39] These doses usually exceed the normal tissue tolerance of organs in which metastases from breast cancer frequently occur. It has been suggested that the TD 5/5, which represents the tolerance radiation dose levels for normal tissues, is 1500 to 2000 rads for the lung, 2500 rads for the liver, 4500 rads for the spinal cord and for the heart, and 5000 rads for the brain and the small intestines.[49] It is, therefore, apparent that the permanent eradication of gross metastatic tumors in these organs is frequently not attainable. Furthermore, although the TD 5/5 of bone tissue exceeds 6000 rads, the frequent proximity of bone metastases to radiation-sensitive organs significantly interferes with the effective management of such tumor deposits with radiotherapy. Nonetheless, the treatment of metastatic breast carcinoma with radiation is still considered effective and useful, since either a temporary eradication or a partial remission of tumor masses in these and other organs can frequently be achieved with relatively low radiation doses, well below the tolerance limits of these organs. Such types of tumor responses often confer effective palliation in symptomatic patients, especially in those with either skeletal or brain metastases.[8,14,15,48] Therefore, radiation is indeed considered one of the more effective palliative treatment modalities for breast cancer metastases into these organs.

PALLIATION OF BONE METASTASES

Nearly 50 percent of patients who present with breast cancer will eventually develop bone metastases.[35] In many patients the skeleton is the only site of recurrence and the disease may remain confined to this organ for long periods.[54] This type of metastatic spread is not necessarily life-threatening, and some patients remain alive for many years before the tumor spreads to other organs. However, metastatic tumors to the bone are often symptomatic and may be debilitating, even in those patients with slowly progressing lesions. The most frequent symptom of osseous metastases is localized pain which can develop gradually over the course of many weeks or months.[31] The pain is frequently positional in nature and is aggravated by shifting weight to the involved area.

While pain is the first and only symptom of most bone lesions, pathologic fractures of long bones may occur when lytic lesions destroy more than 50 percent of the cortex.[16] Most patients show evidence of concomitant multiple bone lesions, but the presence of a solitary lesion as the only evidence for metastatic spread is not infrequent. The most common sites of involvement are the vertebral bodies, the pelvic bones, the proximal third of the femur, and the ribs.[26,59] The scapula, sternum, skull, clavicle, and humerus are less often involved, while the hands, feet, forearms, tibia, and fibula are infrequent sites of metastasis.[26,59] Once bone metastases are suspected, the diagnosis can usually be established by an isotope bone scan and skeletal radiography. Percussion tenderness at the site of involvement is a reliable clinical sign, which often directs the physician to the most symptomatic lesions.

Relief of pain and the prevention of pathologic fractures, while preserving normal tissue integrity, are the radiation therapist's main goals in treating osseous metastases. The treatment is usually highly effective, and published series have reported significant relief of pain in approximately 90 percent of treated patients, and less than 10 percent pathologic fractures occurring in previously treated areas.[16,26,30,56–59,63] The most common treatment technique involves a course of multifractionated irradiation, although some studies have suggested single-fraction radiotherapy. Vargha et al. described the experience with limited field, single-dose treatment for bone pain.[63] Tumor doses in this study ranged from 400 to 1800 rads. Surprisingly, no correlations between dose and response were observed. All 25 patients receiving radiation doses of 400 to 800 rads had satisfactory pain relief with minimal side effects, and a similar response was observed in another 22 patients given 800 to 1400 rads. The duration of palliation and the recurrence rate were not assessed in this study, as the median survival was 4 months only.

The demonstration that low-dose, single-fraction radiotherapy can effectively and safely relieve pain prompted investigators from the Princess Margaret Hospital in Toronto to increase gradually both the doses and field sizes employed in patients with mutiple bone metastases to include simultaneously as many lesions as possible within a single treatment field. These investigators developed a treatment protocol for half-body irradiation (HBI) employing a dose of 600 to 1000 rads given in a single exposure.[20] The body is divided at the level of the umbilicus into the upper half (UHB) and the lower half (LHB), and the more symptomatic half is treated first with a pair of anterior-posterior opposed fields. Following hematologic recovery, which usually occurs 6 to 8 weeks after the first treatment, the other half is treated if indicated. Using high-energy photon beams, midplane tumor doses of 600 to 1000 rads are delivered to the LHB, and 600 to 800 rads to the UHB. In the UHB, the eyes, mucosa of the mouth, and parotid glands are protected with lead shields. Most patients have to be admitted prior to HBI for management of the acute radiation syndrome associated with HBI, consisting of nausea, vomiting, increase in body temperature and pulse rate, and a drop in blood pressure. The syndrome occurs mainly with UHBI and lasts for less than 24 h. Leukopenia and thrombocytopenia are common, occurring usually by the end of the second week after treatment, with recovery by the sixth to eighth week. Radiation pneumonitis occurs in more than 10 percent of patients who received more than 600 rads UHBI, and is another potential serious side effect.[24] This complication usually develops approximately 100 days following treatment and is often irreversible and fatal.

Since the initial introduction of HBI, considerable experience has been accumulated concerning its efficacy.[6,44,46,50,51] Roughly 75 percent of treated patients experience significant subjective or complete pain relief, and nearly one-half of these have demonstrable objective tumor regressions. The relief of pain is most dramatic, with more than one-half of patients responding in 48 h. However, the mean duration until pain relief is achieved is 2 weeks and it then persists for nearly two-thirds of the patient's remaining life. Patients with carcinoma of the breast previously treated with combination chemotherapy tolerate the treatment less well.[6] Irreversible pancytopenia frequently occurs in such patients who usually have low reserves of functional marrow due to previous extensive multiagent chemotherapy, and this complication is often fatal.[6,57]

In summary, although HBI offers a rapid palliation to patients with multiple sites of metastases, it should be reserved for terminally ill patients, as the duration of response is usually short and the complications involved in its application can be fatal.

While single-dose radiation, either for localized or hemibody fields, is indicated in carefully selected patients, multifractionated radiation therapy is the more common practice. There is considerable controversy regarding the total dose, size, and number of fractions, and the total length of time required for multifractionated radiation courses of bone metastases. Several retrospective and nonrandomized prospective studies have compared different low-dose, short-term courses of 500 to 2000 rads given in two to five fractions in less than a week, to more protracted radiation courses involving 2500 to 4500 rads in 12 to 22 fractions, delivered over the course of 2 to 5 weeks.[1,17,38,59] However, most of these techniques were found to be equally effective in palliating symptoms of bone metastases, and a dose-response relationship could not be established. In all reports, approximately 90 percent of treated patients responded with significant pain relief. When the onset of relief was examined, it seemed that a higher proportion of patients who received short-course therapy had a delayed pain relief.[1] The duration of responses and the rates of recurrences were difficult to compare as the median survival of treated patients was often short.

To further address the question of the most optimal treatment technique, the Radiation Therapy Oncology Group (RTOG) conducted a prospectively randomized study to evaluate different dose fractionation schemes.[58] A total of 1016 patients was divided into two groups, depending on whether they had solitary bone metastasis, or multiple metastases. The first group was randomized to receive either 4050 rads/3 weeks or 2000 rads/1 week. Patients in the multiple metastases group were randomized to receive either 3000 rads/2 weeks, 1500 rads/1 week, 2000 rads/1 week, or 2500 rads/1 week. Almost 90 percent of patients in all treatment groups experienced some relief of pain. Eighty-three percent responded with partial relief, and 54 percent had complete pain relief. In the solitary metastasis group the complete response rate was higher in the 4050 rads group than in those receiving 2000 rads, (61 percent versus 53 percent, respectively), but the difference was not statistically significant. Nearly all patients who responded showed some degree of pain relief by 2 to 4 weeks after initiation of radiotherapy. However, approximately 50 percent of those who achieved a complete response did so for the first time more than 4 weeks after initiation of treatment. The median durations of partial and complete response were longer in the solitary than in the multiple metastases group. Although not statistically significant, the longest duration of partial response was obtained in patients who received the highest doses of irradiation in both the solitary and the multiple groups. The relapse rate was high, and 54 percent of those with a complete response eventually had recurrence with pain at the previously treated sites. This recurrence rate is higher than the 0 percent to 22 percent recurrence rate reported by others.[1,56] Although this difference could be related to the low-dose therapy employed in some patients, it is still frustrating for the high-dose group of 4050 rads/3 weeks. However, it should be noted that in this study group approximately 50 percent of patients were lost to follow-up, a fact that could explain a statistical bias in the interpretation of treatment results.

Prevention of pathologic fractures is another important criterion of success when treatment of bone lesions is judged. Some investigators recommend the use of prophylactic internal fixation for high-risk patients with large (more than 2.5 cm) osteolytic lesions involving the cortex of long bones.[7] Other studies suggested that fractures of high-risk long bone lesions may be treated successfully by high-dose radiotherapy with doses of 3000 to 4000 rads.[16] In the RTOG study, prevention of fractures was achieved in 81 percent of all treated sites, with 13 percent of long bone sites fractured and 6 percent of vertebral bodies compression fractures seen. There was no significant difference in fracture rates among the treatment arms in the multiple metastases group, but in the solitary group, fractures occurred in 18 percent of patients receiving 4050 rads, but only in 4 percent of those receiving 2000 rads. The difference may be attributed to the large number of patients lost to follow-up, and to the fact that once a recurrence became evident, 24 percent of patients in the 2000-rads arm were reirradiated, while none in the high-dose group could receive a second course of radiation. When pathologic fractures occur in untreated bones, internal surgical fixation followed by radiation therapy of 3000 to 3500 rads is indicated.[12,25] Excellent palliation and approximately 90 percent of bone healing have been demonstrated in patients surviving for more than 6 months.[25] Only about 65 percent of comparably irradiated fractures healed when immobilized in a cast without an internal fixation.

In view of the controversies and conflicting reports regarding the treatment of metastatic bone disease in breast carcinoma, firm dose/fraction/time schedules and unified radiation field arrangements for the various metastatic sites are not available. However, a few general guidelines should be kept in mind when planning the treatment of the individual patient. Low-dose, short-term treatment is as effective as the high-dose protracted course of irradiation in achieving an acute relief of pain. The duration of response is probably longer and the recurrence rate lower with high-dose regimens. While some areas in the body can tolerate reirradiation without major morbidities (foot, arm), other areas cannot be re-treated without risking severe complications (spine, whole pelvis). Increasing the size of radiation fields to include nonsymptomatic lesions is sometimes advisable to avoid subsequent problems of matching future treatment fields. The selection of a dose/fraction/time schedule should be individualized according to the site of bone metastases and the expected life duration of the treated patient. Whereas low-dose, short-term schedules are recommended for terminally ill patients, higher doses should be employed in patients with relatively long life expectancy, and for areas which cannot be safely re-treated.

PALLIATION OF CENTRAL NERVOUS SYSTEM METASTASES

As previously indicated, metastases of breast cancer to the brain are frequent, and are second only to carcinoma of the lung among metastatic brain tumors.[13] In a large autopsy study of 1044 patients who died of breast cancer, Trukada et al.[60] reported that 309 (29.5 percent) had central nervous system (CNS) involvement at the time of death. The brain was involved in 193 cases, the cranial dura in 167 cases, the leptomeninges in 59 cases, and the spinal cord in 32 of the patients examined. Metastases to the infratentorial regions of the brain were almost as frequent as to the cerebrum. Forty-two percent of patients showed single metastatic lesions. In only 31 percent of cases was CNS involvement clinically diagnosed or suspected prior to death. Headache, loss of motor function, and impaired mentation with lethargy are the most frequent symptoms of cerebral metastases. Seizures, sensory loss, and cerebellar dysfunction are also common. While a careful neurological examination may help in localizing the lesion within the brain, computerized axial tomography (CT) is the most accurate method for establishing the diagnosis. When meningeal carcinomatosis is suspected, cytologic examination of the cerebrospinal fluid (CSF) is essential for diagnosis.

When untreated, brain metastasis is lethal within a relatively short period of time. Lang et al. reported that in 76 untreated patients the mean survival was 2 months, and the median survival was 1 month.[36] While chemotherapy has little or no value in the treatment of brain metastases, and surgery is reserved for highly selected patients, radiotherapy is the principal and often the sole treatment available for the majority of patients. Although prolongation of life is often used as a criterion for the assessment of therapeutic effects in brain metastasis, this should always be coupled with evaluation of the improvement in the functional capacity, and the regaining of intellectual awareness and physical abilities. Using these criteria, many reports have demonstrated the value of radiation therapy for most patients with metastatic brain disease.[29,42,64] While some investigators advocate the use of large single-fraction radiation of 1000 rads,[32,52] most reports recommend fractionated and more protracted treatment courses, delivered to the whole brain. Although no firm conclusions can be made regarding the most optimal dose/fraction/time schedules, available data suggest that 2000 rads in 1 week is as effective as 4000 rads in 4 weeks. About 75 percent of patients treated with such protocols experienced functional improvement and in general survival was prolonged to approximately 6 months.[29,42,64] However, relapse and progression of brain disease was ultimately the cause of death in more than 50 percent of treated patients.[29] In those patients who survived for more than 1 year after treatment, functional improvement decreased as a function of survival duration,[42] resulting from either relapsing disease or from progressive chronic radiation-induced damage. This suggests that, when long-term survival is expected and high tumor doses of radiation are necessary, the combination of whole-brain irradiation and a boost aimed at the tumor bed with as little surrounding normal brain tissue as deemed necessary should be employed. Such boost doses carried to 1500 to 2000 rads are usually given following 4000 rads whole-brain irradiation given in 4 weeks, which has been suggested as safe with regard to long-term toxicity.

Whereas most data available in the literature are based on retrospective studies, two large prospectively randomized studies were conducted by the RTOG to define the most optimal schedules for palliation of metastatic brain cancers.[13] Seventeen percent of the total of 1800 patients studied had breast cancer. Five different radiation fractionation schemes ranging from 2000 rads in 1 week to 4000 rads in 4 weeks were evaluated. As previously shown by others, approximately 75 percent of patients responded with a clinical improvement, regardless of the dose fractionation time scheme used. Some degree of improvement was achieved in approximately two-thirds of patients who had severe limitations of performance, and who required nursing care or hospitalization prior to whole-brain irradiation. The degree of improvement observed in ambulatory patients, and in particular in those who had the brain as the only site of metastases, was significantly higher. Various degrees of improvement in motor function, sensory loss, impaired mentation, cerebellar dysfunction, convulsions, headache, lethargy, and cranial nerve paralysis were observed in 69 to 77 percent of patients, with 32 to 41 percent responding with complete remissions. Breast cancer patients, as a group, had a median survival of 21 weeks, with ambulatory patients surviving longer than nonambulatory patients.

Recurrences of brain metastases were the cause of death in 49 percent of patients in the first study group and 31 percent in the second study group.[13] The palliative index was also evaluated in these studies, and 75 to 80 percent of patients surviving for more than 1 month after treatment entertained either an improved or stable neurological state.

The results of the RTOG studies suggest that a short time/dose/fractionation scheme such as 3000 rads in 10 fractions over 2 weeks may be used with equal efficacy as higher doses given in more protracted treatment courses. However, patients with controlled primary tumor lesions and with the brain as the only site of metastases constitute a prognostically favorable group and may benefit from 4000 rads whole-brain irradiation, and from boost field treatment restricted to the tumor bed only carried to additional 1000 to 1500 rads.

The value of concomitant administration of steroids during brain irradiation has not been completely established. In the RTOG studies steroids were given in an uncontrolled fashion. Patients who received steroids responded more promptly than those who did not receive the drugs. Furthermore, patients with worse initial neurological functions had a higher frequency of improvement when given steroid therapy. However, steroids had no influence on either the time to progression or survival. Hence, steroids seem to be beneficial in the induction of early response to treatment but do not affect the ultimate prognosis of treated patients.

Approximately 5 percent of patients with metastatic breast cancer have leptomeningeal involvement.[33] Nonspecific symptoms of radicular pain, low back pain, headache, and change in the mental state are the most common initial symptoms.[41] Specific cranial nerve involvement, focal extremity weakness, and neck pain are less common. Examination of cerebrospinal fluid is diagnostic, with elevated proteins being the most frequent abnormality, while malignant cells and decreased glucose levels are less common findings.[41] If untreated, these patients die within 6 to 8 weeks from diagnosis. Aggressive treatment is necessary, combining intrathecal chemotherapy and whole-brain irradiation of 2000 to 4000 rads over 2 to 3 weeks. The limited data available in the literature report initial responses in up to 85 percent of treated patients with a median survival of 22 weeks.[33] The radiation fields involved are designed to include the whole cranial leptomeninges and the upper two cervical vertebrae to encompass the maximal volume of CSF in which an optimal distribution of drugs injected to the spinal canal is frequently not achieved.

PALLIATION OF LIVER METASTASES

The liver is a frequent site of metastases in breast cancer, and is frequently associated with widespread metastases to other organs. Usually, multiple metastases are present in the liver, and if untreated the mean survival has been approximately 6 months. Abdominal pain, fatigue, and anorexia are the most common symptoms, and nausea, vomiting, abdominal distension, fever, night sweats, jaundice, and ascites are less common. Since hepatic metastases are frequently accompanied with concomitant metastases to other organs, the treatments of choice have usually been either combination chemotherapy or hormonal manipulation.

The use of whole-liver irradiation is limited by the intolerance of the liver to radiation of doses exceeding 2500 to 3000 rads.[34] When liver tolerance is exceeded, radiation hepatitis develops between 4 to 6 weeks following treatment. The syndrome consists of anorexia, ascites, tender hepatomegaly, jaundice, and elevation of serum liver enzymes. Radiation hepatitis is usually transient and subsides spontaneously in most patients, but can be fatal in some.[34,43] Ingold et al. described a dose-response relationship for radiation injury to the liver.[34] With doses of less than 3000 rads, radiation hepatitis following whole-liver irradiation is uncommon with daily fractions of 200 rads or less. However, with daily fractions greater than 200 rads, the threshold for radiation hepatitis may be as low as 2500 rads, regardless of the fractionation employed. Thrombocytopenia is another potentially serious side effect of hepatic irradiation[55] which may be prolonged and life-threatening, especially in patients receiving chemotherapy.

Liver irradiation has not been routinely used in the past for the treatment of hepatic metastases. The scanty experience reported in the literature has usually involved patients with colorectal cancer, although occasional reports included patients with breast cancer.[37,45,53,61] In most of these reports whole-liver irradiation was delivered through two opposed parallel fields to doses between 2000 to 3000 rads, with daily fractions between 200 to 300 rads, five times per week. Approximately 90 percent of patients had some degree of relief of symptoms, and pain relief usually lasted for nearly the remaining duration of the patient's survival. Nausea and vomiting were the most common side effects and no fatal radiation hepatitis was reported. Most patients ultimately failed with progressive liver disease, and succumbed to this situation. In one report, of 10 patients with metastatic breast carcinoma, three survived for more than 1 year, and one was alive in remission at 36 months.[53]

PALLIATION OF LUNG METASTASES AND OTHER ORGANS

The lung and the pleura are secondary only to the bones as sites of metastatic involvement in patients with carcinoma of the breast.[19,27] The use of radiation for the management of lung metastases has been uncommon. This is related to the restriction of lung tolerance to whole-organ irradiation to 1500 rads only.[49] Therefore, occasionally when a patient has metastatic lesions involving only a small part of one lung, and especially when such lesions produce obstruction of a large bronchus with atelectasis, small-field radiotherapy may be indicated. If the field is small enough, doses of 4000 to 5000 rads can be safely employed and may be beneficial for bronchial obstruction or hemoptysis. Radiation pneumonitis almost invariably develops in such treated volumes, but is well tolerated if the treated volume is indeed small. Bagshaw has suggested a more aggressive approach to pulmonary metastases.[5] He treated patients who developed single or several small asymptomatic lesions, utilizing multiple small portals aimed separately at each tumor. Although there are no studies demonstrating that this approach is superior to watchful waiting without specific therapy, he has nonetheless been successful in achieving long periods of asymptomatic survival.

In addition to the bones, CNS, liver, and the lungs, metastatic breast cancer may occasionally involve any other organ. The choroid and retina of the eye are uncommon sites of involvement and radiotherapy is regarded as the only effective mode of treatment for such metastases.[9] Typically, complaints of a change in visual acuity lead to the diagnosis of this complication. In nearly half the patients, bilateral involvement is found either initially or in subsequent follow-up. Small retinal metastases are best managed with a single lateral field placed posterior to the lens. Doses of 2000 to 2500 rads delivered in 2 weeks are usually effective in restoring vision.[9] In more advanced, neglected tumors, the loss of vision is seldom reversible.

Another site of infrequent dissemination is the pericardium, but radiation has only a limited role in the management of malignant pericardial effusion.[10] Pericardiocentesis is always the first measure to establish the diagnosis and to relieve cardiac tamponade. Local or systemic chemotherapy, pericardiectomy, and radiotherapy can be used as a palliative treatment. Radiation of the entire pericardial sac with doses of 3000 to 4000 rads often prevents reaccumulation of the effusion for the rest of the patient's life.[10]

REFERENCES

1. Allen KL, Johnson TW, Hibbs GG: Effective bone palliation as related to various treatment regimens. *Cancer* 37:984, 1976.
2. American Cancer Society (ACS): *Cancer Facts and Figures*. New York, ACS Inc., 1983.
3. Baclesse F: Roentgen therapy alone in cancer of the breast. *Acta Un Int Cancer* 15:1023, 1959.
4. Baclesse F: Roentgen therapy as the sole method of treatment of cancer of the breast. *Am J Roentgenol* 62:311, 1949.
5. Bagshaw MA: Presumptive palliative irradiation in metastatic carcinomas of the breast. *Cancer* 28:1692, 1971.
6. Bartelink H, Battermann J, Hart G: Half body irradiation. *Int J Radiat Oncol Biol Phys* 6:87, 1980.
7. Beals RK, Lawton GD, Smell WE: Prophylactic internal fixation of the femur in metastatic breast cancer. *Cancer* 28:1350, 1971.
8. Bedwinck J, Venkata R, Perez C, Lee J, Finberg B: Stage III and localized stage V breast cancer: Irradiation alone vs irradiation plus surgery. *Int J Radiat Oncol Biol Phys* 8:31, 1982.
9. Berkeley RG, Fuller LM, Sears ME, Tapely N duV: Orbit, in MaComb WS, Fletcher GH: *Cancer of the Head and Neck*. Baltimore, Williams & Wilkins, 1967, p. 390.
10. Biran S, Brufman G, Klein E et al: The management of pericardial effusion in cancer patients. *Chest* 71:182, 1977.
11. Bonadonna G, Brusamolino E, Valagussa P et al: Most common site for recurrence in bone. *N Engl J Med* 294:405, 1976.
12. Bonarigo BC, Rubin P: Nonunion of pathologic fracture after radiation therapy. *Radiology* 88:889, 1967.
13. Borgelt B, Gelber R, Kramer S et al: The palliation of brain metastases: Final results of the first two studies by the radiation therapy oncology group. *Int J Radiat Oncol Biol Phys* 6:1, 1980.
14. Bruckman JE, Harris JR, Levene MB, Chaffey JT, Hellman S: Results of treating stage III carcinoma of the breast by primary radiation therapy. *Cancer* 43:985, 1979.
15. Brufman G, Weshler Z, Proswitz LR, Fuks Z: Treatment of locally advanced breast carcinoma with high dose external beam supervoltage radiotherapy. *Isr J Med Sci* 17:940, 1981.
16. Cheng DS, Seitz CB, Eyre HJ: Nonoperative management of femoral, humeral, and acetabular metastases in patients with breast carcinoma. *Cancer* 45:1533, 1980.
17. Delclos L: New and old concepts in radiotherapeutic treatment. *Int J Radiat Oncol Biol Phys* 1:1217, 1976.
18. Donegan WL, Lewis D: Clinical diagnosis and staging of breast cancer. *Semin Oncol* 5:373, 1978.
19. Fisher B, Slack N, Cavanaugh PJ et al: Postoperative radiotherapy in the treatment of breast cancer. *Ann Surg* 172:711, 1970.
20. Fitzpatrick PJ, Rider WD: Half body radiotherapy. *Int J Radiat Oncol Biol Phys* 1:197, 1976.
21. Fletcher GH: *Textbook of Radiotherapy*, 3d ed. Philadelphia, Lea & Febiger, 1980.
22. Fletcher GH, Montague ED: Radical irradiation of advanced breast cancer. *Am J Roentgenol* 93:573, 1965.
23. Fox MS: On the diagnosis and treatment of breast cancer. *JAMA* 241:489, 1979.
24. Fryer CJH, Fitzpatrick PJ, Rider WD, Poon P: Radiation pneumonitis: Experience following a large single dose of radiation. *Int J Radiat Oncol Biol Phys* 4:931, 1978.
25. Gainor BJ, Buchert P: Fracture healing in metastatic bone disease. *Clin Orthop* 178:297, 1983.
26. Garmalis CJ, Chu FCH: The effectiveness of radiation therapy in the treatment of bone metastases from breast cancer. *Radiology* 126:235, 1978.
27. Haagensen CD: The choice of treatment for operable carcinoma of the breast. *Surgery* 76:685, 1974.
28. Henderson IC, Canellos GP: Cancer of the breast: The past decade. *N Engl J Med* 302:17, 78, 1980.
29. Hendrickson FR: The optimum schedule for palliative radiotherapy for metastatic brain cancer. *Int J Radiat Oncol Biol Phys* 2:165, 1977.

30. Hendrickson FR, Skehata WM, Kirchner AB: Radiation therapy for osseous metastasis. *Int J Radiat Oncol Biol Phys* 1:275, 1976.
31. Hendrickson FR, Sheinhop MB: Management of osseous metastasis. *Semin Oncol* 2:399, 1975.
32. Hindo WA, DeTrana FA, Lee MS, Hendrickson FR: Large dose increment irradiation in treatment of cerebral metastases. *Cancer* 26:138, 1970.
33. Ingle JM, Tormey DC, Tan HK: The bone marrow examination in breast cancer. *Cancer* 41:670, 1978.
34. Ingold JA, Reed GB, Kaplan HS, Bagshaw MA: Radiation hepatitis. *Am J Roentgenol* 93:200, 1965.
35. Jaffe HL: *Tumors and tumorous conditions of the bones and joints.* Philadelphia, Lea & Febiger, 1958.
36. Lang EF, Slate J: Metastatic brain tumors: Results of surgical and nonsurgical treatment. *Surg Clin North Am* 44:865, 1964.
37. Leibel SA, Order SE, Raminger CJ, Asbell SO: Palliation of liver metastases with combined hepatic irradiation and misonidazole: Results of a radiation therapy oncology group phase I–II study. *Cancer Clin Trials* 4:285, 1981.
38. Martin WMC: Multiple daily fractions of radiation in the palliation of pain from bone metastases. *Clin Radiol* 34:245, 1983.
39. Montague E: Radiation management of advanced breast cancer. *Int J Radiat Oncol Biol Phys* 4:305, 1978.
40. Mueller CB, Awes F, Anderson GD: Breast cancer in 3558 women: Age a significant determinant in the rate of dying and causes of death. *Surgery* 83:123, 1978.
41. Olson ME, Chenik NL, Posner JB: Infiltration of the leptomeninges by systemic cancer. *Arch Neurol* 30:122, 1974.
42. Order SE, Hellman S, Van Essen CF, Kligerman NM: Improvement in quality of survival following whole brain irradiation for brain metastasis. *Radiology* 91:149, 1968.
43. Philips R, Karnofsky DA, Hamilton LD et al: Roentgen therapy of hepatic metastasis. *Am J Roentgenol* 71:826, 1954.
44. Poussin-Rossilo H, Salazar OM, Prempree T, Amin P, Patanophan V, Sewchand W: Systemic half-body irradiation, achievements and perspectives. *Int J Radiat Oncol Biol Phys* 1(suppl 8): 129, 1982.
45. Prasad B, Lee MS, Hendrickson FR: Irradiation of hepatic metastasis. *Int J Radiat Oncol Biol Phys* 2:129, 1977.
46. Qusim MM: Techniques and result of half body irradiation (HBI) in metastatic carcinomas and myelomas. *Clin Oncol* 5:65, 1979.
47. Romsdahl MM, Sears ME, Eckles NE: Post-treatment evaluation of breast cancer, in *Breast Cancer Early and Late. Proc Ann Clin Conferences,* sponsored by the University of Texas, M. D. Anderson Hospital and Tumor Institute. Year Book Medical Publishers Inc., 1970, p. 291.
48. Rubens RD, Armitage P, Winter PJ, Toup D, Hayward JL: Prognosis in inoperable stage III carcinoma of the breast. *Eur J Cancer* 13:805, 1977.
49. Rubin P, Cooper R, Philips TL (eds): *Radiation Biology and Radiation Pathology Syllabus.* Chicago, American College of Radiology, 1975.
50. Salazar AM, Rubin P, Hendrickson FR et al: Single-dose half-body irradiation for the palliation of multiple bone metastases from solid tumors: A preliminary report. *Int J Radiat Oncol Biol Phys* 7:738, 1981.
51. Salazar OM, Rubin P, Keller B, Scarantino C: Systemic (half body) radiation therapy: Response and toxicity. *Int J Radiat Oncol Biol Phys* 4:937, 1978.
52. Shehata WM, Hendrickson FR, Hindo WA: Rapid fractionation technique and re-treatment of cerebral metastases by irradiation. *Cancer* 34:257, 1974.
53. Sherman DM, Weichselbaum R, Order SE, Cloud L, Trey C, Piro AJ: Palliation of hepatic metastasis. *Cancer* 41:2013, 1978.
54. Smalley RV: The management of disseminated breast cancer, in Carter SK, Glatstein E, Livington B (eds): *Principles of Cancer Treatment.* New York, McGraw-Hill, 1982, p. 327.
55. Tefft M, Traggis D, Filler RM: Liver irradiation in children: Acute changes with transient leukopenia and thrombocytopenia. *Am J Roentgenol Radium Ther Nucl Med* 106:750, 1969.
56. Thomas P: Radiotherapy of metastases of mammary carcinoma. *Clin Radiol* 45:306, 1976.
57. Tochner Z, Weshler Z, Rizel S, Fuks Z: Fractionated hemiskeletal irradiation for multifocal skeletal pain in patients with widespread carcinomatous metastases to bone. *Int J Radiat Oncol Biol Phys* 1(suppl 8):128, 1982.

58. Tong D, Gillick L, Hendrickson FR: The palliation of symptomatic osseous metastases; final results of the study by the radiation therapy oncology group. *Cancer* 50:893, 1982.
59. Trodella L, Ausili-Cefaro G, Turriziani A, Marmiroll L, Cellini N, Nardone L: Pain in osseous metastases; results of radiotherapy. *Pain* 18:387, 1984.
60. Trukada Y, Fouad A, Pickren JW, Lane WW: Central nervous system metastasis from breast carcinoma; autopsy study. *Cancer* 52:2349, 1983.
61. Turek-Maischeider M, Kazem I: Palliative irradiation for liver metastases. *JAMA* 232:625, 1975.
62. Valgurra P, Bonadonna G, Keronesi A: Patterns of relapse and survival following radical mastectomy. *Cancer* 41:1170, 1978.
63. Vargha ZO, Glicksman AS, Boland J: Single-dose radiation therapy in the palliation of metastatic disease. *Radiology* 93:1181, 1969.
64. West J, Maor M: Intracranial metastases: Behavioral patterns related to primary site and results of treatment by whole brain irradiation. *Int J Radiat Oncol Biol Phys* 6:11, 1980.

31

Interferon and Other Biological Response Modifiers

Richard V. Smalley, M.D.

INTRODUCTION

The use of biologicals (or biological response modifiers) as a therapeutic modality in patients with carcinoma of the breast remains an area for clinical investigation. The interferons, a prototype for this approach, have a substantial antitumor effect in a number of B-cell tumors, but have shown limited effect as single agents in patients with advanced solid tumors, including breast cancer. The development of recombinant DNA technology has provided the means for the unlimited availability of a large number of cytokines with a potential antitumor effect. Limited amounts of material for either clinical or preclinical testing have hampered development heretofore, but extensive preclinical testing and the subsequent intelligent application of this knowledge in the development of appropriate clinical usage should now be possible. Other promising lymphokines with either cytotoxic or response-modifying capabilities are currently being developed, and monoclonal antibodies, the potential magic bullets, are about to be clinically tested. This chapter will review the clinical potential for biological therapy, with emphasis on the interferons, in patients with carcinoma of the breast.

INTERFERON

The interferons are a family of proteins with potent immunological and cytostatic effects. Some interferon molecules are glycosylated and all are between 145 to 166 amino acids in length, with a molecular weight between 17 and 20,000.[1] Interferons are classified immunologically into three types: alpha, beta, and gamma, and are produced in vivo by mammalian cells in response to either viral or immune stimulation. The alpha and beta interferons, produced primarily by leukocytes and fibroblasts respectively, following viral stimulation, are closely related, with about one-third of each molecule showing homology of amino acids.[2] Gamma interferon, produced by lymphocytes following immune stimulation, is structurally substantially different.[3,4] There are at least 12 alpha interferon molecules differing from each other by about 20 percent of their amino acids, but only one beta and one gamma interferon gene has been identified.[5–7] The in vitro production of natural interferon may be induced by appropriately stimulating peripheral blood leukocytes, fibroblasts, or lymphocytes followed by purification of the supernate.

Purification procedures vary in their approaches and their efficiency, leading to a great degree of variability in the natural materials that are used therapeutically. The original process was developed by Cantell in Finland and until the late 1970s the Finnish Red Cross provided all the therapeutic-grade alpha interferon.[8] Since that time several other laboratories have produced natural alpha interferon for therapeutic trials, all using techniques that are similar in concept but differing in specifics. Subsequent refinements and improvements in production and purification techniques,[9] as well as development of recombinant DNA technology,[2–4,6,10] have combined to substantially increase the availability of a wide variety of interferon molecules for therapeutic trials. Thus, both clinical and preclinical scientists have been given the opportunity to study in depth these various molecules and their ability to alter the host-tumor interface.

The American Cancer Society (ACS) initiated the clinical development of alpha interferon in the United States in the late 1970s by purchasing a large amount of material from the Finnish Red Cross and organizing a number of trials in various diseases, including advanced breast cancer.[11,12] The National Cancer Institute (NCI) in the early 1980s contracted with both Meloy and Warner-Lambert Laboratories to produce a natural alpha interferon for clinical study.[13] Although others have also produced natural alpha interferon, these sources have been used for the three large phase II trials of natural alpha "leukocyte" interferon in patients with advanced breast cancer.[11,12,14] All natural alpha "leukocyte" interferon is produced by stimulating peripheral blood leukocytes, harvested from normal human blood, with Sendai virus. Following a 24-to-48 h stimulation period, the supernate is harvested and partially purified by a variety of techniques. Natural alpha "leukocyte" interferon for therapeutic use is a mixture of interferons and other molecules, is less than 0.1 percent pure interferon, and has a specific activity of 10^6 units per milligram of protein. The three trials which have been performed in patients with breast cancer with this relatively impure material are the two sponsored by the ACS using Finnish Red Cross material and the NCI-sponsored trial using material produced by Warner-Lambert Laboratories.

Scientists at Burroughs-Wellcome Ltd. in the United Kingdom have utilized the Namalwa line, a continuously growing lymphoblastoid cell line obtained from a child with Burkitt's lymphoma, for production of lymphoblastoid interferon, also an alpha interferon.[9] Stimulating these cells with Sendai virus and purifying the material using monoclonal antibody techniques, they have obtained a highly purified product which is 85 to 90 percent pure, has a specific activity of 10^8 units per milligram of protein, and contains 8 of the 12 or more alpha interferon molecules but no other biologically active material. This material has been evaluated in several trials involving patients with advanced breast cancer.[15–18]

Genetic engineering techniques using recombinant DNA technology have evolved following the isolation, sequencing, and cloning of the various alpha interferon molecules, and several pharmaceutical companies have the capability of producing one or more of these molecules for therapeutic use. Two systems of nomenclature for the alpha molecules have evolved: alpha 1, 2, 3, etc. (Schering-Plough Corp.; Biogen); and clone A, B, C, D, etc. (Hoffmann-LaRoche

Co.; Genentech). Alpha 2 and clone A are alleles, differing by one amino acid,[6] and are the two recombinant molecules which have undergone extensive clinical testing and potential commercial development. Alpha 1 and clone D, the names assigned the first alpha molecule sequenced and cloned, have each undergone extensive preclinical testing, while clone D has been compared biologically and clinically with clone A in at least one trial.[6,19,20] The various alpha molecules differ in their functions and in their influence on a variety of in vitro cellular functions, but while their effects may differ substantially on a single cell grown in vitro, their biological effects on the host in vivo may not differ substantially. Of potential clinical interest is the development of hybrid molecules in which desired segments of individual interferon molecules are joined and a hybrid recombinant alpha interferon molecule produced.[6] In this way, it is possible to construct a molecule that will have an increased degree of a particular desired function. It remains to be determined whether these techniques will produce products that will be of clinical interest.

Both beta and gamma interferon molecules have been produced by natural means in vitro and tested clinically.[21–25] Gamma interferon appears to be a more potent immunostimulatory and cytostatic/cytotoxic agent when evaluated in vitro than either alpha or beta interferon,[26] and combinations of gamma with either alpha or beta interferon are synergistic in a number of in vitro situations.[27,28] Whether these in vitro effects will translate into significant clinical benefit is yet to be tested. The beta and gamma interferon molecules have also been sequenced, cloned, and produced by recombinant DNA technology and are, as of 1986, undergoing phase II clinical testing.[29–32] Recombinant beta interferon, cloned and sequenced by Cetus Corporation, is being clinically tested under license to Triton Biosciences, while recombinant gamma interferon, produced by both Genentech and Biogen, is undergoing evaluation in trials sponsored by those companies.

Preclinical Evaluation of Alpha Interferon

A number of experimental situations evaluating the antitumor effect of human alpha interferon against breast cancer cells grown in continuous cell culture,[33–37] in soft agar,[38,39] or in nude mice,[40–46] as well as two experiments evaluating the therapeutic effect of murine alpha interferon against spontaneous murine mammary carcinoma,[47,48] have demonstrated that the alpha interferons have a significant cytostatic effect. This effect is both dose- and schedule-dependent but is invariably reversible following cessation of interferon treatment. Alpha interferon, using either natural or recombinant material in concentrations as low as 50 pg/mL, is nonspecifically inhibitory to the growth of human breast adenocarcinoma or normal mammary epithelial cells grown in continuous cell cultures.[33–37] There was increasing inhibition with increasing concentrations but normal growth patterns were reestablished following removal of the interferon. When established breast carcinoma cell lines or samples obtained from fresh biopsy material were grown in soft agar, both were inhibited by either natural alpha, clone A, or clone D interferon.[38,39] Under these circumstances, permanent inhibition of colony formation in cultures exposed to interferon was demonstrable, suggesting a potential permanent inhibitory effect of interferon on the colony-forming cell. Additionally, the lack of regeneration in colony formation may indicate that interferon is capable of inhibiting the development of metastases. In the soft agar experiments with fresh human breast cancer cells, interferon inhibited growth in about 30 percent of tumor samples to the degree usually associated with clinical antitumor effect. Clone A was somewhat more effective than clone D on a milligram-for-milligram basis. Concentrations effective in these in vitro experiments are well

Table 31-1 Responses Observed in Patients with Advanced Breast Cancer Using Natural Alpha Interferon

	Dose (MU)	Schedule	Evaluable	PR	MR	Reference
1	3–9/TD	Daily IM × 28 days	17	6	1	11
2	3/TD	Daily IM × 28 days	23	5	4	12
3	1–24/m^2	Daily IM × 28 days	16	0	3	14

PR = number achieving a partial response.
MR = number achieving a minor response.
MU/TD = total dose per patient.
MU/m^2 = dose per meter square.

within the range achievable following therapeutic administration.

Additional evidence of the potential cytostatic capabilities of alpha interferons has been obtained from experiments in which implantations of human tumor cells in nude mice have been treated with both human and murine alpha interferon.[40,41] These experiments have demonstrated that alpha interferon from either source will inhibit xenograft growth, although the human alpha interferon is more effective than the murine. Murine interferon will augment murine immunologic responses in these nude mice (other than T-cell responses), whereas the human interferon will not, suggesting that the major effect, at least of interferon in these circumstances, is a direct cytostatic effect rather than an augmented immune response effect. As in the in vitro experiments, both dose and schedule are important. A definitive dose-response was obtained and daily treatment was substantially superior to intermittent or single-dose treatment.

Of significant interest is the observation that in both the in vitro continuous cell culture experiments and the in vivo nude mouse systems, the cytostatic effect of alpha interferon is synergistic with other modalities of treatment. In the cell culture system, dose-related synergism in vitro has been demonstrated between interferon and both 5-fluorouracil and radiotherapy,[49,50] while in the nude mouse system, interferon has been shown to be synergistic with both doxorubicin and cyclophosphamide.[46] The combination of interferon with chemotherapy has led to tumor regression and apparent cures in the nude mouse, something neither agent was able to do alone.[46] There is very little human clinical experience with combination therapy (interferon plus cytotoxic drug therapy) but at least one trial is exploring this in patients with breast cancer.[51]

Clinical Breast Cancer Trials

Tables 31-1 through 31-3 list the responses seen in phase II trials performed with the natural alpha interferon (Cantell) material, with the highly purified natural lymphoblastoid interferon [Wellferon–human lymphoblastoid interferon (HLBI)], and with the recombinant molecule, clone A.

The first two trials, sponsored by the ACS and performed in patients with advanced breast cancer, used Cantell Finnish Red Cross interferon.[11,12] Each demonstrated significant antitumor activity in about 25 percent of patients. The first of these trials was performed in previously heavily treated patients and the second in patients not previously exposed to cytotoxic therapy. Objective antitumor responses were seen in both. These responses predominantly occurred in older postmenopausal individuals and were noted primarily in patients with significant granulocyte depression secondary to interferon therapy. An arbitrarily chosen dose of 3 million units per patient administered

Table 31-2 Responses Observed in Patients with Advanced Breast Cancer Using Natural Human Lymphoblastoid Interferon

	Dose (MU/m^2)	Schedule	Entered	PR	MR	Reference
1	5–20 2	Daily IV × 10 Daily IM	27	1	4	17,18
2	0.5 3.0	Tiw IM Tiw IM	22	1	0	16
3	30	Weekly IM	12	0	0	15

For explanation of abbreviations, see Table 31-1.

daily was used in each trial. A subsequent trial sponsored by the NCI, also using a relatively impure natural alpha interferon, was unable to confirm these results.[13,14] Although this was considered a phase I to II trial, all patients were escalated to a maximally tolerable dose and received treatment for at least 28 days. Most patients received between 12 and 24 MU/m^2 daily. They appeared clinically comparable to the patient population treated in the first ACS trial. Of the 23 patients entered, 7 received an inadequate course (less than 4 weeks of therapy) and were considered inevaluable for response. No objective responses were seen in the remaining 16 evaluable patients. Although these patients had been previously heavily treated with cytotoxic therapy, most were postmenopausal (19 of 23) and most (16 of 23) had only one or two sites involved with metastases. Only 3 of the 23 had hepatic metastases. These were all characteristics that might be expected to be associated with a response.

Three trials have been completed using human lymphoblastoid interferon (HLBI), the pure natural material obtained from lymphoblastoid cells.[15–18] A total of at least 69 previously heavily treated patients were evaluated in these trials in which a variety of schedules and dose ranges were studied. Two low-dose (0.5 MU/m^2 and 3 MU/m^2) daily administration schedules,[16–18] a high-dose weekly schedule (30 MU/m^2),[15] a maximally tolerable three times a week (tiw) schedule (15 MU/m^2 tiw),[16] and a high intermittently administered dose (5 to 25 MU/m^2 daily × 10 every 28 days, administered IV),[17,18] have all been evaluated. Only two objective partial responses have been noted.[16,18] These two responses as well as several minor responses (an objective antitumor effect but less than 50 percent tumor shrinkage) were noted with the

Table 31-3 Responses Observed in Patients with Advanced Breast Cancer Using Recombinant Clone A Interferon

	Dose (MU/m^2)	Schedule	Entered	PR	MR	Reference
1	10–50	Tiw IM	17	0	0	57
2	10–50	Tiw IM	9	0	0	58
3	20 50	Daily IM Tiw IM	15	3	6	59
4	3–50	Daily IM	19	1	5	60
5		Total:	60	4	11	

For explanations of abbreviations, see Table 31-1.

higher dose, more frequently administered regimens.

These disappointing results certainly indicate that HLBI has little antitumor activity as a single agent in advanced breast cancer and then only when higher doses are administered frequently, as suggested by the preclinical studies. The National Surgical Adjuvant Breast Project (NSABP) currently has a trial ongoing in previously untreated patients in which HLBI is administered using both a low and a high dose (3 MU/m^2 daily versus 30 MU/m^2 tiw) to patients at the time of their first recurrence.[52] This trial should indicate whether or not prior cytotoxic therapy is a significant negative factor.

Similar trials with the recombinant materials have been performed with similarly disappointing results. Both high and low doses administered daily, three times a week, or intermittently (daily for 5 days every 21 days) have all been tested.[53–60] All these trials evaluated recombinant interferon in previously heavily treated patients. Very few objective antitumor responses were seen. The only two studies noting antitumor activity at all were those evaluating higher doses administered frequently and regularly (daily or three times a week).[59,60] However, in the one trial in which doses were escalated in groups of patients, no dose effect was noted.[60]

It would seem that an adequate number of trials with a variety of products using a range of doses and schedules have been performed, but have not corroborated the initial encouraging results. Although there is some clinical suggestion that dose and schedule are important, confirming the preclinical experience, the results remain disappointing. The nude mouse experiments indicate that a synergistic beneficial effect may be expected between interferon and cytotoxic chemotherapy. Additionally, interferon increases the expression of antigenic structures on cell surfaces,[61–63] including both tumor-associated antigens and estrogen receptors, and therefore the use of interferon with hormonal or other immunologic approaches may be useful. While alpha interferon has only marginal antitumor activity as a single agent in far-advanced human breast cancer, it may be that its use in combination therapy with cytotoxic drugs, hormonal agents, or other biologicals may yet prove to be clinically beneficial.

Phase I studies with both beta and gamma interferon are under way and at least two exploratory studies evaluating natural beta interferon in breast cancer patients have been performed.[63–65] Results are too preliminary for comment. In vitro studies suggest that gamma interferon may be a more potent immunomodulatory and cytostatic agent than either alpha or beta interferon. Phase I trials with gamma interferon have been completed[32] and phase II studies instituted. Combinations of gamma with either alpha or beta may also be potentially useful.

INTERFERON INDUCERS

A number of agents, both natural and synthetic, capable of inducing interferon production either in vitro or in vivo, have been identified. Some of these have been evaluated in murine and subhuman primate systems for their antitumor and/or immune modulating effects, but very few have been tested in humans. The mechanism(s) by which interferon production is induced by these agents is unknown. In general, the antitumor activity and immunomodulating capabilities of interferon inducers have correlated with their ability to induce demonstrable levels of serum interferon activity, although there are exceptions to this.

In addition to viruses, several other microorganisms, including some bacteria (e.g., *Brucella abortus, Corynebacterium parvum*), protozoa, rickettsiae, and mycoplasmas, as well as bacterial products such as endotoxin and certain antibiotics, are capable of inducing interferon production.[66] However, to date, the most extensively studied agents have been the polyanions, including the synthetic nucleic acids, poly ICLC and polyadenylic acid–polyuridylic acid (poly A:U). In addition, certain low-molecular-weight amines such as the pyrimidinones, the fluorenones, and the lipoidal amines await clinical testing. Most of these agents, in addition to inducing interferon production, also have a profound effect on the immune system. While the unavailability, until recently, of interferon in a sufficient quantity to do all the preclinical and clinical trials desired undoubtedly led to the interest in many of these interferon inducers, it may be that they have sufficient immunomodulating capability of their own. Continued interest in the interferon inducers may therefore be justified despite the current general availability of highly purified interferons. In fact, in many experimental situations inducers have consistently had greater antitumor and antiviral activity than exogenously administered interferon.

Poly ICLC

In 1967 it was reported that both natural and synthetic double-stranded RNA were capable of inducing high titers of interferon in rodents.[67] It has subsequently been demonstrated that these agents are perhaps the most efficient agents capable of interferon induction.[68] Poly I:C, a synthetic double-stranded RNA, has demonstrable antitumor and immune augmentating activity in several rodent systems[69] and has become the most widely studied interferon inducer. It has been shown, however, that this agent is not very efficient at inducing interferon production in primates,[68] presumably because it is neutralized by the hydrolytic activity present in human and other primate plasma. Various complexes have been formed in attempts to counteract this hydrolysis. One such formulation, a complex of poly-L-lysine and carboxymethylcellulose followed by the addition of poly I:C, provides an opalescent but soluble complex—poly-ICLC.[70] This material is relatively resistant to hydrolysis by primate sera and is capable of inducing detectable interferon production in both monkeys and humans.

Clinical toxicity following administration of poly ICLC can be significant but is dose-related. A dose above 12 mg/m^2 is intolerable, while doses between 6 and 12 mg/m^2 cause some potential concern. Doses of 4 mg/m^2 or less, however, appear tolerable and most current studies are using doses in this range. Results from preliminary immunologic evaluations have been variable but suggest augmentation of monocyte-mediated cytostatic activity, despite the inability to detect substantial amounts of induced circulating interferon activity.

Extensive immunological monitoring was performed on patients receiving poly ICLC in two studies in which patients received weekly or biweekly doses of 1 and 4 mg/m^2 intramuscularly or intravenously.[71] These studies demonstrated sustained augmentation of monocyte-mediated cytostatic activity and 2′-5′A synthetase expression (a marker of interferon induction) which were *not* clearly dose-related. Augmentation of NK activity was seen only occasionally. T-cell subset evaluation revealed consistent elevation in the percentage of cells expressing the surface antigen OKT10 (normally found on NK cells and activated T and B lymphocytes) and an increase in the ratio of helper to suppressor cells.

In summary, objective antitumor responses (complete, partial, or minor) have been noted in a few patients in these preliminary trials, all in malignancies also responsive to exogenous interferon. Currently, there are ongoing phase II studies evaluating poly ICLC in patients with a variety of tumors, including advanced breast cancer.[72]

Polyadenylic Acid–Polyuridylic Acid (Poly A:U)

Polyadenylic acid–polyuridylic acid (poly A:U) is a double-stranded synthetic polynucleotide. In a recent review of the available preclinical data, Johnson reported that poly A:U had demonstrable immune-augmenting capabilities similar to other polynucleotides, despite the fact that it is a very poor inducer of interferon.[73] It does, however, have a profound augmenting effect on murine macrophage activity, increasing antigen processing ability and cytotoxicity following in vitro stimulation.

Poly A:U has been shown to have demonstrable antitumor activity in at least three rodent systems. A dose of 250 μg per mouse reduced the number of subsequent metastases and prolonged life when administered as an adjuvant to the complete surgical removal of the primary spontaneous mammary tumor of C3H mice.[74] Three doses of 15 μg given soon after birth also delayed and/or prevented the development of spontaneous mammary tumors in a significant number of genetically susceptible C3H mice.[75] Also, in this spontaneous C3H mammary tumor system, the combination of poly A:U with cyclophosphamide has been shown to be synergistic in both an antitumor effect and in augmenting NK cytotoxicity. Smaller tumors, fewer animals with tumors, and prolongation of life were all noted following the use of combined treatment and were associated with an augmentation of NK cytotoxicity.[76]

In a large controlled clinical trial for which the C3H studies served as a model, poly A:U has been reported to have improved the overall survival of patients (5-year follow-up) with operable breast cancer.[77,78] Patients with stage I or II adenocarcinoma of the breast were randomized following mastectomy to receive either 30 mg poly A:U intravenously weekly for 6 weeks or no further therapy. All patients subsequently determined to have histologic node involvement also received postoperative radiation therapy. Three-year and 5-year analyses reveal that the group receiving poly A:U survived longer than those receiving no adjuvant immunostimulatory therapy.[77,78] Subset analysis indicated that nearly all the therapeutic benefit from poly A:U was confined to those patients with only one to three nodes involved. Poly A:U therapy was also associated with an augmentation of NK cytotoxicity and with an increase in protein kinase and 2′-5′A synthetase activity, even though circulating interferon was not detectable in the serum.[79,80]

In a series of studies evaluating the effect of poly A:U on NK cytotoxicity and on the induction of interferon-induced enzyme activity, Hovanessian et al. have reported that augmentation of NK cytotototoxicity and induction of protein kinase and 2′-5′A synthetase occurred in both tumor-bearing rodents and humans.[81–83] In another interesting series of experiments, nude mice, carrying a xenograft of HeLa cells, were treated with either poly A:U, murine alpha/beta interferon, or human beta interferon.[83] Murine interferon stimulated protein kinase and 2′-5′A synthetase activity in the host cells, human beta interferon stimulated similar activity in the human xenograft, while poly A:U stimulated enzyme activity and demonstrable interferon production in both murine and human (HeLa) cells. Thus, human tumor cells may be induced to produce interferon following poly A:U stimulation with subsequent interferon induction of both protein kinase and 2′-5′A synthetase activity.

In summary, this synthetic polynucleotide, although a relatively poor inducer of interferon, has demonstrable antitumor activity in several murine systems; has been associated with prolongation of survival in one human clinical trial; has variable immune-augmenting effects on the immune systems of both rodents and humans; and appears to be nontoxic. As a result, more extensive clinical testing is planned.

MONOCLONAL ANTIBODIES

Several laboratories have recently produced monoclonal antibodies to a variety of breast cancer-associated antigens. Ceriani and colleagues originally produced a polyclonal heterologous antisera to human milk fat globules.[84,85] As milk is secreted, the breast epithelial cell encases the fat globule in the plasma membrane. Thus, a polyclonal antisera produced with milk fat globule would also contain antibodies that would recognize components of the plasma membrane. Using this polyclonal heterologous antiserum, three antigenic structures within the plasma membrane were demonstrated with molecular weights of 150,000, 75,000, and 45,000. Most patients with breast cancer were also shown to have circulating tumor-associated antigens recognized by this polyclonal antisera. More recently, monoclonal antibodies have been produced which recognize these membrane components.[86,87] These are undergoing development for potential clinical use. Recent preclinical experiments revealed enhanced effects using combinations of these antibodies.[88]

Vitteta and her group have produced a monoclonal antibody to cultured breast cancer cells which recognizes a subset of ER+ malignant cells. They have tagged this monoclonal, an IgM, with the toxin ricin and have demonstrated in vitro cytotoxicity.[89,90] Further development of this immunoconjugate is under way.

Schlom and associates at the NCI initially produced human monoclonal antibodies by hybridizing lymphocytes, obtained from axillary lymph nodes of patients with primary mammary carcinoma, with a murine myeloma cell line.[91] Subsequently, they have also used metastatic tumor cells as immunogens and produced a number of murine monoclonal antibodies which recognize a number of tumor-associated antigenic determinants on a variety of malignant breast cells.[92–94] One of these monoclonal antibodies has been shown to recognize human breast cancer tissue in the nude mouse model and one or more may prove useful diagnostically or therapeutically.

IMMUNOBIOLOGY OF BREAST CANCER

Relatively little is known of the immunobiology of adenocarcinoma of the breast. During the time of peak interest in nonspecific immunostimulation therapy, several studies were performed evaluating the general immunocompetence of patients with breast cancer.[95–104] These studies established that there is a tendency to an increase in immunoincompetency as the tumor burden increases; patients with carcinoma of the breast generally remain immunocompetent throughout the natural history of their disorder. Some decrease in responsiveness to dinitrochlorobenzene (DNCB) was frequently demonstrated, but very few other consistent abnormalities, either in delayed hypersensitivity, the absolute number of lymphocytes or E-rosette-positive cells, the blastogenic response to phytohemagglutinin, or in immunoglobulin levels were demonstrable. Further, no correlation between prognosis and immunocompetence or lack thereof in patients with any stage of disease was shown. (See Chap. 10 for other viewpoints.)

Immunoreactivity to tumor-associated antigens has been demonstrated by a number of techniques in patients with all stages of breast cancer. In vitro, using both the leukocyte migration inhibition (LMI) assay and the leukocyte adherence inhibition (LAI) assay, a number of investigators have demonstrated immunoreactivity to tumor-associated antigens using tumor cell extracts, soluble membrane extracts of MCF-7 cells, and soluble membrane extracts of fresh tumor tissue obtained by biopsy.[105–109] Associated with several of these studies has been the demonstration of serum blocking factors.[110–112] An inverse correlation between the stage of tumor and the degree of cellular immunity to tumor-associated antigens demonstrated in vitro by either the LAI or the LMI and a direct correlation between clinical stage and the quantity of serum blocking factors with stage of tumor can be demonstrated. Nearly 80 percent of patients with stage I or II disease have demonstrable in vitro cell-mediated immunity, but fewer than 30 percent with more advanced disease do.

Circulating immune complexes have frequently been demonstrated in patients with all stages of adenocarcinoma of the breast.[113,114] One prospective study evaluated the potential for immune complex determination as a diagnostic tool and demonstrated that, while levels of complexes were increased in many patients, none of the assays had sufficient discriminatory capacity to warrant serious attention to this approach as a diagnostic tool.[113]

The demonstration of delayed hypersensitivity (in vivo) to tumor-associated antigens has not been particularly successful. Most studies have used crude membrane-soluble extracts of fresh tumor cells and/or of cultured breast carcinoma cells (MCF-7), and the results have been variable and poorly discriminatory. However, by using crude membrane extracts prepared from cultured breast tumor cells (MCF-7) which had been infected with vesicular stomatitis virus, augmentation of antigenicity was demonstrable. Using these crude membrane extracts, 85 percent of patients with breast cancer demonstrated positive delayed hypersensitivity.[115] This augmenting approach could conceivably be evaluated as an immunodiagnostic test.

Lastly, the T antigen, a precursor of the M and N blood group antigens, has been demonstrated on the cell surface of nearly all breast and other adenocarcinoma tissues examined. This antigen is not expressed on normal cells (it is masked) and as a result, all normal individuals have demonstrable circulating anti-T (an IgM) antibody. When the T antigen becomes unmasked in adenocarcinoma tissues, patients mount a strong cellular immune reaction to it. Eighty-five percent of such patients have demonstrable delayed hypersensitivity and over 40 percent have demonstrable in vitro leukocyte migration inhibition induced by the T antigen. About 20 percent of patients will also have severely depressed anti-T immunoglobulin levels.[116]

NONSPECIFIC IMMUNOTHERAPY

Nonspecific immunotherapy in the form of bacillus Calmette-Guérin (BCG), *Corynebacterium parvum*, and levamisole has been evaluated in a number of studies.[117] BCG has been studied in three randomized studies: one in combination with cytotoxic chemotherapy in patients with stage II disease, a second in combination with radiation therapy of primary breast carcinoma, and a third in combination with cytotoxic chemotherapy in patients with stage IV disease. In none of these studies was clinical benefit associated with nonspecific therapy.[118–120] *Corynebacterium parvum* has also been studied in patients with stage IV disease in combination with chemotherapy. Again, in no study was clinical benefit demonstrable.[121,122] Levamisole was initially shown to prolong survival following radiation therapy in patients with stage III carcinoma and was also beneficial when given in combination with cytotoxic chemotherapy, but three subsequent studies using levamisole in combination with chemotherapy in patients with stage II and stage IV disease have demonstrated no survival benefit.[123–127] Thus, in only 2 of 10 studies evaluating these nonspecific agents could any benefit be shown.

A number of studies using animal models have demonstrated therapeutic efficacy using an ex vivo exposure of plasma to staphylococcal protein A.[128] Staph protein A (SPA) is a polypeptide with a molecular weight of about 42,000 and is produced by most staphylococcal organisms. It has a strong affinity for the Fc fragment of mammalian IgG and may therefore bind circulating Ig and/or immune complexes. These in vivo animal studies demonstrated therapeutic effect using both a spontaneous mammary carcinoma system in dogs and a chemically induced mammary carcinoma in rats.

Investigators have demonstrated an immune complex decrease in plasma following exposure to protein A and simultaneously demonstrated an increase in tumor-specific cytotoxic antibodies. It was felt that the removal of immune complexes which may have been immunosuppressive allowed the release of, or at least allowed tumor-cytotoxic antibodies to become effective. In a pilot study performed in five patients with advanced carcinoma of the breast therapeutic efficacy was demonstrable following repeated exposure of plasma to SPA embedded in a colloidal charcoal mixture.[128] Several studies attempting to confirm these results have been and are being performed.[128] To date, results have been variable. Responses have been seen but not in all studies and not to the degree originally reported. Further investigation continues.

CONCLUSION

The era of immunotherapy during the 1970s produced much hope and no clinical benefit. The era of the interferons during the late 1970s and early 1980s produced more hope but also some demonstrable clinical effect, even in patients with advanced breast cancer. Problems with dose, scheduling, and use in appropriate combination therapy must now be worked out. Approaches using other lymphokines are being developed preclinically while monoclonal antibody therapy with its ability to select tumor cell targets for cytotoxic therapy has begun being clinically tested. Interest in the area of biological therapy remains high and its potential is real.

Acknowledgment

The author acknowledges with appreciation the secretarial assistance of Randi Sigal.

REFERENCES

1. Krim M: Towards tumor therapy with interferons, Part 1. Interferons: Production and properties. *Blood* 55:711, 1980.
2. Taniguchi T, Mantei N, Schwarzstein M, Shigekazu N, Muramatsu M, Weissmann C: Human leukocyte and fibroblast interferons are structurally related. *Nature* 285:2848, 1980.
3. Gray PW et al: Expression of human immune interferon cDNA in *E. coli* and monkey cells. *Nature* 295:503, 1982.
4. Fiers W et al: Molecular-biological studies on human fibroblast interferon, immune interferon and interleukin-2 genes, in DeMaeyer E, Schellekens H (eds): *The Biology of the Interferon System 1983.* Amsterdam, Elsevier, 1983, p. 3.
5. Allen G, Fantes KH: A family of structural genes for human lymphoblastoid (leukocyte-type) interferon. *Nature* 287:408, 1980.
6. Weissmann C et al: Structure and expression of human a-interferon genes, in Miwa M et al (eds): *Primary and Tertiary Structure of Nucleic Acids and Cancer Research.* Tokyo, Japan Sci. Soc Press, 1982, p. 1.
7. Rubinstein M: The structure of human interferons. *Biochim Biophys Acta* 695:5, 1982.
8. Cantell K, Hirvonen S: Preparation of human leukocyte interferon for clinical use. *Tex Rep Biol Med* 35:138, 1977.
9. Finter NB, Fantes KH: The purity and safety of interferons prepared for clinical use: The case of lymphoblastoid interferon, in Gresser I (ed): *Interferon 2.* London, Academic Press, 1980, p. 65.
10. Goeddel DV et al: Human leukocyte interferon produced by *E. coli* is biologically active. *Nature* 287:411, 1980.
11. Gutterman JU et al: Leukocyte interferon-induced tumor regression in human metastatic breast cancer, multiple myeloma, and malignant lymphoma. *Ann Intern Med* 93:399, 1980.
12. Borden EC et al: Leukocyte-derived interferon (alpha) in human breast carcinoma. *Ann Intern Med* 97:1, 1982.
13. Smalley RV: Anti-tumor effects of natural alpha (leukocyte) interferon, in Finter NB, Oldham RK (eds): *Interferon—In Vivo Use.* Amsterdam, Elsevier, p.251, 1985.
14. Henderson IC, Frei E: Personal communication, 1984.
15. Sarna GP, Figlin RA: Phase II trial of alpha-lymphoblastoid interferon (Wellferon) given weekly as treatment of advanced breast cancer. *Cancer Treat Rep*, 1985.

16. Goodwin BJ et al: Phase II trial of human lymphoblastoid interferon (Wellferon) in metastatic breast cancer. *Proc ASCO* 3:60, 1984.
17. Silver HKB et al: Effect of lymphoblastoid interferon of lymphocyte subsets in cancer patients. *J Biol Resp Modif* 2:428, 1983.
18. Silver HKB, Connors JM, Salinas FA: A prospectively randomized phase I study of high versus low dose lymphoblastoid interferon. *Cancer Treat Rep*, 1985.
19. Masucci MG et al: Effect of interferon-A-1 from *E. coli* on some cell functions. *Science* 209:1431, 1980.
20. Hawkins MJ, Borden EC, Fein S, Simon KJ: Evaluation of the clinical and biological effects of recombinant human interferon alpha rD. *Proc ASCO* 2:50, 1983.
21. Hawkins MJ et al: American Cancer Society phase I trial of human interferon beta (IFN-B). *PROC AACR* 23:246, 1982.
22. Horoszewicz JS et al: Human fibroblast interferon in human neoplasia: Clinical and laboratory study. *Cancer Treat Rep* 62:1899, 1978.
23. Dianzani F, Fleischmann WR, Georgiades JA, Monahan TM: Immune interferon: Potential for cancer therapy, in Hersh EM et al (eds): *Augmenting Agents in Cancer Therapy*. New York, Raven Press, 1981, p. 239.
24. Osther K et al: Phase I and phase II trials with human gamma interferon, in DeMaeyer E, Schellekens H (eds): *The Biology of the Interferon System 1983*. Amsterdam, Elsevier, 1983, p. 527.
25. Sherwin SA et al: A preliminary phase I trial of partially purified interferon-gamma (IFN-y) in patients with cancer. *J Biol Resp Modif* 3:599, 1984.
26. Blalock JE, Georgiades JA, Langford MP, Johnson HM: Purified human immune interferon has more potent anticellular activity than fibroblast or leukocyte interferon. *Cell Immunol* 49:390, 1980.
27. Fleischmann WR Jr: Potentiation of the direct anticellular activity of mouse interferons: Mutual synergism and interferon concentration dependence. *Cancer Res* 42:869, 1982.
28. Weigent DA, Langford MP, Fleischmann WR Jr, Stanton GJ: Potentiation of lymphocyte natural killing mixtures of alpha or beta interferon with recombinant gamma interferon. *Infect Immun* 40:35, 1983.
29. Borden EC et al: Phase I trial of serine substituted recombinant interferon beta. *Proc ASCO* 3:58, 1984.
30. Devos R, Cheroutre H, Taya Y, Degrave W, Van Heuverswyn H, Fiers W: Molecular cloning of human immune interferon cDNA and its expression in eukaryotic cells. *Nucleic Acids Res* 10:2487, 1982.
31. van der Burg M et al: A phase I clinical study of recombinant interferon gamma (r-IFN-gamma) in cancer patients. *PROC ASCO* 3:64, 1984.
32. Smalley RV, Oldham RK: Phase I trials of biologic response modifers, *Drugs Exptl Clin Res*, 1986, in press.
33. Balkwill FR, Oliver RTD: Growth inhibitory effects of interferon on normal and malignant human haemopoietic cells. *Int J Cancer* 20:500, 1977.
34. Taylor-Papadimitriou J: Effects of interferons on cell growth and function, in Gresser I (ed): *Interferon 2*. London, Academic Press, 1980, p. 13.
35. Balkwill FR: Review: Interferons as cell-regulatory molecules. *Cancer Immunol Immunother* 7:7, 1979.
36. Shibata H, Taylor-Papadimitriou J: Effects of human lymphoblastoid interferon on cultured breast cancer cells. *Int J Cancer* 28:447, 1981.
37. Balkwill F, Watling D, Taylor-Papadimitriou J: Inhibition by lymphoblastoid interferon of growth of cells derived from the human breast. *Int J Cancer* 22:258, 1978.
38. Von Hoff DD, Gutterman J, Portnoy B, Coltman CA Jr: Activity of human leukocyte interferon in a human tumor cloning system. *Cancer Chemother Pharmacol* 8:99, 1982.
39. Salmon SE, Durie BGM, Young L, Liu RM, Trown PW, Stebbing N: Effects of cloned human leukocyte interferons in the human tumor stem cell assay. *J Clin Oncol* 1:217, 1983.
40. Balkwill F, Taylor-Papadimitriou J, Fantes KH, Sebesteny A: Human lymphoblastoid interferon can inhibit the growth of human breast cancer xenografts in athymic (nude) mice. *Eur J Cancer* 16:569, 1980.
41. Taylor-Papadimitriou J, Shearer M, Balkwill FR, Fantes KH: Effects of HuIFN-Alpha 2 and HuIFN-Alpha (Namalwa) on breast cancer cells grown in culture and as xenografts in the nude mouse. *J Int Res* 2:479, 1982.

42. Balkwill FR, Moodie EM, Freedman V, Fantes KH: Human interferon inhibits the growth of established human breast tumours in the nude mouse. *Int J Cancer* 30:231, 1982.
43. Balkwill FR, Moodie EM, Freedman V, Lane EB, Fantes KH: An animal model system for investigating the antitumor effects of human interferon. *J Int Res* 3:319, 1983.
44. Sebesteny A, Taylor-Papadimitriou J, Ceriani R, Millis R, Schmitt C, Trevan D: Primary human breast carcinomas transplantable in the nude mouse. *J Natl Cancer Inst* 63:1331, 1979.
45. Borden EC, Balkwill FR: Preclinical and clinical studies of interferons and interferon inducers in breast cancer. *Cancer* 53:783, 1984.
46. Balkwill FR, Moodie EM: Positive interactions between human interferon and cyclophosphamide or Adriamycin in a human tumor model system. *Cancer Res* 44:904, 1984.
47. DeClercq E, Zhang ZX, Huygen K, Leyten R: Inhibitory effect of interferon on the growth of spontaneous mammary tumors in mice. *J Natl Cancer Inst* 69:653, 1982.
48. Came PE, Moore DH: Effect of exogenous interferon treatment on mouse mammary tumors. *J Natl Cancer Inst* 48:1151, 1972.
49. Namba M, Miyoshi T, Kanamori T, Nobuhara M, Kimoto T, Ogawa S: Combined effects of 5-fluorouracil and interferon on proliferation of human neoplastic cells in culture. *GANN* 73:819, 1982.
50. Gould MN, Kakria RC, Olson S, Borden EC: Radiosensitization of human bronchogenic carcinoma cells by interferon beta. *J Interf Res* 4:123, 1984.
51. Priestman TJ: The present status of clinical studies with interferon in cancer in Britain. *Philos Trans R Soc Lond* [*Biol*] 299:119, 1982.
52. Wolmark N, Whisnant JK: Personal communication, 1984.
53. Horning SJ, Levine JF, Miller RA, Rosenberg SA, Merigan TC: Clinical and immunologic effects of recombinant leukocyte A interferon in eight patients with advanced cancer. *JAMA* 247:1718, 1982.
54. Gutterman JU et al: Recombinant leukocyte A interferon: Pharmacokinetics, single-dose tolerance, and biologic effects in cancer patient. *Ann Intern Med* 96:549, 1982.
55. Sherwin SA et al: A multiple-dose phase I trial of recombinant leukocyte A interferon in cancer patients. *JAMA* 248:2461, 1982.
56. Muss H et al: Intravenous interferon alpha-2 in patients with advanced breast cancer. *Proc ASCO* 2:99, 1983.
57. Sherwin SA et al: Recombinant leukocyte A interferon in advanced breast cancer. *Ann Intern Med* 98:598, 1983.
58. Neefe JR: Personal communication, 1984.
59. Nethersell A, Smedley H, Katrak M, Wheeler T, Sikora K: Recombinant interferon in advanced breast cancer. *Br J Cancer* 49:615, 1984.
60. Quesada JR: A collaborative phase I–II study of recombinant DNA-produced leukocyte interferon (clone A) in metastatic breast cancer, malignant lymphoma, and multiple myeloma. *AM J Med* 77:427, 1984.
61. Dimitrov NV, Meyer CJ, Strander H, Einhorn S, Cantell K: Interferon as a modifier of estrogen receptors. *Ann Clin Lab Science* 14:32, 1984.
62. Greiner JW, Horan Hand P, Noguchi P, Fisher PB, Pestka S, Schlom J: Enhanced expression of surface tumor-associated antigens on human breast and color tumor cells after recombinant human leukocyte alona-interferon. *Cancer Res* 44:3208, 1984.
63. Pouillart P et al: Administration of fibroblast interferon to patients with advanced breast cancer: Possible effects on skin metastasis and on hormone receptors. *Eur J Cancer* 18:929, 1982.
64. Lucero MA et al: Comparison of effects of leukocyte and fibroblast interferon on immunological parameters in cancer patients. *Eur J Cancer Clin Oncol* 18:243, 1982.
65. Quesada JR, Gutterman JU, Hersh EM: Clinical and immunological study of beta interferon by intramuscular route in patients with metastatic breast cancer. *J Interf Res* 2:593, 1982.
66. Sehgal PB, Pfeffer LM, Tamm I: Interferon and its inducers in chemotherapy of viral infections, in Came PE, Caliguiri LA (eds): *Handbook of Experimental Pharmacology*, vol. 61. Berlin, Springer-Verlag, 1982, p. 205.
67. Field AK, Tytell AA, Lampson GP, Hilleman MR: Inducers of interferon and host resistance. II. Multistranded synthetic polynucleotide complexes. *Proc Natl Acad Sci* 58:1004, 1967.

68. Levy HB: Induction of interferon by polynucleotides, in Stringfellow DA (ed): *Interferon and Interferon Inducers: Clinical Applications*. New York, Marcel Dekker, 1980, p. 167.
69. Levy HB, Stephen EB, Harrington D, Engel K, Riley F, Lvovsky E: Polynucleotides in the treatment of disease, in Hersh EM, Mastrangelo M, Chirigos M (eds): *Augmenting Agents in Cancer Therapy*. New York, Raven Press, 1981, p. 135.
70. Levy HB et al: A modified polyriboinosinic-polyribocyticylic acid complex that induces interferon in primates. *J Infect Dis* 132:434, 1975.
71. Stevenson HC, Abrams PG, Schoenberger CS, Smalley RV, Herberman RB, Foon KA: A phase I evaluation of Poly (I,C)-LC in cancer patients. *J Biol Resp Modif* 4:650, 1985.
72. Smalley RV, Stringfellow DA: Interferon inducers for clinical use, in Finter NB, Oldham RK (eds): *Interferon—In Vivo Use*. Amsterdam, Elsevier, 1985, p.337.
73. Johnson AG: Modulation of the immune system by synthetic polynucleotide. *Semin Immunopathol* 2:149, 1979.
74. Lacour F, Spira A, Lacour J, Prade M: Polyadenylic-polyuridylic acid, an adjuvant to surgery in the treatment of spontaneous mammary tumors in C3H/He mice and transplantable melanoma in the hamster. *Cancer Res* 32:648, 1972.
75. Lacour F, Delage G, Chianale C: Reduced incidence of spontaneous mammary tumors in C3H/He mice after treatment with polyadenylate-polyuridylate. *Science* 187:256, 1975.
76. Youn JK, Lacour F, Hue G: Inhibition of C3H/He mouse mammary tumor growth by combined treatment with cyclophosphamide and polyadenylic-polyuridylic acid. *Cancer Res* 42: 4706, 1982.
77. Lacour J et al: Adjuvant treatment with polyadenylic-polyuridylic acid (poly A-poly U) in operable breast cancer. *Lancet* 2:161, 1980.
78. Lacour J et al: Adjuvant treatment with polyadenylic-polyuridylic acid in operable breast cancer—updated results of a randomized trial. *Br Med J* 288:589, 1984.
79. Hovanessian AG et al: Enhancement of natural killer cell activity and 2-5A synthetase in operable breast cancer patients treated with polyadenylic-polyuridylic acid. *Cancer* 55:357, 1985.
80. Hovanessian AG, Riviere Y, Montagnier L, Michelson M, Lacour J, Lacour F: Enhancement of interferon-mediated protein kinase in mouse and human plasma in response to treatment with polyadenylic-polyuridylic acid. *J Interf Res* 2:209, 1982.
81. Youn JK, Hovanessian AG, Riviere Y, Hue G, Lacour F: Enhancement of natural killer cell activity and 2-5A synthetase in mice treated with polyadenylic-polyuridylic acid. *Cell Immunol* 79:298, 1983.
82. Hovanessian AG et al: Protein kinase (pp67-Ifn) in plasma and tissues of mice with high levels of circulating interferon. *Ann Virol* 132:175, 1981.
83. Riviere Y, Hovanessian AG: Direct action of interferon and inducers of interferon on tumor cells in athymic nude mice. *Cancer Res* 43:4596, 1983.
84. Ceriani RL, Thompson K, Peterson JA, Abraham S: Surface differentiation antigens of human mammary epithelial cells carried on the human milk fat globule. *Proc Natl Acad Sci* 74:582, 1977.
85. Sasaki M, Peterson JA, Ceriani RL: Quantitation of human mammary epithelial antigens in cells cultured from normal and cancerous breast tissues. *In Vitro* 17:150, 1981.
86. Taylor-Papadimitriou J, Peterson JA, Arklie J, Burchell J, Ceriani RL, Bodmer WF: Monoclonal antibodies to epithelium-specific components of the human milk fat globule membrane: Production and reaction with cells in culture. *Int J Cancer* 28:17, 1981.
87. Ceriani RL, Sasaki M, Sussman H, Wara WM, Blank EW: Circulating human mammary epithelial antigens in breast cancer. *Proc Natl Acad Sci* 79:5420, 1982.
88. Ceriani RL, Peterson JA, Blank EW: Experimental immunotherapy of human mammary tumors with monoclonal antibodies against normal breast epithelial cell surface components. Abstract E1. Conference on Immunity to Cancer, Williamsburg, Va., September, 1984.
89. Krolic KA, Yuan D, Vitetta ES: Specific killing of a human breast carcinoma line by a monoclonal antibody coupled to the A-chain of ricin. *Cancer Immunol Immunother* 12:39, 1981.
90. Yuan D, Hendler FJ, Vitetta ES: Characterization of a monoclonal antibody reactive with a subset of human breast tumors. *J Natl Cancer Inst* 68:719, 1982.

91. Schlom J, Wunderlich D, Teramoto YA: Generation of human monoclonal antibodies reactive with human mammary carcinoma cells. *Proc Natl Acad Sci* 77:6841, 1980.
92. Colcher D, Horan Hand P, Nuti M, Schlom J: A spectrum of monoclonal antibodies reactive with human mammary tumor cells. *Proc Natl Acad Sci* 78:3199, 1981.
93. Horan Hand P, Nuti M, Colcher D, Schlom J: Definition of antigenic heterogeneity and modulation among human mammary carcinoma cell populations using monoclonal antibodies to tumor-associated antigens. *Cancer Res* 43:728, 1983.
94. Colcher D, Zalutsky M, Kaplan W, Kufe D, Austin F, Schlom J: Radiolocalization of human mammary tumors in athymic mice by a monoclonal antibody. *Cancer Res* 43:736, 1983.
95. Wanebo HJ, Rosen PP, Thaler T, Urban JA, Oettgen HF: Immunobiology of operable breast cancer: An assessment of biologic risk by immunoparameters. *Ann Surg* 184:258, 1976.
96. Bolton PM et al: Immune competence in breast cancer—relationship of pretreatment immunologic tests to diagnosis and tumor stage. *Cancer Immunol Immunother* 1:251, 1976.
97. Stein JA, Adler A, Efraim SB, Maor M: Immunocompetence, immunosuppression, and human breast cancer. I. An analysis of their relationship by known parameters of cell-mediated immunity in well-defined clinical stages of disease. *Cancer* 38:1171, 1976.
98. Weese JL et al: Immunologic monitoring in carcinoma of the breast. *Surg Gynecol Obstet* 145:209, 1977.
99. Wanebo HJ et al: Immunologic reactivity in patients with primary operable breast cancer. *Cancer* 41:84, 1978.
100. Krown SE, Pinsky CM, Wanebo HJ, Braun DW, Wong PP, Oettgen HF: Immunologic reactivity and prognosis in breast cancer. *Cancer* 46:1746, 1980.
101. Humphrey LJ, Humphrey MA, Singla OM, Volenec J: Immunologic responsiveness of patients with cancer. Relationship to tumor type, stage and prognosis. *Ann Surg* 193:574, 1981.
102. Levine PH et al: Studies on the role of cellular immunity and genetics in the etiology of rapidly progressing breast cancer in Tunisia. *Int J Cancer* 27:611, 1981.
103. Hortobagyi GN et al: Prognostic value of prechemotherapy skin tests in patients with metastatic breast carcinoma. *Cancer* 47:1369, 1981.
104. Hager JC, Rudczynski AB, Mortensen RF, Heppner GH, Furmanski P, Rich MA: Is tumor-associated immunologic reactivity in breast cancer patients prognostically significant? *Proc AACR* 22:145, 1981.
105. Black MM, Leis HP Jr, Shore B, Zachrau RE: Cellular hypersensitivity to breast cancer. Assessment by a leukocyte migration procedure. *Cancer* 33:952, 1974.
106. Cannon GB et al: Use of the leukocyte migration inhibition assay to evaluate antigenic differences in human breast cancers and melanomas. *J Natl Cancer Inst* 60:969, 1978.
107. McCoy JL et al: Inhibition of leukocyte migration by tumor-associated antigen in soluble extracts of human breast carcinoma. *J Natl Cancer Inst* 53:11, 1974.
108. Rudczynski AB, Dyer CA, Mortensen RF: Detection of cell-mediated immune reactivity of breast cancer patients by the leukocyte adherence inhibition response to MCF-7 extracts. *Cancer Res* 38:3590, 1978.
109. Lopez M, O'Connor R, MacFarlane JK, Thomson DMP: The natural history of antitumour immunity in human breast cancer assayed by tube leucocyte adherence inhibition. *Br J Cancer* 38:660, 1978.
110. Fujisawa T, Waldman SR, Yonemoto RH: Leukocyte adherence inhibition by soluble tumor antigens in breast cancer patients. *Cancer* 39:506, 1977.
111. Yonemoto RH, Fujisawa T, Waldman SR: Effect of serum blocking factors on leukocyte adherence inhibition in breast cancer patients. Specificity and correlation with tumor burden. *Cancer* 41:1289, 1978.
112. Tanaka F, Yonemoto RH, Waldman SR: Blocking factors in sera of breast cancer patients. *Cancer* 43:838, 1979.
113. Herberman RB et al: Report on international comparative evaluation of possible value of assays for immune complexes for diagnosis of human breast cancer. *Int J Cancer* 27:569, 1981.
114. Salinas FA, Wee KH, Silver HK, Ragaz J: Circulating immune complexes (CIC) and associated

antigen in breast carcinoma (BC) (meeting abstract). *Proc AACR* 23:986, 1982.

115. Austin FC et al: Breast cancer skin test antigens of increased sensitivity prepared from vesicular stomatitis virus-infected tumor cells. *Cancer* 49:2034, 1982.
116. Springer GF, Murthy MS, Desai PR, Scanlon EF: Breast cancer patient's cell-mediated immune response to Thomsen-Friedenreich (T) antigen. *Cancer* 45:2949, 1980.
117. Smalley RV, Oldham RK: Biological response modifiers: Preclinical evaluation and clinical activity. *CRC Critical Rev Oncol Hematol* 1:259, 1984.
118. Buzdar AU et al: Adjuvant chemotherapy with 5-fluorouracil, doxorubicin (Adriamycin) and cyclophosphamide, with or without BCG immunotherapy in stage II or III breast cancer, in Terry W, Rosenberg SA (eds): *Immunotherapy of Human Cancer*. Amsterdam, Elsevier North Holland, Inc., 1982, p. 175.
119. McCulloch PB, Poon M, Dent PB, Dawson P: A stratified randomized trial of 5-fluorouracil, doxorubin (Adriamycin), and cyclophosphamide alone or with BCG in stage IV breast cancer, in Terry W, Rosenberg SA (eds): *Immunotherapy of Human Cancer*. Amsterdam, Elsevier North Holland, Inc., 1982, p. 183.
120. Serrou B et al: Inefficacy of postradiotherapeutic BCG immunotherapy in T3-T4 breast cancer patients: A randomized trial, in Terry W, Rosenberg SA (eds): *Immunotherapy of Human Cancer*. Amsterdam, Elsevier North Holland, Inc., 1982, p. 195.
121. Pinsky C et al: *Corynebacterium parvum* as adjuvant to combination chemotherapy in patients with advanced breast cancer, in Crispen RG (ed): *Neoplasm Immunity: Solid Tumor Therapy*. Philadelphia, Franklin Institute Press, 1977, p. 145.
122. Haskell C, Ossorio R, Sarna G: Cyclophosphamide, methotrexate, and 5-fluorouracil with and without *Corynebacterium parvum* in the treatment of metastatic breast cancer, in Crispen RG (ed): *Neoplasm Immunity: Solid Tumor Therapy*. Philadelphia, Franklin Institute Press, 1977, p. 153.
123. Rojas AF, Mickiewicz E, Feierstein JN, Glait H, Olivari AJ: Levamisole in advanced human breast cancer. *Lancet* 1:211, 1976.
124. Klefstrom P, Holsti P, Grohn P, Heinonen E: Combination of levamisole immunotherapy with conventional treatments in breast cancer, in Terry W, Rosenberg SA (eds): *Immunotherapy of Human Cancer*. Amsterdam, Elsevier North Holland, Inc., 1982, p. 185.
125. Kay RG et al: Levamisole in primary breast cancer. A controlled study in conjunction with L-phenylalanine mustard. *Cancer* 51:1992, 1983.
126. Executive Committee of the Danish Breast Cancer Cooperative Group: Increased breast-cancer recurrence rate after adjuvant therapy with levamisole. A preliminary report. *Lancet* 2:824, 1980.
127. Smalley RV et al: Southeastern Cancer Study Group: Breast Cancer Studies 1972-1982. *Int J Radiat Oncol Biol Phys* 9:1867, 1983.
128. Oldham RK: Proceedings of symposium on ex vivo plasma immunoabsorption and protein A in cancer therapy. *J Biol Resp Modif* 3:229, 1984.

32

Interscapulomammothoracic Amputation

Irving M. Ariel, M.D.

INTRODUCTION

The purpose of this chapter is twofold:

1 An operative procedure is described for patients whose breast cancer has spread to the axillary lymph nodes, which have enlarged and fixed. The fixation of metastases to the axilla precludes performance of the usual radical mastectomy.

2 Also discussed is how the procedure applies to those cancers which remain localized and have spread to local-regional areas, but which have not produced any discernible distant metastases. Certain cancers do remain localized, spread through the regional lymph nodes, but do not spread to distant sites.

This is contrary to some current teachings of certain authors that all breast cancers are widely disseminated when first diagnosed and that attention should be directed to the metastases. These authors state that it does not matter what is done for the local cancer.[2]

INTERSCAPULOMAMMOTHORACIC AMPUTATION

Indications

Patients with extensive cancer of the breast with fixed axillary metastasis, often with ulceration, a mutilated and useless arm which is usually lymphedematous, who are otherwise in fair-to-good nutritional state and have exhausted all other therapeutic measures, are candidates for interscapulomammothoracic amputation.

Skin invasion of the breast with ulceration is no contraindication. However, if there is skin invasion by the cancer in the sites where the incision will be made, then the operation is contraindicated. Other contraindications to this radical operation are (1) distant metastases from the cancer, (2) deep infiltration in the chest wall with involvement of the ribs and musculature of the chest wall, and (3) fixed metastases to the supraclavicular region. If there are movable metastases to the

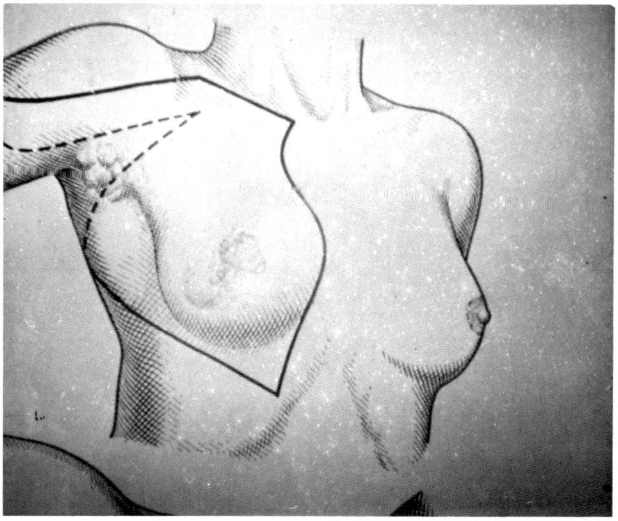

Figure 32-1 Lines of incision. The cephalic vein is exposed between the deltoid and pectoralis major muscles.

supraclavicular area, they can be handled by a low neck dissection.

The operation carries a relatively low mortality. Prudente experienced only 2 of 28 patients who expired, and these were the second and third patients on whom the operation was performed. We had no mortality in the four patients on whom we have performed the operation.

Technique of Interscapulomammothoracic Amputation

The technique is that originally developed by Prudente.[4]

Skin Incision

The incision starts at the internal border of the deltoid muscle at the level of its humeral insertion, following the deltopectoral space up to the coracoid process, and extends to the clavicle as far as its sternal attachment. The incision then makes an acute angle and descends circumferentially to the internal and inferior border of the breast, then ascends along the lateral mammary margin and crosses the lateral wall of the thorax toward the medial part of the latissimus dorsi (Fig. 32-1).

At the posterior wall of the thorax, the incision extends diagonally in a cephalad direction. It extends along the posterior axillary line and over the posterior edge of the deltoid as far as the humeral insertion, where it changes abruptly in direction, extending around the arm to reach its starting point. A generous flap is left on the posterior and superior part of the arm to cover the defect, as described by Ariel.[1]

Cleidectomy

This first portion of the incision with subsequent excision of the platysma muscle exposes the clavicle, the deltoid, and the pectoralis major muscle, as well as the clavicular insertion of the sternocleidomastoid and trapezius muscles. The cephalic vein is seen in the deltopectoral space. The periostium is elevated from the anterior surface of the clavicle, thereby removing the muscular insertions, and the cleidosternal and cleidocostal disarticulations are carefully made. The clavicle is severed close to the acromion with a Gigli saw.

Ligature of the Subclavian Vessels

The subclavian vessels and the brachial plexus are thus exposed. Ligature of the transverse

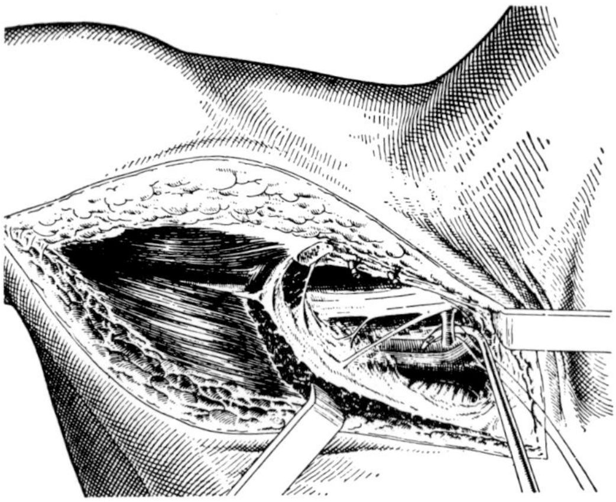

Figure 32-2 Disarticulation of the clavicle.

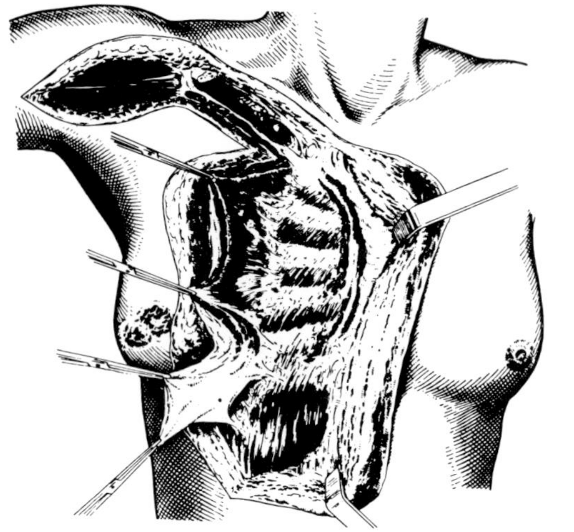

Figure 32-4 The incision has been made around the internal border of the breast. The pectoralis major muscle and anterior rectus sheath are divided and lifted, exposing the costal insertion of the pectoralis major.

cervical artery is easily performed as it crosses transversely through the superior part of the operative field (Fig. 32-2). The subclavian artery is then ligated in its extrascalenic portion as close as possible to the external edge of the anterior scalenus muscle. The subclavian vein is doubly ligated and brachial plexus are then severed (Fig. 32-3).

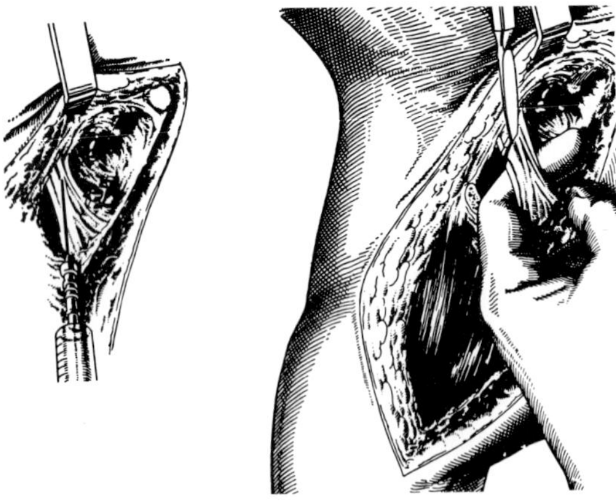

Figure 32-3 The brachial plexus is severed. Insert shows infiltration of brachial plexus with 2% procaine before severing the plexus.

Mastectomy

Resuming the cutaneous incision, one curves it around the inner aspect of the breast (Fig. 32-4). The dissection is continued, exposing the pectoralis major and anterior rectus sheath, as in a Halsted radical mastectomy. The pectoralis major is divided from the chest wall. The upper part of the rectus fascia is retracted. The exposed pectoralis minor muscle is severed off the chest wall (Fig. 32-5), which permits the resection of the breast and both pectoral muscles (Fig. 32-6).

Posterior Dissection

The patient's arm is rotated and placed in abduction. The cutaneous incision is then completed. A skin flap from the region of the deltoid is developed (Fig. 32-7). The muscles that arise from the thoracic wall and insert into the humerus and scapula can be exposed. The trapezius muscle, the levator scapulae, the rhomboideus, and the latissimus dorsi are

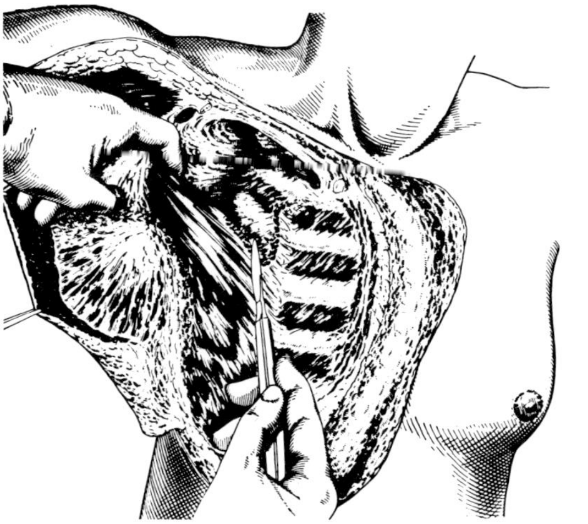

Figure 32-5 The pectoralis minor is dissected off the chest wall.

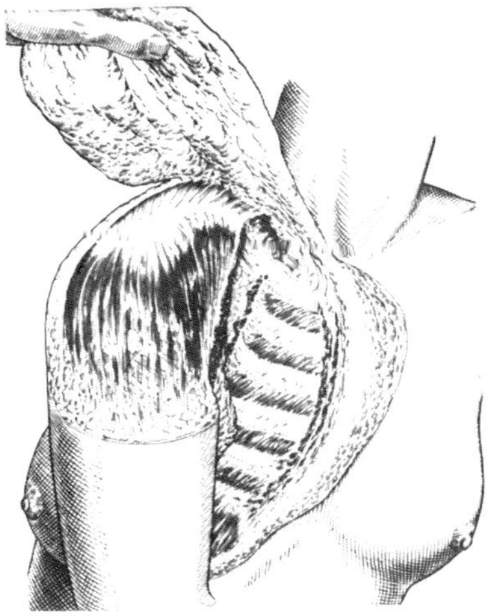

Figure 32-7 The arm is placed in abduction and the incision completed.

divided from above (Fig. 32-8), which permits removal of the whole member (Fig. 32-9). Several Hemovac drains are placed posteriorly, attached to suction.

Technical Variations

In some cases it is necessary to increase the scope of the operation by including a low neck (supraclavicular) dissection. Silva Neto and Abrao published a case of extension of the operation to the supraclavicular area as well as the internal mammary lymph nodes.[5]

RESULTS

This operation has been performed on four patients for breast cancer, as depicted in Table

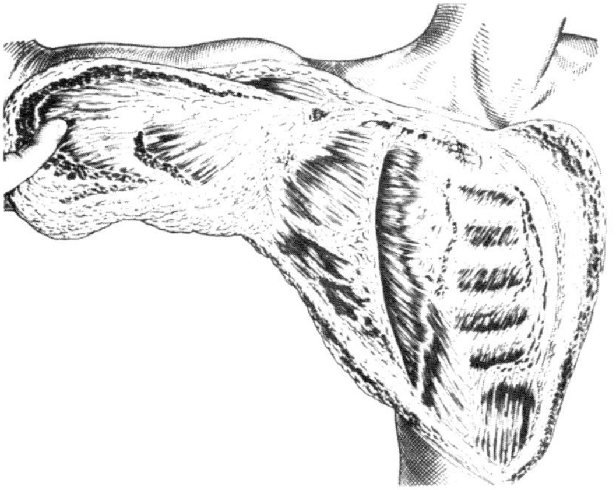

Figure 32-6 Breast and both pectoralis muscles swing to lateral side of chest.

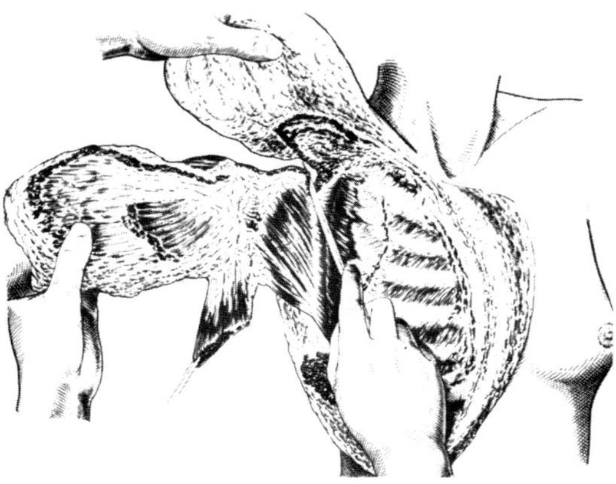

Figure 32-8 The trapezius and levator scapulae muscles are sectioned.

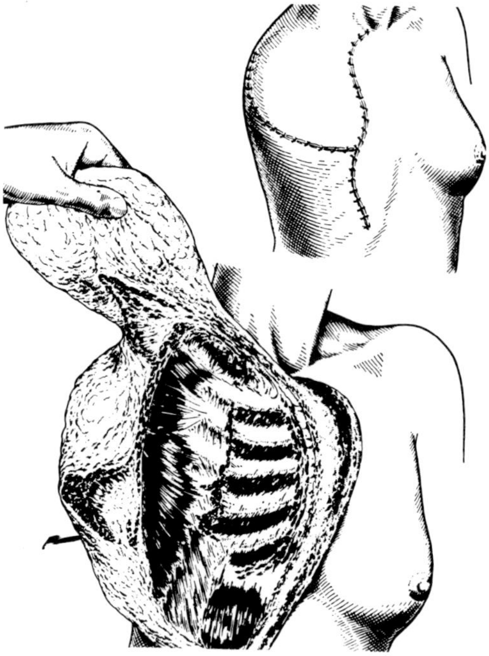

Figure 32-9 After removing the upper extremity, including the breast, skin flaps from the doomed extremity will cover the defect. In the upper part of the figure is seen the completed operation. Hemovac drains are inserted posteriorly.

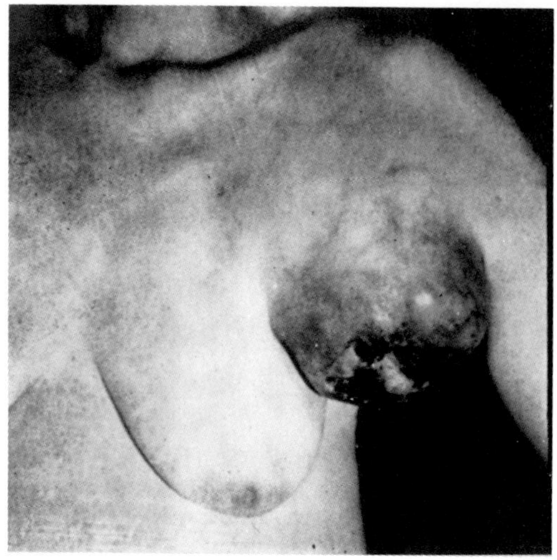

Figure 32-10 Clinical photograph of a 42-year-old female with a huge, fixed, ulcerated, and painful metastasis in the axilla. This represents a typical indication for interscapulo-mammothoracic amputation.

32-1. (Four additional operations were performed for sarcomas not arising in the breast and will not be discussed further in this presentation.)

Two of the patients succumbed 6 and 9 months after the operation—one due to metastasis to the brain and the other from generalized metastases. In these two patients, the operation was performed for palliation. Both were extremely grateful for the relief of excruciating pain due to involvement of the brachial plexus. The two other patients were followed—one for 5 years and the other for 6 years—and then were lost to follow-up. They remained free of evidence of metastases at the time of the last follow-up. They both moved out of our vicinity (one came from Venezuela), and despite exhaustive attempts to locate them, our efforts failed (Figs. 32-10, 32-11, and 32-12).

Prudente[4] reported that 27 percent survival of 5 years or longer occurred in 22 patients. One patient died 9 years after the amputation, and one died 11 years after the operation without evidence of recurrence. In other patients, recurrences developed at varying periods after the operation, varying from 5 to 9 months. These data indicate that breast cancer can grow to extensive proportions regionally, without concomitant distant metastases.

Holleb and Lucas[3] have had experience with six patients, five of whom had excellent palliation lasting from 8 months to 5 years. They stress that one must exclude those patients whose cancers are so extensive as to suggest a poor immediate prognosis and that proper selection of patients will usually provide worthwhile palliation and even, although rarely, a cure. Prudente stated that during a period from 1943 to 1947, the radical operation was almost completely abandoned in favor of therapeutic

Table 32-1 Summary of Patients Treated by Interscapulomammothoracic Amputation

Patient	Age	Indications for operation	Results and remarks
AB	35	Fixed axilla, severe pain. Status postmastectomy	Died 9 months from brain metastases; excellent palliation
RB	40	Severe ulceration due to breakdown of axillary metastases; excruciating pain	Died 1 year from disseminated metastases; extremely grateful for palliation
GR	42	Hard, fixed mass in axilla plus an edematous breast producing severe pain. Soft, mobile node in supraclavicular region	Well 5 years after operation; lost to follow-up
RZ	50	Severe pain in axilla due to ulcerated, impacted lymph nodes which measured 10 cm in diameter	Well 6 years after operation; lost to follow-up

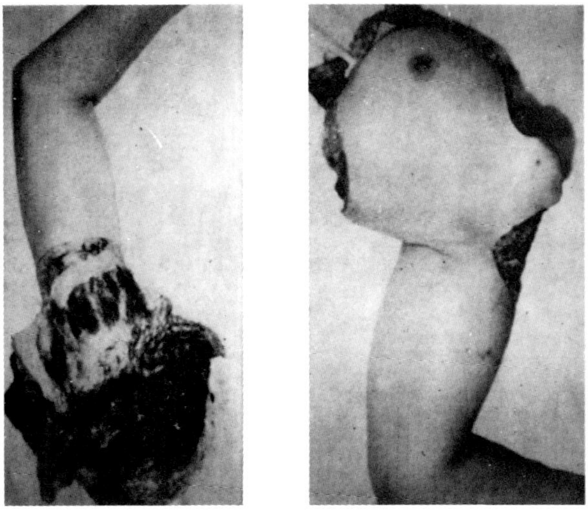

Figure 32-11 Surgical specimen removed by interscapulomammothoracic amputation. A. Anterior view. B. Posterior view. Patient remained well for 5 years with marked palliation.

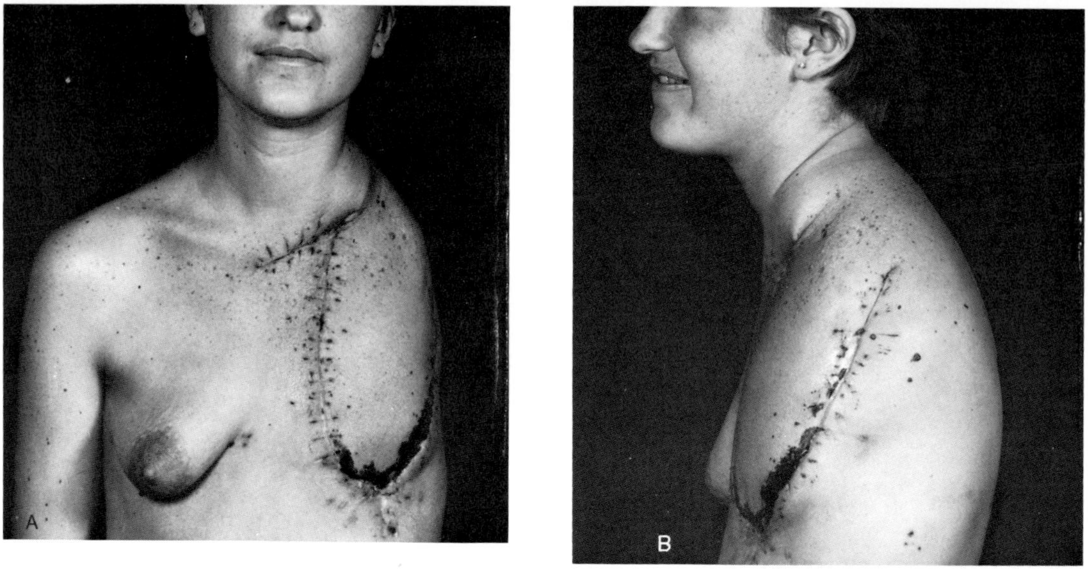

Figure 32-12 Anteroposterior view of a patient after interscapulomammothoracic amputation.

tests of treating these advanced carcinomas with hormone therapy. Although the initial results were encouraging, the duration of symptomatic relief was so short-lived that he was forced to return to the interscapulomammothoracic amputation.

CONCLUSION

Patients with fixed axillary metastases, marked lymphedema of the upper extremity, a mutilated and useless arm as a result of the pathologic involvement, who are otherwise in good nutritional state and have no evidence of distant metastases, are suitable candidates for the interscapulomammothoracic amputation. It will cure the cancer in a selected few instances and will offer worthwhile palliation in others. Other treatment modalities (radiation therapy, chemotherapy, and hormone therapy) had been administered and failed.

The fact that some, albeit a few, patients may be cured and others will have a worthwhile prolongation of their lives emphasizes the need for adequate local-regional therapy. All breast cancers have not become disseminated when the patient is first seen by the surgeon. In fact, some cancers may remain localized to a given anatomic region for prolonged periods before generalized dissemination occurs. This observation is emphasized by two of the patients of this report, and those reported by Prudente where marked increased survival was obtained despite the very extensive cancers necessitating so radical a procedure as interscapulomammothoracic amputation.

REFERENCES

1. Ariel IM: The use of flaps from the doomed extremities for closing defects after major amputations. *Clin Orthop* 26:128, 1963.
2. Fisher B, Wolmark N, Bauer M, Redmond C, Gebhardt N: The accuracy of clinical nodal staging and of limited axillary dissection as a determinant of histological nodal status of carcinoma of the breast. *Surg Gynecol Obstet* 152:765, 1981.

3. Holleb AI, Lucas JC Jr: Palliative interscapulothoracic amputation in the management of breast cancer patients. *Cancer* 12:643, 1959.
4. Prudente A: Interscapulomammothoracic amputation, in Pack G, Ariel I (eds): *Treatment of Cancer and Allied Diseases*. Paul Hoeber, New York, 1964, Vol. IV, p. 133.
5. Silva Neto JB, Abrao A: Supraclavicular resseccao de cadeia gangliomas mamaria interna por cancer da mamma. *Per Brasil Cir* 35:205, 1958.

Part Seven

Reconstruction

33

Breast Reconstruction

Francis J. Gillen, M.D.

INTRODUCTION

As alternatives in the treatment of breast cancer have evolved during the past 20 years, so has reconstruction of the breast. Patients have become more aware of the availability of reconstructive procedures and now seek from their surgeons information regarding this phase of treatment. In a population that has become more knowledgeable and, in a society concerned with esthetics and choices, it has become natural for patients to seek information regarding reconstruction (Fig. 33-1). With the experience gained over the past decade, reconstructive techniques have improved dramatically. The original idea of reconstruction to create an acceptable mound[26] has evolved to construct for the patient a chest wall that is esthetically pleasing.[14]

There has been a marked increase in the number of breast reconstructions in recent years. Those seeking reconstruction are self-referrals. Physicians still hesitate to refer patients for breast reconstruction. The patient is breaking the barrier between the ablative surgeon and the reconstructive surgeon.

The relationship between physician and patient is important.[13] The physician should know the patient, what she does, who she is, who is at home, how she feels about herself, and how she and her husband relate. This can be very time-consuming. Some doctors are not sensitive to this particular need of the breast cancer patient and are never able to bridge the gap between authoritative decision making and the role of the advisory physician who consoles, guides, and helps the patient toward decisions during this crisis situation.

It is estimated that less than 5000 mastectomy patients seek reconstruction per year. The conjecture is that few are referred, and the usual reason from referring physicians is that the reconstructive results are not good. (For whom?)

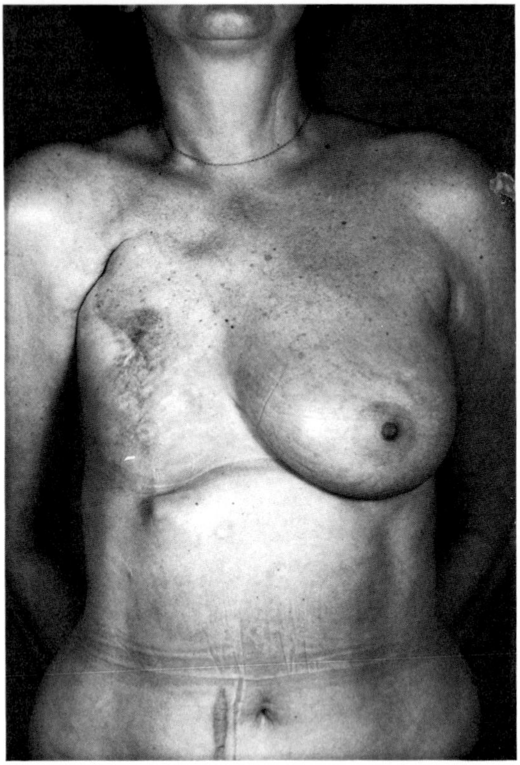

Figure 33-1 A typical defect 3 years following radical mastectomy. Notice flattening in the infraclavicular area and obliteration of the axillary fold.

With the expanded experience gained from the number of recent reconstructions, the results have also improved, resulting in satisfaction by the average patient.

EVALUATION

The reconstructive surgeon must obtain as much information as possible concerning treatment up to the time of consultation. The operative and pathology reports should be reviewed and adjuvant forms of therapy noted, whether current or planned for the future. In reviewing operative notes, the following points should be checked: (1) extent of dissection, (2) thickness of flaps, (3) amount of skin removed, (4) weight and size of the specimen, and (5) how the thoracodorsal bundle was handled (seen or unseen, dissected or not, ligated). The thoracodorsal bundle can play an important role in reconstruction and, if at all possible, should be preserved. From the pathology report, one checks (1) the histologic type, (2) location of the lesion, (3) size of specimen, (4) weight, (5) measurements of the skin in two dimensions, and (6) the number and level of nodes.

By knowing the primary tumor size and nodal involvement, the physician can estimate chances of local recurrence.[3] The amount of skin removal at ablation is important in determining the techniques for reconstruction.[19] Breast cancer is not a skin disease and should not be treated as such.[19]

MASTECTOMY INCISIONS

Ideally, a low oblique incision at the time of mastectomy is most favorable from a reconstructive point of view.[19] This incision can provide adequate access to the axilla, yet is concealed beneath a bra (Fig. 33-2). The incision should not compromise the surgical procedure, and should include the biopsy site and nipple area. It should be planned so that unnecessary scarring is prevented and optimum healing is obtained. Axillary scars are difficult to conceal, and scars approaching the sternum tend to hypertrophy (Fig. 33-3). If possible, incisions should be angled away from these two areas.

TYPES OF RECONSTRUCTION

Reconstruction is individualized and depends on the type of mastectomy, position of scars, adjuvant therapy, and the needs of the patient.[24,27,28] The aim of reconstruction should be an attractive chest wall with minimal scarring, that is pleasing when uncovered, and which shows symmetry and naturalness in size and shape.[10] The surgery itself should be

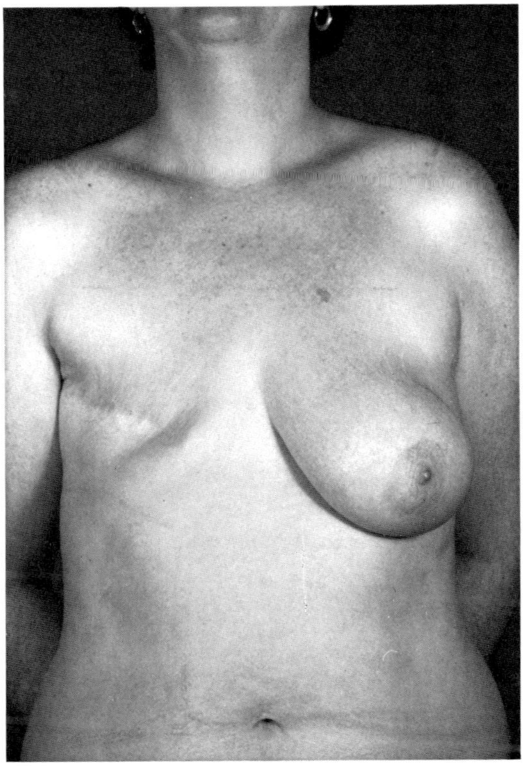

Figure 33-2 A low oblique incision is easily concealed.

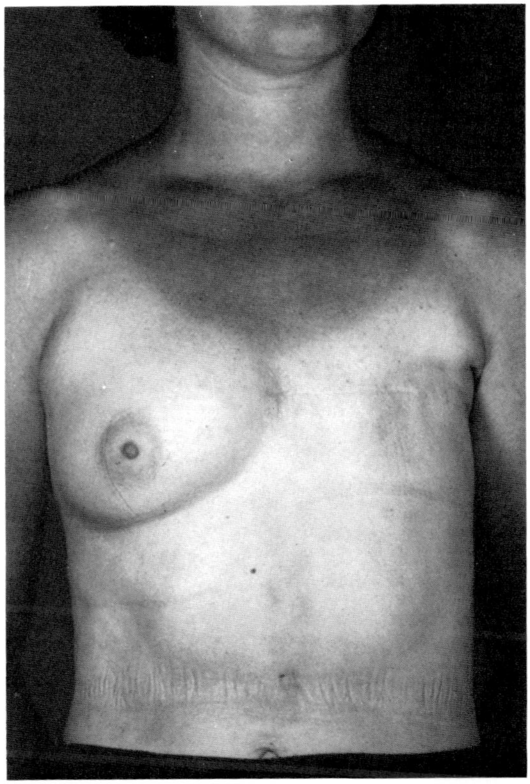

Figure 33-3 A well-healed scar would have avoided the midline.

nonthreatening to the patient and create minimal distortion to other parts of the body.

The simplest reconstruction involves the insertion of a prosthesis beneath the skin. This is what has been described as a breast mound.[26] This type of reconstruction, which can be done easily and is the least taxing to the patient, generally does not give a satisfactory result. After reconstruction, the breast should be attractive, natural in appearance, and symmetrical[9]; the simple insertion of a prosthesis beneath the skin does not provide for symmetry in most cases. The prosthesis becomes encapsulated and at times distorted, and the cosmetic result is not pleasing (Fig. 33-4).[17] The choice for reconstruction is with available local tissue or with tissue brought from a distant site.

Over a 15-year period nationwide, over 80 percent of breast cancer operations performed are now modified mastectomies.[2] At Memorial Sloan-Kettering Cancer Center in New York City, the ratio of radical to modified mastectomy has been reversed. The modified radical mastectomy makes for a better situation for reconstruction. The defects following modified mastectomy should be classified so that efforts to correct them can be devised.[6] For example, damage to the pectoral nerves will cause atrophy of the pectoralis major muscle (Fig. 33-5).

If sufficient skin, soft tissue, and preserved pectoral muscle are present, and if the defect present measures less than 6 cm, an implant

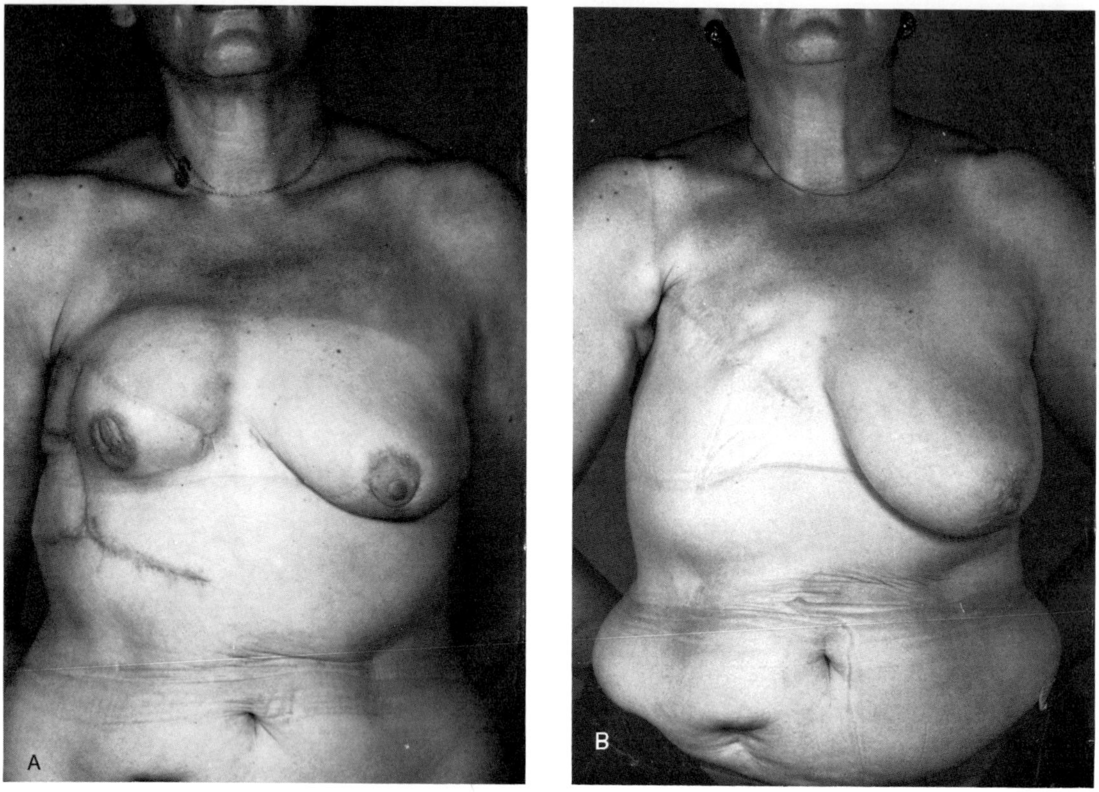

Figure 33-4 Local tissue reconstruction with implant beneath skin. A. Preoperative appearance. B. Appearance after a subcutaneous prosthesis.

placed beneath the muscles of the chest wall will give excellent results.[1,10] The implant is inserted in a submuscular fascial pocket beneath the pectoral muscles and those muscles below and lateral to the fifth rib (serratus anterior, external oblique, and rectus abdominis) which are raised as a unit to the sixth intercostal space, inferiorly, and the midaxillary line.[20] Submuscular placement provides good coverage for the implant, limits the incidence of exposure, and provides a more satisfactory symmetry.[25] Any theoretic objections to reconstruction on the grounds that recurrence can be masked by implant coverage is answered by this technique.[29] Another advantage is that subsequent biopsies can be performed without danger of implant exposure. This technique by itself is unsuitable if a large amount of skin has been removed or if the opposite breast is large.

Another method of reconstruction is replacing tissue removed at ablation by either local or distant flaps.[18,26] Replacement via local flaps has proved unsuccessful in my hands. Extensive scarring, inadequate available tissue, and asymmetry are a few of the problems.

One of the advances in plastic surgery in recent years has been use of the musculocutaneous flap. In this technique, muscle with overlying skin can be freed from its attachment, supported by its neurovascular bundle and moved to a new location. At present, the latissimus dorsi musculocutaneous flap is very popular.[7] The latissimus dorsi muscle is similar

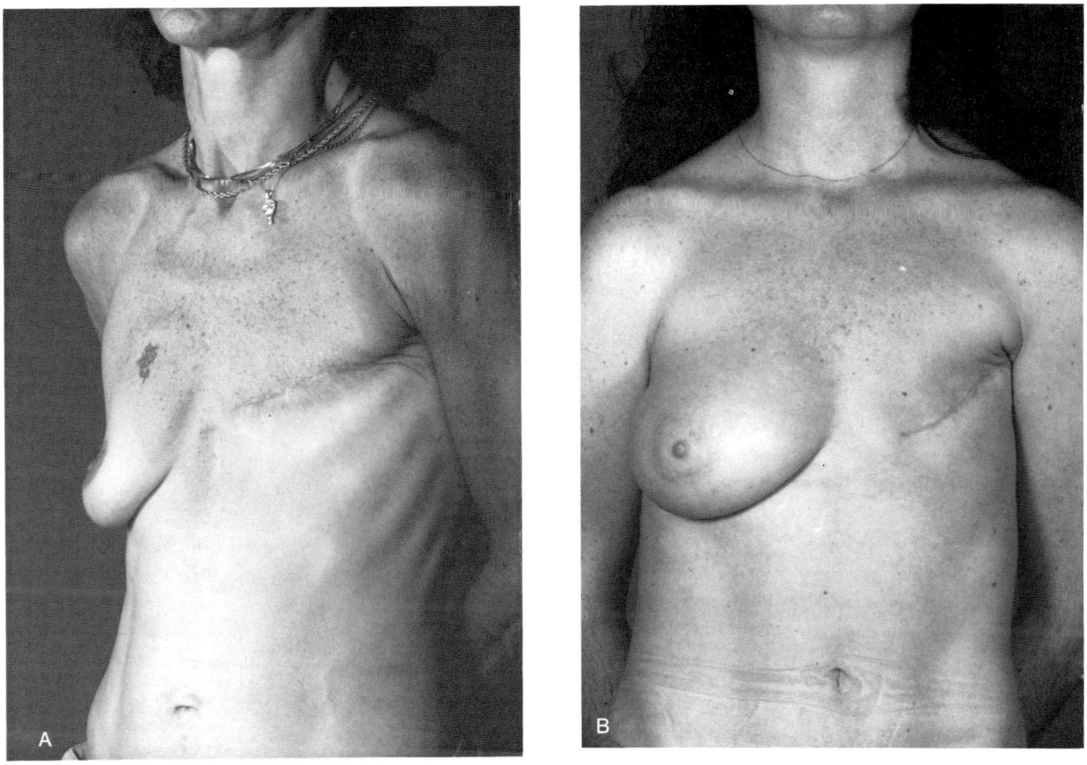

Figure 33-5 Modified mastectomy demonstrating variation in technique. Notice flatness inferior to suture line indicating damage to pectoral nerves.

in thickness to the pectoral muscle and, through its blood supply, can provide nourishment to a large portion of overlying skin and subcutaneous tissue.[5] The defect on the back can be closed primarily and the loss of the latissimus leaves little morbidity or long-term disability. It is a method of choice following standard radical mastectomies; one can replace missing skin, soft tissue, and muscle without need for delay.[8] Its use provides symmetry with the opposite breast, even if there is moderate ptosis (Figs. 33-6 and 33-7). The importance of the preservation of the blood supply to this muscle cannot be overemphasized. If the thoracodorsal bundle has been compromised, the muscle can still be used as a carrier for skin and soft tissue (based on lateral circulation from the serratus),[16] but the muscle is atrophic, easy to disrupt, and its reliability is lessened (Fig. 33-8).

Following radical mastectomy, this skin-muscle flap can be used to provide tissue for filling the infraclavicular area left hollow by removal of the pectoralis major muscle.[23] The axillary insertion of the latissimus dorsi muscle can be moved around to the divided pectoralis major insertion, thus simulating an anterior axillary fold (the normal swing of the pectoralis muscle across the axilla).

Most recently, the rectus abdominis muscle has been used as a source for a musculocutaneous flap.[14,15,18] This flap provides sufficient bulk so that a prosthesis is not needed. This flap is technically more difficult to obtain, takes twice as long to accomplish as the latissimus flap, and is less reliable. The contralateral rectus

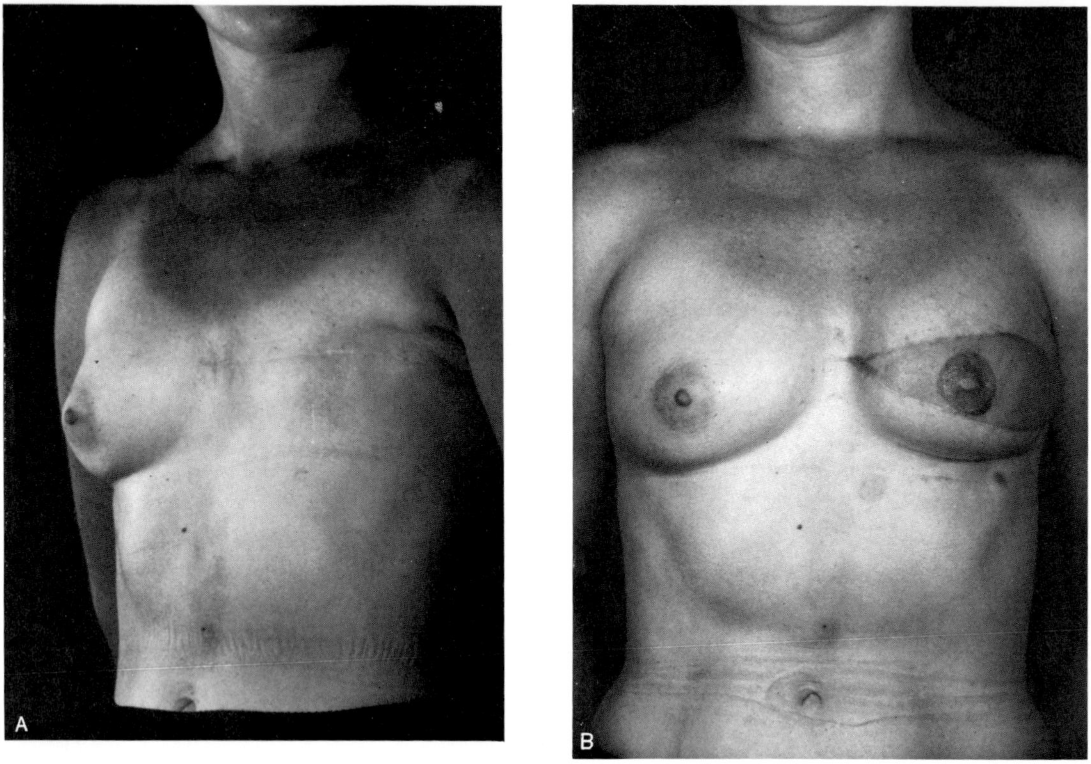

Figure 33-6 Latissimus dorsi reconstruction. The tanned ellipse of back skin gradually faded. A. Preoperative appearance. B. Appearance 1 year after a latissimus dorsi musculocutaneous flap.

muscle is used with the skin and subcutaneous tissue coming from the vertical, or transverse direction. If the skin and subcutaneous tissue is taken in a transverse fashion, it may be taken from above or below the umbilicus. This technique is challenging, but excellent results can be obtained. Patients should be chosen carefully. Those who have had previous abdominal surgery (more than half my patients), mediastinal radiation, or smokers should be carefully screened.

Removing the rectus below the arcuate line promotes a portal for a hernia to develop. This problem has been avoided by reinforcing this area with prolene mesh.

TIMING

Breast reconstruction can be performed at any time, even at the same time as the ablative surgery, except during chemotherapy. Submuscular fascial implantation at the conclusion of a modified mastectomy appears to provide the simplest and yet most satisfying reconstruction. There is no increase in morbidity or hospital stay, nor need for later readmission. It can be performed prior to the start of chemotherapy so that there is no prolonged waiting period. Positive nodes should not be a contraindication. In fact, some would argue that these patients should have immediate reconstruction since their time span may be less.

To accomplish the goal of immediate reconstruction, there must be a good working

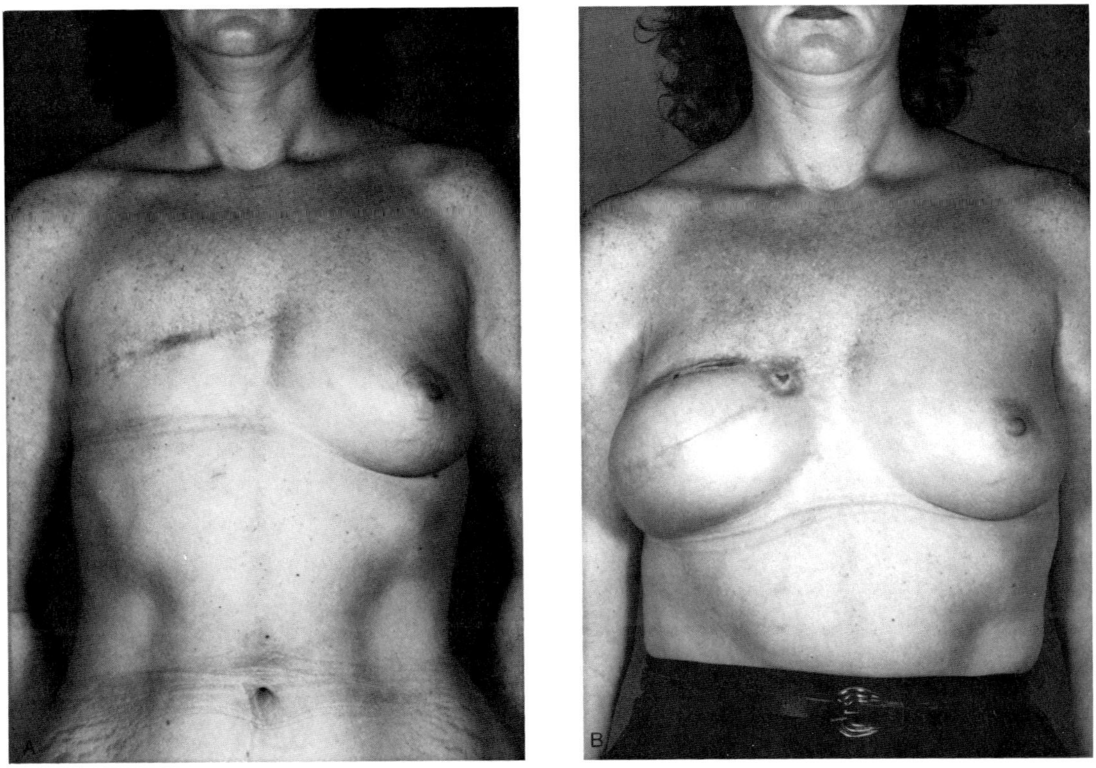

Figure 33-7 A. The latissimus flap provides cover and protection to the prosthesis, even when healing is delayed. B. Preoperative appearance.

relationship between the ablative and reconstructive surgeons, as it has to be a team effort.

If nothing else is accomplished, we have to lay to rest the ancient axiom that reconstruction should only be attempted after the patient has been able to experience the loss. Similarly, the statement that to overcome successfully the effects of mastectomy a patient must undergo a period of mourning for the amputated breast is barbaric and crude.

Delayed reconstruction, if immediate reconstruction is contraindicated, can be performed when the skin and soft tissue over the chest wall has softened, which is generally 3 to 6 months following mastectomy. At present, most patients are seen at this interval and with proper evaluation and selection of reconstructive techniques, a satisfactory result can be obtained.

THE OPPOSITE BREAST

In the age group with which we are dealing, it is not uncommon to have a ptotic opposite breast. If satisfactory symmetry cannot be obtained through the reconstructive procedures previously mentioned, then surgery on the remaining breast should be discussed with the patient and the surgeon. The options are many, including the need for prophylactic mastectomy and immediate reconstruction. Commonly, the opposite breast is usually reduced in size and elevated (reduction mammoplasty).

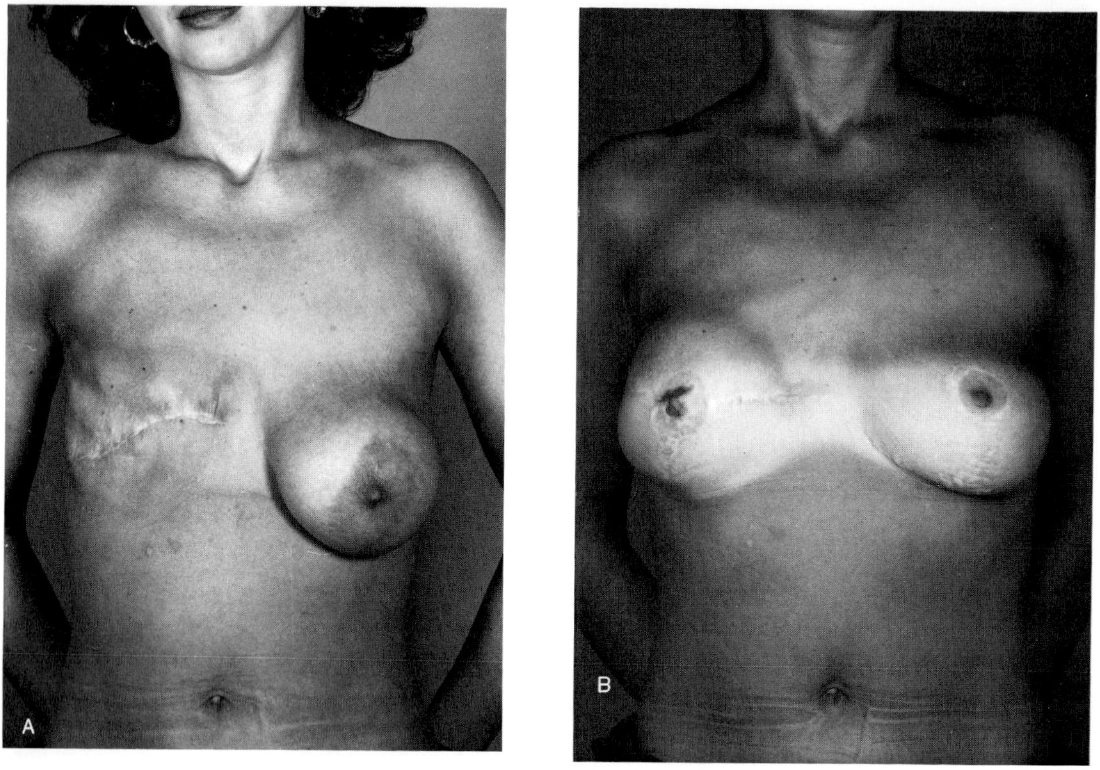

Figure 33-8 A. An unfavorable result with extensive scarring. The neurovascular bundle to the latissimus had been compromised at mastectomy. B. Appearance after modified radical mastectomy.

NIPPLE-AREOLAR RECONSTRUCTION

An acceptable nipple-areolar complex can now be satisfactorily reconstructed. At present, any breast reconstruction is performed in two stages. The breast mound is first established and subsequently, when the mound becomes stable, generally 3 months following the initial procedure, nipple-areolar reconstruction can be performed locally as an outpatient procedure. At the same time, any minor adjustments in breast mound size or position can be accomplished. As techniques for breast mound reconstruction have improved, more patients are pleased with the symmetry and now request the final phase, nipple-areolar reconstruction. Nipple-areolar reconstruction must provide a complex similar in appearance, color, diameter, and projection as its opposite (Fig. 33-9). If nipple-areolar tissue is available from the opposite breast, it should be considered the prime source of reconstructive material. If this source is not available, the upper medial thigh crease[12] or retroauricular skin can be utilized.

To create a nipple, local flaps,[21] composite flaps,[4,11] toe pulp, and the opposite nipple have been used. I have found it difficult to retain permanent projection and all have limitations. Selection should be made on an individual basis.

At one time, the nipple-areolar complex was removed at the time of ablation as a composite graft and stored in the groin crease or suprapubically. This technique has been abandoned for oncological and esthetic reasons. There have

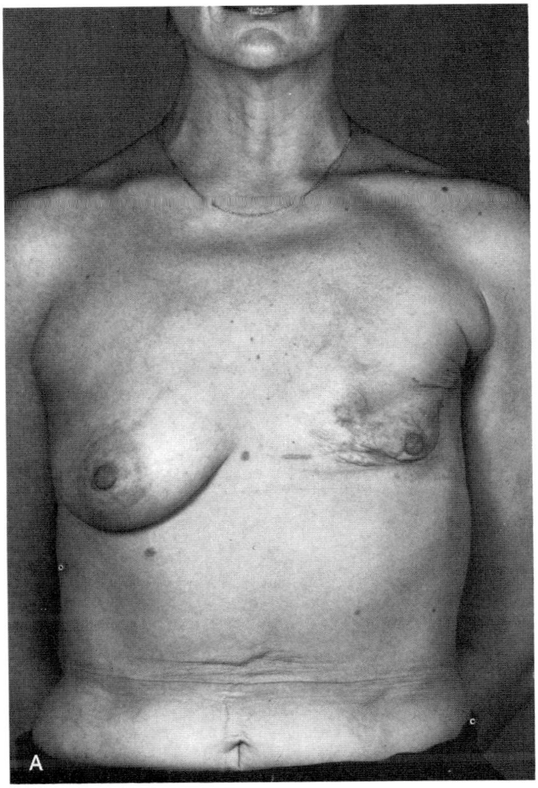

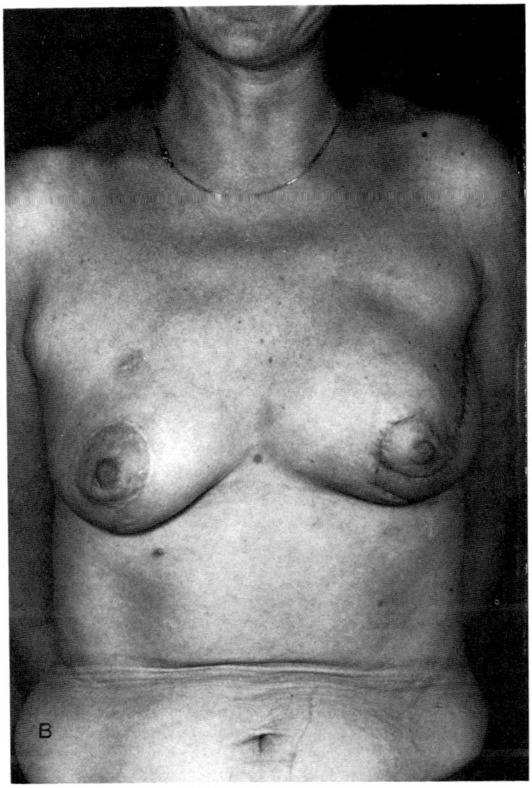

Figure 33-9 Nipple-areolar preservation compromises the ablative procedure and is of limited usefulness in reconstruction. Its use is contraindicated. A. Appearance after reconstruction with reapplication of the nipple-areolar complex. B. Appearance after mastectomy with preservation of the nipple-areolar complex.

been a few reported cases of tumors transferred to the groin. Esthetically, the transferred composite graft loses pigment and projection.

Full-thickness grafts of labia have not proven satisfactory since they tend to hyperpigment and hypertrophy.

SELECTION OF PATIENTS

It is estimated that less than 5 percent of mastectomy patients in the United States have reconstruction. Each patient should be made aware that reconstruction is available, and encouraged at least to seek consultation in which the various procedures, types of reconstruction, and expectations can be discussed. There is no absolute contraindication. The patient with positive nodes should not be denied any procedure that may enhance the quality of life. Fear of recurrence should not postpone reconstruction (2 years, 5 years post-ablation). The breast surgeon, oncologist, and reconstructive surgeon must discuss the treatment, goals, expectations, and quality of life that can be expected.

TISSUE EXPANSION

Tissue expansion is to be considered as an alternate means of treatment. If there is a deficit of

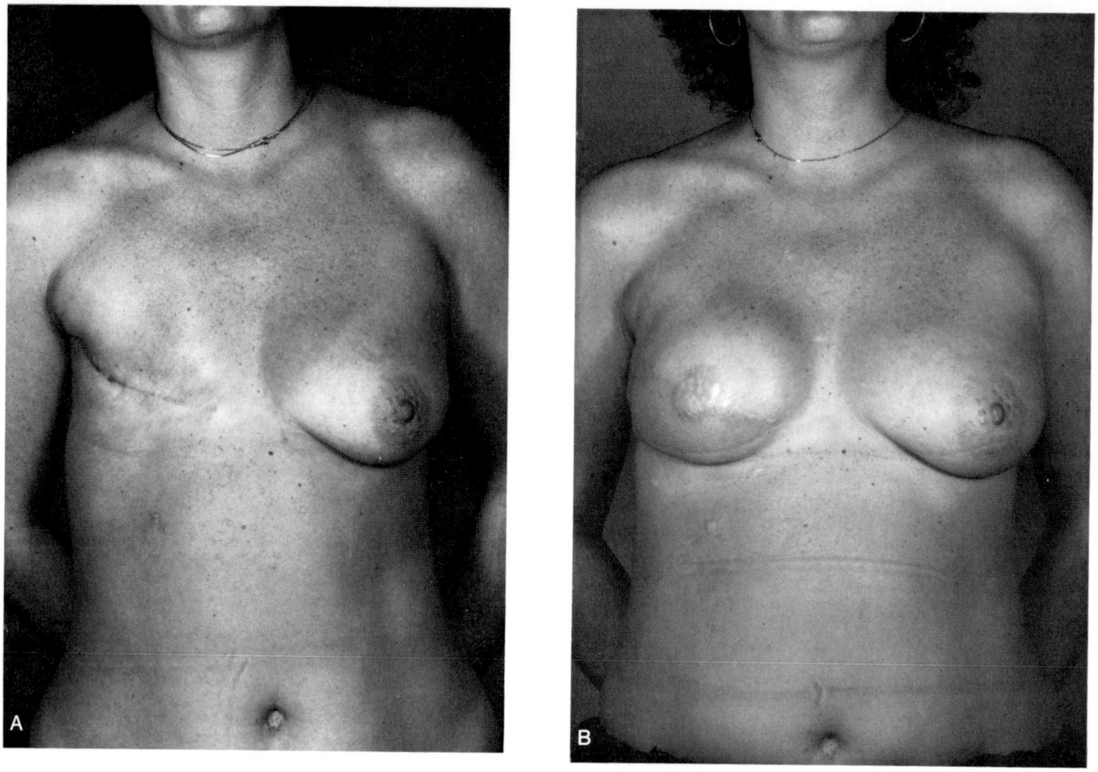

Figure 33-10 A. A satisfactory reconstruction obtained by means of a latissimus myocutaneous flap. B. Appearance after modified radical mastectomy.

skin on the mastectomy side, greater than 5 cm, and other forms of correction are inadvisable or unacceptable, a tissue expander may be placed beneath the skin, through the mastectomy scar and over a two to three month period the overlying skin can be stretched sufficiently, so that an adequate prostheses can later be inserted and acceptable symmetry may be obtained.

CONCLUSION

Satisfactory breast reconstruction can be accomplished (Fig. 33-10). The type of procedure performed is selected on an individual basis and influenced by the ablative procedure. If the physician strongly believes that ablative surgery is the best treatment for breast cancer, then he or she must be able to present to the patient satisfactory means of reconstruction at the time of ablation, or the patient will select an alternate means of therapy which will spare her breast. Immediate reconstruction, unless there are contraindications, provides an alternative to the patient. It causes no discomfort, the operating time is not considerably prolonged, and there is no additional hospital admission. It will not interfere with any future therapy or surgery, and the patient is given back her symmetry.

REFERENCES

1. Apfelberg DB, Laub DR, Master MR, Lash H: Submuscular breast reconstructions and technique. *Ann Plast Surg* 7(3):2, 1981.

2. Ashikari RH: Modified radical mastectomy. *Surg CNA* 64(6):1095, 1984.
3. Auchincloss H: Significance of location and number of axillary metastases in carcinoma of the breast. *Ann Surg* 158:37, 1963.
4. Barton FE: Latissimus dermal–epidermal nipple reconstruction. *Plast Reconstr Surg* 70:234, 1982.
5. Biggs TM, Cronin ED: Technical aspects of the latissimus dorsi myocutaneous flap in breast reconstruction. *Ann Plast Surg* 6:381, 1981.
6. Bostwick J: Breast reconstruction; a comprehensive approach. *Clin Plast Surg* 6:143, 1979.
7. Bostwick J III, Jurkiewiez MJ: Recent advances in breast reconstruction: Transposition of the latissimus dorsi muscle singly or with the overlying skin. *Ann Surg* 46(10):537, 1980.
8. Bostwick J III, Scheflan M: The latissimus dorsi musculocutaneous flap: A one-stage breast reconstruction. *Clin Plast Surg* 7:71, 1980.
9. Bostwick J: Colloquium: Total breast reconstruction. *Ann Plast Surg* 7(1):62, 1981.
10. Bostwick J III: *Aesthetic and Reconstructive Breast Surgery*. St. Louis, C. V. Mosby, 1983.
11. Bostwick B, Bostwick J: Nipple areolar reconstruction with auricular tissues. *Plast Reconstr Surg* 60:353, 1977.
12. Broadbent TR, Metz PS, Woolf RM: Restoring the mammary areola by a skin graft from the upper inner thigh. *Br J Plast Surg* 30:22, 1977.
13. Budoff PW: Breast cancer as viewed by the family physician. *Surg Clin North Am* 64(6):1209, 1984.
14. Dinner MI, Labandter HP, Dowden RV: The role of the rectus abdominis myocutaneous flap in breast reconstruction. *Plast Reconstr Surg* 69:209, 1982.
15. Drerer JM: Total breast reconstruction. *Ann Plast Surg* 7:54, 1982.
16. Maxwell GP, McGibbon BM, Hoopes JE: Vascular considerations in the use of latissimus dorsi myocutaneous flap after mastectomy with axillary dissection. *Plast Reconstr Surg* 64:771, 1979.
17. Gruber RP, Kahn RA, Nash H, Master MR, Apfelberg DB, Laub DR: Breast reconstruction following mastectomy: A comparison of submuscular and subcutaneous techniques. *Plast Reconstr Surg* 67(3):312, 1981.
18. Hartrampf CR, Scheflan M, Block PW: Breast reconstruction following mastectomy with a transverse flap. Anatomical and clinical observations. *Plast Reconstr Surg* 69:216, 1982.
19. Lewis JR Jr: Use of a sliding flap from the abdomen to provide cover in breast reconstruction. *Plast Reconstr Surg* 64:491, 1979.
20. Little JW III, Golembe EV, Fisher JB: The "living bra" in immediate and delayed reconstruction of the breast following mastectomy for malignant and non-malignant disease. *Plast Reconstr Surg* 68(3):392, 1981.
21. Little JW, Munasifi T, McCullogh DT: One stage reconstruction of projecting nipple: The quadrapod flap. *Plast Reconstr Surg* 71:126, 1983.
22. Maxwell GP: Latissimus dorsi breast reconstruction: An aesthetic assessment. *Clin Plast Surg* 8(2):373, 1981.
23. Pers M: The selection of patients for reconstruction following mastectomy for carcinoma of the breast. *Br J Plast Surg* 34(1):58, 1981.
24. Rosato FE, Horton EE, Maxwell GP: Postmastectomy breast reconstruction. *Curr Probl Surg* 17(11):585, 1980.
25. Ryan JJ: A lower thoracic advancement flap in breast reconstruction after mastectomy. *Plast Reconstr Surg* 70:153, 1982.
26. Snyderman RK, Gutherie RH: Reconstruction of the female breast following radical mastectomy. *Plast Reconstr Surg* 47:565, 1971.
27. Snyderman RK: Alternatives in reconstruction surgery after mastectomy. *Cancer* 46(suppl 4):1053, 1980.
28. Woods JE: Breast reconstruction after mastectomy. *Surg Gynecol Obstet* 150(6):869, 1980.
29. Woods JE, Irons GB Jr, Arnold PG: The care for submuscular implantation of prosthesis in reconstructive breast surgery. *Ann Plast Surg* 5(2):115, 1980.

Part Eight

Specific Clinical Considerations

34

The Nipple

Robert E. Rothenberg, M.D.

ANATOMY

The nipple, or mammilla, is composed of a circumscribed region of thickened, pigmented skin containing 15 to 20 various-sized ducts through which milk or other secretions pass as they exit the breast. At their point of origin within the acinar lobules, the ductules are microscopic in size and as they course toward the nipple they coalesce and become larger, terminating in so-called milk sinuses. Although one duct or sinus may predominate in size within the nipple and serve as the main conduit for the passage of milk, there is no set anatomical pattern. Often the exit of the central duct is located eccentrically in the nipple (Fig. 34-1).

The nipple is surrounded by a lighter-colored pigmented skin, the areola, within which are Montgomery glands, seen as small follicles arising from the skin's surface. These glands do not connect with the lactiferous ducts nor do they secrete milk. They are modified sebaceous glands.

NIPPLE DISCHARGE

Normally, during the fertile years of a female's life, there may be a small amount of light amber secretion from the nipple, manifesting itself as a stain on a brassiere or nightgown, or when a woman practices self-examination of her breasts. Women who take contraceptive medications are likely to have this type of discharge and it may also be seen from the stimulation of suckling or intercourse. Generally, this discharge has no pathologic significance.[1] Nipple discharge is an indication of cancer in approximately 10 percent of cases. Papanicolaou and coworkers[2] discovered only one carcinoma in 613 clinically normal breasts from which secretions had been elicited by manual pressure.

Rothenberg and coworkers,[3] in an attempt to retrieve malignant cells from the nipple of cancer-bearing breasts, curetted the mammary ducts down to a depth of 3 to 4 cm. They inserted a 1 mm eye curette through the aperture of the central mammary duct prior to beginning

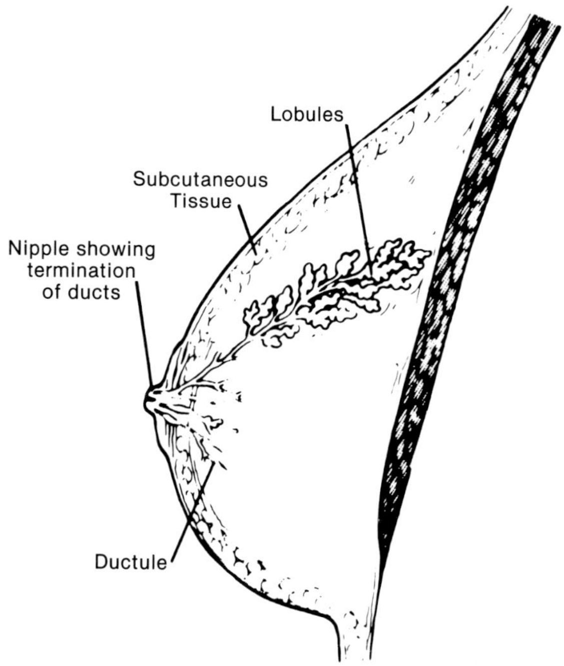

Figure 34-1 Schematic drawing showing multiple apertures of ducts in the nipple.

surgery, after the patient had been anesthetized (Fig. 34-2). In 32 instances of carcinoma, not a single curetting revealed identifiable malignant cells. Microscopic examination of the curettage did show some clusters of cuboidal cells which line the ducts, and in several cases they displayed focal atypia (Fig. 34-3).

Leis and Pilnik[4] found that in 1868 consecutive breast operations for all types of pathology, there were 152 (8.14 percent) patients with spontaneous nipple discharge. Of those, 19 patients (12.5 percent) had cancer. Of the 19 patients with cancer, 6 had a bloody discharge, 7 had a serosanguineous discharge; in 4 the discharge was serous, and in 2 it was watery. Thus, it can be seen that *a bloody discharge* was present in less than one-third of the cancer cases who also presented with nipple discharge. This is important because there is a tendency among some physicians to conclude that a nonbloody discharge signifies benign pathology. Conversely, many physicians tend to think that a bloody discharge is indicative of a malignancy when, in reality, it is often associated with a benign intraductal papilloma.

There are certain types of discharge that are considered "surgical," i.e., they warrant a biopsy to rule out malignancy: nipple discharge that is bloody, serosanguineous, serous, or watery falls into this category and cytology, mammography, and biopsy should be done. When there is no associated palpable mass, or when mammagraphy shows no suspicious area, the biopsy procedure is the *central duct excision.* In this technique, a 180° circumareolar incision is made, following the areolar margin. The areolar skin is lifted up as a skin flap, and then the coalescing terminal central ducts are coned out from the undersurface of the nipple. This entire terminal portion of the central duct system represents the specimen sent for pathologic examination. Of course, breast-feeding is no longer possible from the breast that underwent this procedure. Occasionally during surgery the in-

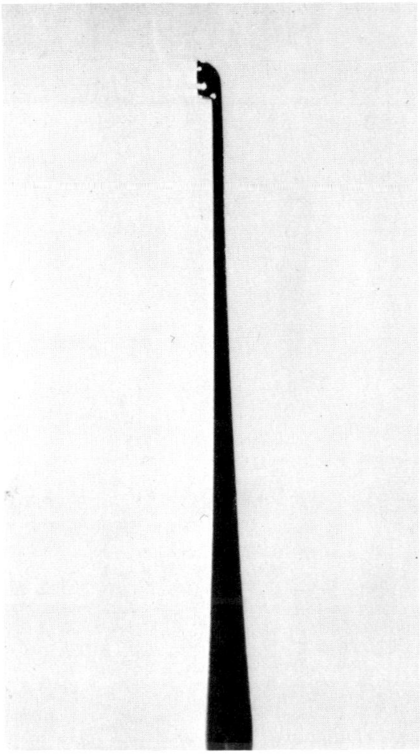

Figure 34-2 Photograph of eye curette used in curetting mammary ducts. Magnification ×4.

volved duct or ducts appears obvious and the excision may be limited to this segment of the central duct, thus preserving lactational function.

A milky discharge from the nipple (*galactorrhea*) may have causes; however, when present alone without other symptoms or signs, it represents a "nonsurgical" condition, i.e., biopsy is not required. Galactorrhea may be due to prolonged lactation, to a variety of drugs including phenothiazines, *Rauwolfia* alkaloids, and methyldopa, as well as being secondary to a prolactin-secreting pituitary tumor.

The third general category of nipple discharge is the sticky multiduct discharge. This is most often due to an underlying duct ectasia with associated inflammation. Cytologic examination and mammography should be done. Nipple cleansing with a mild antibacterial solution and avoidance of nipple manipulation will usually suffice as treatment. If a mass is present, if mammography shows a suspicious area, or if a chronic low-grade inflammatory condition persists, biopsy is warranted.

NONCANCEROUS LESIONS

The nipple is a rather amazing structure in that it is rarely the site of a purulent infection, despite the fact that it undergoes repeated trauma from suckling and biting, and infrequently becomes irritated or inflamed because of friction caused by brassieres. Moreover, though the ducts coursing through the nipple are patent until long after menopause, when they tend to become stenosed, infection seldom gains entrance to the interior of the breast except during periods of nursing. There are a number of lesions affecting the nipple that must be recognized and differentiated from cancer. These are the following:

1 Crusts. Women who normally secrete from the nipple are frequently unaware of the phenomenon and permit discharge to coagulate and form crusts. When the crust is scraped away, normal underlying nipple epithelium is uncovered.

2 Psoriasis. Although the nipple and areola are not common locations for psoriatic lesions, nevertheless they can occur there. Usually, the lesion also involves the skin beyond the areola.

3 Infected ulcerations. Most bites of the nipple heal without infection, unlike human bites elsewhere on the body.

4 Keratoses. These are seen not infrequently on the areola, and sometimes encroach upon the nipple itself.

5 Keloid. Occurs occasionally after a deep abrasion or laceration, or following an operative procedure upon the nipple.

6 Chancre. A primary syphilitic lesion of the nipple may be confused with a Paget's erosion.

7 Intraductal papilloma of the nipple. A solitary papilloma of a nipple duct may extrude through the nipple and appear on the surface as

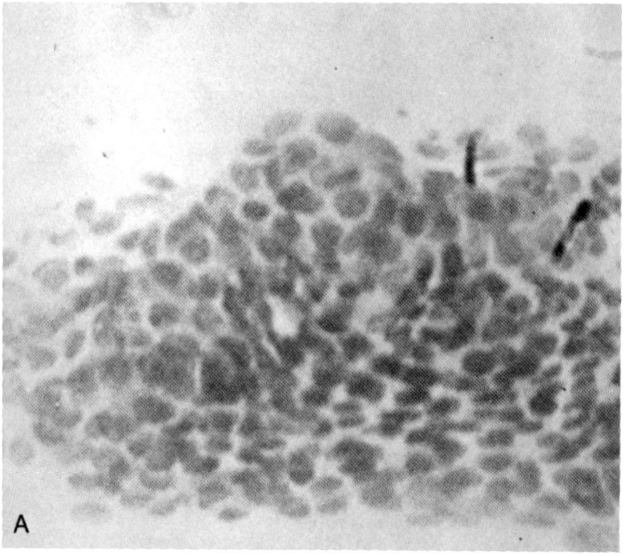

Figure 34-3 A. Curettings showing normal cuboidal cells lining the mammary ducts. B. Curettings showing focal atypia of cuboidal cells.

oozing, ulcerating lesions. A biopsy of the lesion invariably differentiates a papilloma from Paget's carcinoma.

RARE NEOPLASMS

Leiomyoma and neurofibroma These are two lesions rarely encountered beneath the nipple or in the areola. The absence of skin ulceration or inflammation helps to distinguish them from Paget's carcinoma.

Basal cell and squamous cell carcinoma Both of these lesions have been known to occur within the skin of the nipple, and in most instances have been diagnosed erroneously as Paget's disease. Paget cells are not present in basal or squamous cell carcinomas. Treatment of these lesions requires wide local excision.

Melanoma Since Paget cells on microscopic examination sometimes contain melanin, a diagnosis of melanoma of the nipple may be entertained. However, true melanoma of the nipple has not been reported in the literature, despite the fact that there is no reason why this area should be exempt from the possibility of involvement. Certainly, the nipple contains more pigment than most other surfaces of the body.

Whenever there is doubt about the diagnosis of a lesion on the nipple, a biopsy is mandatory. The nipple has extraordinary healing power and usually heals without scarring even when a generous portion of its substance has been excised.

PAGET'S CARCINOMA

Paget's carcinoma of the nipple constitutes approximately 2.5 percent of all breast cancers. There are approximately 2800 to 3000 new cases of Paget's carcinoma in the United States each year.[5] Pathologists have debated the question whether Paget's carcinoma results from the migration of intraductal carcinoma cells of the breast into the epidermis of the nipple, or whether the malignant Paget cells that originate in the nipple subsequently invade the lactiferous ducts of the breast. The treatment for the disease is the same no matter what the origin of the Paget cell. Perhaps the most clear-cut statement is that of Haagensen,[7] "... the fact is now established beyond any reasonable doubt

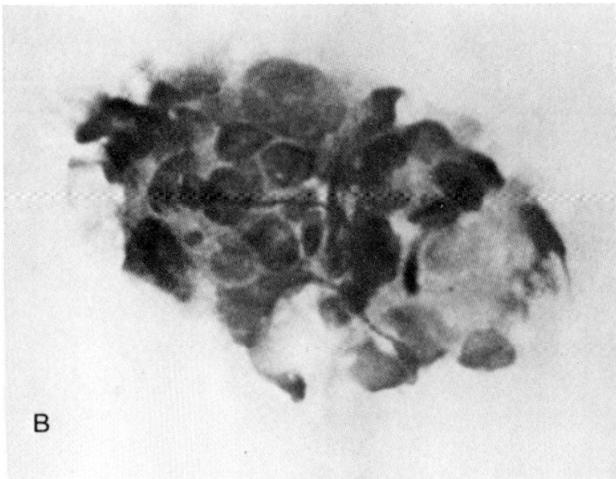

that they are carcinoma cells that have invaded the epidermis of the nipple from carcinoma in the subjacent *nipple ducts*."

The sine qua non for the diagnosis of Paget's carcinoma is the presence of the typical malignant Paget cells. These are recognized readily on histologic examination because of their large size, location in the epidermis of the nipple, compressed, pale-staining cytoplasm, and prominent, irregularly shaped nuclei. They are sometimes seen as single cells but may appear in clusters, and in more advanced cases, they tend to form acini. Mitotic figures are encountered frequently within the nuclei (Fig. 34-4).

Symptoms

The vast majority of patients with Paget's carcinoma have typical onsets with similar developing symptoms and signs. The initial incorrect diagnosis is made most often by the patient herself who, upon noting a change in the nipple, concludes that this is due to an irritation, an inflammation, an infection, an abrasion, or trauma. As the condition undergoes few visible changes during the ensuing weeks or months, the patient may become convinced that the condition is innocuous and will eventually disappear spontaneously. If she practices self-examination of her breasts during the early stages of the disease, it is likely she will not palpate a mass. Thus, her belief that the lesion is of little consequence is bolstered. Unfortunately, on consulting a physician some weeks or months later, the suspicion that the lesion is merely a skin irritation or inflammation is often confirmed. More time elapses, during which appropriate therapy is delayed. The diagnosis of Paget's carcinoma is considered only after prolonged, unsuccessful treatment with sundry, locally applied medications. During this period, the process usually spreads.

Haagensen[8] stresses the fact that in Paget's carcinoma the cancer is found not only in the epidermis of the nipple but in the nipple ducts, and that in most cases there is also invasive ductal carcinoma within the breast itself. Of 148 cases of Paget's disease, he found intraductal carcinoma within the breast in 131 (88.5 percent) of patients.

Itching or burning sensations in the nipple may be the first symptoms of Paget's carcinoma, having their onset prior to changes in the appearance of the nipple. Some weeks thereafter a smooth redness of the nipple may be noted, leading to the self-diagnosis of an irritation. The nipple may next take on roughness of its

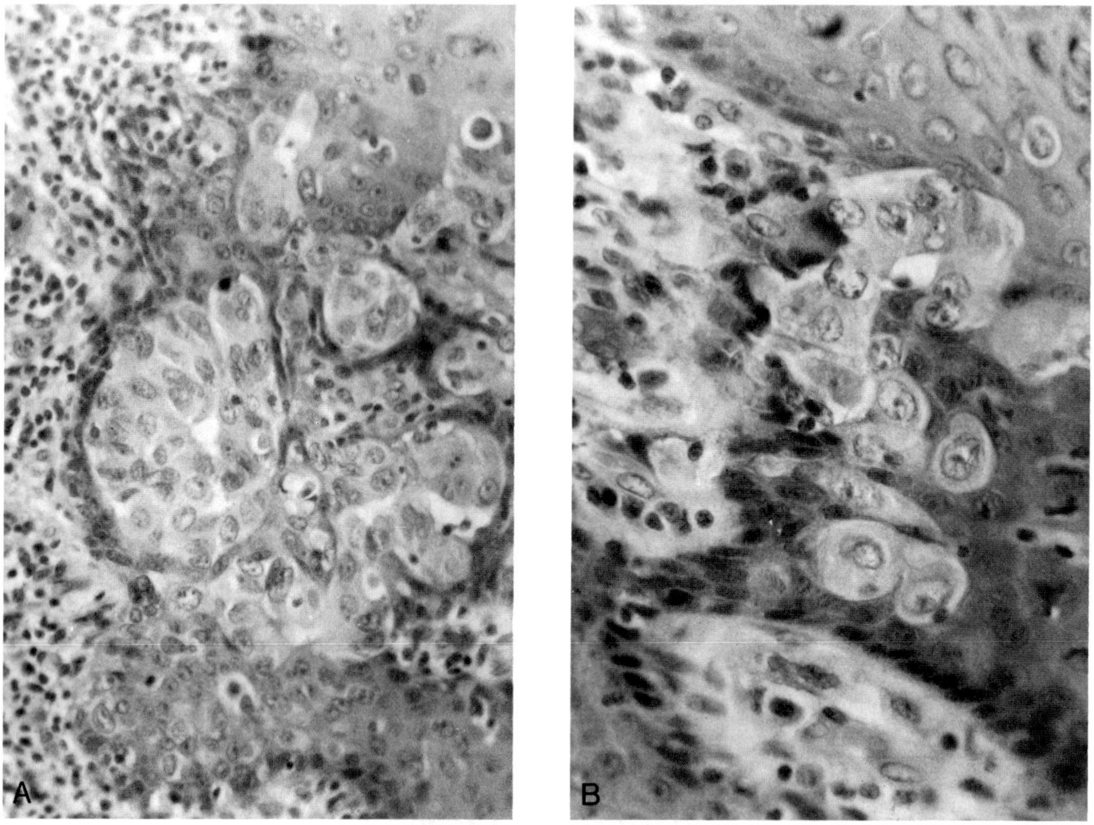

Figure 34-4 A. Photomicrograph of typical malignant Paget cells grouped in clusters, seen within the epidermis. ×100 B. High-powered view of malignant Paget cells showing atypical nuclear features. The cells lie in approximation to the basal membranes of the epidermis. × 400

surface, flatten, become distorted in shape, and eventually a small erosion appears. The stage of erosion may not ensue for several months after the first symptoms and signs have been recognized (Fig. 34-5).

Twenty years ago, the average interval between the onset of overt symptoms and signs of Paget's carcinoma and consultation with a physician or surgeon was estimated to be approximately 1 year. This interval has been reduced somewhat since women are now more aware of the dangers of breast lesions. However, it is estimated that the time it takes a patient with Paget's carcinoma to seek medical advice at present is almost double that of a woman who notes a lump in her breast.

Signs

The slow progression and paucity of the external signs of Paget's carcinoma and its apparent indolence belie what is going on in the deeper substance of the breast. Although no breast mass may yet have become palpable, the mammary ducts may be extensively involved in a carcinoma that is markedly invasive. In some instances, axillary node metastases may have occurred long before the presence of a mass within the breast.

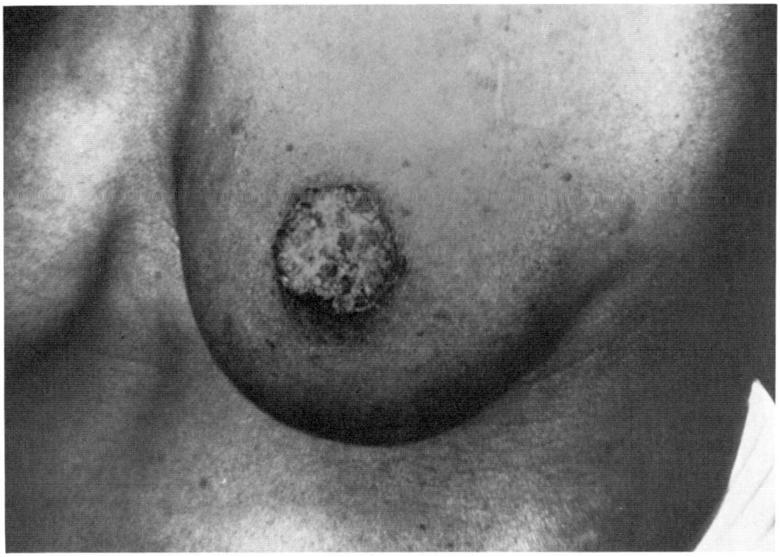

Figure 34-5 Photograph showing flattened, distorted appearance of nipple involved in Paget's carcinoma.

Delay in Treatment

If the public, and the medical profession, too, were more alert to the possibility of a malignancy when nipple changes take place, many patients would start treatment before a mass in the breast became palpable. This group, however, according to Kister and Haagensen,[9] represented 42.7 percent of the total number of Paget's carcinoma seen at Columbia-Presbyterian Medical Center from 1920 to 1969. The other 57.3 percent of cases presented for treatment only after a breast mass had already formed. Sadly, two-thirds of those with nipple changes and a palpable breast mass had axillary lymph node metastases by the time surgical treatment was instituted. Paone and Baker[10] reviewed 50 cases of Paget's carcinoma seen at the Johns Hopkins Hospital during a 30-year period and found that in 19 patients (38 percent), the disease was confined to the nipple and was unassociated with a palpable breast tumor.

Treatment Policies

Since fully developed Paget's carcinoma is accompanied by infiltrating ductal carcinoma within the breast in approximately 90 percent of cases, its treatment should be similar to that for any invasive ductal carcinoma. The 10 percent of patients in whom the lesion is limited to the nipple might receive special consideration.

To determine the category into which a patient with Paget's carcinoma falls and the type of treatment that should be instituted, the following approach is recommended:

1 A small elliptical biopsy of the nipple lesion is taken, utilizing local anesthesia.

2 If the biopsy shows Paget's carcinoma and there is no palpable breast mass, a large elliptical, vertical excision of the nipple, the areola, and the underlying central duct system of the breast should be performed. This excisional biopsy should be made perpendicularly to the nipple and should extend down to the pectoral muscle fascia. The excised material should be sent to the pathology

laboratory with the request that the depth of the carcinoma in relation to the pectoral fascia be measured.

3 If the lesion is less than 6 months old, if the examination of the material submitted to the laboratory shows that the lesion is superficial and is limited to the nipple itself, and if no axillary nodes are palpable, simple mastectomy with sampling of axillary nodes might be the appropriate operation. Unfortunately, because of the late appearance of patients with Paget's carcinoma for treatment, very few will fall into this category. Too few reports on 10-year survival rates have appeared in the literature to justify use of breast-preserving operations to judge its role. The large excisional biopsy that must be carried out to discover that the lesion is limited to the nipple and has not invaded the ducts will alter the appearance of the remaining breast to such a great extent that it may not be worthwhile salvaging.

4 If examination of the excisional biopsy material shows that the carcinoma is invasive but its lowermost extent is more than 2.0 cm distant from the pectoral muscle fascia, then a modified radical mastectomy should be performed. On the other hand, if the carcinoma has approached within 1 to 2 cm of the pectoral fascia or has invaded the fascia or muscle, a radical mastectomy or one which includes removal of a generous portion of the underlying pectoral muscle, is recommended. In Rothenberg and coworkers'[12] series of 100 consecutive cases of all types of cancer, 22 lesions were within 1 cm of the pectoral fascia or had invaded the pectoral muscle.

Results

Survival rates after surgery for Paget's carcinoma have been reputed to be lower than those for ordinary infiltrating ductal carcinoma of the breast. This finding is in all probability due to the fact that patients with Paget's carcinoma seek treatment later than those whose first sign of trouble is a lump in the breast. Also, lower survival rates may have eventuated because surgeons heretofore have treated Paget's carcinoma as a less dangerous malignancy than the ordinary ductal carcinomas of the breast. Therefore, they performed less extensive surgery and paid less attention to the importance of postoperative therapy.

Table 34-1 Five- and Ten-Year Survival Rates for Various Stages of Paget's Carcinoma

			Overall survival rate, %		Survival rate, no mass, %		Survival rate with mass, %	
Author	Year of report	Number of cases	5 years	10 years	5 years	10 years	5 years	10 years
Ashikari et al.[14]	1970	209	NR	60	92	87	42	NR
Freund et al.[15]	1977	29	74	69	94	91	40	33
Kay[17]	1966	23	NR	NR	83	NR	19	NR
Haagensen and Kister[16]	1971	158	NR	58	NR	81	NR	47
McGregor and McGregor[18]	1959	27	NR	NR	100	NR	50	NR
Paone and Baker[10]	1981	50	NR	NR	NR	100	NR	33
Rissanen and Holsti[19]	1969	NR	47	43	83	75	NR	NR
Salvadori et al.[20]	1976	91	59	44	92	82	38	22

NR = Not recorded.

Haagensen[13] reported 83 percent of 10-year survivals in Paget's carcinoma among patients who had not yet developed a breast mass or axillary metastases and who had undergone radical mastectomy. This compares most favorably with survival rates for non-Paget's carcinoma of the breast. The survival rate drops markedly for those who present with a mass or axillary metastases. In recent years, it has been recognized that Paget's carcinoma is in every sense as virulent a carcinoma as any other breast malignancy, and it is now treated as vigorously as any other breast cancer. Five- and ten-year survival rates for the various stages of Paget's carcinoma are now quite comparable to those of other types of cancer (see Table 34-1).

Acknowledgment

We should like to express our thanks to the medical student, Dagna Skoog, who helped in the preparation of this manuscript.

REFERENCES

1. Gremer H, Paulussen F: *Geburtshilfe Frauenheilkd* 42:590, 1982.
2. Papanicolaou GN, Holmquist OG, Bader GN, Falk EA: Exploratory cytology of the human mammary gland. *Cancer* 11:337, 1968.
3. Rothenberg RE, Sabatini MT, LaRaja RD, Lobbato V: Mammary duct curettage for early detection of breast disease. *Breast* 8:2, 1982.
4. Leis HP Jr, Pilnik S: Nipple discharge. *Hosp Med* 6:11, 1970.
5. Haagensen CD: Incidence of Paget's carcinoma, in *Diseases of the Breast.* Philadelphia, W. B. Saunders Co., 1970, p. 546.
6. Silverberg E: American Cancer Society: Estimated new breast cancer cases–1984. *CA* 34(1):Jan./Feb. 1984.
7. Haagensen CD: The nature of the Paget cell, in *Diseases of the Breast.* Philadelphia, W. B. Saunders Co., 1970, p. 533.
8. Haagensen CD: The morphology of Paget's disease of the breast. *Am J Surg* 119:606, 1970.
9. Kister SJ, Haagensen CD: Paget's disease of the breast. *Am J Surg* 119:606, 1970.
10. Paone JF, Baker R: Pathogenesis and treatment of Paget's disease of the breast. *Cancer* 48:825, 1981.
11. Shah JP, Rosen PP, Robbins GF: Pitfalls of local excision in the treatment of carcinoma of the breast. *Surg Gynec Obstet* 136:5, 1973.
12. Rothenberg RE, LaRaja RD, Sabatini MT, Cruz E, Sheth N: Proximity of breast cancer to the underlying pectoralis major fascia and muscle: Surgical implications. *Breast* 7:4, 1981.
13. Haagensen CD: The surgical treatment of Paget's carcinoma, in *Diseases of the Breast.* Philadelphia, W. B. Saunders Co., 1970, p. 567.
14. Ashikari R, Park K, Huvos AG, Urban JA: Paget's disease of the breast. *Cancer* 26:680, 1970.
15. Freund H, Moydovnik M, Laufer N: Paget's disease of the breast. *J Surg Oncol* 9:93, 1977.
16. Haagensen CD: *Diseases of the Breast,* 2d ed. Philadelphia, W. B. Saunders Co., 1971.
17. Kay S: Paget's disease of the nipple. *Surg Gynecol Obstet* 123:1010, 1966.
18. McGregor JK, McGregor DD: Paget's disease of the breast. *Surgery* 562, 1959.
19. Rissanen PM, Holsti P: Paget's disease of the breast. *Oncology* 23:209, 1969.
20. Salvadori B, Farigelli G, Roberto ST: Analysis of 100 cases of Paget's disease of the breast. *Tumors* 62:529, 1976.
21. Sinha MR, Prassad SB: Bilateral Paget's disease of the nipple. *J Indian Med Assoc* 80:2, Jan. 16, 1983.

35

Inflammatory Breast Cancer

Ezra M. Greenspan, M.D.

DESCRIPTION AND DIAGNOSIS

Inflammatory breast cancer is a discrete, life-threatening, nosologic and clinicopathologic entity occurring in 1 to 2.5 percent of new patients with breast cancer, or in approximately 15 percent of stage III cases. Its classic form is characterized by the rapid, florid development within several weeks of a diffuse erythematous infiltration and thickening of a substantial portion, at least one-third, of the superficial breast tissue. This is often associated with pain, tenderness, warmth, erythema, axillary node involvement, and *peau d'orange*. A substantial enlargement of the entire breast may occur. At times, irregular areas of thickened tumor nodulation may appear. The pathologic hallmark of inflammatory cancer is neoplastic infiltration and blockage of the dermal and subdermal lymphatics with high-grade undifferentiated cancer cells.[1] Invasion of blood vessels is common. The peak incidence is in the early postmenopausal age group, in most series between 51 and 54 years. Inflammatory breast cancer is a subgroup of stage III disease with the most dire prognosis.

Primary lesion ulceration is rare except in atypical indolent cases. Axillary node involvement is common pathologically in 80 percent, but is clinically apparent in less than 50 percent of cases. Distant metastases at presentation are infrequent (less than 20 percent). The carcinoembryonic antigen (CEA) and the estrogen receptor (ER) determinations are usually negative or low. Mammography is usually positive but often is initially nonspecific. The left breast is involved almost twice as frequently as the right breast.[2] In one study survival was better in left-sided cases.[3] Frequently, after the first chemotherapy-induced regression, the mammogram becomes obviously positive within one or two circumscribed areas of residual tumor induration. Subsequent biopsies and mammograms will be normal if complete regression has been induced. Virtually complete regressions may be associated with hyalinized tumor cells and nodes.

An erroneous clinical diagnosis of mastitis or cellulitis has been made in as many as 19 percent of patients.[2] This may result in prolonged treatment with antibiotics and a consequent delay in diagnosis. Surgeons are likely to confront patients who are under the mistaken assumption that the "inflammation" of the breast is infectious. A representative ellipse of skin and subcutaneous tissues must be removed for pathologic demonstration of dermal lymphatic involvement. A single random incisional biopsy may miss the characteristic lesion if the biopsy site is not carefully selected. Two needle biopsies should suffice to fulfill the necessary pathologic criteria for "inflammatory" cancer. A single inadequate needle biopsy may be misleading. No patients should be treated without pathologic confirmation.

TREATMENT

The inherent incurability of the extensive infiltration has been obvious to surgeons[4] for many years. The dismal results of radical mastectomy as initial therapy has caused the abandonment of the procedure, even in those presenting with only a partial involvement of the breast. Effective therapy must be directed against occult systemic metastases as well as the local neoplastic process. Some have viewed inflammatory cancer as an advanced form of a more indolent ductal breast cancer, but most patients with classic features represent an acute process characterized by rapid cell proliferation (doubling time). Yet some patients insist that they first noticed breast changes a year or more prior to diagnosis. This is unlikely except in improperly classified indolent atypical stage III cases.

In quickly diagnosed cases, increasing data confirm the prospects for superior long-term control and even "cure" after sustained treatment with combination chemotherapy. Prior to the era of systemic therapy before 1955, the median life expectancy was 4 to 9 months[5] regardless of radiotherapy and surgery in either order. The median duration of remission was only 6 months in 77 inflammatory breast cancer patients treated at the M. D. Anderson Hospital[6] from 1948 to 1970. A large review of 346 combined cases from various institutions treated before 1976 reported a median survival of 12 to 18 months and a 5-year survival of only 3.7 percent.[5] The disease remained dormant or suppressed for 2 to 3 years in a small cohort of perhaps 10 percent.

The optimum method of integrating local-regional therapy, i.e., surgery and/or radiotherapy, with chemotherapy has not been precisely established. There are no recent randomized studies with patients in a no-radiotherapy or no-surgery arm. Thus, the survival benefits, if any, are not accurately definable from local-regional therapy whether surgery follows or precedes radiotherapy.

Methotrexate was the first agent to demonstrate the rapid exquisite inhibition of inflammatory cancer by cytotoxic drugs. Complete remissions could be induced within 5 to 7 days after oral tablet therapy (2.5 mg tid for 3 to 4 days) among one-third of patients. When combined with thiotepa, quick regression was induced in 15 of 16 patients.[7] However, despite induction of complete regressions in many of these patients, and cycles of methotrexate every 3 weeks, tumor recurrence due to drug resistance occurred in 75 percent of patients within a year after the onset of the methotrexate plus thiotepa therapy. Despite quick crossover to cyclophosphamide (Cytoxan) and fluorouracil after 1962, the number of 2-year survivors was small, only 3 of 16 cases in the author's experience.[8] The lack of optimum use of combination chemotherapy by most oncologists continued into the early 1970s. In addition, patients continued to be operated at various intervals after diagnosis and/or were given radiotherapy and surgery in several different sequences.

In the last decade, cellular kinetic theory has modulated the timing and focused on early use of polychemotherapy. The optimum timing for attempts at local-regional control must vary for each individual patient. An intact blood supply in the first few months of therapy is obviously needed to permit maximum drug accessibility for local control by chemotherapy. Prompt prior resort to systemic therapy can exert quick inhibition of distant metastases. For these reasons, radiotherapy and/or surgery have been empirically deferred until three, four, or more cycles of chemotherapy have induced maximal inhibition of tumor growth.

The advent of polychemotherapy in the early 1970s and particularly the addition of doxorubicin (Adriamycin) after 1974 to the armamentarium of three to six drug combinations heralded the marked improvement in the prognosis of inflammatory breast cancer. Because of the steady improvement in the prognosis with the combination chemotherapy employed since then, the possibility of long-term "cure" has become real. Data suggest that best results are obtained in early-diagnosed cases. For these reasons, confirmation of the diagnosis of inflammatory cancer should be promptly made on an emergency basis by biopsy. In a recent French study an apparent clinical cure was achieved in a major fraction of patients associated with a median survival of 56 months after onset of this clinical entity.[9] This occurred after sustained use of aggressive polychemotherapy and bacillus Calmette-Guérin (BCG) immunotherapy on a long-term basis. Surgery was employed on all patients in this study but only a few were given radiotherapy.

Immunotherapy appears to play some role in the treatment of inflammatory cancer. Response to immunotherapy is more likely to occur in "out front" skin and subcutaneous metastases in contrast to visceral metastases, particularly in patients with some degree of immunocompetence. The prompt recognition and therapy of inflammatory breast cancer as a true clinical emergency could result in significant prolongation of life.

Although progress in increased survival has become apparent, each report of improved results with polychemotherapy has involved a small number of cases, usually from 12 to 32 patients. At the M. D. Anderson Hospital, Blumenschein et al.[6] and Hortobagyi et al.[10,11] employed a regimen of 5-fluorouracil, doxorubicin, cyclophosphamide (FAC) given for 3 months with or without methotrexate and vincristine. Chemotherapy was routinely and arbitrarily interrupted after 3 months when radiotherapy was given, then resumed until relapse.[11] An 89 percent complete remission rate was induced (16/18) with only one failure, but 2 of the 16 complete responders did not complete the response until radiotherapy was given after the third course of chemotherapy. BCG was also given by scarification between the 3-week cycles of chemotherapy. Although the median survival exceeded 2 years, the 5-year survival did not exceed 15 percent. A cumulative updated series from M. D. Anderson Hospital (32 cases) in 1981 showed a mean disease-free interval of 16 months for FAC-BCG compared to 9 months for a radiotherapy-alone group (historical control) and a median survival of 24 months compared to 18 months for the radiotherapy-alone group.[12]

In most studies of chemoradiotherapy for inflammatory carcinoma, the radiotherapy is arbitrarily administered after 3 months of chemotherapy have been given.[11,12] However, Zylberberg et al. in Paris[9] employed thermography as a guide to determine how long to continue initial chemotherapy. In most of their 15 patients, the thermographic findings did not reach normal levels until the fourth or fifth cycle of chemotherapy. This study achieved an apparently superior long-term median survival of 56 months. It should be noted that the polychemotherapy employed was complex, including doxorubicin 45 mg/m^2 IV on day 1; vincristine 1 mg/m^2 IV on day 2; cyclophosphamide

500 mg IV, and 5-fluorouracil 500 mg IV in 250 mL of glucoserum (5%) (per day on day 3 and day 4); melphalan per os (4 mg per day), from day 3 to day 9. This protocol was repeated every 28 days. Intensive BCG was employed in-between chemotherapy cycles. Mammographies were done before surgery, which preceded radiotherapy. No radiotherapy was given unless incomplete removal occurred or residual tumor was found histopathologically at operation. When chemotherapy was resumed it included a maintenance regimen for 1 year, including methotrexate and cyclophosphamide. BCG immunotherapy was administered for 3 years in all patients. The impact of the immunotherapy was not established per se.

Intraarterial infusion chemotherapy was employed in 25 patients with inflammatory breast cancer from 1969 to 1982 in Osaka, Japan[13] in a further attempt at combining local-regional and systemic methods. Mitomycin and 5-fluorouracil were given from 1969 to 1978 and doxorubicin thereafter. One-third of each drug was given via the internal thoracic artery and two-thirds via the subclavian artery. Severe local side effects such as dermatitis occurred in 27 percent, shoulder pain and retarded wound healing in 16 percent, and an occasional case of pleural effusion ensued. Adriamycin caused fewer local side effects. The vasoactive drug angiotensin II was also employed to increase drug accessibility. Response rates locally were enhanced with this technique. Mastectomy was performed on all patients 1 month after termination of intraarterial chemotherapy. Good pathohistologic responses were produced with marked cell degeneration and fibrosis. One year of postoperative chemotherapy with cyclophosphamide, tegafur, and tamoxifen was given after surgery. Five-year survival time was 59 percent with median survival time of 56 months, a result similar to the French study.

Hormonal treatment has been tried in treating inflammatory cancer. Adrenalectomy in several dozen cases (collected) failed to provide any noteworthy increase in survival.[14–16] Since most inflammatory cancers are estrogen and progesterone receptor-negative, it should be expected that antiestrogen therapy with tamoxifen or ablative procedures would not be of major benefit. The conventional approach of surgery, followed by radiotherapy and oophorectomy/adrenalectomy employed immediately after diagnosis without antiestrogen, is unwarranted, except in a locally advanced case probably erroneously classified as inflammatory cancer with a very high progesterone receptor (PR) and estrogen receptor (ER) titer. If such a unique case exists, it would be expected to show a well-differentiated carcinoma pathologically, itself a feature which normally would exclude it from the designation of inflammatory cancer. The largest series of inflammatory cancer cases recently reported involved 66 consecutive patients seen between 1977 and 1983 in Milan by the Bonadonna group.[17] Initial cytoreductive chemotherapy involved cyclophosphamide 100 mg/m^2 per os days 1 to 14, doxorubicin 30 mg/m^2 IV days 1 and 8, 5-fluorouracil 500 mg/m^2 IV days 1 and 8, prednisone 40 mg/m^2 IM days 1 to 14 (CAFP) administered on a monthly schedule for 6 cycles. The initial complete plus partial response rate was 80 percent. Median age was 49 years and ER was "positive" in 50 percent. In patients with complete response, additional chemotherapy with cyclophosphamide, methotrexate, 5-fluorouracil (CMF), and prednisone was planned for 6 to 12 months. The median recurrence-free interval of all patients was only 14 months and the median survival only 23 months. It is not clear why so many patients were ER-positive. They could represent the 20 percent who survived 5 years. Among the first 36 cases, full-dose local-regional radiotherapy was randomized. Local-regional recurrence was reduced from 50 percent to 11 percent, but 5-year survival was not statistically different from those receiving chemotherapy alone (35 versus 29 months).

CONCLUSION

Inflammatory cancer is a subgroup comprising 5 to 15 percent of stage III breast cancer. This cohort can be used as a template to improve therapy in all locally advanced breast cancer patients. The prospects for continuing the improvement in long-term disease-free survival with inflammatory cancer appear to rest upon continuation of innovative sequential polychemotherapy and new drug development. Cyclical reinstitution of induction therapy every 3 to 4 months for many years would seem worthy of investigation in these high-risk patients. Whether use of tertiary drugs such as mitomycin is warranted prior to relapse remains to be established. A role for antiestrogen (tamoxifen) has not been established. Late metastatic relapse patterns do not differ from those of other patients with more common presentations of breast cancer. When to interdigitate surgery and radiotherapy in a multimodality program remains to be determined by randomized phase III therapeutic trials.

REFERENCES

1. Taylor GW, Meltzer A: "Inflammatory carcinoma" of the breast. *Am J Cancer* 33:33, 1938.
2. Meyer AC, Dockerty MB, Harrington SW: Inflammatory carcinoma of the breast. *Surg Gynecol Obstet* 87:417, 1948.
3. Loprinzi CL, Carbone PP, Tormey DC, Rosenbaum PR et al: Aggressive combined modality therapy for advanced local-regional breast carcinoma. *J Clin Oncol* 2:157, 1984.
4. Treves N: The inoperability of inflammatory carcinoma of the breast. *Surg Gynecol Obstet* 109:240, 1959.
5. Camp E III: Inflammatory carcinoma of the breast. *Am J Surg* 121:583, 1976.
6. Blumenschein GR, Montague ED, Eckles NE, Hortobagyi GN, Barker JL: Sequential modality therapy for inflammatory breast cancer. *Breast, Dis Breast* 2:16, 1976.
7. Greenspan EM, Fieber M, Lesnick G, Edleman S: Response of advanced breast carcinoma to the combination of the antimetabolite methotrexate and the alkylating agent thiotepa. *J Mt Sinai Hosp* 30:246, 1963.
8. Greenspan EM: Combination cytotoxic chemotherapy in advanced disseminated breast carcinoma. *J Mt Sinai Hosp* 33:1, 1966.
9. Zylberberg B, Salat-Baroux J, Ravina JH, Dormont D et al: Initial chemoimmunotherapy in inflammatory carcinoma of the breast. *Cancer* 49:1537, 1982.
10. Hortobagyi GN, Gutterman JU, Tashima CK: Combination chemotherapy immunotherapy of metastatic breast cancer with 5-fluorouracil, Adriamycin, cyclophosphamide and BCG. *Cancer* 43:1225, 1979.
11. Krutchik AN, Buzdar AU, Blumenschein GR, Hortobagyi GN et al: Chemoimmunotherapy and radiation therapy of inflammatory carcinoma. *J Surg Oncol* 11:325, 1979.
12. Buzdar AU, Montague ED, Barker JL et al: Management of inflammatory carcinoma of breast with combined modality approach: An update. *Cancer* 47:2537, 1981.
13. Koyama H, Nishizawa Y, Wada T, Kabuto T et al: Intra-arterial infusion chemotherapy as an induction therapy in multidisciplinary treatment for locally advanced breast cancer. A long-term follow-up study. *Cancer* 56:725, 1985.
14. Pollak EW, Getzen LC: Inflammatory carcinoma of the breast. A therapeutic approach followed by improved survival. *Am J Surg* 136:722, 1978.
15. Dao TL, McCarthy JD: Treatment of inflammatory carcinoma of the breast. *Surg Gynecol Obstet* 105:289, 1957.
16. Yonemoto RH, Keating JL, Byron RL Jr, Riihimaki DU: Inflammatory carcinoma of the breast treated by bilateral adrenalectomy. *Surgery* 68:461, 1970.
17. Rossi A, Brambilla C, Zucali R, Valagussa P, Bonadonna G: Five-year results of a combined chemo-radiotherapy (CT + RT) program in inflammatory breast cancer. *Proc Eur Soc Med Oncologists* No. 214:S54, 1984.

36

The Opposite Breast

Hiram S. Cody III, M.D.
Jerome A. Urban, M.D.

INTRODUCTION

The most frequent second cancer to develop in patients treated for breast carcinoma is a cancer of the other breast. Early in this century, when relatively few patients were cured of their first cancers, little importance was attached to the diagnosis and treatment of second primaries. Three developments have changed this pattern. First, a strong emphasis on early detection (by frequent self- and physician examination, identification of high-risk groups, and the use of screening mammography); second, the consistent application of an adequate local therapy to the first cancer; and third, complete investigation of the other breast (particularly by mammography and contralateral biopsy), coincident with therapy for the primary disease. The first two are widely accepted and practiced: The third remains the subject of considerable anxiety to patients and controversy (as well as confusion) among their doctors.

METASTASES VERSUS SECOND PRIMARY

Any consideration of cancer in the second breast must first distinguish between metastases from the first cancer and a true second primary. Any noninvasive carcinoma (either intraductal or lobular carcinoma in situ) or invasive cancer of a histologic type or nuclear grade distinct from the first cancer, may be considered a second primary. Otherwise, the pertinent criteria are clinical and histopathologic, and have been well summarized previously by Leis and Urban[1] as noted in Table 36-1. On occasion, the distinction between metastatic disease and a true second primary may be quite difficult or become apparent only in retrospect. These pa-

Table 36-1 Primary versus Metastatic Lesions

	Metastatic origin	Primary origin
Stage	Always invasive	May be noninvasive or invasive
Histologic type	Usually similar to first carcinoma	May be different from first carcinoma
Nuclear grade	Usually similar to first carcinoma	May be different from first carcinoma
Configuration of invasive mass	Ill-defined; no consistent characteristics	One of classical patterns: stellate, multinodular, comedo carcinoma
Site	Medial part of breast or fatty tail	Most often upper outer quadrant
Tissue relationships	Often discrete nodules in adipose tissue	In mammary tissue; may extend to adipose tissue
Multiple invasive nodules	Frequently present	Occasionally present
Carcinoma in situ or epithelial atypia adjacent to invasive mass	Rarely present	Usually present
Intramammary and subcutaneous lymphatic vessels	Often contain neoplastic cells	Rarely contain neoplastic cells
Appears more than 5 years after first carcinoma	Rarely	Commonly

tients should probably be treated with curative intent as second primary cancers.

SYNCHRONOUS VERSUS METACHRONOUS DISEASE

Second primary breast cancers may be either synchronous (found simultaneously with the first cancer) or metachronous (detected subsequent to the development of the first cancer). The reported incidence of synchronous bilateral breast cancer varies widely and depends highly on the diagnostic approach taken. If clinical criteria alone are used (i.e., the presence of a mass), perhaps 0.5 percent of breast cancers are bilateral. Much of the vast literature on the bilaterality of breast cancer falls into this category. If mammographic screening is added,[2] 3 to 4 percent of patients will be found to have contralateral cancers. Finally, if screening biopsy of the opposite breast is routinely performed at the time of treatment for the first cancer, as many as 12.5 percent of biopsied patients will be found to have a cancer of the other breast. These figures are derived from the personal experience of Urban[3] with 1204 breast cancer patients treated between 1964 and 1975, among whom contralateral breast biopsy was performed in 80 percent (954 patients), and cancer found in 12.5 percent of these. Some 6.7 percent of patients had noninvasive disease (intraductal or lobular carcinoma in situ), and 5.8 percent had invasive cancer. Contralateral cancers were found more often in patients with primary noninvasive than with primary invasive cancer. Among the 119 patients found to have contralateral cancers, suspicious physical findings were present in only 18.5 percent. Among the patients found on contralateral biopsy to have cancer in whom preoperative mammography had been performed, only 34 percent had suspicious mammograms. In other words, of all the contralateral cancers detected by routine screening biopsy, *more than 80 percent would have been missed on physical examination, and two-thirds undetected by mammography.*

Furthermore, of patients found unexpectedly to have invasive cancer in the other breast, 8.5 percent had axillary nodal metastases: During the same period, 41 percent of all patients with primary invasive cancers had positive axillary nodes. Clearly, contralateral breast biopsy is the best screening test available for early detection of cancers in the second breast.

Another major advantage of contralateral breast biopsy is the assessment of risk for a later development of a second breast cancer. In an exhaustive analysis of bilateral breast cancers, following 1458 breast cancer patients over 20 years, Robbins and Berg[4] estimated the risk of a second breast cancer at 0.7 percent per year after treatment of the first cancer, or eight to ten times that normally expected. Among these patients, the risk of metachronous contralateral disease is greatest in premenopausal patients with multicentric or prognostically favorable first cancers (lobular carcinoma in situ, intraductal carcinoma, and node-negative invasive cancers), a family history of breast cancer (particularly if it was bilateral and premenopausal), and atypical ductal or lobular hyperplasia. The latter were found in about 10 percent of benign contralateral biopsies done by Urban, and 15.3 percent of patients reported by Leis.[1] Particularly careful surveillance is required for this subgroup, with physical examination and mammography performed more frequently than would otherwise be required.

CLINICAL APPROACH TO THE OTHER BREAST

All patients with a clinical cancer in one breast should undergo mammography preoperatively. This is particularly important to evaluate the second breast and rule out the presence of suspicious but clinically occult densities or microcalcifications and is a useful guide for localization of the contralateral biopsy.

Three approaches are possible for management of the other breast at the time of treating the first cancer: (1) observation only (serial physical examinations and mammography), (2) contralateral biopsy, and (3) a prophylactic mastectomy. None is appropriate for all patients, and each should be used selectively.

Observation alone is preferable for patients who are elderly, who have serious underlying medical conditions, or who have locally advanced (stages III and IV) cancers, which would dominate the prognostic picture. The survival advantage of detecting an early cancer in the opposite breast would be minimal for each of the above groups.

Contralateral biopsy should be performed for the vast majority of clinically unilateral breast cancers. Urban found that 40 percent of cancers in the second breast were at mirror image locations, almost as often as would be expected by chance. Robbins and Berg[4] have also shown that the location of contralateral breast cancers bears no relationship to the quadrant of the first cancer, and thus there is no need to "mirror" the site of the first lesion. A generous biopsy of the contralateral breast should be taken of (1) any mammographically questionable area (with specimen x-ray if necessary to confirm excision), (2) any area of increased thickening, or (3) in the event of a clinically and radiographically normal breast, of the upper outer quadrant. The biopsy should be as generous as possible, consistent with a good cosmetic result (approximating 20 to 25 percent of the breast parenchyma), the defect should be carefully palpated for additional suspicious areas, and a careful layered closure done. In most cases, further surgery is deferred pending results of the final pathologic report.

If intraductal or lobular carcinoma in situ is found, total mastectomy with a low axillary dissection (preserving both pectoralis major and minor) is normally done, although some patients with lobular carcinoma in situ will elect observation alone. For infiltrating cancers, a Patey-type modified radical mastectomy with excision of the pectoralis minor and full axillary dissection is performed. Radical mastectomy is usually reserved for patients with large cancers and gross axillary nodal disease, and hence only applied to patients with bilateral clinically obvious stages II to III disease.

The third option, prophylactic mastectomy, is most controversial, necessitates a careful and honest dialogue with the patient, and is probably applicable to only a minority of patients. As noted, the overall risk of developing a second breast cancer is about 0.7 percent per year of follow-up,[4] and, even for young patients, when projected for entire life expectancy, is in the range of 10 to 15 percent. The other risk factors of multifocal primary, noninvasive primary, adverse family history (premenopausal and/or bilateral), and presence of atypical duct or lobular hyperplasia, may or may not increase this figure. In a series of 101 high-risk patients, Leis performed prophylactic mastectomy, finding cancer in 16.8 percent of patients.[1] Other factors may occasionally lead to the recommendation of prophylactic mastectomy. The contralateral breast may be extremely dense or nodular, precluding accurate physical or mammographic examination. Occasionally, extreme anxiety will lead patients to request contralateral mastectomy. Finally, in patients planning to undergo breast reconstruction, surgery is often recommended for the other breast, either augmentation mammoplasty, mastopexy, or reduction mammoplasty. If marked asymmetry is anticipated, or if many of the above factors are present, the option of contralateral total mastectomy with immediate reconstruction should be considered. "Subcutaneous mastectomy" is less desirable than a total mastectomy with full excision of the breast parenchyma.

It should be noted that frequent use of contralateral screening biopsy (and appropriate treatment of any cancer found) will reduce, but not eliminate, the risk of second breast cancers. In Urban's experience to date, about 2 percent of patients with negative biopsies subsequently developed cancers in that breast. Clearly, a negative biopsy in no way reduces the need for lifetime surveillance of the other breast. Regardless of findings on the contralateral biopsy, all treated breast cancer patients should undergo examinations of the other breast at least every 6 months, with screening mammography done every 1 to 2 years (depending on the number of risk factors present).

CONCLUSION

Management of the other breast in most patients with clinically unilateral breast carcinoma should consist of (1) preoperative mammography; (2) a generous contralateral biopsy of any dominant thickening, mammographically suspicious area, or of the upper outer quadrant; (3) appropriate surgery for any cancers found (with extent of operation based on tumor type); (4) close lifetime surveillance of the remaining breast (with frequent physical examination and mammography); and (5) consideration of prophylactic mastectomy for patients felt to be at highest risk of second breast cancer.

REFERENCES

1. Leis HP, Urban JA: The other breast, in Gallager HS, Leis HP, Snyderman RK, Urban JA (eds): *The Breast.* St. Louis, C. V. Mosby, 1978, p. 487.
2. Egan RL: Roles of mammography in the early detection of breast cancer. *Cancer* 24:1197, 1969.
3. Urban JA, Papachristou D, Taylor J: Bilateral breast cancer: Biopsy of the opposite breast. *Cancer* 40: 1968, 1977.
4. Robbins GF, Berg JW: Bilateral primary breast cancers: A prospective clinicopathological study. *Cancer* 17:1501, 1964.

37

Breast Diseases in Children

John H. Seashore, M.D.

INTRODUCTION

The child's breast is subject to a variety of disorders which may arouse considerable concern in parents and in adolescent patients. A thorough history, gentle examination, and full understanding of these disorders are important to allay anxiety, to avoid unnecessary surgery, and to choose appropriate treatment. Diffuse enlargement of the breast(s) usually represents normal breast tissue which has hypertrophied in response to a systemic stimulus. Biopsy is rarely indicated and in young children may irrevocably damage the breast bud. Breast cancer is extremely rare in children (under 21 years) but persistent, localized masses, seen mostly in adolescent girls, should usually be excised to prevent damage to the breast from secondary infection or progressive enlargement.

This chapter begins with a brief description of breast development, then presents breast pathology in neonates, prepubertal children, and adolescents. While many of the conditions can occur at any age, this format serves to emphasize the most common problems in each age group.

THE DEVELOPING BREAST

Bilateral ectodermal thickenings, known as milk streaks, are first seen in the sixth week of fetal life. These normally regress except in the thoracic area, where they differentiate into recognizable mammary tissue. By the fifth month, nipple, areola, and a branching mass of cells with primitive duct formation are present.[1] Further breast growth commences at about 32 weeks gestation, presumably under the influence of maternal hormones, so that a breast bud with an average diameter of about 8 mm is palpable at term.[2]

The breast continues to enlarge for 2 to 3 weeks after birth, mostly due to accumulation of a colostrum-like substance ("witches' milk"). The average maximum size is 14 mm but enlargement to 2 to 3 cm is not uncommon (Fig. 37-1). The breast bud then slowly

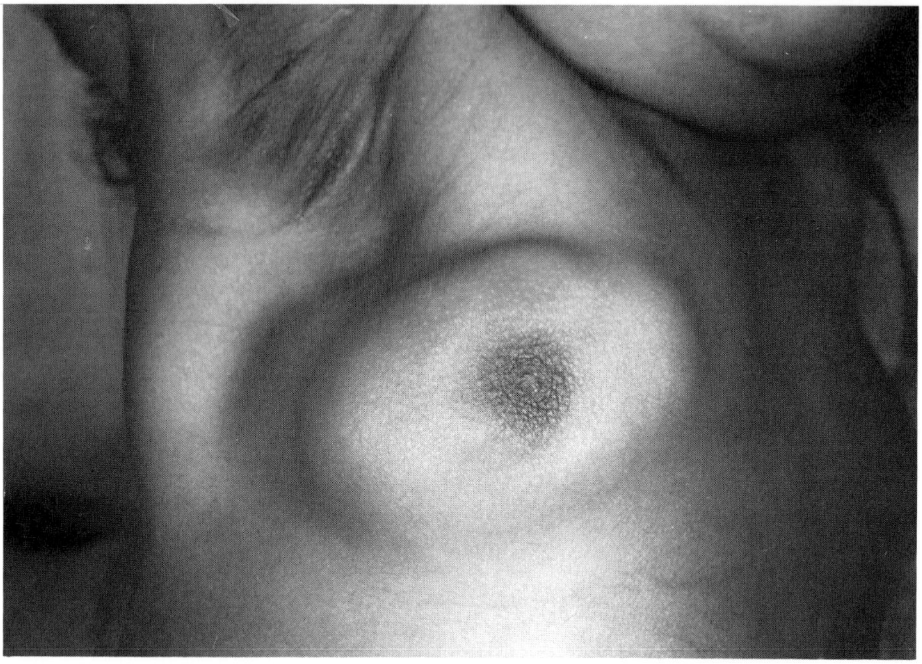

Figure 37-1 Marked breast bud enlargement in a neonate. (*Reproduced with permission from Pediatric Annals.*)

decreases in size to about 1 cm and remains quiescent until puberty.[2]

Breast growth is usually the first sign of puberty and may begin as early as age 8. Estrogen, growth hormone, corticosteroids, and prolactin contribute to the growth and branching of ducts and development of alveoli. Following menarche, the cyclic secretion of progesterone probably influences lobular development.[3] There is a striking increase in the connective tissue stroma which accounts for the firm and often nodular character of developing breasts.

NEONATES

Congenital Anomalies

Supernumerary nipples (polythelia) occur in 1 to 3 percent of the population and may be anywhere along the milk lines.[4] They have no functional significance but may be excised for cosmetic reasons. Polymastia is rare. The extra breast may be rudimentary or well developed and capable of secretion.

Amastia (absence of the breast) is also uncommon. Bilateral amastia occurs in children with ectodermal dysplasia. Absence or hypoplasia of the breast and pectoralis muscles, often associated with deficiencies of underlying costal cartilages and ribs and with ipsilateral syndactyly, is known as Poland's syndrome, and may require extensive reconstruction. The best treatment for amastia is placement of a subcutaneous implant once full growth is achieved. Iatrogenic amastia due to overzealous biopsy of putative breast masses in young girls should be avoided.

Inflammatory Masses

If the normal postpartum breast enlargement is excessive, the breast bud may become tense

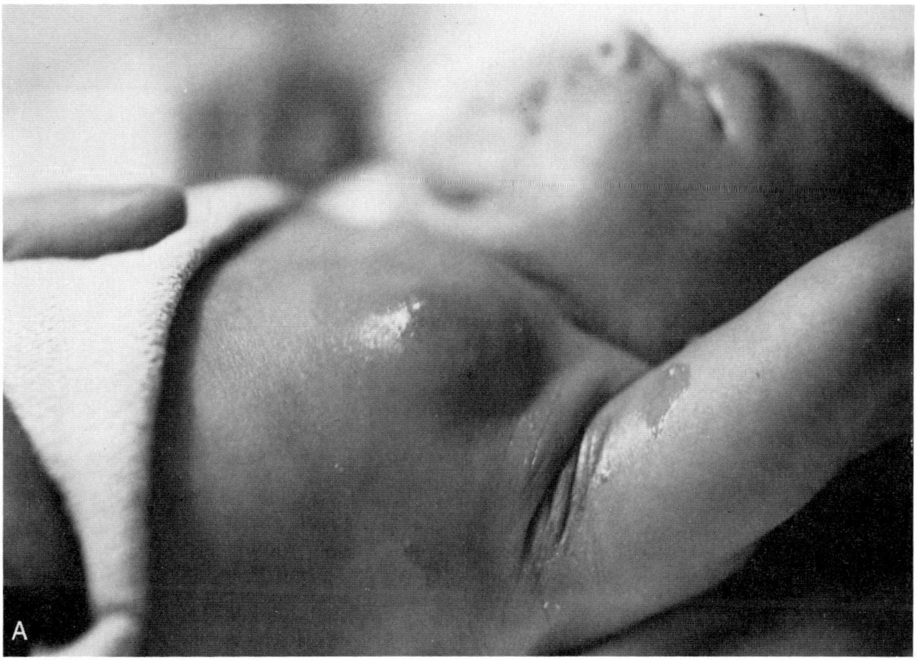

Figure 37-2 A. Breast abscess (mastitis neonatorum) in the enlarged breast bud of a neonate. Note the thin, shiny skin. (*Reproduced with permission from the C.V. Mosby Co.*) B. Incision and drainage, using local anesthesia, yielded 10 mL of creamy white pus.

and tender with shiny red skin, a condition known as *mastitis neonatorum* (Fig. 37-2). Attempts to express the fluid in the breast are likely to worsen the infection, which is usually caused by *Staphylococcus aureus*. Simple cellulitis can be treated with an appropriate oral antibiotic and warm soaks. Fever and other systemic manifestations require vigorous intravenous antibiotic therapy. Abscess formation is common and prompt drainage of pus through a circumareolar incision is indicated. Reduction in adult breast size following neonatal breast abscess has been reported, but the incidence of this complication is not known.[5]

Other Masses

Cysts and tumors of the infant breast are very rare. Capillary hemangiomas appear in early infancy, enlarge for a few months, then involute spontaneously. Surgery is contraindicated. Cavernous hemangiomas and cystic hygromas may need to be excised, but dissection should be very limited to avoid permanent injury to the breast bud.

PREPUBERTAL CHILDREN

Diffuse Breast Enlargement

Premature thelarche, the growth of normal breast tissue in girls before age 8 years, is by far the most common breast problem in this age group. The pediatrician or endocrinologist is likely to see 15 or 20 girls with premature thelarche for every prepubertal child with a pathologic lesion intrinsic to the breast. Breast growth is usually bilateral but onset may be asynchronous and there may be some

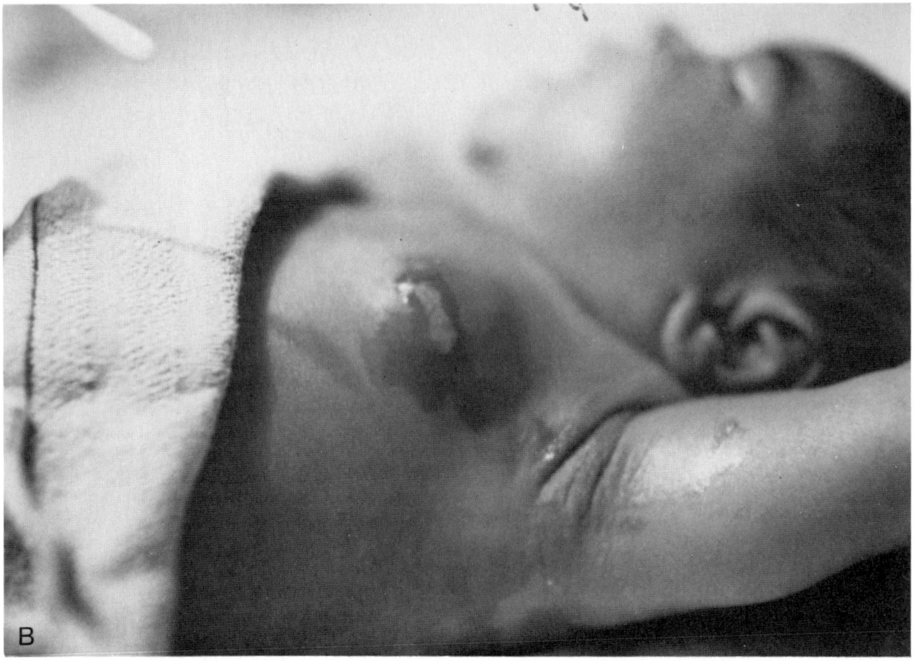

Figure 37-2 B

asymmetry. The breasts are perfectly normal in appearance and by palpation. Biopsy or excision of breast tissue is contraindicated.

Table 37-1 lists the various known causes of premature thelarche. While the majority are idiopathic, a careful history and physical examination are essential to rule out other causes. Estrogen-containing creams or drugs may have been taken deliberately or accidentally. Various medications, including digitalis and isoniazid, have been implicated as causing premature thelarche. Hormone-secreting tumors usually produce multiple signs of precocious puberty, but breast growth may be the first manifestation. The mechanism(s) by which diseases of the central nervous system, lungs, and thyroid cause premature thelarche is not known but does not appear to be related to measureable hormonal abnormality.[6] Chronic liver disease interferes with the normal catabolism of sex steroids.

Girls who have premature thelarche should be examined and followed carefully for other evidence of precocious puberty, including axillary and pubic hair, increased growth velocity, increased bone age, evidence of estrogen effect on vaginal mucosa, vaginal bleeding, and, less frequently, ovulation. Adrenal or ovarian tumors are found in about 20 percent of cases.[7,8] Several cases of follicular cysts of the ovary associated with precocious puberty have been reported and can be treated by simple excision of the cyst and preservation of the ovary.[9] In the McCune-Albright syndrome, precocious puberty is associated with polyostotic fibrous dysplasia. Most of the rest are thought to be of central origin, a supposition borne out by a recent study in which CT scans demonstrated small hypothalamic lesions in 50 percent of girls with precocious puberty.[10] Management of these children is difficult and clearly requires counseling and emotional support. Ovulation can be suppressed with progestational agents. Cyproterone acetate and a luteinizing hormone-releasing hormone analogue have been somewhat effective

Table 37-1 Known Causes of Diffuse Breast Enlargement

Known Causes
Exogenous estrogen: creams, oral medications
Drugs: digitalis, isoniazid, amphetamines
Tumors: CNS, adrenal, ovarian, testicular
Klinefelter's syndrome
Neurologic disorders: hamartomas, trauma, syringomyelia, transverse myelitis
Pulmonary disease: TB, bronchitis, bronchiectasis
Chronic liver disease

Adapted from Brambilla et al.[6]

experimentally in reversing the signs of precocious puberty.[11]

If all other causes of breast enlargement have been excluded, a diagnosis of idiopathic premature thelarche is made. Onset is during the first year or two of life in most cases. In about half these girls, the breasts enlarge for a number of months then stabilize until puberty. In somewhat less than half, breast growth regresses during follow-up. Only a few have continued growth through the prepubertal years.[12] In all cases, breast growth at puberty is entirely normal and these children do not have other medical or sexual problems. Reassurance and emotional support are indicated.

Gynecomastia in prepubertal males is uncommon but several small series have been reported.[13,14] Most cases are idiopathic but the conditions listed in Table 37-1 must be considered. Precocious puberty is much less common in boys than in girls. On the other hand, adrenal or testicular tumors are relatively more common causes of gynecomastia in prepubertal boys than in adolescent males.[15,16] Spontaneous regression of idiopathic gynecomastia occurs in most cases. If enlargement persists, subcutaneous mastectomy may be indicated for cosmetic reasons.

Discrete Masses

Localized breast masses are uncommon in this age group. Infection and abscess are most likely related to trauma. Granular cell myoblastoma is a peculiar tumor of neural origin which occurs in the breast fairly frequently in adults and occasionally in children. It is stony hard; grossly and on frozen section it is often thought to be malignant. Therapeutic decisions about breast masses in children should always be made after review of paraffin-embedded sections. Keratomas and

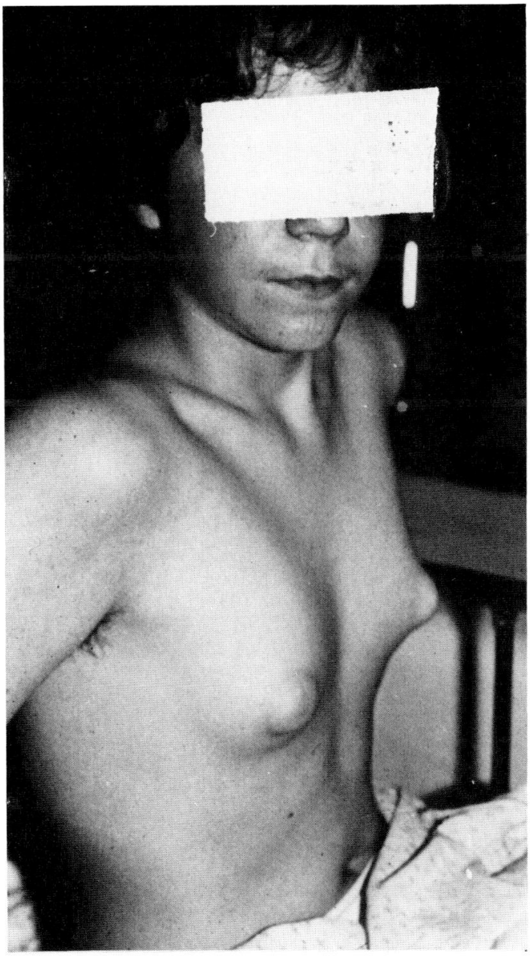

Figure 37-3 Extreme adolescent gynecomastia in a 15-year-old boy. Bilateral subcutaneous mastectomy produced an excellent cosmetic result. *(Reproduced with permission from Year Book Medical Publishers, Inc.)*

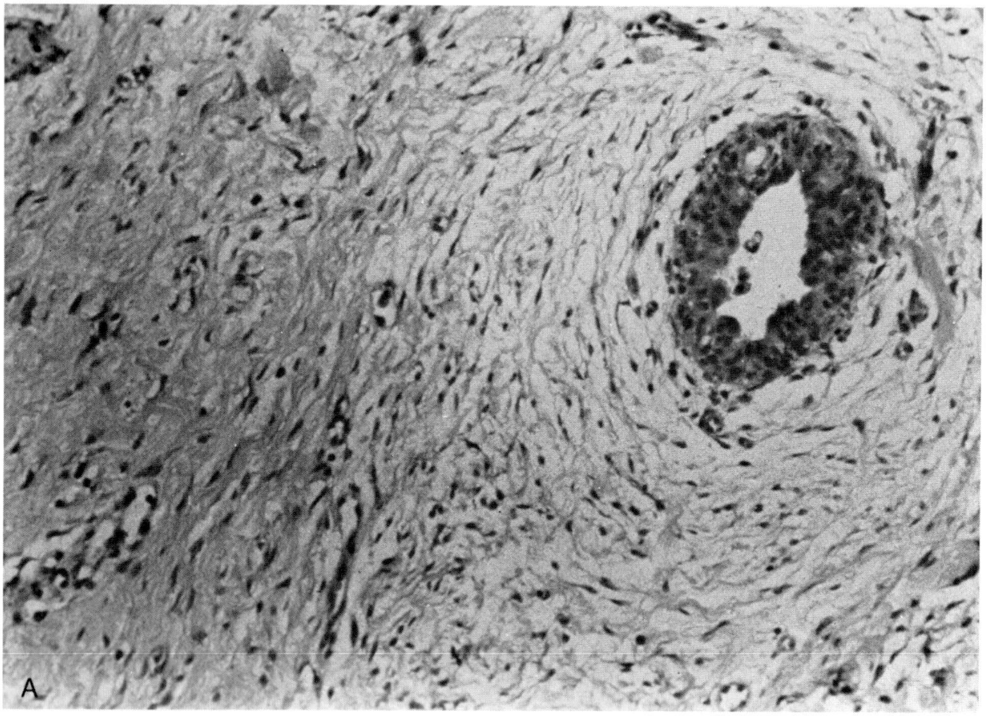

Figure 37-4 High-power photomicrographs of gynecomastia, juvenile hypertrophy, and fibroadenoma. Although these lesions are clearly different, they have in common a striking degree of stromal and ductular proliferation. A. Gynecomastia. This section shows an enlarged duct surrounded by dense hypertrophied stroma. The area on the left is normal breast tissue. B. Juvenile hypertrophy. There is moderate proliferation of ducts and massive hypertrophy of a relatively acellular stroma. C. Fibroadenoma. This discrete tumor is always surrounded by a dense fibrous capsule. Marked stromal proliferation and variable degrees of ductal development are characteristic findings. (*Reproduced with permission from Year Book Medical Publishers, Inc.*)

papillomas of the nipple or areola are occasionally seen.

ADOLESCENTS

Diffuse Enlargements

Gynecomastia

About 70 percent of teenage boys have a 1-to-2-cm disklike nodule of breast tissue beneath the areola of one or both breasts. This typically appears about a year after onset of puberty, enlarges for 1 to 2 years, then regresses and is gone by age 17 or 18.[17] Gynecomastia persists into early adulthood in 10 to 15 percent of males and may never disappear in a small number. One or 2 percent of boys develop more significant breast enlargement which is unilateral in about 80 percent of these.[18] Occasionally, gynecomastia is so extreme that it resembles normal adolescent female breasts (Fig. 37-3). Pain and tenderness are common complaints but nipple discharge does not occur.

The histologic appearance of gynecomastia is one of overgrowth of normal breast tissue, particularly the fibrous stroma and ducts. There is some ductal branching but no lobule formation (Fig. 37-4 A). These findings are consistent with stimulation by estrogen and growth hormone but not progesterone. Some studies have

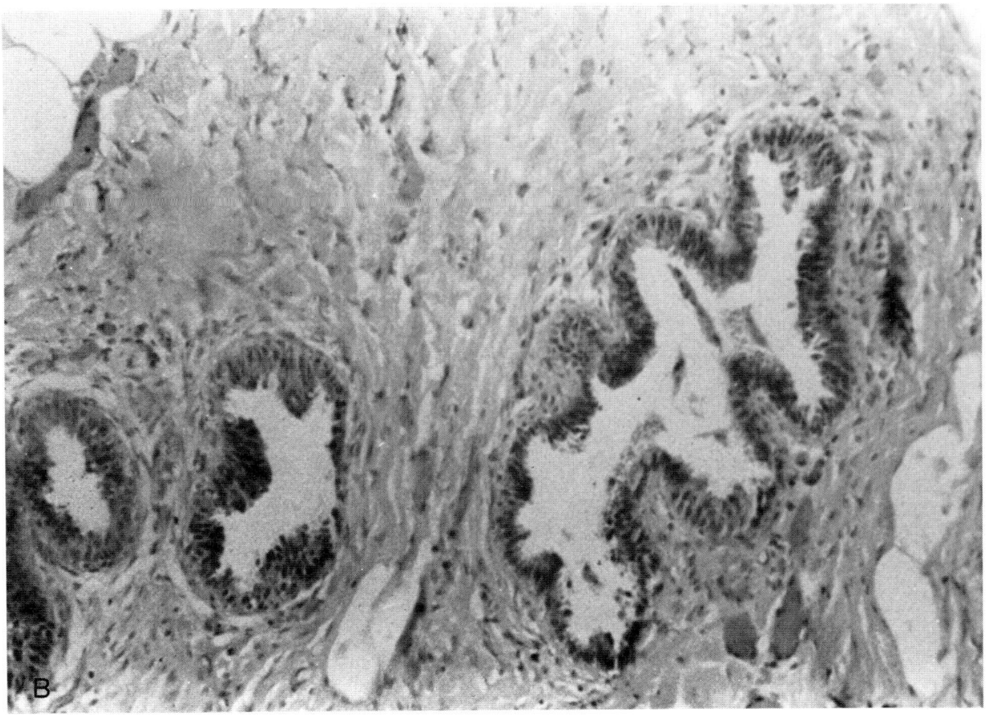

have demonstrated a slight imbalance between estrogen and testosterone or subtle abnormalities in the diurnal secretion of androgens in boys with gynecomastia.[19,20] Other studies have failed to confirm these findings, however.[21]

Adolescent gynecomastia is almost invariably idiopathic—in fact, a normal variant. The causes of breast enlargement shown in Table 37-1 should be considered but the only disorder which occurs with any frequency is Klinefelter's syndrome. These boys are easily identified by their female body habitus and hypoplastic genitalia. Complete endocrine evaluation is not indicated in boys who have typical adolescent gynecomastia.

Since gynecomastia is a normal variant and usually self-limited, reassurance is adequate treatment for most boys. If the breast enlargement is noticeably excessive or persists into late adolescence, it can be very emotionally disturbing. These boys may benefit from subcutaneous mastectomy and are often our most grateful patients. Removal of all breast tissue is performed through a circumareolar incision. It is particularly important to shave breast tissue off the undersurface of the areola to eliminate the protrusion of nipple and areola which is so disconcerting to these boys (Fig. 37-5). It is equally important to preserve the normal fat around the breast and approximate it beneath the areola to prevent adherence of the areola to pectoral fascia.

Obese boys may have prominent breasts due to fat deposition which may be misdiagnosed as gynecomastia. Fat is much softer to palpation than breast tissue. Weight reduction is more effective than mastectomy.

Macromastia

Some adolescent girls have unusually large breasts which nonetheless have normal contours and are composed of normal breast tissue histologically. More and more teenage girls are seeking reduction mammoplasty for

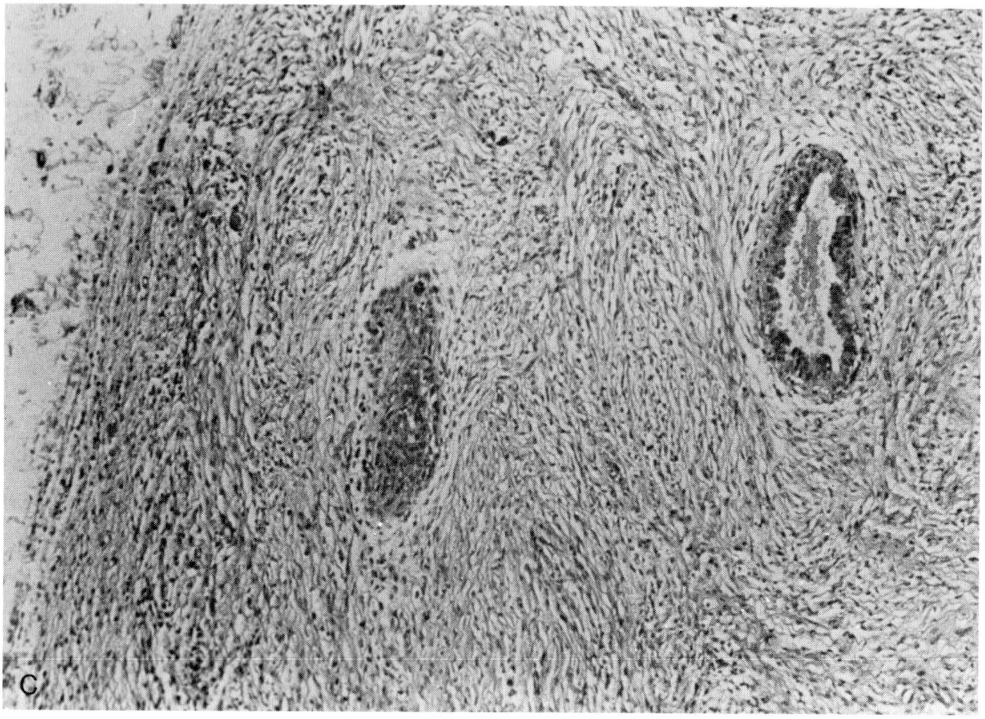

Figure 37-4 C

macromastia. What constitutes excessive size is clearly a subjective and personal judgment. Given the emotional lability of adolescents, prudence is advisable in recommending this operation. Certainly fatigue, poor posture, and skin irritation from bra straps are problems for some girls but most desire mammoplasty for cosmetic reasons. The girl's reasons for wanting an operation and the risks and implications of surgery should be thoroughly discussed by a sensitive physician on at least two separate visits. The effects of partial mastectomy on subsequent lactation have not been well studied. Reduction mammoplasty should not be performed until full growth has been achieved.

Juvenile Hypertrophy

This rare pathologic condition is characterized by extreme overgrowth of the breasts which may reach gargantuan proportions and be a severe physical and emotional handicap.[1,22] Histologically there is a tremendous amount of loose, relatively acellular connective tissue stroma and a more modest proliferation of ducts (Fig. 37-4 B). As in gynecomastia, there is no lobule formation. Juvenile hypertrophy is thought to result from an excessive response to estrogen during adolescent growth but this has not been documented. The only effective treatment for extreme juvenile hypertrophy is total mastectomy. Reduction mammoplasty may be helpful for lesser degrees of hypertrophy, but regrowth is common. Medroxyprogesterone has been reported to slow the rate of hypertrophy and to prevent regrowth following partial mastectomy.[23,24]

Discrete Masses

Inflammatory masses

Breast abscess occurs most commonly in the

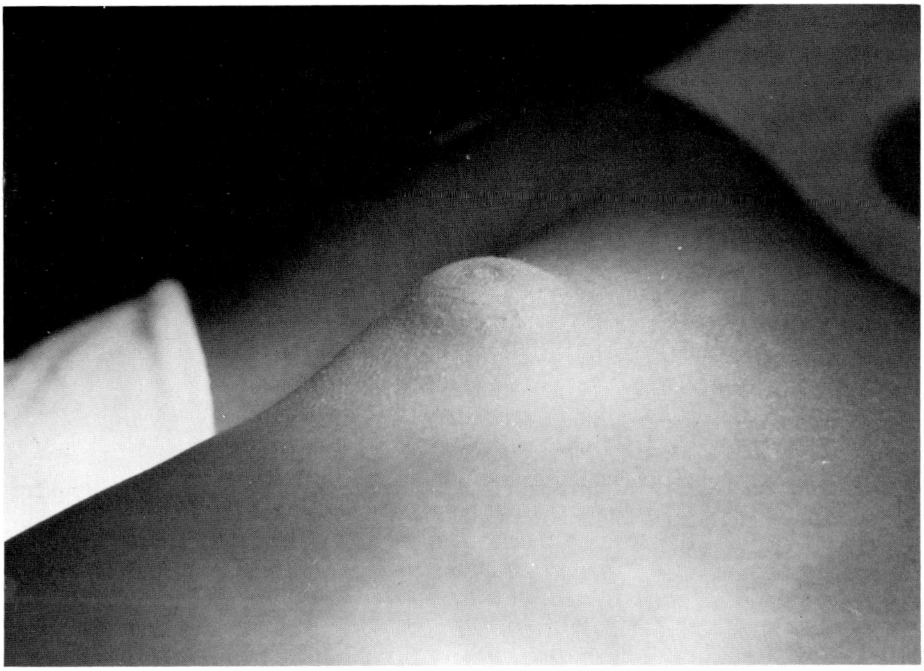

Figure 37-5 Typical unilateral idiopathic adolescent gynecomastia. This 16-year-old boy requested subcutaneous mastectomy particularly because of the degree of areolar protrusion. (*Reproduced with permission from Pediatric Annals.*)

lactating breast but may be seen at any age. It is usually centrally located and can be drained through a circumareolar incision to minimize scarring. Antibiotic therapy is indicated only if there is significant cellulitis. The breasts of active adolescent girls are frequently subject to trauma, which may cause hematoma or fat necrosis. Occasionally these may present months later as an irregular hard mass, the history of trauma long since forgotten.[25] Excisional biopsy is indicated for persistent masses.

Mastopathies

Fibrous mastopathy, lobular hyperplasia, sclerosing adenosis, periductal fibrosis, and cystic ductular hyperplasia have all been reported in adolescent girls.[25] These usually present as discrete masses whose borders are less well defined than fibroadenomas. They are usually mobile but may have some fixation to skin or fascia. Tenderness may be present. If these masses do not regress after a period of observation, excisional biopsy is performed.

Cysts

Simple cysts, blue-domed cysts, and galactoceles may occur at any age but are most common in adolescent girls. They are usually subareolar and often tender. There may be a watery or milky discharge. Excision is indicated since cysts are prone to infection and progressive enlargement.

Fibrocystic disease appears to be increasing in frequency among adolescent girls. The disease may be localized or involve both breasts diffusely. The characteristic ropelike thickenings are due to increased fibrous tissue while the larger irregular masses represent cysts or clusters of cysts. Since the cysts are often deep and tense with fluid, they are easily mistaken for solid tumors. Fine-needle aspiration of fluid will confirm the cystic character of the mass in selected patients. Pain and tenderness are almost always worse before and during menses and the physical findings usually change from month to month as cysts collapse and new ones form. The inflammatory nature of fibrocystic disease and its relationship to the menstrual cycle are evident. It is logical to assume a relationship to the cyclic secretion of hormones but this has not been demonstrated.

Since the risk of cancer is negligible in adolescent girls, biopsy is rarely indicated. The diagnosis can usually be made by repeated examination over several menstrual cycles. Biopsy is considered only if a particularly large and firm mass persists for several months. Mammography is of limited value in teenage girls because of the large amount of fibrous stroma in their breasts. Since this disease is likely to persist into adult life, these girls should be taught the technique of self-examination of the breasts.

Tumors

Fibroadenoma is by far the most common breast lesion in adolescent girls, accounting for 60 to 90 percent of all surgically excised masses in various series.[25,28] The diagnostic features of fibroadenomas on physical examination are their sharp, smooth borders and their mobility. They are hard but not stony and usually are not tender. They may be anywhere in the breast but most commonly are in the upper outer quadrant. Multiple or bilateral tumors occur in 15 to 20 percent of patients.[25,29] Fibroadenomas usually grow slowly and have an average size of 2 to 3 cm at the time of discovery. Growth may be more rapid at times of intense hormonal stimulation. Occasionally, giant fibroadenomas may fill an entire quadrant of the breast.

The most striking histologic feature of fibroadenoma is the dense, fibrous capsule which surrounds and demarcates it from the adjacent breast tissue. The tumor itself resembles gynecomastia and juvenile hypertrophy though it tends to be more compact. There is an abundant fibrous stroma and branching ducts without lobule formation. (Fig. 37-4 C).

Fibroadenomas are benign although there is some evidence that long-standing neglected tumors may degenerate into fibrosarcomas. Excision is indicated to prevent progressive enlargement and destruction of breast tissue. Removal is facilitated by the dense capsule; the tumor "shells out" easily. Whenever possible, a circumareolar incision is used. If the tumor is located peripherally, a short, curved incision following skin lines gives satisfactory cosmetic results.

Cystosarcoma phyllodes is a large, irregular, rapidly growing tumor which is often fixed to skin or fascia. Histologically it resembles fibroadenoma but has a larger amount of very cellular fibrous stroma. Despite its name, most are benign. In about 25 percent the fibrous component is frankly malignant but even then the tumor tends to be locally aggressive and metastasizes late.[30] Only four cases of malignant cystosarcoma phyllodes have been reported in girls under age 20.[31,32] One died of metastatic disease while the others were apparently cured by *simple* mastectomy, which is generally considered to be the treatment of choice.

Cancer of the breast in children is extremely rare. An extensive literature review in 1974 yielded 33 well-documented cases in the English literature.[28] Ten additional cases have been reported since then.[33–39] About half the children were prepubertal and most of these had the type of "secretory carcinoma" first described by McDivitt and Stewart.[40] Most were treated by local resection or simple mastectomy and all but one survived. Adolescent children had a variety of types of carcinoma similar to those seen in adults. Treatment ranged from local resection to radical mastectomy with radiotherapy and about 50 percent survived. The number of patients is too small to draw any conclusions about therapy but it is probably appropriate to treat these adolescents as adults. Three of the prepubertal children were boys and two of the adolescents were males, or 12 percent of the entire group, which is a much higher incidence than is seen in adult males.

The breast is occasionally the site of *metastatic tumors*, especially ovarian tumors and lymphomas. Primary sarcomas have also been described.[41]

CONCLUSION

Abnormalities of the breast are relatively common in children. Most diffuse enlargements occur because of excessive circulating estrogens or an exaggerated response to normal hormone concentrations. Careful evaluation for estrogen-secreting tumors or cysts is indicated in prepubertal children. Surgery is not indicated except for severe cases of male gynecomastia or juvenile hypertrophy. Discrete breast masses should usually be removed after a period of observation. Normal breast tissue should be carefully preserved, especially in prepubertal children.

REFERENCES

1. Geschickter CF: *Diseases of the Breast.* Philadelphia, J. B. Lippincott Co., 1943, p. 7.
2. McKiernan JF, Hull JD: Breast development in the newborn. *Arch Dis Child* 56:525, 1981.
3. Porter JC: Hormonal regulation of breast development and activity. *J Invest Dermatol* 63:85, 1974.
4. de Cholnoky T: Supernumerary breast. *Arch Surg* 39:926, 1939.
5. Rudoy RC, Nelson JD: Breast abscess during the neonatal period. *Am J Dis Child* 129:1031, 1975.
6. Brambilla F, Epstein JA, Kupperman HS: Intermittent precocious breast development associated with mild bronchitis. *J Clin Endocrin Metab* 21:80, 1961.
7. Drop SLS, Bruining GJ, Visser HKA, Sippel WG: Prolonged galactorrhea in a 6 year old girl with isosexual precocity due to a feminizing adrenal tumor. *Clin Endocrinol* 15:37, 1981.
8. Lack EE, Perez-Atayde AR, Murthy ASF, Goldstein DP, Crigler JF, Vawter GF: Granulosa theca cell tumors in premenarchal girls. *Cancer* 48:1846, 1981.
9. Kosloske AM, Goldthorn JF, Kaufman E, Hayek A: Treatment of precocious pseudopuberty associated with follicular cysts of the ovary. *Am J Dis Child* 138:147, 1984.
10. Cacciari E, Frejaville E, Cicognani A: How many cases of true precocious puberty are idiopathic? *J Pediatr* 102:357, 1983.
11. Comite F, Cutler GB, Rivier J, Vale WW, Loriaux DL, Crowley WF: Short term treatment of idiopathic precocious puberty with a longacting analogue of luteinizing hormone-releasing hormone—a preliminary report. *N Engl J Med* 305:1546, 1981.
12. Mills JL, Stolley PD, Davies J, Mostrang T: Premature thelarche. *Am J Dis Child* 135:743, 1981.
13. August GP, Chandra R, Hung W: Prepubertal male gynecomastia. *J Pediatr* 80:259, 1972.
14. LaTorre H, Kennem FM: Idiopathic gynecomastia in seven pre-adolescent boys. *Am J Dis Child* 126:771, 1973.
15. Itami RM, Amundson GM, Kaplan SA, Lippe BM: Prepubertal gynecomastia caused by an adrenal tumor. *Am J Dis Child* 136:584, 1982.
16. Johnstone G: Prepubertal gynecomastia in association with an interstitial cell tumor of the testis. *Br J Urol* 39:211, 1967.
17. Jung FT, Shafton AL: Mastitis, mazoplasia, mastalgia and gynecomastia in normal adolescent males. *Ill Med J* 73:113, 1938.
18. Geschickter CF: *Diseases of the Breast.* Philadelphia, J. B. Lippincott Co, 1943, chap. 4.
19. LaFranchi SH, Parlow AF, Lippe BM, Coyotupa J, Kaplan SA: Pubertal gynecomastia and transient elevation of serum estradiol level. *Am J Dis Child* 129:927, 1975.
20. Large DM, Anderson DC: Twenty-four hour profiles of circulating androgens and oestrogens in male puberty with and without gynecomastia. *Clin Endocrinol* 11:505, 1979.
21. Marynick SP, Nisula BC, Pita JC, Loriaux DL: Persistent pubertal macromastia. *J Clin Endocrinol Metab* 50:128, 1980.
22. Goodman BA: Mastitis gargantuan: An unusual case of puberty hypertrophy of breasts. *JAMA* 103:335, 1934.
23. Mayl N, Vasconez LO, Jurkiewicz MJ: Treatment of macromastia in the actively enlarging breast. *Plast Reconstr Surg* 54:6, 1974.

24. Sperling RL, Gold JJ: Use of an anti-estrogen after a reduction mammoplasty to prevent recurrence of virginal hypertrophy of the breast. *Plast Reconstr Surg* 52:439, 1973.
25. Farrow JH, Ashikari H: Breast lesions in young girls. *Surg Clin North Am* 49:261, 1969.
26. Daniel WA, Matthews MD: Tumors of the breast in adolescent females. *Pediatrics* 41:743, 1968.
27. Bowers R, Bell MJ, Ternberg JL: Management of breast lesions in children and adolescents. *J Pediatr Surg* 11:337, 1976.
28. Seashore JH: Breast enlargements in infants and children. *Pediatr Annals* 4:542, 1975.
29. Sandison AT, Walker JC: Diseases of the adolescent female breast. *Br J Surg* 55:443, 1968.
30. Treves N, Sunderland DA: Cystosarcoma phyllodes of the breast: A malignant and a benign tumor. *Cancer* 4:1286, 1954.
31. Hoover HC, Trestioreanu A, Ketcham AS: Metastatic cystosarcoma phyllodes in an adolescent girl. *Ann Surg* 181:279, 1975.
32. Iverson RE, Hegg SI: Cystosarcoma phyllodes presenting as massive unilateral breast hypertrophy in an adolescent. *Ann Plast Surg* 4:315, 1980.
33. Deutsch M, Altomare FJ, Mastrian AS, Chervenak JP: Carcinoma of the male breast following thymic irradiation. *Radiology* 116:413, 1975.
34. Gogas J, Sechas M, Skalkeas G: Surgical management of diseases of the adolescent breast. *Am J Surg* 137:634, 1979.
35. Hammar B: Childhood breast carcinoma: Report of a case. *J Pediatr Surg* 16:77, 1981.
36. Heydenrych JJ, Villet WT, Vonder Heyden V: Carcinoma of the breast in children. *S Afr Med J* 57:1005, 1980.
37. Massi SR, Rioux A, Beauchessone C: Juvenile carcinoma of the breast. *Human Pathol* 12:1044, 1981.
38. Stone AM, Shenker IR, McCarthy K: Adolescent breast masses. *Am J Surg* 134:275, 1975.
39. Tavassoli FA, Norris HJ: Secretory carcinoma of the breast. *Cancer* 45:2404, 1980.
40. McDivitt RW, Stewart FW: Breast carcinoma in children. *JAMA* 195:338, 1966.
41. Hermann JB: Tumors and other enlargements of the breast, in Ariel IM, Pack GT (eds): *Cancer and Allied Diseases of Infancy and Childhood.* Boston, Little, Brown and Co., 1960, chap.7, p. 115.

38

Cancer of the Breast and Pregnancy

Leonid J. Deemarsky, M.D.*
V. F. Semiglazov, M.D.

INTRODUCTION

Breast cancer has two age peaks: one in women between 45 to 50 years, and one in women between 55 to 60 years (Table 38-1). However, the number of patients aged 35 to 45 has been increasing, a factor associated with a more active search for tumors among "healthy" asymptomatic women. Thus, more patients who may be or may become pregnant are anticipated. The influence of pregnancy (whether terminated or permitted to go to natural termination) and lactation upon the course of a breast cancer would depend on whether the breast cancer was diagnosed (1) in a parous woman, (2) simultaneous with the pregnancy, (3) during lactation, or (4) in a woman whose pregnancy occurred after treatment of the breast cancer.

Statistical data from the United States and the Soviet Union show that about 17 to 22 percent of newly diagnosed breast cancer patients are in the third to fourth or early fifth decade of life, i.e., at the age when pregnancy (terminated or resulting in delivery) could coincide with development of breast cancer[19,41,62] (Fig. 38-1).

INCIDENCE

The incidence of breast cancer diagnosed in pregnant women is approximately 0.03 percent, (Lewison,[37] 1 per 1360 deliveries; F White,[71] 25 per 1547 deliveries). The incidence of pregnancy occurring after treatment of a breast cancer ranges from 0.75 to 3.1 percent. This rate seems constant for the United States, Soviet Union, Egypt, and Western Germany. In a few women (7 percent), the cancer occurred during the first pregnancy. The remainder shows numerous (up to 19) pregnancies but few deliveries before the onset of the breast cancer.

*Deceased.

When staging is referred to, both the older system and the recent TNM system of classification are used.

Table 38-1 Breast Cancer Incidence among USSR Females in Different Age Groups (1974)*

Age in years	Ratio
Under 30	1: 1,700,000
30–39	1: 55,000
40–49	1: 2200
50–59	1: 1650
60–69	1: 2000
70 and onwards	1: 2500

*Navarina et al.[44]

Incidence of Breast Cancer in the Parous Woman

In 91 percent of cases, the interval between a previous pregnancy and pregnancy accompanied by cancer was 5 or more years. In two-thirds of patients, induration indicative of cancer in the breast was revealed either before pregnancy or in the first trimester. In one-third of patients, it was noted after delivery, either during or immediately after lactation (Table 38-2). Tumors were detected in 14.4 percent of all cases in the second and third trimesters.

HORMONAL CHANGES

In the first trimester, hormonal changes associated with breast cancer are influenced by a sharp rise in levels of corticosteroids, estriol, and estrone (Fig. 38-2).[13,48] Increased levels of prolactin and growth hormone occur in cases of pregnancy interruption within this period.[34] At the end of the third trimester, the levels of corticosteroids, estriol, and estrone become higher[30] against the background of decreasing cellular immunity (a diminution of T lymphocytes).[33,63]

In the postpartum period and during lactation, the activating factors are high levels of prolactin and growth hormone,[1] estrone, and estradiol. Maximal values are seen by 36 to 38 weeks.[12] During pregnancy, a diabetes-like condition often develops, which

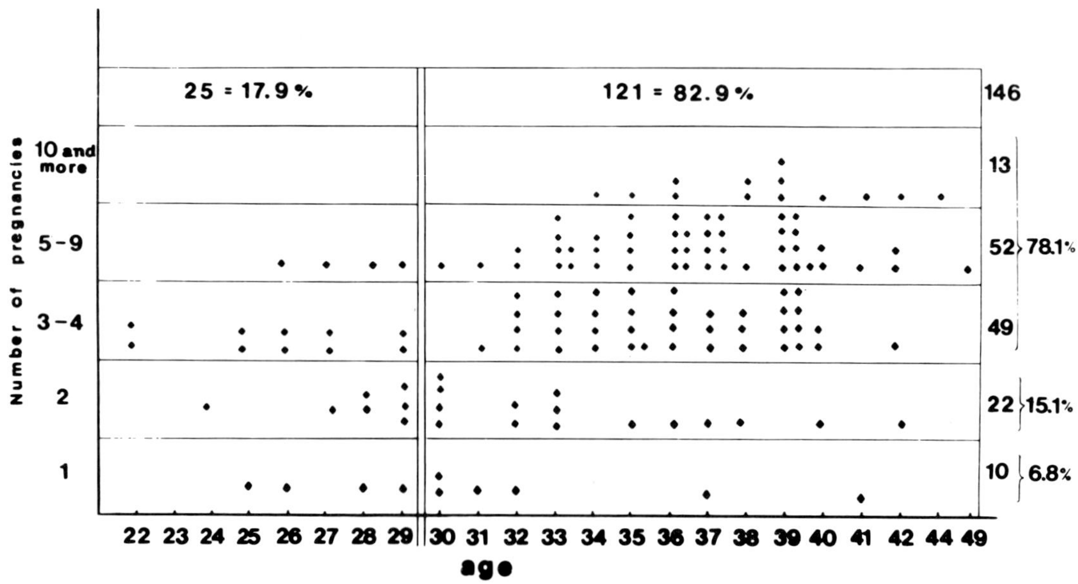

Figure 38-1 Age of patients and number of pregnancies.

Table 38-2 Time of Tumor Detection and Clinical Signs of Tumor Progression

		Tumor progression is noted					
Time of tumor detection	Number of observations	After pregnancy termination in the first trimester	During pregnancy in the second to third trimester	After delivery (cesarean section)	During lactation	After lactation	Absence of progression signs
Prior to pregnancy	32	22	—	2	2	3	3
First trimester of pregnancy	56	51	—	—	3	—	2
Second to third trimesters of pregnancy	21	—	5	4	6	—	6
Immediately after delivery	7	—	—	2	4	1	—
During lactation period	20	—	—	—	8	6	6
After lactation period	10	—	—	—	—	8	2

is associated with an increase of chorionic somatotropin-physiological analogue of growth hormone. There is a sharp rise in these hormones when pregnancy is interrupted at an early phase (Fig. 38-3).[18,34]

The middle of pregnancy (from the early second to third trimester) is characterized by a decrease in the level of corticosteroids, growth hormone,[4,17,19] and by the so-called "mitotic rest of epithelium" of the breast associated with a high level of progesterone[1] and low DNA synthesis under the influence of estriol. Based on this, we can make an assumption about the protective effects of pregnancy against breast tumors.[64,69] The ratio of estriol (noncarcinogenic agent)[63] to estrone (carcinogenic agent) and estradiol (relative carcinogen) in healthy women does not exceed 1:3 in premenopausal women and 1:2 in postmenopausal women. However, in patients with breast cancer accompanied by pregnancy, this ratio decreased to 0.5 to 0.8. The ratio of estriol to estrone plus estradiol increases in early pregnancy and, hence, the latter "protects" breast tissue from carcinogenic effects which may lead to malignancy. In women aged 30 or more, there is an opposite effect when the level of estradiol sharply increases, whereas the ratio of estriol to estrone plus estradiol decreases substantially.[39]

HISTOLOGIC CHANGES

Tumor histology suggests the presence of occult foci of rapid proliferation of epithelium including preinvasive cancers prior to pregnancy (Table 38-3). Of significance is the frequency of lobular cancer and proliferative changes of myoepithelium in the tissues around the tumor.

Studies by Morozova and Anokhina[43] demonstrated disappearance of undifferentiated structures, stroma edema, and small cystic mastopathy after normal delivery and lactation. In patients over 30 years of age, pronounced ductal and lobular proliferation not only persists after pregnancy (especially when the latter

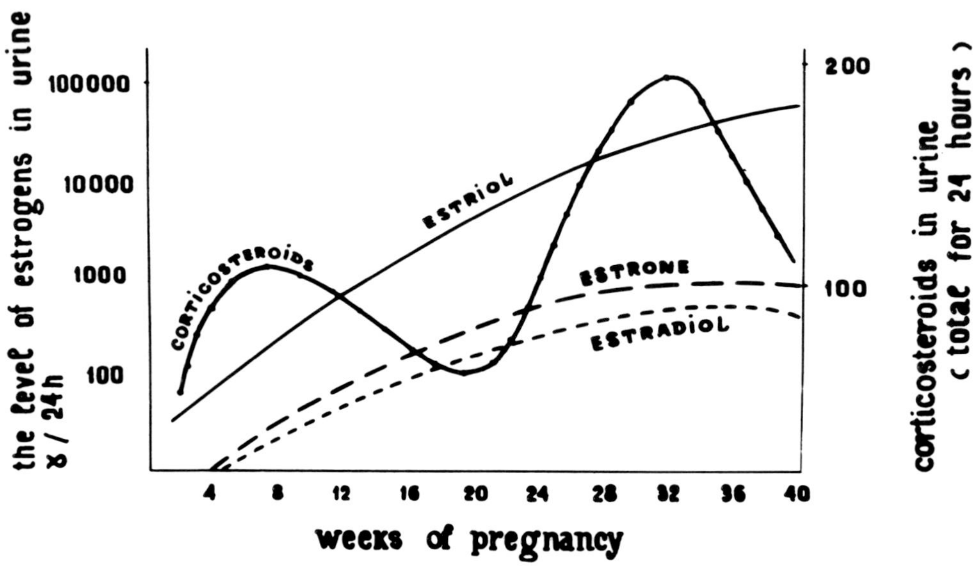

Figure 38-2 Level of estrogens and corticosteroids in the course of normal pregnancy.

is interrupted at the end of the first trimester) but progresses.

Thus, it is concluded that in women with multiple pregnancies but few deliveries, and in late pregnancy (in the fourth to fifth decade) occurring many years after a previous childbirth, there develops microscopic foci of malignancy. Therefore, it seems justified to attribute these tumors to the so-called "ovarian forms of cancer"[14] described by Semiglazov.[61] These patients are characterized by a high incidence of previous hyperplastic processes in the mammary tissue, late (over 30 years) first delivery, aborted last pregnancy, and hyperestrogenemia.

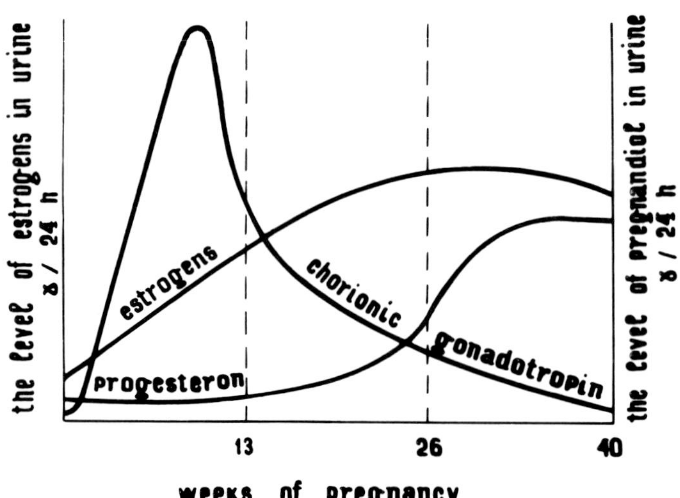

Figure 38-3 Correlation of hormones during pregnancy.

Table 38-3 Morphological Pattern and Tissue Proliferation Associated with Pregnancy

		Invasive carcinomas of mixed and undifferentiated type		Lobular, ductal, comedo, cystadenocarcinomas and carcinomas in situ	
Term of pregnancy	**Number of patients**	**With intra-canalicular or intralo-bular prolif-eration, grades 2–3**	**Without proliferation**	**With intracana-licular or myo-epithelial proliferation, grades 2–3**	**Without proliferation**
Tumor detected in the first trimester (pregnancy inter-rupted)	70 (+7)	6	49	11 (9, lobular carcinomas)	4
Tumor detected in the second-third trimester (normal delivery or cesarean birth)	22 (+1)	—	13	8 (7, lobular carcinomas)	1
Tumor detected during or immediately after lactation	45 (+1)	9	23	9 (10, lobular carcinomas)	4
Total	137 (+9 -after radiotherapy histo-logic form was not specified)	15	85	28	9

DELAY IN DIAGNOSIS

The correlation between poor prognosis and late detection of breast cancer patients has been repeatedly reported. Some authors believe that the prognosis is worsened with the duration of the pregnancy and is especially unfavorable in the second and third trimesters and during lactation. Donegan[19] determined the time from the development of a mass in pregnant women 35 years of age or less and the diagnosis of a tumor to be 11 to 15 months. Only one-third of patients were admitted to the hospital for treatment of the cancer within a 6-to-7-month period. Byrd[6] presents even more disappointing data. Two-thirds of women of the same age with a tumor detected during pregnancy were advised to defer treatment until after delivery.

The diagnosis of cancer in the lactation period is unsatisfactory. Ratner,[54] Byrd et al.,[6] and Lernoud[36] explain the delay in diagnosis by the fact (1) that it is generally believed that breast cancers are found predominantly in pre- and postmenopausal women and not during pregnancy or the postpartum period; (2) that hyperplasia of lobules, galactostasis, and enlarging breasts in pregnancy, and particularly in lactation hide a tumor and hinder its detection; and (3) that lactating breasts are unusually dense and their palpation is sometimes painful, mammography or thermography being of little value in these cases, whereas biopsy is rejected by many doctors due to the possible hazard of infection and possible formation of mammary fistulas. An example of delayed diagnosis is presented from the Petrov Research Institute of Oncology where, of 37 patients with cancer diagnosed in the lactation period, 17 underwent earlier antiinflammatory treatment in an outpatient clinic for 3 to 5 months, and 10 patients were not given any treatment for prolonged periods since a painless induration did not cause any anxiety to either the patient or the doctor.

Cytologic study is mandatory. Byrd et al.[6] performed aspiration biopsies of the breast in 135 pregnant women and found 29 cancers with the average rate of one cancer per 4.6 biopsies. In nonpregnant women with an obscure mass in the breast, one out of 5.4 aspirations is reported as being suspicious for malignancy. Hence, the difference is not great.[32] Risk from such procedures is minimal since even in diagnostic sectoral resections and mastectomies performed in the first or second trimester of pregnancy the number of spontaneous abortions does not exceed 1 per 86 operations (1.2 percent).[6,19] Biopsy is indicated in all cases of obscure thickening in the breast irrespective of the term of pregnancy and during lactation.

TREATMENT POLICIES AND PROGNOSIS

Patients with breast cancer were previously and erroneously declared incurable. As a general proposition, breast cancer diagnosed in a pregnant female should be treated by the same oncologic principles as if she were not pregnant. The risk of spontaneous abortion after mastectomy is approximately 1 percent. Cheek,[9] in a review of 47 authorities, reported instances of results as good as in the nonpregnant female and in some improved end results in pregnant patients were recorded. Hornstein et al. reported similar results.[28]

The choice of treatment in patients with breast cancer coincident with pregnancy is determined by two major factors: (1) spread of the tumor process, i.e., size, involvement of regional lymph nodes, and absence of detectable distant metastases; and (2) the term of pregnancy or lactation. In the first half of pregnancy, the predominant motive is "to treat the breast cancer with minor emphasis on pregnancy," while in the second half, efforts should be made to avoid damage to the fetus.

Treatment during the First Trimester of Pregnancy

Therapeutic Abortion

An unexpected observation were the poor results in patients on whom a therapeutic abortion was performed before treatment of the breast cancer (Table 38-4). *Accordingly, a therapeutic abortion is not indicated.*

Oophorectomy

Despite innumerable hormonal and metastatic consequences subsequent to an oophorectomy, including the fact that the blood level of estrone is higher than estradiol during this period, prophylactic castration does not improve survival and is not indicated (Table 38-5).

Mastectomy

The best treatment is an immediate mastectomy and axillary dissection. When the lymph nodes are positive on histologic analysis, the use of local radiation therapy or adjuvant chemotherapy must be carefully evaluated regarding potential harmful effects upon the fetus. Numerous instances are recorded where both irradiation and chemotherapy were given without any effects upon the fetus. In view of the current multimodality protocols for treating breast cancer, the effect on ontogenesis awaits the results of a double-blind study.

In patients who present with a severe form of cancer or if distant metastases exist, an abortion is indicated.

Prognosis

Prognosis of patients with breast cancer accompanied by pregnancy had in the past been considered worse than that for other patients with cancer of this site. Recent reports demonstrate

Table 38-4 Effects of Therapeutic Abortion before Treatment of Cancer in First Trimester of Pregnancy

Authors	Number of treated patients	Five-year results without recurrences and metastases: Treatment after therapeutic abortion		Five-year results without recurrences and metastases: Treatment begun without abortion	
Peete et al.[49]	13	$\frac{2}{7}$	(29%)	$\frac{3}{6}$	(50%)
Clark and Reid[11]	26	$\frac{9}{18}$	(50%)	$\frac{5}{8}$	(62.5%)
Helman and Benett[25]	10	$\frac{4}{7}$	(57%)	$\frac{3}{3}$	(100%)
Hochman and Schreiber[27]	16	$\frac{4}{6}$	(67%)	$\frac{4}{10}$	(40%)
Rissanen[56]	14	$\frac{3}{4}$	(75%)	$\frac{8}{10}$	(80%)
Deemarski and Neishtadt[16]	26	$\frac{6}{15}$	(40%)	$\frac{9}{11}$	(81.8%)
Total	105	$\frac{38}{100}$	(38%)	$\frac{32}{48}$	(66.6%)

the results to be as good, or even better, in the pregnant female than for women who are not pregnant when analyzed according to age and stage of the cancer (Table 38-6). The fate of patients depends not so much on the pregnancy itself, but primarily on timely diagnosis of tumors, which in 30 percent of cases is delayed. Therefore, the frequency of metastases in regional lymph nodes is high, 72 to 95 percent versus 50 to 55 percent in nonpregnant breast cancer patients.[28,60] If the diagnosis of the cancer is not delayed,[5] the prognosis should be as good as for the nonpregnant female.

Cancer Discovered during the Second and Third Trimester of Pregnancy

Treatment of patients with tumors detected in the late second or in the third trimester (Table 38-7) should have surgical intervention plus postoperative radiation treatment. The stage of pregnancy is no contraindication for radiation therapy. Cesarean section (if the term of pregnancy is not less than 34 to 35 weeks) is indicated, or waiting for full-term delivery (in late pregnancy) are the choices for the conduct of pregnancy. Subsequently, it is necessary to continue adjuvant chemotherapy and/or

Table 38-5 Results of Oophorectomy in Pregnant Patients with Breast Cancer

Term of pregnancy	Number of patients	Five-year survival: With oophorectomy		Five-year survival: Without oophorectomy	
First trimester (after abortion)	53	$\frac{6}{19}$	(31.6%)	$\frac{21}{34}$	(61.7%)
Second, third trimesters (postpartum or after cesarean birth)	14	$\frac{4}{4}$		$\frac{7}{10}$	
Lactation period	32	$\frac{2}{13}$	(15.4%)	$\frac{8}{19}$	(42.1%)

Table 38-6 Results of Treatment of Patients Coincident with Pregnancy and Lactation*

Authors	Years of follow-up	Number of patients	Patients subjected to mastectomy, %	Survival: Five and more years after radical treatment, % — With metastases in regional lymph nodes	Without metastases in lymph nodes
Harrington[23]	1910–1933	92	100	6	62
Hochman and Schreiber[27]	After 1953	20	90	42	75
White[71]	After 1956	37	100	8	50
Byrd et al.[6]	1925–1960	29	72	33	100
Holleb and Farrow[29]	1920–1953	133	—	17	65
Peters[50]	1938–1961	187	—	—	—
Horsley et al.	1921–1962	17	71	100	100
Earley et al.	1930–1984	46	83	28	68
Applewhite[3]	1948–1967	48	69	18	56
Hernandez[26]	—	23	74	—	87
Clark and Reid[11]	1931–1975	330	—	36.2	63.4
Deemarsky[15,16]	1926–1972	100	91	39.2	69.2

*After Donegan.[19]

Table 38-7 Results of Treatment of Patients Concurrent with Pregnancy and Lactation at the Petrov Research Institute of Oncology (1926–1978)

Stage and lymph node involvement (after histologic study of specimen)	Total number, treated patients	Five-year survival	Including: Tumors detected in the first trimester (after abortion)	Tumors detected in the second to third trimester (after normal delivery or cesarean birth)	Tumors detected in lactation period
p $T_{1-3}N_0M_0$ (lymph nodes negative)	32	23 71.8 %	$\frac{14}{17}$	$\frac{6}{6}$	$\frac{3}{9}$
p $T_{1-3}N_{1-2}M_0$ (lymph nodes positive)	66	25 37.8 %	$\frac{14}{33}$	$\frac{4}{6}$	$\frac{7}{24}$
$T_4N_3M_x$ (locally advanced tumors, untreated)	10	—	$\frac{0}{6}$	—	$\frac{0}{4}$

postoperative radiation therapy. Immediate suppression of lactation is necessary. In our series of 55 patients treated according to the above stated scheme, not a single one was found to have relapse within a 5-year follow-up. *It is emphasized that treatment should never be postponed until after delivery of the baby.* Definitive treatment should commence as soon as diagnosis is made by a team familiar with the problem of cancer in the pregnant female.

Pregnancy Subsequent to Mastectomy for Cancer

Patients subjected to radical treatment for breast cancer are usually informed about the danger of future pregnancy and are often advised to undergo tubal ligation or castration for the purpose of sterilization.[9] Despite this, 7 to 10 percent of all women treated for breast cancer become pregnant and in 70 percent, pregnancy occurs within the first 5 years after mastectomy.[19,24,28]

There are numerous data[2,50,52] showing a normal course of pregnancy and its favorable outcome, especially in patients who became pregnant 3 to 5 years after mastectomy. According to Schweppe et al.,[60] pregnancy which occurs after breast cancer treatment, if not beneficial, exerts no unfavorable effect upon the prognosis. Data reported by Harrington[23] from New York hospitals in 1937 are impressive: of 53 patients followed with delivery subsequent to radical treatment, 42 (79 percent) survived 5 years and 40 (76 percent) survived 10 years. Our experience (23 patients, Table 38-8) reaffirms that pregnancy is less hazardous when it occurs 3 or more years after mastectomy and that women who have delivered prove to have a better prognosis than those with interrupted pregnancies. There is no justification for recommending pregnancy termination in women apparently cured by mastectomy. The incidence of transplacental metastatic spread is extremely low (22 reliable observations are described in literature for all cancers).[31]

Transplacental effects of carcinogenic and mutagenic agents (i.e., methotrexate, cyclophosphamide in chemotherapy, low doses of

Table 38-8 Fate of Patients with Pregnancy and Delivery Subsequent to Mastectomy for Cancer

Status of regional lymph nodes (histologic data)	Number of observations: Alive without metastases 5 and more years	Number of observations: Number of operated patients	Period between mastectomy and subsequent pregnancy: Up to 1 year	From 1 to 2 years	From 2 to 3 years	More than 3 years
Absence of metastases	$\frac{6}{7}$		$\frac{2}{3}$	$\frac{1}{1}$	—	$\frac{3}{3}$
Presence of metastases	$\frac{10}{16}$		$\frac{1}{3}$	$\frac{3}{6}$	$\frac{4}{5}$	$\frac{2}{2}$
Total	$\frac{16}{23}$ (69.5 %)		$\frac{3}{6}$ (terminated pregnancy)	$\frac{4}{7}$ (terminated pregnancy)	$\frac{4}{5}$ (all had delivery, 1 developed carcinoma of contralateral breast after 9 years)	$\frac{5}{5}$ (2 out of 5 had delivery, 1 developed carcinoma of contralateral breast after 3 years)

irradiation in radiotherapy) are presumed to increase the risk of congenital malformations and prenatal tumor induction, but this incidence is very low. Other extraneous factors may contribute to an increased risk to the embryo[8,32] but they do not present a known hazard. Accordingly, except for the risk of the mother eventually dying from her cancer, there is no contraindication to her becoming pregnant.

CONCLUSION

Patients with breast cancer diagnosed during pregnancy and lactation largely belong to women in the fourth and early fifth decades of life. They have had multiple pregnancies but relatively few deliveries, usually with a rather long (5 or more years) interval since a previous pregnancy or childbirth. The frequency of lobular and ductal cancers in situ, which is nearly ten times higher than in nonpregnant patients with cancer of this particular site, allows us to assume that proliferating hyperplastic processes and preinvasive multicentric carcinomas existed prior to the pregnancy. Changes in the endocrine system seem to stimulate progression and metastatic spread of already existing tumors in pregnancy interruption in the first trimester, in the postpartum period, and during lactation. Delayed diagnosis of tumors related to difficulties in differentiating them from galactostasis and chronic mastitis worsens the prognosis and is a continuing problem. The outcome seems to be unfavorable for patients with abortion performed in the first trimester and for lactating patients.

Biopsy is an obligatory differential diagnostic procedure in the presence of persistent indurations of the breast in pregnant and lactating women. Treatment (including radiation and chemotherapy, if necessary) should be initiated before pregnancy termination (or delivery), in the first and second trimesters. In the third trimester, treatment procedures do not impede normal delivery and can be continued immediately after childbirth. Lactation must be interrupted and bottle feeding begun. Adjuvant chemotherapy by repeated courses of the cyclophosphamide-methotrexate-5-fluorouracil (CMF) or CFMVP programs with intervals of 28 to 45 days is carried out after mastectomy. Subsequent pregnancy and delivery are allowable after 3 or more years of the relapse-free period following mastectomy, mainly in patients with limited forms of tumors (without regional lymph node involvement). However, the probability of genetic predisposition and mutation in the progeny of patients treated for cancer is not excluded.

REFERENCES

1. Afonina LI: The level of progesterone in blood during physiologic pregnancy. *Obstet Gynecol* 5:16, 1978.
2. Anderson JM: Mammary cancers and pregnancy. *Br Med J* 1:1124, 1979.
3. Applewhite RR, Smith LR, Di Vincenti F: Carcinoma of breast associated with pregnancy and lactation. *Am Surg* 39:101, 1973.
4. Averbach MM: Pathology of dishormonal hyperplasies diseases and cancer of the breast. *Moscva Medgiz Publ* 28, 1958.
5. Beryoskin DP: Significance of some peculiarities of the organism in prognosis of breast cancer. *News in Oncology*, Petrov Research Inst Oncol, the USSR Ministry of Health, Leningrad, 1971, p. 191.
6. Byrd BF Jr, Bayer DS, Robertson JC, Stephenson SE Jr: Treatment of breast tumors associated with pregnancy and lactation. *Ann Surg* 155:940, 1962.
7. Campion PD, Currey HLF: Cell-mediated immunity in pregnancy. *Lancet* 2:830, 1972.
8. Chakrov AM: "Milk factor" as a factor of risk for dissemination of breast cancer in females. *J Exper Klin Med* 21(4):391, 1981.
9. Cheek JH: Survey of current opinions concerning carcinoma of the breast occurring during pregnancy. *CA* 33(4):244, 1983.
10. Chomette G, Auriol M, Delcourt A, Tereau Y: Contribution àláistogeńesé du cancer lobulaire du sein. *Ann Anat Pathol* 25(2):85, 1980.

11. Clark RM, Reid J: Carcinoma of the breast and pregnancy and lactation. *Int J Radiat Oncol Biol Phys* 4(7–8):693, 1978.
12. Coats P, Walker E, Voussefnejadian E, Craft JL: Variations in plasma steroid and prostaglandin concentrations during human pregnancy. *Acta Obstet Gynecol Scand* 56(5):153, 1977.
13. Davis ME, Plotz EJ: *Obstetrics*, 13th ed. Philadelphia, W. B. Saunders, 1965, p. 233.
14. Deemarsky LJu, Semiglazov VF: Pathogenic factors and formation of the groups at "high risk" for breast cancer. *Soviet Med* 6:77, 1976.
15. Deemarsky LJu: Cancer of the breast and pregnancy, in Napalkov NP (ed): *Malignant Tumours and Pregnancy*. Leningrad, Petrov Research Inst Oncol, 1981, p. 1.
16. Deemarsky LJu, Neishtadt EL: Breast cancer and pregnancy. *Breast. Diseases of the Breast* 7(2):17, 1981.
17. Dessaive P: Le prognostic des cancers de la glande mammaire. *Acta Chir Belg* 60(9):957, 1961.
18. Dilman VM: Mechanisms of inter-relations between pregnancy and tumour processes, in Napalkov NP (ed): *Malignant Tumours and Pregnancy*. Leningrad, Petrov Research Inst Oncol, 1981, p. 38.
19. Donegan WL: Management of pregnancy and lactation, in Stoll B (ed): *Breast Cancer Management, Early and Late*. London, Heinemann, 1977, p. 195.
20. Fournier VD, Kubli F, Klapp J, Weber E, Schneider-Affeld F: Infrared thermography and breast cancer doubling time. *Acta Thermogr* 3:107, 1978.
21. Fracchia AA, Farrow JH, De Palo AJ, Connolly DP, Huvos AG: Castration for primary inoperable or recurrent breast carcinoma. *Surg Gynecol Obstet* 128:1226, 1969.
22. Gregl A, Krack UYuD, Timmirmann S, Stankovic P, Wellmer H-K: Brustkrebs und Schangeerschaft. *Deutsch Med Wochenschr* 95(39): 1951, 1970.
23. Harrington SW: Carcinoma of the breast: Results of surgical treatment when the carcinoma occurred in the course of pregnancy or lactation and when pregnancy occurred subsequent to operation. *Ann Surg* 106:690, 1937.
24. Harvey JC, Rosen CC, Ashikari R, Robbins GF, Kinne DW: The effect of pregnancy on the prognosis of carcinoma of the breast following radical mastectomy. *Surg Gynecol Obstet* 153(5):723, 1981.
25. Helman P, Benett MB: Breast cancer and pregnancy. *S Afr Med J* 37:1236, 1963.
26. Hernandez MG: Cancer de mama y embarazo. *Ginedips* 8(2):115, 120, 124, 1977.
27. Hochman A, Schreiber H: Pregnancy and cancer of the breast. *Obstet Gynecol* 2:268, 1953.
28. Hornstein F, Skornick Y, Rozin R: The management of breast carcinoma in pregnancy and lactation. *J Surg Oncol* 21(3):179, 1982.
29. Holleb AJ, Farrow JH: Breast cancer and pregnancy. *Acta Union Inter Contra Cancr* 20(6):29, 1964.
30. Inde S: A study of blood hormone levels in normal menstrual cycle and normal early pregnancy. *Acta Obstet Gynecol Jpn* 30(3):261, 1978.
31. Jones EM: Cancer and the fetus. *Br Med J* 6250:1227, 1980.
32. Kholdin SA: Malignant tumours of the breast, in Petrov NN, Kholdin SA (eds): *Malignant Tumours*. Leningrad, Vol. 3, 1962, p. 31.
33. Klinda K, Bek E, Runnebaum B: Material peripheral testosterone levels during the first half of pregnancy. *Am J Obstet Gynecol* 131(1):60, 1979.
34. Kononova ES, Savchenko ON, Stepanov GS, Sokolov EG: Peculiarities of hypophyseal-ovarian correlations in women suffering with spontaneous abortions. *Obstet Gynecol* 8:37, 1977.
35. Kovalyova LG, Isajev WG, Soboleva SS, Fyodorova TB: On treatment tactics in combination of acute leukemia and pregnancy. *Obstet Gynecol* 5:24, 1978.
36. Lernoud M: Cancer genitomamario y embarazo. *Rev Argent Cancerol* 17(3):62, 1979.
37. Lewison EF: Breast cancer and pregnancy or lactation. *Surg Gynecol Obstet* 99:417, 1954.
38. Logan WPD: Cancer of the breast: No decline in mortality. *WHO Chronicle*, 12:462, 1975.
39. McMahon B et al: Oestrogen profiles of Asian and North American Women. *Lancet* 2:900, 1971.
40. *Manual of Clinical Oncology*, 3d ed. Berlin, Springer-Verlag, International Union Against Cancer, 1982.
41. Merabishvili VM, Deemarsky LJu: The main trends of cancer of the breast mortality and morbidity among the USSR populations. *Vopr Oncol* 8:8, 1978.
42. Merabishvili VM, Serova LS: Evaluation of efficacy of treatment of breast cancer patients in the USSR. *Proc Symp* Comparative evaluation of

breast cancer patients survival in different methods of treatment, Leningrad, 1983, p. 27.

43. Morozova MG, Anokhina MA: Morphologic changes in the mastopathy foci in pregnancy and lactation. *Vopr Oncol* Voronezh University, 1974, p. 230.
44. Navarina SV, Demin VN, Shalnevy TS: On the volume of surgical intervention for ovariectomy in patients with breast cancer. *Vopr Oncol* 23(11):39, 1977.
45. Neishtadt EL: Morphological criteria of risk for development of breast cancer in patients with mastophaty, in *Early Diagnosis of Breast Cancer.* Leningrad, Petrov Research Inst Oncol, 1980, p. 35.
46. Noyes R, Spanos W, Montague E: Breast cancer in women aged 30 and under. *Cancer* 49(6):1302, 1982.
47. Olinya AY, Vitola GY: Endocrine aspects of breast cancer. "*Zinatne*," Riga, 1981, p. 57.
48. Palladi GA, Poklitar MG, MukuTse EB: Glucocorticoids in the system mother-placenta-fetus. "*Shtiintsa*," Kishinev, 1978, p. 32.
49. Peete CH Jr, Hunelycutt HC Jr, Cherny WB: Cancer of the breast in pregnancy. *NC Med J* 27:514, 1966.
50. Peters M: The effect of pregnancy in breast cancer, in Forrest APM, Kukler PB (eds): *Prognosis Factors in Breast Cancer.* London, 1968, p. 65.
51. Petrov YuV: Cancer of the breast. "*Medicina*," Leningrad, 1964, p. 176.
52. Prodan I, Letica D, Majerović M: Rak dojke u trudnoci. *Libri Oncol* 10(2–3):143, 1981.
53. Purtilo DT, Hallgren HM, Yunis ES: Depressed material lymphocyte response to PHA in human pregnancy. *Lancet* 1:769, 1972.
54. Ratner LM: Diagnostic errors and diagnosis of breast cancer. "*Medgis*", Sverlovsk, 1949, p. 108–113.
55. Remy Sola E: Carcinoma de mama y emberazo. *Rev Argent Cancerol* 17:(3–4):58, 1979.
56. Rissanen PM: Pregnancy following treatment of mammary carcinoma. *Acta Radiol Ther* 8:415, 1962.
57. Robbins GF, Berg J: Curability of patients with invasive breast cancer based on 30 year study. *World J Surg* 1:284, 1977.
58. Sahni K, Sanyal B, Agrawal MS, Pant GC, Khanna NN, Khanna S: Carcinoma of the breast associated with pregnancy and lactation. *J Surg Oncol* 16(2):167, 1981.
59. Schottenfeld D, Nach AG, Robbins GF, Beattie EJ: Ten year results of primary operable breast carcinoma. *Cancer* 8:1001, 1976.
60. Schweppe K-W, Möhlen KH, Beller FK: Mammakarzinom und Schwangerschaft. *Geburtshilfe Frauenheilkd* 39(12):1083, 1979.
61. Semiglazov VF: Current principles of early detection and treatment of breast cancer. *Chirurgia,* 11:38, 1983.
62. Serov VV, Zolotorevsky BV: Clinical morphology of early breast cancer. *Arch Pathol* 41(1):3, 1979.
63. Shubic P, Hartwell JL: *Survey of compounds which have been tested on carcinogenic activity,* Washington, NIH, 1957.
64. Smith SR, Woods KL, Morrison JM, Howell A: An association between parity and age of presentation in human breast cancer. *Br J Cancer* 42(1):201, 1980.
65. Spitalier JM, Santamaria F et al: Infrared thermography and non-palpable breast cancer. *Acta Thermogr* 3(1):34, 1978.
66. Stone DA: Carcinoma of the breast in women under 30 and during pregnancy. *J Am Osteopathol Assn* 79(2):91/71–97/77, 1979.
67. Tannerich DT: Pregnancy, breast cancer risk, and maternal-fetal genetics. *Lancet* 8111:327, 1979.
68. Vorherr H, Messer RH: Breast cancer: Potentially predisposing and protecting factors. *Am J Obstet Gynecol* 130:335, 1978.
69. Vorherr H: Pregnancy and lactation in relation to breast cancer risk. *Semin Prinatol* 3(3):299, 1979.
70. Vrousos C, Bolla M: Les facteurs de prognostic du cancer du sein chez la femme. *Rev Franc Gynecol Ostét* 72(11):729, 1977.
71. White TT: Prognosis of breast cancer for pregnant and nursing women. Analysis of 1413 cases. *Surg Gynecol Obstet* 100(6):661, 1955.
72. Wiesner-Bornstein R, Niesen M, Grole-Einsler K, Schulte-Holtey M: Zytosta tica-Therapie bei Morbus Hadgkin in der Schwangerschaft. *Geburtshilfe Frauenheilk* 43(6):373, 1983.

EDITORIAL ADDENDUM

In the past, any patient whose cancer of the breast was discovered at the time she was pregnant was looked upon as having undue risk, and the prognosis was considered uniformly poor. The same was considered for a patient who became pregnant after a mastectomy. Cancers discovered at the time of pregnancy have the same cure rate as those in women who are not pregnant. A major reason for suspecting that pregnancy adversely affected the clinical course of a woman with breast cancer is the observation of the effects both conditions have on the immunologic tolerance of the patient. Gleicher et al.[6] have pointed out that "Normal pregnancy and cancer are the only two biologic conditions in which antigenic tissue is tolerated by a seemingly intact immune system."

Manifestations of immunologic intolerance in the two conditions include[4]:

1 Depression of cellular immunity
2 Presence of circulating serological blocking factors that permit the tolerance of antigen tissue, probably an immunoglobulin (IgG)
3 Immunosuppressive effect of various hormones such as estrogen, progesterone, and human chorionic gonadotropin
4 Presence of suppressive T cells
5 Presence of a leukocyte migration enhancement factor
6 Decreased red blood cell immune adherence

Donegan[4] states "unfortunately, the mechanism that ensures the survival of the fetus during pregnancy presumably also favors the progress of the neoplasia."

Contributing influences attributed for the believed poor results of breast cancer diagnosed during pregnancy include (1) increased vascularity and lymphatic permeability of the breast, (2) stimulation by the sex steroids of what is known to be a hormone-dependent tumor, and (3) a depressed immune response associated with pregnancy. The poor results of previous years have also been erroneously attributed to the histologic type of tumor which is now shown to be the same as for the nonpregnant woman. Contrary to an earlier belief, the frequency of inflammatory carcinoma is not increased during pregnancy.

Emphasis now is on early diagnosis and prompt treatment. The diagnosis should be established with dispatch without consideration for the pregnancy. Biopsy as an outpatient practice is the indicated procedure for the pregnant woman.[2] Although the risk of radiation from mammography is extremely slight for the fetus, the dense breast of the pregnant patient makes this test less reliable. Isotope scanning should be completely avoided. Other methods for detecting cancer, such as sonography, etc., are now available.

There have been only six reported instances of breast cancer believed to have been transmitted to the placenta in a report from 1866 to 1973.[9] Of these six cases, the placenta was involved in all cases and no evidence of fetal involvement was ever encountered. The fetus and placenta are remarkably resistant to metastasis as noted in animal models and human experience. The possibility of placental fetal involvement should not enter into the decision for treatment of the breast cancer.[11]

TREATMENT

Dependence on surgery for the pregnant female harboring breast cancer is advisable. Although conservative alternatives are available for nonpregnant patients, the effects of such procedures upon the fetus are largely unknown. Local excision of the tumor followed by intensive irradiation may be harmful to the fetus. A fetus located 25 cm below the base of the radiation field to which 7500 rads has been delivered would receive approximately 30 rads.[3]

During the second half of pregnancy, the fetus is larger and lies higher in the abdomen, and would be at greater exposure. The risk of teratogenic or mutagenic effects on the fetus has been estimated at 1/1000 per cGy.[7]

Women with nodal metastases have accounted for 75 percent of treated cases and are candidates for chemotherapy. Most chemotherapeutic drugs are teratogenic. Near term, chemotherapy might be delayed until after delivery and, if indicated, a cesarean section might be performed. There have been reports of normal infants delivered following chemotherapy. The alkylating agents seem safer, whereas methotrexate is highly mutagenic. The incidence of malformation in the neonate after chemotherapy is +5 percent.[8]

In patients with advanced cancer diagnosed in the first or second trimester, palliative therapy ordinarily requires termination of pregnancy. Effective systemic chemotherapy or radiation and the administration of endocrine therapy would be risky for the fetus, and the pregnancy should be terminated during the first and second trimester. If the diagnosis is made in the third trimester, it would be wise to delay adjuvant therapy for 3 to 4 weeks to permit the fetus to grow to 1500 g in size, which would ensure neonatal survival. Donegan states that "delaying palliative treatment until the fetus is viable when a cancer diagnosis is made late in pregnancy is a decision that must be discussed by the patient and the physician."[4]

The question of subsequent pregnancy must be carefully discussed with the patient. Approximately 7 percent of fertile women become pregnant after treatment, usually within the first 5 years. The overall survival rate is the same as for patients who have no history of pregnancy. If the pregnancy can be delayed for 3 years, this is a wise procedure to follow. If the patient becomes pregnant within the 3-year period, the pregnancy should be permitted and the patient watched.

PROGNOSIS

Ribeiro and Palmer[10] reported 5-year survival rates of 90 percent for stage I cancers, 37 percent for stage II cancers, 15 percent for stage III cancers, and 0 percent for stage IV cancers in pregnant females. An overall survival of 70 percent was obtained at 5 years. Similar reports have been reported by others.[1–5]

REFERENCES

1. Anderson JM: Mammary cancers and pregnancy. *Br Med J* 1:1124, 1979.
2. Cheek JH: Cancer of the breast in pregnancy and lactation *Am J Surg.* 126:729, 1973.
3. Denoix P: Recent results in cancer research. *Cancer Res* 31:83, 1970.
4. Donegan WL: Breast cancer and pregnancy. *Obstet Gynecol* 50:244, 1977.
5. Gleicher N, Siegel I: Common denominators of pregnancy and malignancy, in Gleicher N (ed): *Reproductive Immunology.* New York, Alan R. Liss Inc., 1981, p. 339.
6. Gleicher N, Deppe G, Cohen CJ: Common aspects of immunologic tolerance in pregnancy and malignancy. *Obstet Gynecol* 54:335, 1979.
7. Mossman KL, Hill LT: Radiation risks in pregnancy. *Obstet Gynecol* 60:237, 1982.
8. Murray CL, Reichert JA, Anderson J, Twiggs LB: Multimodal cancer therapy for breast cancer in the first trimester of pregnancy: A case report. *JAMA* 252(18):2607, 1984.
9. Potter JF, Schoeneman M: Metastasis of maternal cancer to the placenta and fetus. *Cancer* 25:380, 1970.
10. Ribeiro GG, Palmer MK: Breast carcinoma associated with pregnancy: A clinician's dilemma. *Br Med J* 2:1524, 1977.
11. Rothman LA, Cohen CJ, Astarloa J: Placental and fetal involvement by maternal malignancy: A report of rectal carcinoma and review of the literature. *Am J Obstet Gynecol* 116:1023, 1973.

39

Sarcomas and Other Unusual Cancers of the Breast

Irving M. Ariel, M.D.
Arthur S. Caron, M.D.

INTRODUCTION

Breast sarcomas form a rare and complicated group of neoplasms. Within this category are the largest cancers (cystosarcomas) and the most malignant tumors (hemangiosarcomas) afflicting the breast. From a historic standpoint intriguing situations arise, inasmuch as most of these tumors were originally considered benign, but as more was learned about them some (cystosarcomas) or all (hemangiosarcomas) have been classified as malignant.[60–64]

From a histologic viewpoint the origin of some of these lesions elicits questions; for example, the origins of such lesions as leiomyosarcomas or rhabdomyosarcomas present interesting dilemmas, inasmuch as there are no muscular structures in the breast with the exception of the nipple (unless the myoepithelial cells play a role).

This chapter addresses the problems associated with this perplexing group of neoplasms from a nosologic and clinical standpoint.[10,31] Although the supporting structures of the breast constitute over three-quarters of the tissue of the organ, tumors arising from these structures constitute approximately 1 percent of all breast malignancies. They will be described as follows:

1 Tumors containing both epithelial and mesodermal histologic elements—cystosarcoma phyllodes
2 Tumors arising from an apparently specialized form of connective tissue—stromal sarcomas
3 Specific sarcomatous types—hemangiosarcomas, etc.
4 Miscellaneous cancers—malignant melanomas arising from the skin of the breast, lymphomas, etc.
5 Metastatic tumors to the breast

Anatomy of the Supporting Structures of the Adult Female Breast

The breast is ensheathed in the superficial fascia, except for the axillary tail of Spence, which pierces the deep fascia through an opening known as Langer's foramen to extend well up into the axilla. The breast's characteristic shape is due to fat which lies for the most part anterior to the secreting tissue, presumably for protection. Thick, irregular strands and septa of fibrous tissue run from the pectoral or deep fascia to the skin. This fibrous tissue is known as *suspensory ligaments of Cooper*. Handley likens this arrangement to a sea sponge "whose intraces are filled with fat, secreting tissues and vascular pipe-lines."[34]

The Cooper's ligaments are both interlobular and interlobar and are interposed with fat and a few elastic fibers. The *intra*lobular connective tissue is much more delicate, more cellular, and free from fat. Free cells—lymphocytes, histiocytes, and fibroblasts—are present in the intralobular connective tissue. The large mammary ducts are supported by sheaths of dense fibrous tissue which, in the nipple, is interspersed with bundles of smooth-muscle fibers. In the nipple the fibrous sheaths contain no fat.

Blood vessels, nerves, and lymphatics are dispersed generously throughout the breast. Cancer may arise from each of the supporting structures by means of metaplasia; complex, bizarre histologic forms may be produced.

CYSTOSARCOMA PHYLLODES

Cystosarcoma phyllodes was so named by Müller who, in 1838, described a fleshy tumor, as implied by the German word "sarkom." Müller regarded the cystosarcoma as entirely benign.[62] Although the term "sarcoma" is incorrect from a nosologic standpoint, its popular use for both the benign and malignant forms for over 100 years favors its continued use. "Benign" or "malignant" should always accompany the term cystosarcoma phyllodes. This tumor constitutes 50 to 60 percent of mammary tumors arising from the supporting structures exclusive of fibroadenoma.[16] Malignant changes have been observed in about 30 percent of all cystosarcoma phyllodes.[2] Pathologic criteria are often unreliable; some tumors diagnosed as "benign" may behave as malignant neoplasms.

Martin and Gallager state that their experience has led them to believe that cystosarcoma phyllodes is almost always a malignant neoplasm capable of widely varying behavior.[56] They further state that no clinical or pathological criteria or set of criteria are "reliably capable of predicting what individual behavior may be. . . . We believe therefore that surgical treatment should be aggressive. Partial mastectomy may be suitable for small (under 4 cm) masses with low mitotic indices and little or no anaplasia. In all other cases total mastectomy is the treatment of choice. There is no advantage in adding an axillary dissection unless it is necessary to encompass the mass and a reasonable margin of uninvolved tissue."[56]

The benign nature of the tumor was stressed by Lee and Pack who, in 1931, collected a series of 105 reported cases from the literature, and added 77 cases of their own.[47] Although they considered the tumor benign, five of their patients developed regional metastases and one died from pulmonary metastasis, thus indicating the malignant nature of the tumor.

Symptoms and Signs

The age of patients varies greatly. These tumors have been observed in youths as young as 16 years of age,[4,30] and the oldest patient observed with cystosarcoma phyllodes was 75 years of age.[37] Age cannot be used to separate the benign from the malignant variety. In a series of patients at Memorial Hospital, New York City, the average age of patients with benign cystosarcomas was 43 years and of those with malignant cystosarcomas was 46 years.[16] Occasionally cystosarcoma phyllodes may be bilateral.[69]

The almost universal reason that patients seek treatment is because of the presence of a palpable breast mass.[9] Patients have noticed a mass for an average of 1 year before seeking treatment. They give a history of either latent growth followed by periods of rapid growth or rapid growth from the onset. There is no difference between a benign and a malignant tumor if it is judged by its growth characteristics. Furthermore, the size of the tumor is not related to whether it is benign or malignant. The mass is usually mobile and rounded or lobulated. Pain and tenderness are very rare. The skin is mobile over the mass, and the nipple is usually not retracted.[29] A rather common finding is dilated veins associated with the presence of the mass. With continued growth the skin becomes pale and thin and often shows a dusky discoloration. Ulceration is a late manifestation.

The mammographic appearance is similar to that of a fibroadenoma, which is sharply demarcated from the surrounding breast tissue. If the patient has delayed seeking treatment, a large tumor, not demonstrating infiltration to the surrounding breast tissue, is characteristic of cystosarcoma phyllodes.

Gross Appearance

There is usually a sharp demarcation between the tumor and surrounding breast tissue, which is generally compressed. A cut section usually presents a leaflike pattern with fingerlets spreading from a central mass. These are formed by coarse fibrotic papillations; they give the tumor its name. The tumor is usually gray-white, often with hemorrhagic foci. Cavity formation is common as a result of central degeneration and necrosis.[37] The large size is more or less characteristic. In Lee and Pack's report, the average size was 7.6 lb (3.5 kg) and tumors were frequently as big as an adult's head.[47] In the report by Treves and Sunderland in 1951, the average size was about 15 cm.[92] Ribbert reported one weighing 20 kg.[70] In view of public awareness, smaller tumors are now being treated.[8,9] Variations in color or texture are related to size rather than aggressiveness. (See Fig. 39-1.)

Microscopic Characteristics

A unique feature of this cancer is the fact that the epithelial elements are always benign. The only hyperplastic elements arise from the fibrous tissue stroma. The tumors are roughly the same as fibroadenomas but contain a cellular hyperplastic stroma.[2] The proliferating stroma compresses the epithelial components and protrudes into their lumen, causing compression of the epithelial elements from columnar to cuboidal to completely flat. The hyperplastic stroma contains mixtures of fibrous, fatty, and myxoid tissue, one or all of which may be malignant.[38] Depending upon the preponderance of such mixed hyperplastic tissue in the stroma, myxoliposarcomas may occur, as well as occasional transformation into chondroids or osteoids.[43] The overgrowth of the fibrous tissue may be so great as to simulate stromal sarcomas; the distinction may be made by finding epithelium-lined canaliculae within the cystosarcoma. [63] Focal calcification is seen in both benign and malignant cystosarcoma; it is of no prognostic significance. There have been attempts to separate cystosarcoma phyllodes into benign, borderline, and malignant varieties, dependent upon such factors as size, encapsulation, cyst formation, necrosis and/or hemorrhage, cellularity, and atypia with mitoses, with little success. The more the atypia and number of mitoses, the more malignant is the tumor.[9]

Treatment

If the pathologic diagnosis is *benign* cystosarcoma phyllodes, a wide segmental resection is all that is required. However, treatment must be individualized. If the tumor exists in a small breast, in order to get a wide enough margin and not leave behind the fingerlike projections, it may be necessary to remove the entire breast.[52] Resection of the axillary lymph nodes is not indicated, inasmuch as these tumors rarely metastasize to lymph nodes. Depending on the location and the degree of infiltration of underlying tissue, it may at times be wise to

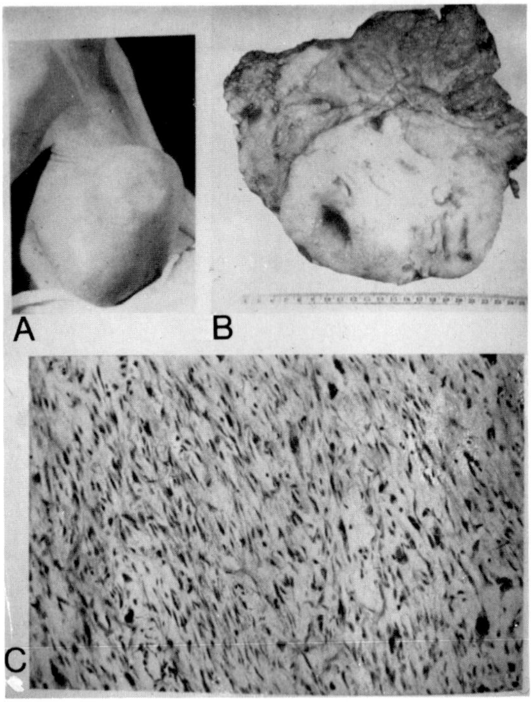

Figure 39-1 A. Cystosarcoma phyllodes (malignant variant) in a 58-year-old woman in whom a walnut-sized nodule increased slowly in size over a 10-year period and then grew rapidly. Simple mastectomy was performed. The patient failed to return for follow-up care. B. Operative specimen after a total mastectomy of the neoplasm shown in A. C. Microscopic appearance of the tumor shown in A and B. The stroma has undergone malignant change, as evidenced by cell pleomorphism, nuclear hyperchromatism, and presence of multinucleated cells.

extirpate part of the pectoralis major, although complete removal of this muscle is seldom indicated.

If the pathology report indicates that the tumor is malignant, a total mastectomy should be performed.[66] Recurrences are common after local excision, occurring in as much as 50 percent of reported cases.[38,52,94] Recurrences contain the same histologic degree of atypia as the primary lesion. Malignant transformation was not observed in recurrences when the original tumor was benign.[52,56]

Metastases are characterized by the bizarre locations in which they may occur. Although the most frequent sites are the liver and lungs, such sites as the gingiva, the vulva, and the brain have been reported. Unlike local recurrence, the degree of anaplasia in metastases is usually greater than in the original tumor.[53,56] Most metastases appear within 2 years of the initial treatment, but there have been reports of metastases occurring as long as 10 years after treatment of the primary tumor.

In view of the propensity of these tumors to spread by the hematogenous route, it is appropriate to consider some form of chemotherapy. No established studies have been performed to indicate what value chemotherapy has for the malignant variant of cystosarcoma phyllodes.

Prognosis

Prognosis is related more to the stage of the disease than to the type of treatment, as claimed by McDivitt, Stewart, and Berg.[60] At the M. D. Anderson Hospital, four patients were treated by local excision; there were no 5-year survivors. Of 21 patients treated by simple or extended simple mastectomy, 11 of 19 (58 percent) survived 5 years, and 7 of 13 (54 percent) survived 10 years. In 10 patients a radical mastectomy was performed; 50 percent survived 5 years and 33 percent survived 10 years. The poor results for the radical mastectomy group are attributed to the greater extent of the disease when the patient was first treated.[56] Excision of the chest wall has been reported because of infiltration of the tumor.[58]

Since some authorities believe that cystosarcoma may arise from preexisting fibroadenomas, it is wise to excise all fibroadenomas before they can degenerate into cystosarcoma phyllodes. In 1951 Treves and Sunderland stated: "Take care of the fibroadenomas and the cystosarcomas will take care of themselves."[92] While many cystosarcoma phyllodes may arise in fibroadenomas, they may also have an independent origin.[54]

Carcinoma of the breast occurs in patients with cystosarcoma phyllodes more frequently than in the general population.[61,71] Mammography is necessary to detect the carcinoma before surgery.

MAMMARY SARCOMAS

The tendency to lump all sarcomas into one group, similar to that generalizing which has occurred for sarcomas of the extremities and trunk, is a throwback to the time before proper nosology became available.[20,21,25,73,83]

The tumors frequently listed under breast sarcoma include stromal sarcoma, fibrosarcoma, liposarcoma, undifferentiated high-grade sarcoma, leiomyosarcoma, malignant fibrous histiocytoma, dermatofibrosarcoma protuberans, and sarcoma with bone and cartilage.[7,13,14] Barnes and Pietruszka make an appeal to avoid use of the term "stromal sarcoma" as a pathologic entity including all sarcomas and to limit its application to the specialized supportive tissue peculiar to the breast.[6]

As more is learned about each of the specific types and a better understanding of them becomes more accessible, individual diagnostic criteria, as well as clinical behavior of the tumors and methods of treatment and prognosis, may become more apparent.[93]

Clinical Features of Breast Sarcomas

The rarity of breast sarcomas is stressed by the fact that at Memorial Hospital, New York, only 32 patients with sarcomas of the breast were encountered,[16] and at the M. D. Anderson Hospital only 16 patients with sarcomas were seen.[56] The clinical features are not characteristic; the patients reported ranged in age from 22 to 80 years, with an average age at diagnosis of 49 years.[7] All but a few cases have been in white women. The usual sign is the presence of a painless mass, and in only an exceptional case has there been a history of rapid growth. Axillary nodes may be enlarged due to an inflammatory reaction, but are almost never invaded by metastases.[41] The masses can range in size from 2 to 20 cm; on cut section they are composed of firm or rubbery gray-white or yellow-gray tissue with small cystic spaces. Necrosis and hemorrhage are common.[15]

Histologic appearance varies greatly.[55] Breast sarcomas may be essentially spindle cell neoplasms, but metaplasia, with foci resembling liposarcoma, myxosarcoma, chondrosarcoma, or osteosarcoma present throughout, may be intermingled or even dominate the histologic appearance.

Treatment is usually simple mastectomy without attention to the axilla because metastases to the axillary nodes rarely occur.[49,93] Attention should be paid to the underlying pectoral muscle. Mortality at 5 years, as judged by reports in the literature, varies from 30 to 40 percent,[6,16,32,76] although a recent report from Memorial Hospital presented a survival rate of over 90 percent.[16] Most of the patients who died did so within 2 years.

The size of the mass and other variables have been found to be unreliable as prognosticators. A high histologic grade suggests a poor prognosis.[55] An interesting phenomenon of possible prognostic significance is the "pushing" margin with minimal cytologic atypia, which is a relatively favorable sign.

Adequate surgery is the treatment of choice. Radiation therapy and chemotherapy have not been employed sufficiently to permit comment on their efficacy.

TUMORS OF FIBROUS TISSUE ORIGIN

In this category fall a host of neoplastic entities including fibromatosis[3,17] infiltrative fibromatosis, desmoid tumors,[80] fibrous histiocytomas,[45] stromal sarcoma,[16] and fibrosarcoma.

The high incidence with which fibrous tissue occurs in sarcomas of the breast is exemplified in the Memorial Hospital, New York City series, where 19 of the 25 tumors initially treated were of fibrous tissue type; these tumors were categorized as follows: fibrosarcoma, nine patients; malignant fibrous histiocytoma, five patients; desmoid tumor, three patients; and dermatofibrosarcoma protuberans, two patients.[16] The other sarcomas of that series were diagnosed as follows: hemangiopericytoma, one patient; leiomyosarcoma, two patients; stromal sarcoma, two patients; and liposarcoma, one patient.

Fibromatosis

Fibromatosis arising in the breast can be locally relentless but it will never metastasize. It thus becomes imperative to distinguish fibromatosis from fibrosarcomas, which do metastasize to other organs.[3] In view of the rarity of this lesion (about 25 cases have been reported to date),[17] little is known about the biologic behavior of fibromatosis except that it is notorious for its ability to infiltrate the surrounding tissue, resulting in severe mutilation and even death.[80] It almost always recurs after a conservative local excision and reexcision is usually followed by additional recurrences. One case infiltrated the entire thickness of the chest wall to involve the lung, with eventual death of the patient. This case is similar to one recorded by Chen.[17]

Fibromatosis usually occurs in women between 21 and 65 years of age. There is one report of a 13-year-old girl whose 3-cm lesion was widely excised; she remains alive and free of disease 3 years later.[17] The average tumor size in reported cases is 6 cm. Gross section reveals extension into the pectoral fascia and the muscle in one-fourth of cases. Extension into the dermis was recorded in three instances by Chen: one patient belonged to a family with "familial multicentric fibromatosis" and two patients had Gardner's syndrome.

Microscopically, the tumor is poorly circumscribed, composed of fascicles of spindle-shaped cells as well as intercellular collagenous fibrous tissue. Nuclear pleomorphism is minimal; only occasional mitoses (one per ten high-power fields) are present. Adipose tissue is infiltrated by tumor cells and breast ducts and lobules are incorporated in the lesion.[3] Some of the reported cases were initially diagnosed as stromal sarcomas. The differential diagnosis from other fibrous tissue tumors, such as the "benign spindle cell breast tumor" reported by Toker et al., is often difficult.[89] Making the exact diagnosis is important because a sarcoma is best treated by mastectomy. Inasmuch as fibromatosis is not multicentric, a wide excision should suffice. If margins of the excised specimen reveal tumor cells, a wider excision is indicated. Recurrent tumors are much more difficult to manage and may require a mastectomy.

Radiation therapy and/or hormone manipulation may prove useful in the treatment of breast fibromatosis as they are for fibromatoses elsewhere. Use of these treatments has not been reported to date.

According to Callery et al., "these tumors should not be underestimated no matter how innocent they may look."[16]

Malignant Fibrous Histiocytoma

Only 23 cases of malignant fibrous histiocytoma of the breast have been reported to date. When this entity was first described by O'Brien and Stout, of 53 malignant lesions, five occurred in the female breast.[67a] It may occur as a separate independent lesion, associated with another neoplasm (i.e., cystosarcoma phyllodes), or after irradiation[45]. It generally occurs in the fourth to sixth decade, exhibits a storiform morphology, and contains from 10 to 50 mitoses per 50 high-power fields. The lesions vary in size from 5 to 10 cm in diameter. Metastases to regional lymph nodes occur in less than 10 percent of cases.[45]

The treatment for malignant fibrous histiocytoma is total mastectomy; in view of the dearth of metastases to the axilla, axillary dissection is not indicated. Because recurrences have been recorded in 40 percent of patients subjected to wide excision, mastectomy is the treatment of choice.[45,46,48]

Overall mortality is 25 percent, similar to fibrous histiocytoma occurring elsewhere in the body.[21] Of three patients on whom a radical mastectomy was performed at Memorial Hospital, all remained well from 1 year to 54 months later.[16]

The role of radiation therapy remains uncertain. A recent randomized study suggested that adjuvant chemotherapy using doxorubicin, cyclophosphamide, and high-dose methotrexate with leucovorin rescue is useful for treating malignant fibrous histiocytoma of the extremities. Such treatment might also be useful for this disease of the breast.[32,45]

Stromal Sarcoma

The term *stromal sarcoma* of the breast as originally described by Berg et al. in 1962 has erroneously come into usage to describe all sarcomas of the breast, with the exclusion of cystosarcoma phyllodes and angiosarcoma.[12] This is unfortunate, because the breast is composed of specialized hormone-responsive stroma[16] as well as fibrous, adipose, and other mesenchymal elements. Thus, in a strict sense, the term stromal sarcoma (or sarcoma of mammary stroma) should be reserved for those tumors arising from the specialized stroma of the breast.[16]

Their rarity was stressed by the fact that only two such cases were seen of 32 sarcomas in the Memorial Hospital series.[16] One patient, a 49-year-old woman with a 4-cm sized lesion of intermediate tumor grade was treated by a modified radical mastectomy and she remained well 122 months later. Another 41-year-old lady with an 8-cm sized tumor was located by a radical mastectomy and she was free of cancer 63 months later. Because of the rarity of stromal sarcomas, nothing can be said of their biologic behavior and the best possible treatment for this disease.

Fibrosarcoma

It is impossible to determine the exact incidence of fibrosarcoma because many reports include subvarieties (fibromatosis, malignant fibrous histiocytoma), "spindle sarcoma," stromal sarcoma, etc.

Fibrosarcomas are metastasizing cancers, usually of a high tumor grade. The average age of patients in the Memorial Hospital series was 49 years. The youngest patient was 20 years old and the oldest was 65. Average tumor size was 5 cm in diameter.[16] There was a tendency for the smaller tumors to have a higher tumor grade. Metastases are usually to lungs, liver, and brain, but metastases to unusual places (stomach, intestines, etc.) have been reported.

Fibrosarcoma may be treated by a wide excision or, preferably, a mastectomy. The fact that the tumor may infiltrate the underlying pectoral muscle makes it imperative that the pectoral fascia be removed. If there is a question of invasion of the pectoral muscle, it too should be removed. Recurrence rate is high and there have been reports in the literature of tumor recurrences removed from six to twenty times over a period of 10 years. Some of the fibrosarcomas show cartilage or osteoid metaplasia; at one time this was considered a sign of increased malignancy, but is not believed to be so at present. (See Fig. 39-2).

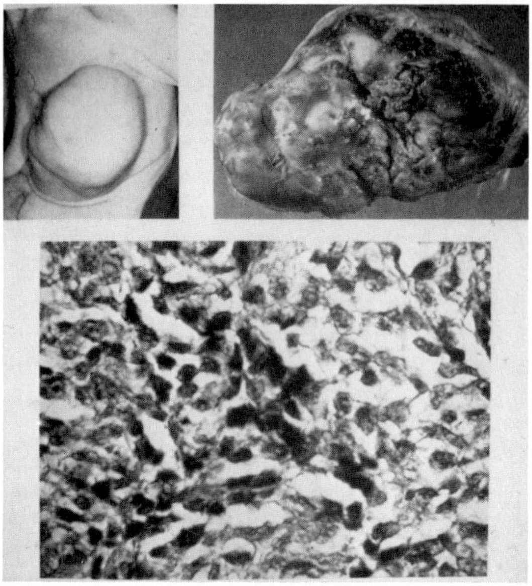

Figure 39-2 Fibrosarcoma of the breast. A. The tumor in this 62-year-old woman grew to the size shown within a period of 5 years. The breast measured 25 × 18 × 15 cm, was ulcerated on its undersurface, and was partially fixed to the chest wall. A mastectomy with resection of two underlying involved ribs was performed. The patient died 3 months later of metastases. The abdominal scar is from a colonic resection for carcinoma done a short time previously. B. The excised tumor is seen to be lobular and nodular. C. Photomicrograph showing the fibrosarcomatous structure of the tumor.

In the Memorial Hospital series, all eight patients with fibrosarcoma initially treated there were cured of their cancers an average of 98 months after operation.[16] Three patients had undergone a modified radical mastectomy; three had been subjected to a simple mastectomy, and two had received a radical mastectomy. Since none of the patients manifested metastases to the regional lymph nodes, resecting these nodes is not indicated. Three patients with fibrosarcoma originally treated elsewhere and referred to Memorial Hospital all died shortly after salvage mastectomy (one patient) and radiation therapy.

Tumor grade and number of mitoses per high-power field are important prognostically; size of tumor and method of treatment (if adequate) play minor roles.

Radiation-Induced Sarcoma

A feature which warrants discussion is the report of radiation-induced fibrosarcoma and fibrous histiosarcoma following treatment of breast cancer. Sixteen such cases have been reported.[14] Of nine patients with fibrosarcoma for whom follow-up was obtained, seven died within 1 year after diagnosis and two are living, but with tumor recurrences. No cures are recorded.[35,44,67] One such case caused erosion of the subclavian artery, requiring that the patient have an interscapulothoracic amputation.[1]

Three cases of malignant fibrous histiocytoma arising after irradiation for breast cancer have been reported.[45] The histiocytomas developed from 44 to 138 months after irradiation and were treated by wide local excision. One patient died from dissemination of the cancer; one remains well 68 months later; there is no follow-up report on the third.[45]

LIPOSARCOMA

Mammary liposarcomas as well as mammary lipomas are rare; approximately 50 cases have been reported.[68] In a series of 32 cases of sarcoma, two were liposarcomas.[16] The average age of patients was 45 years. Liposarcomas differ from other sarcomas in that they may metastasize both to the axilla and via the hematogenous route. They may arise from a preexistent lipoma, but more commonly they arise de novo.

Treatment of liposarcoma is wide excision of small tumors of low-grade malignancy. Recurrences are not unusual and should be treated by a mastectomy with an axillary lymph node dissection.

Radical mastectomy is indicated for the more malignant liposarcomas because metastases occur by way of the lymphatics in about 40 percent of patients. The tumors are relatively radiosensitive.

Prognosis

Reports regarding prognosis have been mixed. Geschickter[29] reported on three patients with liposarcomas, all of whom died within a very short time after diagnosis. Hermann[39] reported an average 5-year survival of 75 percent. Of the two patients with mammary liposarcoma treated at Memorial Hospital, one is living and well 14 years after a simple mastectomy and the other is alive and well 25 years after a radical mastectomy performed for a recurrence.[16]

RHABDOMYOSARCOMA

Rhabdomyosarcoma is a rare form of sarcoma. It may occur either in pure form or, rarely, as a stromal component of a cystosarcoma phyllodes. Only 25 cases of pure rhabdomyosarcoma have been reported.[6] This sarcoma is characterized by its large size, rapid growth, and very poor prognosis. Average time from diagnosis to death is approximately 2.5 years. Two long-term survivors have been reported.[6]

An unusual feature of rhabdomyosarcoma of the extremities is its proclivity to metastasize to the breast. This occurred in 7 of 108 consecutively diagnosed patients with rhabdomyosarcoma of the trunk and extremities.[41] It is believed that the physiologic state of the breast is an important determining factor in the development of such metastases.[41]

Treatment for rhabdomyosarcoma is total mastectomy. The value of radiation therapy and chemotherapy has not been evaluated to date.

LEIOMYOSARCOMA

Leiomyosarcomas have been reported rarely. One patient reported by Chen et al. was treated by mastectomy but died of hepatic metastases which occurred 15 years after surgery.[19] These authors suggest that tumors with three or more mitoses per ten high-power fields are leiomyosarcomas, and those with fewer mitoses should be labeled *leiomyomas*. However, smooth-muscle tumors in general may be diagnosed as benign on histologic criteria but clinically can behave as malignant tumors and metastasize. It is believed that leiomyosarcomas originate in the myoepithelium. One originating in the nipple arose from the muscle at that site, the only place where smooth muscle exists in the breast.[38]

HEMANGIOPERICYTOMA

Hemangiopericytoma is an entirely different entity from hemangiosarcoma. It behaves like a benign lesion. Two cases have been reported by Donnell et al.[24] One, measuring 5 cm in diameter, was treated by local excision; the patient remains free of disease 12 years later. In the other the tumor measured 11 cm in diameter; the patient was treated by total mastectomy and she remains well 23 years after surgery. A comparable benign sequence has been described by Tavassoli and Weiss.[88]

GRANULAR CELL MYOBLASTOMA

Granular cell myoblastoma is rare; only 100 cases have been reported in various locations including the breast. It occurs mostly in black women. It can be confused with carcinoma on physical examination and on mammography. Biopsy is imperative because these lesions can be cured by local excision. Five cases reported by Townsend and Stellato were so treated and each patient remains cured. Granular cell myoblastomas may be multiple, may recur after excision, and rarely metastasize.[90]

HEMANGIOSARCOMA

This tumor is considered separately because the breast is a most frequent site for this unusual neoplasm and because the tumor, although apparently benign and small, is frequently fatal (Fig. 39-3). It is so rapidly progressive that it may kill from 2 to 4 months after its discovery. The lesions metastasize widely and rapidly and cause death often from massive bleeding from the metastases. Hemangiosarcomas generally occur in younger women, some as young as 18 years of age, but have been described in an 82-year-old woman.[18] Incidence varies markedly between different institutions. Thus, at the M.D. Anderson Hospital only three cases have been reported,[56] whereas at the Memorial Hospital in New York more than 60 patients with mammary angiosarcoma have been seen.[24] In 1980 Chen culled 87 cases from the literature.[18] When first described, hemangiosarcomas were called "benign metastasizing angiomas" because of the benign appearance of the tumors. Other synonyms for this lesion include angiosarcoma, hemangioblastoma, hemangioendothelioma,[87] and perithelial angiomyosarcoma. Their site of origin is unknown, but McDivitt et al. express the possibility that they may arise in a perilobular capillary angioma.[60] These authors cite the following to aid in the diagnosis:

> To distinguish the malignant counterpart from a capillary or perilobular angioma: (1) The malignant capillary tumor is lined by cells too large, too hyperchromatic, and too numerous to be endothelium of an innocent vessel. (2) There are sprouts and the vessels may be purely separated or may fuse. (3) There are regions in which the capillaries are reduced to strands or the cells become fusiform and lumina are lacking. (4) In the surrounding fat or within the tumor one may find thick-walled vessels which are probably not part of the tumor itself but are similar to those found in arterial venous aneurysms.

They further state that in the differential diagnosis it is important to separate the hemangiosarcomas from the associated vascularity of juvenile hypertrophy.

Clinically, hemangiosarcomas may be small or may fill the entire breast parenchyma, producing a "veritable vascular sponge." They present clinically as rapidly enlarging, painless masses of brief duration, sometimes presenting a bluish hue.[74] Bilateral tumors are not uncommon, believed to be due to metastases rather than multicentricity.

Figure 39-3 A. Malignant hemangiosarcoma of the breast in a 26-year-old woman. Enlargement of the right breast and a region of purplish discoloration of the skin are present. The patient died of visceral and osseous metastases 11 months after a total mastectomy. B. Photomicrograph of tumor in A, illustrating poorly differentiated blood sinuses.

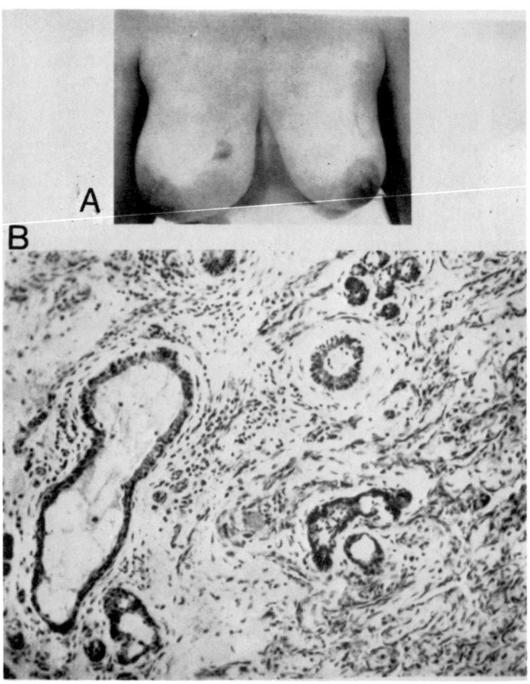

The basic histologic structure is a meshwork of interconnecting irregular vascular spaces lined by atypical endothelial cells and surrounded by a delicate reticulum.[23] Often the neoplastic cells extend well beyond the apparent gross margins.[24] A tumor factor responsible for angiogenesis may play a role in the rapid growth.[27]

Local recurrence is frequent after attempts at local excision.[59] Treatment is a mastectomy with attention given to the underlying pectoral fascia and muscle. Unlike other hemangiosarcomas, those of the breast rarely metastasize to the regional lymph nodes. Four cases of metastases to regional lymph nodes have been reported.[18] This unusual oncologic phenomenon accentuates the difference between breast angiosarcomas and angiosarcomas of other locations, where metastases to the lymph nodes occur in from 60 to 70 percent of the cases.[21] Efforts at radiation therapy for recurrences have been rewarding for brief periods,[24] but its use as a primary form of treatment has been disappointing. In one case in which the patient was given multiple courses of chemotherapy consisting of vincristine, doxorubicin hydrochloride (Adriamycin), and cytoxan after mastectomy and radiation therapy, the patient has remained well for a period of 2 years.[56] Of the reports in the literature, the 5-year survival is calculated to be 7 percent. The average duration of life of those who have died is 22 months.

MELANOMA OF THE SKIN OF THE FEMALE BREAST

Malignant melanoma arising in the skin of the female breast is an unusual lesion (Fig. 39-4).[42,51] Only eight cases were observed in a series of 3305 patients bearing malignant melanoma on all parts of the body, an incidence of 0.24 percent.[5] At the University of Iowa six women presenting with melanoma arising from the skin of the breast were reported.[42] There have been several reports of melanoma aris-

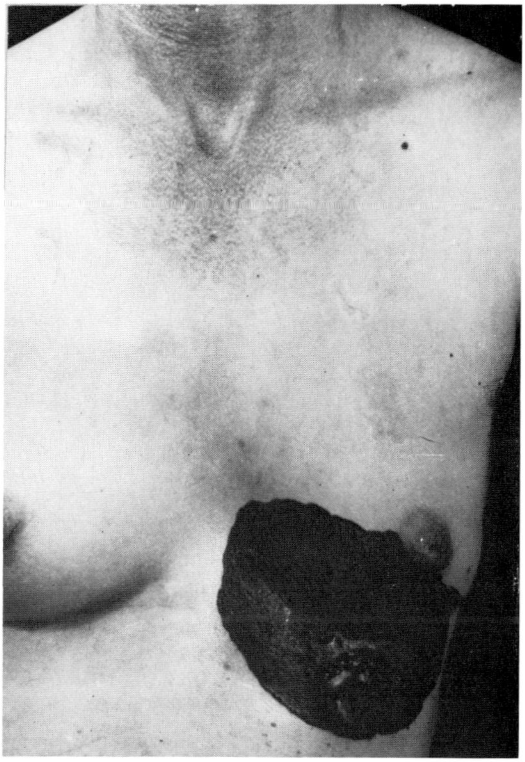

Figure 39-4 A huge malignant melanoma of the skin of the breast, which developed during pregnancy. The tumor was treated by radical mastectomy and skin grafting. The patient later died.

ing from the parenchyma of the breast,[28] but the validity of this is doubtful as there are no melanocytes in the breast. Their treatment involves the breast, hence this entity is included in this chapter.

Malignant melanoma may metastasize to the breast (Fig. 39-5). In a report by Hajdu and Urban it was noted that the tumor that most frequently metastasizes to the breast is malignant melanoma after excluding lymphomatous and leukemic infiltration of the breast tissue.[36]

Treatment

Melanomas have been classified according to the depth of invasion. They are divided by the

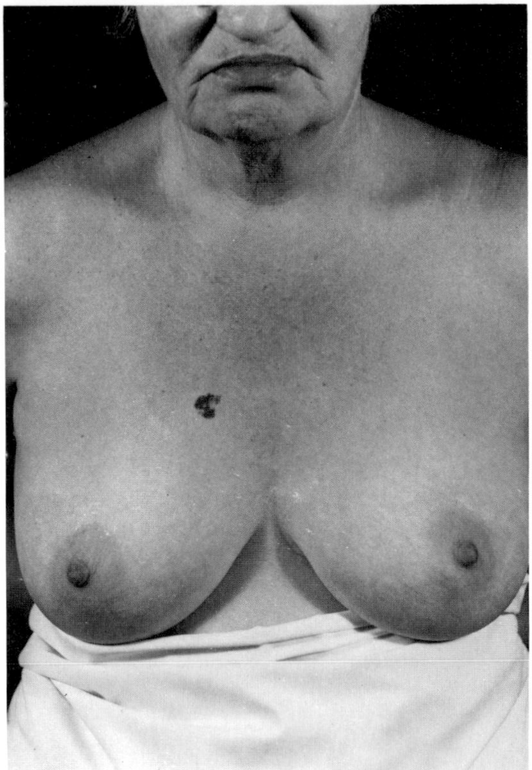

Figure 39-5 Deeply infiltrating malignant melanoma in a 41-year-old woman treated by radical mastectomy with internal mammary node dissection. The patient is alive and well 15 years after mastectomy.

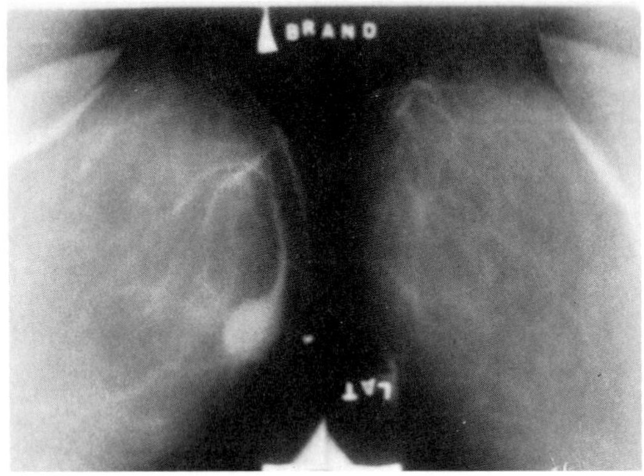

Figure 39-6 Mammogram showing metastatic melanoma in the left breast.

Clark Classification into levels. Level I is most superficial and level V has the deepest infiltration. The level of a given melanoma determines treatment policies. Melanomas of level I require only a wide local incision.

When the melanoma is deeper (Clark levels II and III), a wide, tridimensional excision of the skin in-continuity with an axillary dissection is the indicated procedure (Fig. 39-6). One patient so treated remains well after excision. Treatment in seven patients consisted of radical mastectomy because of deep infiltration of the malignant melanoma (Clark levels IV and V).

There is an elaborate communication between the lymphatic vessels of the skin of the breast and lymphatics of the breast per se. The lymphatic vessels of the mammary skin form a complex network, communicating freely with the lymphatic vessels of the chest and with the skin of the opposite breast. In view of this situation, in patients with infiltrating melanomas (levels IV and V), a mastectomy, either radical or modified, is indicated. In those patients who had infiltrating melanoma involving the inner aspect of the breast, an extended radical mastectomy was performed with resection of the internal mammary nodes. Of three patients, one patient remains well but the other two died (Fig. 39-7).

HODGKIN'S DISEASE AND NON-HODGKIN'S LYMPHOMA

Hodgkin's disease and non-Hodgkin's lymphoma may present as a localized expression of a generalized process by means of a mass in the breast. They are extremely rare, constituting approximately 0.25 percent of all breast lesions.[22,26] Mehrota et al. found five cases of non-Hodgkin's lymphoma in nearly 11,000 breast neoplasms;[57] non-Hodgkin's lymphoma

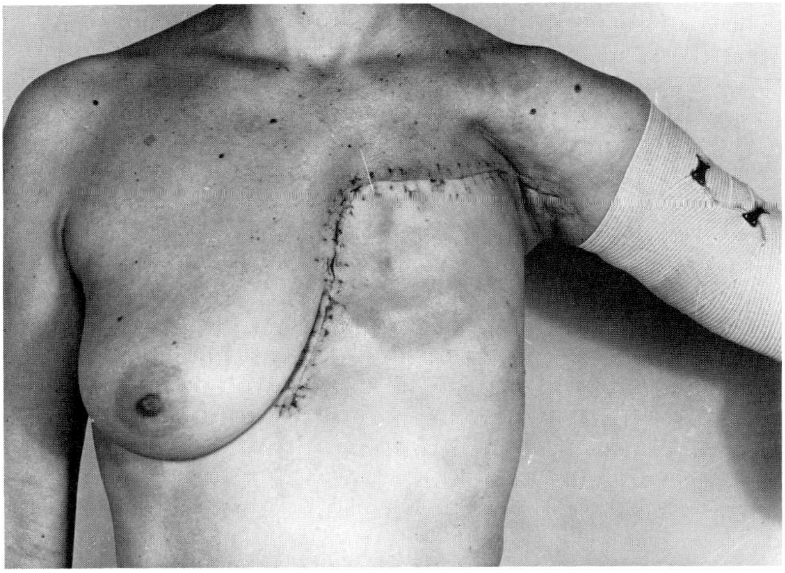

Figure 39-7 Surgical scar after radical mastectomy and internal mammary node dissection for an infiltrating melanoma. The patient died 2 $\frac{1}{2}$ years later from extensive abdominal metastases.

has been found to represent 0.04 percent of malignant breast tumors.[33,57,65,72] These entities are included in this chapter because occasionally they may represent the only presenting sign of the generalized sarcomatous process.[77,79] A characteristic of the local tumor is that, unlike carcinoma, it never becomes adherent to the overlying skin or to the deeper fascia, even in advanced cases.[85] An aid to diagnosis, besides biopsy, is the fact that a gallium scan will often show increased uptake of the isotope by the mass. When diagnosed, with biopsy confirmation and after complete systemic investigation, primary radiation therapy is the treatment of choice; the tumors then will "melt away."[95] This should be followed by a course of chemotherapy, for systemic involvement. When treated exclusively by surgery of the breast only 3.4 percent of 205 cases were disease-free after 5 years and only 2 percent were disease-free after 10 to 15 years, both for the 57 percent of patients who had a mastectomy as well as the 43 percent who had lesser surgical procedures. These data prove that breast lymphoma is not limited to the breast.[26]

LYMPHANGIOSARCOMA

Although lymphangiosarcoma of the arm is not a cancer of the breast it occurs most often in a chronically edematous arm following treatment of breast cancer, as first described by Stewart and Treves.[86] Woodward et al. in 1972 collected 186 reports of such cases from the literature.[96] Of these, 162 occurred following mastectomy and 24 arose from other miscellaneous cancers. Age ranged from 44 to 84 years with a mean age of 63 years. The tumor can be identified as early as 1 year and as late as 26 years after surgery. Prognosis is poor. In 129 cases available for follow-up, the median survival period was 19 months. All types of treatment have been attempted, including surgery, radiation, and chemotherapy,[75,78] Five instances of long-term survivors have been reported following interscapulothoracic amputation.[86] Hermann and Ariel reported a 5-year cure for a patient with lymphangiosarcoma treated by the intraarterial administration of radioactive yttrium microspheres.[40]

It is expected that with the decreased use of radical mastectomy the future incidence of postmastectomy lymphangiosarcoma will be drastically reduced.

CANCER METASTATIC TO THE BREAST

Metastases from other primary sites may occur in the breast.[11,36] Although rare, metastases from lung, stomach, ovary, kidney, and carcinoid tumors have been reported. The most common site of origin is the opposite breast. The metastasis is identical to the tumor of the primary site. If poorly differentiated, identification of a tumor as a metastasis may not be obvious. A tumor metastatic to the breast is characteristically periductular and/or perilobular in location; the duct and lobule cells themselves show no malignant change.[11] Treatment is based on management of the primary site of origin.

REFERENCES

1. Adam YG, Reif R: Radiation induced fibrosarcoma following treatment for breast cancer. *Surgery* 4:421, 1977.
2. Agnantis NJ and Apostolikas N: Histologic classification of cystosarcoma phyllodes: A study of 33 cases. *Breast* 7:24, 1981.
3. Ali M, Fayemi AO, Braun EV, Remy R: Fibromatosis of the breast. *Am J Surg Pathol* 3:501, 1979.
4. Amerson JR: Cystosarcoma phyllodes in adolescent females: a report of seven patients. *Ann Surg* 171:849, 1970.
5. Ariel IM, Caron AS: Diagnosis and treatment of malignant melanoma arising from the skin of the female breast. *Am J Surg* 124:384, 1972.
6. Barnes L, Pietruszka M: Rhabdomyosarcoma arising within a cystosarcoma phyllodes. *Am J Surg Pathol* 2:423, 1978.
7. Barnes L, Pietruszka M: Sarcomas of the breast. A clinicopathologic analysis of 10 cases. *Cancer* 40:1577, 1977.
8. Barnhart GR, Georgean GD, Kay S, Neifield JP: Management of cystosarcoma phyllodes: A reassessment. *Breast* 2:17, 1985.
9. Bleckert-Taft, Hansen JPH, Hansen OH, et al: Clinical course of cystosarcoma phyllodes related to histologic appearance. *Surg Gynecol Obstet* 140:929, 1975.
10. Benediktsdottir K, Lagerberg F, Lundell L, Thulin A: Osteogenic sarcoma of the breast. Report of a case. *Acta Pathol Microbiol Scand* (Sect. A) 88:161, 1980.
11. Benjamin I: Diagnostic problems of metastatic tumors in the breast. *Breast* 7:2, 1981.
12. Berg JW, De Cosse JJ, Fracchia´AA, Farrow J: Stromal sarcomas of the breast: A unified approach to connective tissue sarcomas other than cystosarcoma phyllodes. *Cancer* 15:418, 1962.
13. Borrmann R: Metastasenbildung bei histologisch gutartigan geschwulsten. *Beitr Pathol Anat* 40:373, 1907.
14. Botham RJ, McDonald JT, Clagett OT: Sarcoma of the mammary gland. *Surg Gynecol Obstet* 107:55, 1958.
15. Brennan MJ: Breast cancer, in Holland JF, Frei E III (eds): *Cancer Medicine*. Philadelphia, Lea & Febiger, 1973, p. 1786.
16. Callery CD, Rosen PP, Kinne D: Sarcoma of the breast: A study of 32 patients with reappraisal of classification and therapy. *Ann Surg* 20:527, 1985.
17. Chen KTK: Fibromatosis of the breast. *Breast* 10:25, 1984.
18. Chen KTK, Kirkeguard DD, Bocian JJ: Angiosarcoma of the breast. *Cancer* 46:368, 1980.
19. Chen KTK, Kuo TT, Hoffman KD: Leiomyosarcoma of the breast. A case of long-term survival and late hepatic metastasis. *Cancer* 47:1883, 1981.
20. Costa J, Wesley RA, Glastein E, Rosenberg SA: The grading of soft tissue sarcomas. Results of a clinicopathologic correlation in a series of 163 cases. *Cancer* 53:530, 1984.

21. Das Gupta TK: *Tumors of the Soft Tissue*. Norwalk, Conn., Appleton Century Croft, 1983, pp. 66, 610.
22. De Cosse JJ, Berg JW, Fracchia AA, Farrow JH: "Primary" lymphosarcoma of the breast. A review of 14 cases. *Cancer* 15:1264, 1962.
23. Donegan, LJ, Tobon H, Watson WG: Angiosarcoma of the breast. A report of two cases and a review of the literature. *Surgery* 79:57, 1976.
24. Donnell RM, Rosen PP, Kay S, Lieberman PH, et al: Angiosarcoma and other vascular tumors of the breast. Pathologic analysis as a guide to prognosis. *Am J Surg Pathol* 5:629, 1981.
25. Eilber FR, Morton DL, Eckardt J, et al: Limb salvage for skeletal and soft tissue sarcomas. *Cancer* 53:2579, 1984.
26. Fischer MG, Chideckel NJ: "Primary" lymphoma of the breast. *Breast* 10:7, 1984.
27. Folkman J, Mesler E, Abernathy C, Williams G: Isolation of tumour factor responsible for angiogenesis. *J Exp Med* 133:275, 1981.
28. Gatch WD: A melanoma apparently primary in the breast. *Arch Surg* 73:266, 1956.
29. Geschickter CF: *Diseases of the Breast*. 2d ed. Philadelphia, J. B. Lippincott, 1945, p. 385.
30. Gibbs BF Jr, Roe RD, Thomas DF: Malignant cystosarcoma phyllodes in a prepubertal female. *Ann Surg* 167:229, 1968.
31. Gisser SD, Toker C: Chondroblastic sarcoma of the breast. *Mt Sinai J Med* 42:232, 1975.
32. Glenn J, Kinsella T, Glatstein E, et al: Multimodality treatment of sarcomas of the head, neck, breast, and trunk. *Proc Soc Surg Oncol* 32:271, 1984.
33. Green MR, Kroener JF: Hodgkin's disease and the non-Hodgkin's lymphomas, in Pilch YH (ed): *Surgical Oncology*. New York, McGraw-Hill, 1984, p. 904.
34. Handley RS: The surgical anatomy of the breast, in Lewisohn EF: *Breast Cancer*. Baltimore, Williams & Wilkins, 1955, p. 30.
35. Hatfield PM, Schulz MD: Postirradiation sarcomas. *Radiology* 96:593, 1970.
36. Hajdu SI, Urban JA: Cancers metastatic to the breast. *Cancer* 29:1691, 1972.
37. Hajdu SI, Espinosa MH, Robbins GF: Recurrent cystosarcoma phyllodes: A clinicopathologic study of 32 cases. *Cancer* 38:1402, 1976.
38. Hernandez FJ: Leiomyosarcoma of the male breast originating in the nipple. *Am J Pathol* 2:299, 1978.
39. Hermann JB: Sarcoma of the breast, in Pack GT, Ariel IM (eds): *Treatment of Cancer and Allied Diseases*. New York, Hoeber, Harper & Row, 1960, vol 4, p. 214.
40. Hermann JB, Ariel IM: Therapy for lymphangiosarcoma of the chronically edematous limb. Five-year cure of a patient treated by intra-arterial radioactive yttrium. *Am J Roentgmol* 99: 393, 1967.
41. Howarth CB, Cacec JN, Pratt CB: Breast metastases in children with rhabdomyosarcoma. *Cancer* 46:2520, 1980.
42. Jochimsen PR, Pearlman NW, Lawton RL, Platz CE: Melanoma of the skin of the breast: Therapeutic considerations based on six cases. *Surgery* 81:583, 1977.
43. Kay S: Light and electron microscopic studies of a malignant cystosarcoma phyllodes featuring stromal cartilage and bone. *Am J Clin Pathol* 55:770, 1971.
44. Kim K, Tidrick RT, Skeel RT, et al: Fibrosarcoma of the chest wall following mastectomy and radiation therapy for mammary carcinoma. *Breast* 6:26, 1980.
45. Langham MR, Mills AS, DeMay RM, et al: Malignant fibrous histiocytoma of the breast. A case report and review of the literature. *Cancer* 54:558, 1984.
46. Lattes R: Sarcomas of the breast. *J Am M Assoc* 201:531, 1967
47. Lee BJ, Pack GT: Giant fibroadenomyxoma of the breast. *Am J Cancer* 15:2583, 1931.
48. Lee Y-TN, Chandrasoma P, Craig JR: Sarcoma of the breast. *Contemp Surg* 24:27, 1984.
49. Lee Y-TN, Moore TM, Schwinn CP: Metastasis of sarcomatous lesion to regional lymph node. *J Surg Oncol* 20:53, 1982.
50. Lee Y-TN, Markland FS: Steroid receptors study in breast carcinoma. *Med Ped Oncol* 5:153, 1978.
51. Lee Y-TN, Sparks FC, Morton DL: Primary melanoma of skin of the breast region. *Ann Surg* 185(1):17, 1977.
52. Lindquist KD, van Heerden JA, Weiland LH, Martin JK: Recurrent and metastatic cystosarcoma phyllodes. *Am J Surg* 144:341, 1982.

53. Lubin J, Rywlin AM: Cystosarcoma phyllodes metastasizing as a mixed mesenchymal sarcoma. *South Med J* 65:636, 1972.
54. Maier WP, et al: Cystosarcoma phyllodes mammae. *Oncology* 22:145, 1968.
55. Martin RG: Sarcomas of the breast, in *Breast Cancer Early and Late*, Chicago, Year Book Medical Publishers, 1970, p. 268.
56. Martin RG, Gallager HS: Sarcomas of the breast, in Gallager HS, Leis HP Jr, Snyderman RK, Urban JA (eds): *The Breast*. St. Louis, C.V. Mosby, 1978, p. 539.
57. Mehotra RML, Wahl KM, Abarwal PK: Lymphoma of the female breast. *Indian J Pathol Bact* 17:54, 1974.
58. Mendelko AN, Alktan M: Recurrent cystosarcoma phyllodes of breast excision full thickness of chest wall with immediate repair using steel mesh and a latissimus dorsi myocutaneous flap. *Brit J Plastic Surg* 36:519, 1983.
59. McClanahan BJ, Hogg L Jr.: Angiosarcoma of the breast. *Cancer* 7:586, 1954.
60. McDivitt RW, Stewart FW, Berg JW: *Atlas of Tumor Pathology*. second series: Tumors of the breast. Washington, D.C., Armed Forces Institute of Pathology, 1968, p. 117.
61. McCormick MV, Pillay SP: Malignant cystosarcoma phyllodes associated with scirrhous carcinoma of the breast: A case report. *S Afr Med J* 52:893, 1977.
62. Müller J: *Uber den feinern Bau und die Formen der Krankhaften Geschwulste*. Berlin, G. Reimer, 1838, p. 54.
63. Norris HJ, Taylor HB: Relationship of histologic features to behavior of cystosarcoma phyllodes: Analysis of ninety-four cases. *Cancer* 20:2090, 1967.
64. Norris HJ, Taylor HB: Sarcomas and related mesenchymal tumors of the breast. *Cancer* 22:22, 1968.
65. Novas JJ, Battifora H: Primary lymphoma of the breast. Ultrastructural study of two cases. *Cancer* 39:2025, 1977.
66. Oberman HA: Cystosarcoma phyllodes. *Cancer* 18:698, 1965.
67. Oberman HA: Sarcomas of the breast. *Cancer* 18:1233, 1965.
67a. O'Brien JE, Stout AP: Malignant fibrous xanthomas. *Cancer* 17:1445, 1964.
68. Rasmussen J, Jensen H: Liposarcoma of the breast. Case report and review of the literature. *Virchows Arch* (Pathol Anat) 385:117, 1979.
69. Reich T, Solomon C: Bilateral cystosarcoma phyllodes: Malignant variant with 14 year follow-up. *Ann Surg* 147:39, 1958.
70. Ribbert H: *Geschwulstlehre*, 2d ed. Bonn, S. Conn, 1914, p. 520.
71. Rosen PP, Urban JA: Coexistent mammary carcinoma and cystosarcoma phyllodes. *Breast* 1:9, 1975.
72. Ross CF, Elez A: Lymphosarcoma of the breast. *Brit J Surg* 62:651, 1975.
73. Russell WO, Cohen J, Enzinger F, et al: A clinical and pathological staging system for soft tissue sarcomas. *Cancer* 40:1562, 1977.
74. Saha SP, Thompson R, Still R: Angiosarcoma of the breast. *South Med J* 64:1376, 1971.
75. Salm R: The nature of so-called postmastectomy lymphangiosarcoma. *J Pathol Bacteriol* 85:445, 1963.
76. Salvadori B, Greco M, Galluzzo D, et al: Surgery for malignant mesenchymal tumors of the breast: A series of 31 cases. *Tumori* 68:325, 1982.
77. Sanyai B, Pant GC, et al: Hodgkin's disease of the breast. *Cancer* 11:382, 1974.
78. Schafler K, McKenzie CG, Salm R: Postmastectomy lymphangiosarcoma: A reappraisal of the concept—a critical review and report of an illustrative case. *Histopathol* 3:131, 1979.
79. Schouten JT, Weise JL, Carbone PP: Lymphoma of the breast. *Ann Surg* 194:749, 1981.
80. Schwartz IS: Infiltrative fibromatosis (desmoid) of the breast. *Breast* 9:2, 1983.
81. Shehata WM, Panke TW, Schlueter JA: Hodgkin's disease of the breast: A case report and review of the literature. *Breast* 11:19, 1985.
82. Shiu MH, Castro EG, Hajdu SI, Fortner JG: Surgical treatment of 297 soft tissue sarcomas of the lower extremity. *Ann Surg* 182:597, 1975.
83. Shiu MH, Turnbull AD, Hajdu SI, Hilaris B: Control of locally advanced soft tissue sarcoma by function-saving resection and brachytherapy. *Cancer*, in press.
84. Steingaszner LC, Enzinger FM, Taylor HB: Hemangiosarcoma of the breast. *Cancer* 18:352, 1965.
85. Stephenson SE, Byrd BF: Malignant melanoma of the breast. *Am J Surg* 97:232, 1959.

86. Stewart FW, Treves N: Lymphangiosarcoma in postmastectomy lymphedema: A report of six cases in elephantiasis chirurgica. *Cancer* 1:64, 1948.
87. Stout AP: Hemangioendothelioma: A tumor of blood vessels featuring vascular endothelial cells. *Ann Surg* 116:445, 1943.
88. Tavassoli FA, Weiss S: Hemangiopericytoma of the breast. *Am J Surg Pathol* 5:715, 1981.
89. Toker C, Tang C, Whitely JF: Benign spindle cell breast tumor. *Cancer* 48:1615, 1981.
90. Townsend MC, Stellato TA: Granular cell myoblastoma of the breast: A report of five cases and a review of the literature. *Breast* 11:12, 1985.
91. Treves N: A study of cystosarcoma phyllodes. *Ann NY Acad Sci* 114:922, 1964.
92. Treves N, Sunderland DA: Cystosarcoma phyllodes of the breast: A malignant and a benign tumor. A clinicopathological study of 7 cases. *Cancer* 4:1286, 1951.
93. Vezeridis MP, Moore R, Karakousis CP: Metastatic patterns in soft tissue sarcomas. *Arch Surg* 118:915, 1983.
94. West TL, Weiland LH, Clagett OT: Cystosarcoma phyllodes. *Ann Surg* 173:520, 1971.
95. Wiseman C, Liao KT: Primary lymphoma of the breast. *Cancer* 29:1705, 1972.
96. Woodward AH, Inins JC, Soule EH: Lymphangiosarcoma arising in chronic lymphedematous extremities. *Cancer* 30:562, 1972.

40

Postmastectomy Edema

John M. Edwards, M.S., F.R.C.S.

INTRODUCTION

The incidence of edema after mastectomy is now diminishing. The highest incidence and the greatest severity of presentation occurred within or just after the era when radical mastectomy was the most common treatment applied for carcinoma of the breast, and particularly when mastectomy was combined with radiation treatment of the skin flaps and axilla. At that time the incidence of severe edema of the upper limb was of the order of 10 percent and of mild to moderate edema up to 60 percent.[7] This complication developed early after radical mastectomy or, occasionally, some years after the treatment, particularly after mastectomy combined with radiation therapy.

The modifications of the classic Halsted radical mastectomy, such as the Patey procedure with preservation of the pectoral muscles, did not seem to protect against the development of edema. The relevant aspect of treatment leading to edema was axillary lymph node dissection aggravated by radiation. Other factors which had a deleterious effect included postoperative lymphatoma, sepsis, and loss of flap tissue by necrosis (Fig. 40-1).

The more recent trend toward conservative measures of treatment such as simple mastectomy, partial mastectomy, or simple removal of the tumor followed by radiation has led to a lower incidence of edema. Other modifications of surgical technique have also played a significant role.

DEVELOPMENT OF COLLATERAL CIRCULATION

The development of collateral circulation is, of course, of utmost importance whenever any circulatory pathway is interrupted. This is just as

The current TNM system of classification is used throughout.

POSTMASTECTOMY EDEMA
Factors Encouraging Edema
Axillary node dissection
Seratoma formation
Sepsis
Necrosis of skin flaps
Incisions across anterior shoulder
Radiotherapy

Figure 40-1 Factors encouraging edema after mastectomy.

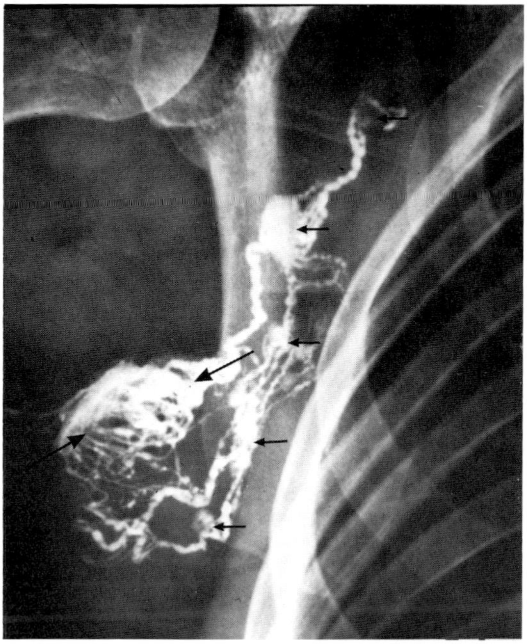

Figure 40-2 Lymphangiogram. Position of large collecting node shown by arrows, with other communications to nodes beginning to show. Later x-rays show nodes more clearly (lymphadenograms).

true after axillary interruption of the lymphatics as after blockage of major arteries or veins.

The axilla is the regional collecting area for lymph from the upper limb, shoulder, and pectoral areas. It is the major drainage area for lymph from the breast; the other avenues of lymph flow are to the internal mammary chain and supraclavicular areas.

The axillary lymph nodes are numerous. By oil contrast lymphography as many as 40 to 50 lymph nodes can be identified. Lymphography by the arm route identifies most of these nodes, but further nodes can be shown if lymphography is subsequently performed by injecting the lymphatics over the back. Many of these nodes are very small and not identified in the routine pathological examination of the dissected axillary specimen. As shown by brachial lymphography there is a large "collecting lymph node" in the axilla which leads on to the apical nodes and then, via the subclavian lymph trunk, to enter the great veins in the root of the neck. Posteriorly a conglomeration of lymph nodes group around the subscapular vessels; anteriorly there are nodes along the pectoral fold. Free communications occur between the nodes; variations are numerous, with little evidence of the orderly arrangements neatly set down in anatomy textbooks (Fig. 40-2). Removal of the bulk of these nodes means that alternative pathways must be found for the lymph from the upper limb. These pathways open up over the shoulder region, either passing directly to the ipsilateral supraclavicular areas or, via the back, eventually entering the contralateral axilla (Fig. 40-3). These routes have been shown in this author's studies and were also well-documented by Bobbio et al. in 1962.[1] The circulation can also be restored by collateral vessel formation within the incised axilla. Subcutaneous severed lymphatics can redevelop circulation with enlarged dermal lymphatics.

Given all these considerations, the choice of incision sites and provision of further treatment such as radiation therapy can have a profound effect on the development of lymphedema. An additional mechanism which may help to limit the severity of edema is the formation of lymphovenous shunts at the axillary level, either as a result of surgery or spontaneously (Fig. 40-4).

Other extra lymphatic channels which may be beneficial and important are the so-called perivenous spaces. These "channels" were noted

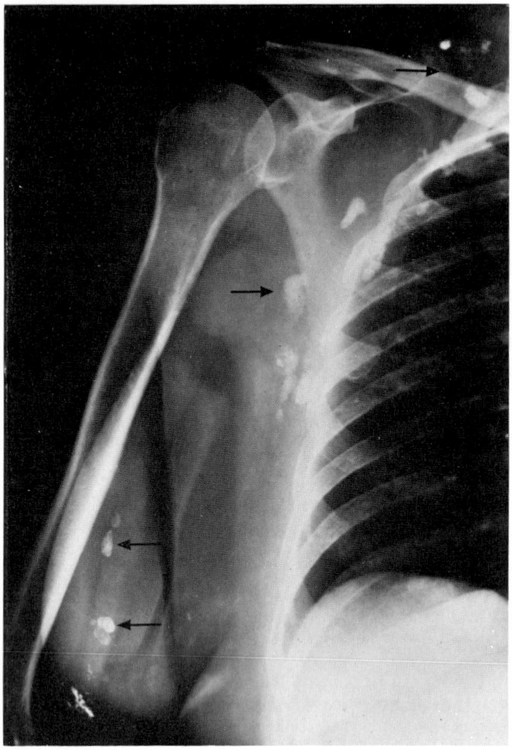

Figure 40-3 Lymphadenogram of arm axilla and supraclavicular areas. Ectopic nodes in arm, a not uncommon variant, are shown. Supraclavicular nodes (arrows) are a very important collateral route for arm lymphatics if axillary nodes are removed.

many years ago in the process of lymphographic investigations using oil contrast media (Fig. 40-5). Ultrafluid lipiodol (UFL) injected subcutaneously in close proximity to a vein can reveal these potential spaces, along which lymph may pass even more readily than oil, and can reach areas where the lymphatic drainage is intact. It is important if axillary dissection is employed not to expose the axillary vein too cleanly and thereby destroy the fat "space" around the vein. Recommendations to protect the developing collaterals after axillary dissection are

1 Use of transverse surgical incisions rather than old-fashioned oblique and extensive incisions

2 Prolonged closed suction drainage to prevent lymphatoma and consequent sepsis

3 Avoidance of radiotherapy if possible

4 Protection with dissection below the vein of the perivenous fat space around the axillary vein

EVALUATION OF THE SWOLLEN ARM

Investigation of the swollen limb after mastectomy requires a detailed clinical examination of the patient followed by special tests of the lymphatic and venous circulations. The most obvious etiological factor may be lymphatic but occasionally obstruction of the axillary vein by fibrosis or tumor may play a significant role or predominate. Some indication that venous obstruction exists is provided by the sudden development of a swollen, erythrocyanotic limb, with later appearance of obvious collateral veins over the anterior shoulder area down to the chest wall. There is nearly always a lymphatic element to the edema, however, even in the presentation; the approach to treatment may require consideration of both lymphatic and venous etiological factors. Thus, in addition to lymphographic investigations by direct oil contrast medium injection, investigation by phlebography and manometry is required.

Lymphography is performed in all cases. A characteristic picture is shown in Fig. 40-6. It presents the appearance of obstructive lymphedema with distended dermal lymphatics and a network of subcutaneous vessels. The lymphatics proximal in the limb are usually not visible due to atrophy ("die-back"). Atrophy is a continuous process and eventually may lead to all the subcutaneous vessels becoming obliterated, leaving only the dermal plexus. Exploration of the subcutaneous tissue may reveal strands of tissue which, if removed and examined by microscopy, show obliterated lymphatics.

In patients with venous edema as suggested by phlebography, the water-soluble contrast media may reveal kinks, constrictions, and irregu-

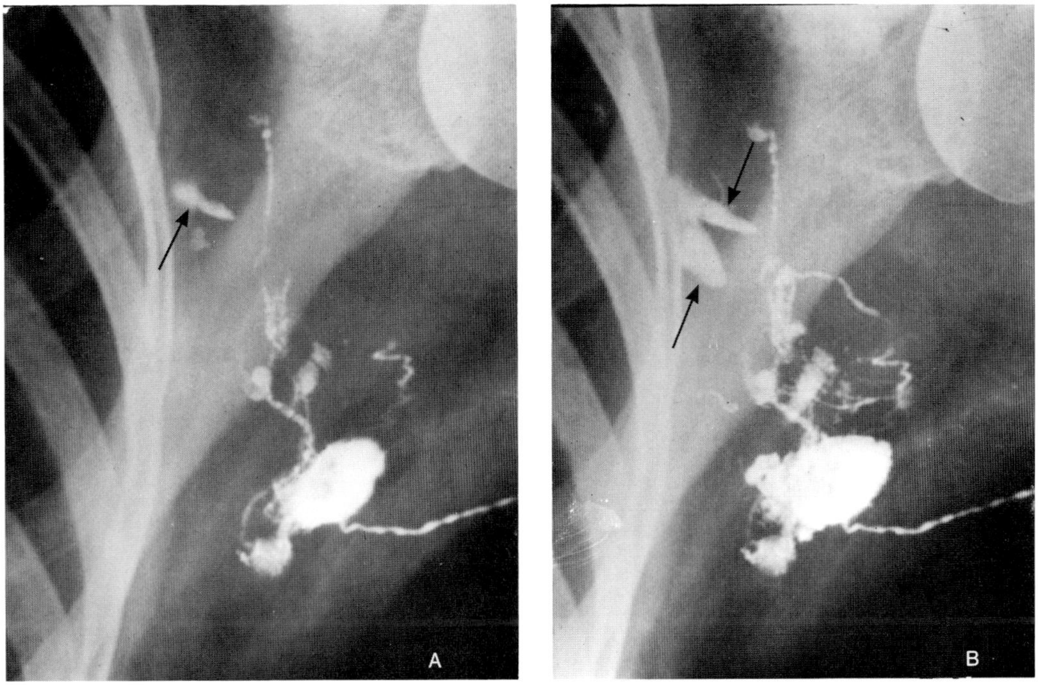

Figure 40-4 Lymphovenous shunt. These x-rays show large "collecting" lymph node in axilla with delineation of lymphovenous shunt. Oil contrast material ultrafluid lipiodol (UFL) is trapped behind a venous valve in the axillary vein. Later radiography showed complete clearance of the contrast material from this site.

larity of the axillary vein, progressing to complete obliteration with development of collateral vessels. Manometry is occasionally of help in establishing that venous obstruction exists, especially when phlebograms are not conclusive. Comparison of the pressures in similar veins in both upper limbs is of more significance than absolute measurements; similar arm positions must be considered in recording the findings. If it is decided that a venous obstructive element which requires surgical treatment exists, then an axillary operation is required.

TREATMENT OF POSTMASTECTOMY EDEMA

Most patients with edema are not affected badly enough to warrant surgery; they are treated by nonsurgical measures. These include meticulous attention to support of the limb with a custom-fitted elastic bandage and repeated prescription at three-month intervals (Fig. 40-7). There is a definite place for intermittent air compression treatment, but it should be performed on a daily basis. This means that the patient has to purchase a machine, an expense which most patients cannot meet.

Surgical Treatment

Indications[6] for surgery are

1 Limitation of function. Lymphedema of such dimensions as to preclude or severely handicap normal activities.

2 Pain and recurrent attacks of cellulitis. The swollen, heavy limb can be painful both from the feeling of distention of the arm and also from

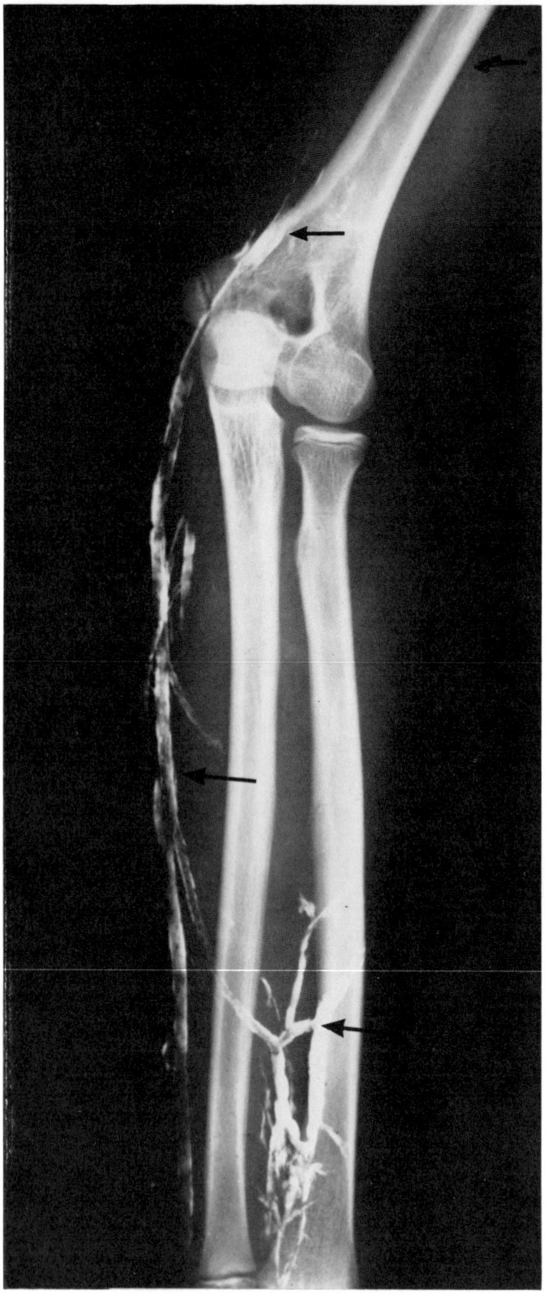

Figure 40-5 Perivenous "spaces" shown using UFL, extravasating after lymphography, and tracking around the veins of the arm.

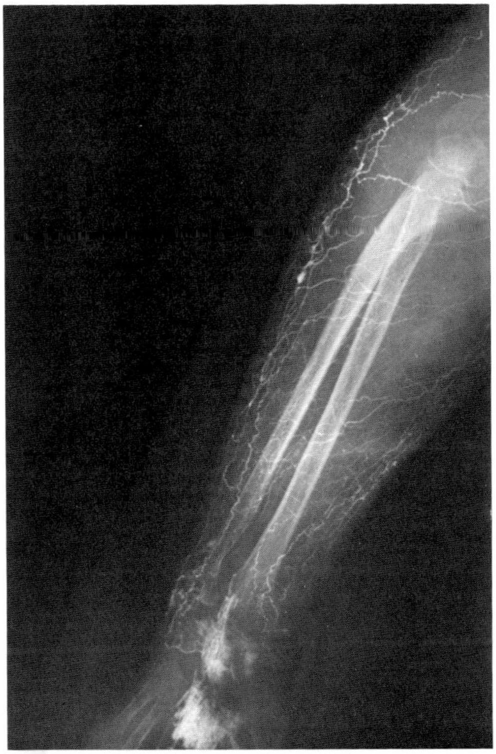

Figure 40-6 Obstructive lymphedema of upper limb after mastectomy and radiotherapy. The tortuous, distended network of lymphatics is visible.

the traction effect on the brachial plexus. Paresthesia and even paralysis due to traction damage to motor nerves can occur. Recurrent attacks of cellulitis due to bacterial infection may produce debilitating symptoms; some of these patients with lymphedema have deficient fibrinolysis leading to chronic cellulitis[2] which would more correctly be described as liposclerosis.

3 Cosmetic appearance. This alone is rarely an absolute indication for operation, although some minor surgical procedures, such as excision of "flabby" edematous tissue on the posterior upper arm, can be considered purely cosmetic.

4 Malignant change. It must always be remembered that apart from the above factors, lymphangiosarcomatous change may occur in the grossly lymphedematous limb.

TREATMENT - EDEMA OF UPPER LIMB

A. Conservative measures:

Support
Elevation
Compression. Lympha press.

B. Operative:

Venous edema:	Bypass Phlebolysis
Lymphatic edema:	Reducing operations Physiological operations

Figure 40-7 Treatment of edema of upper limb.

Surgical treatment can be classified into two types according to whether it involves a purely excisional procedure to remove the mass of lymphedematous tissue or a "physiological procedure" designed to restore lymphatic flow.[4,5]

Excisional operations include the *buried dermal flap procedure* and minor procedures to remove subcutaneous edematous fat in certain areas, particularly the posterior upper arm where the fat "hangs" and makes clothing fit poorly. Physiological operations consist of procedures designed to establish lymphovenous shunts. All other procedures, including pedicle skin flap operations, buried artificial conduits, or operations involving natural materials, have been given trials and may be considered to have failed.

Excisional operations currently practiced consist mainly of buried dermal flap procedures or modifications of the Homans procedure. The Charles operation has been abandoned, largely because the edema in the hand is aggravated due to interference with venous drainage. Ablation of the superficial tissues in the course of the Charles operation destroys the superficial veins of the arm, which are more important to venous drainage than are the superficial veins in the leg. Venous congestion in the hand is uncomfortable for the patient and produces a poor cosmetic result. The replaced skin after a Charles operation also eventually becomes verrucose and unstable.

Far better results are obtained with the buried dermal flap procedure, with improved cosmetic appearance and better resulting function. The operation is particularly indicated where there is no possibility of a physiological procedure with direct lymphovenous shunts. The results of the latter procedure have in the main been disappointing.

Buried Dermal Flap Operation

The original concept of this procedure was to produce lymphatic anastomosis between dermal lymphatics in the buried skin flap and deep lymphatics, presuming that the subcutaneous lymphatics were deficient.[4,8,11] In other respects the operation could be represented as a modification of Kondoleon's operation. In an attempt to maintain continuity between the superficial and deep compartments of the limb, instead of merely excising skin and deep fascia, a flap of skin is buried traversing the two compartments. The shaved flap of skin is implanted between the muscles and near the deep lymphatic vessels so that physiological drainage may be improved. This concept could be more realistically applied to the lower limb as opposed to the upper limb. Usually in the upper limb the flap is merely double-breasted. This buried flap of skin tends to anchor enveloping skin; tissue tension is consequently increased. There is also, of course, an excisional element to the operation: fat is cleared from the medial aspect of the limb. The operation can be repeated if necessary on the lateral aspect. In most patients seen here a one-stage procedure has been performed on the medial aspect of the limb.

The steps of a buried flap operation on the medial aspect of the limb are described below.

First, the limb is prepared. The skin of the entire upper limb including the axilla and shoulder area is thoroughly bathed with antiseptic soap prior to the procedure. Following this the entire upper limb is prepared with surgical antiseptic. The limb is isolated by sterile drapes and a bloodless field established. As it is best to reduce the whole length of one aspect of the limb in one operation, the exposure of the limb should be maximal. Exsanguination of the limb by an Esmarch bandage is performed initially. Soft rubber tubing is then bound around the base of the limb and held in place by a clamp; tubing takes up less room than a pneumatic cuff.* The line of incision as shown in Fig. 40-8 A is made with a sterile pen. The main longitudinal incision is drawn so that the line is just anterior to the edge of the ulna, the medial epicondyle of the humerus, and the medial edge of the arm. This is to produce as inconspicuous a scar as possible. The lines of the transverse incisions are drawn at each end of the longitudinal one. Drawing the line of incision, assessing the amount of fat to be removed, and trimming the skin edges improve with experience. Care must be taken not to cut the flaps too thin as necrosis may occur. It is best to be on the conservative side regarding the tension of the flaps. Trimming can be done, if necessary, later in the operation.

An electric dermatome is used to shave the posterior flap, as shown in Fig. 40-8. A graft of split thickness only is removed so as not to damage the dermal lymphatics unduly. It is necessary to remove the epidermis, otherwise unshaven buried skin may cause problems, which may include sinuses. The skin flaps are raised with care to preserve their blood supply. They should taper from the cut edge posteriorly, to become thicker at the base; overthinning near the base may lose the blood supply. Near the base the incision is deepened down to the muscle; then the entire wedge of fat and deep fascia is removed (Fig. 40-8 B).

Following removal of fat the tourniquet is released and hemostasis is effected. It is important to have adequate suction drainage to prevent seratoma; several suction tubes are inserted through the base of the flaps. It is best to position the tubes at spaced intervals in the

*This technique of using the rubber tubing is practiced in Great Britain.

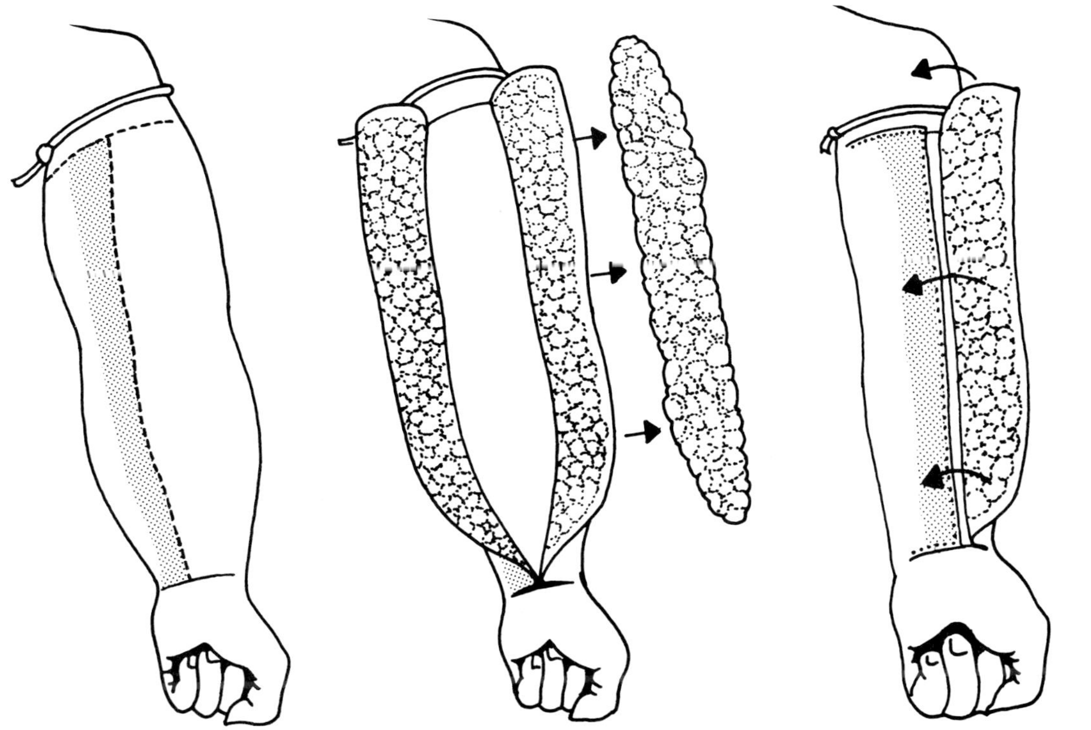

Figure 40-8 Buried flap procedure. A. Lines of incision. Posterior flap shaved with split skin graft removed. B. Removal of wedge fat and deep fascia. C. Posterior flap sutured down and overlapped by anterior flap.

fold and then retain the placement by means of catgut sutures. At this stage the flaps may need to be trimmed. It is better not to have too great a length of overlap at the elbow level, as the thickness may limit joint movement. The posterior flap is then sutured down to muscle and overlapped by the anterior flap (Fig. 40-8 C). Nylon sutures are used to hold the flap down to the edge of the deep fascia. The anterior flap should lie on the posterior without undue tension, kept in place by interrupted sutures supplemented by skin clips. Support to the wound is given by interrupted steristrip "sutures." The wound is dressed with a nonadhesive dressing and cotton batting and a cloth bandage applied. The multiple suction drainage tubes should avoid hematoma; there should not be too much need for compressive bandaging. Elevation of the limb should be maintained for the early postoperative period, but active exercises to preserve joint mobility and function should start as soon as possible after the operation.

When the wound is healed elastic support is continued on the limb with a measured appliance (arm support).

Complications of this procedure include necrosis of the buried flaps and the usually associated sepsis and seratoma. The occurrence of these complications should be reduced with increasing experience.

Direct Lymphovenous Anastomosis (Microsurgical Techniques)

Attempts to construct lymphovenous anastomosis in the obstructed limb would seem to offer a more logical approach to treatment than excisional procedures. Lymph node-to-vein shunt (Nielubowicz) procedures would be

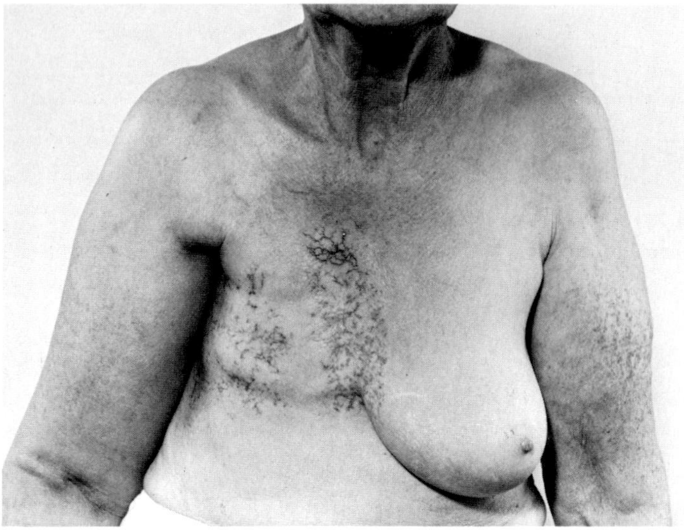

Figure 40-9 Venous edema and lymphatic edema after mastectomy and radiotherapy. Development of both venous and lymphatic collaterals hampered by radiotherapy over the chest wall area. Photograph shows telangiectasis at radiotherapy site.

impractical due to the nature of the initial operation. Lymph vessel-to-vein procedures have not, to date, given uniform satisfaction, possibly because the lymphatics in the patients who present late show irreversible changes. The Degni implantation technique[3] is less useful than in the lower limb; probably direct end-to-side lymphovenous anastomosis as originally described by O'Brien and Shafiroff in 1979[9] will have greater application.

Operations for Venous Occlusion

Most operations for venous occlusion have been performed when there was evidence of kinks or constriction of the axillary vein. Usually a venous decompression with excision of fibrous tissue has been performed. Active attempts to relieve vein obstruction are described in Hughes and Patel's work in 1966.[7] Manometry and phlebography investigations combined should point to this diagnosis in association with clinical features suggesting venous obstruction. The capacity of the venous system to develop collaterals may be hampered by the same factors that affect lymphatic collaterals, the main culprit being radiotherapy as opposed to surgery (Fig. 40-9). The operation is performed through an incision in the skin overlying the vessels. The outcome is best when there is a localized band of fibrous tissue which can be removed. The results of these procedures are very variable. There can be improvement in shoulder mobility previously inhibited by fibrous tissue but restoration of function of the vein is unusual. Venous bypass procedures may have more place, especially when combined with the Palma shunt type of operation.[10]

The use of myocutaneous flaps using the latissimus dorsi muscle is being developed; their application will be observed with interest.

REFERENCES

1. Bobbio P, Perracchia G, Pellegrino F: La circolazione linfatica secondaria di mastectomia radicale. *Ateneo Parmense* 33 (suppl 3):110, 1962.
2. Burnand K, Stewart G, Pattison M: Abnormal fibrinolysis: The cause of lipodermatosclerosis or "chronic cellulitis" in patients with primary lymphoedema. *Lymphology* 17:23, 1984.
3. Degni M: New technique of lymphatico venous anastomosis. *J Cardiovasc Surg* (Milano)19:577, 1979.

4. Edwards JM: Surgery of the lymphatics, in Bevan PG (ed): *Reconstructive Procedures in Surgery.* Oxford, Blackwell, 1982.
5. Edwards JM, Kinmonth JB: Lymphovenous shunts in man. *Brit Med J* 4:579, 1969.
6. Edwards JM, Negus D, Kinmonth JB: Review of operations for lymphoedema. *J Cardiovasc Surg* XVII Cong, Eur Soc Cardiovasc Surg:110, 1969.
7. Hughes JL, Patel AR: Swelling of the arm following radical mastectomy. *Brit J Surg* 53:4, 1966.
8. Kinmonth JB: Lymphatic diseases of the upper limb, in *The Lymphatics.* London, Edward Arnold, 1982.
9. O'Brien BM, Shafiroff BB: Lymphatico venous and resectional surgery in obstructive lymphoedema. *World J Surg* 3:3, 1979.
10. Palma CE, Esperon R: Vein transplants and grafts in the surgical treatment of the postphlebitic syndrome. *J Cardiovasc Surg* 1:94, 1960.
11. Thompson N: The late results of operative treatment of chronic lymphoedema using buried dermis flap procedure. *J Cardiovasc Surg* XVII Cong, Eur Soc Cardiovasc Surg:92, 1969.

41

Cancer in the Male Breast

Robert W. Crichlow, M.D.
Douglas B. Evans, M.D.

INTRODUCTION

Carcinoma is an uncommon occurrence in the breast in men. Early signs are commonly misinterpreted by patient and physician alike, leading to a delay in diagnosis. Management decisions, based on scanty experience with men, have been heavily influenced by an experience with women which is not necessarily transferable.

INCIDENCE

Carcinoma of the male breast constitutes only 1 percent of all breast cancer and less than 1.5 percent of all malignant tumors in men. Age at detection of breast cancer averages just under 60 years for males, 6 to 11 years later than the average age in women.[1] Only 1 percent of carcinomas in men occur before the age of 30[2] and only 6 percent before the age of 40.[3] The bimodal curve of age distribution for women with breast cancer[4] is not seen in men, whose risk increases exponentially through life. There is a predilection for the left breast (1.07/1) similar to that in women, which is unexplained. Breast cancer is less often bilateral in men than in women; the frequency of bilaterality was only 1.4 percent in a collected series of 1158 men.

RISK FACTORS

Although the etiology of breast cancer is as obscure in the male as in the female, there are factors which appear to be associated with an increased risk for men of developing breast cancer.

Hormonal Factors

In searching for an explanation for the hundredfold difference in breast cancer incidence

---

The current TNM system of classification is used throughout.

between men and women, the hormonal milieu is an obvious point to begin. Estrogen has a profound effect on male breast tissue and is able to stimulate formation of acini and true lobules identical to those of the mature female breast. However, evidence to suggest that such hormonal stimulation is of significance in the etiology of male breast cancer is weak. Only 3 of 487 men with breast cancer on whom reported information was adequate had received prior estrogen treatment.[5,6] Of approximately 20,000 males with prostatic carcinoma who were treated with estrogens, only three subsequently developed breast cancer.[3,7] Of the few other reports associating exogenous estrogen with male breast cancer, the most convincing is a report of two transsexual males who developed carcinoma of the breast 5 years after orchiectomy, penectomy, creation of a provagina, and intensive estrogen therapy by multiple routes.[8]

There have been many reports of breast tumors developing in men with prostatic carcinoma while on estrogen therapy in which the tumors proved to represent secondary involvement of an estrogen-altered breast by metastatic prostatic carcinoma. Distinction between primary and secondary breast carcinoma requires demonstration of morphologic and histochemical differences between the tumors, such as the absence of acid phosphatase in the breast tumor.[9,10]

Alterations of hormonal metabolism in men with breast cancer have been demonstrated, but no consistent pattern has emerged. The association of testicular abnormalities with male breast cancer is implied by several studies. For example, prior orchitis occurred more frequently among 120 American men with breast cancer than among controls.[11] Following the original observation by Jackson et al. of an association of breast cancer with Klinefelter syndrome,[12] larger studies have established the risk of breast cancer in the Klinefelter syndrome for men to be one-fifth that for women and 20 times that for normal men,[13] but to date only 15 such instances have been documented.[13,14]

Gynecomastia

That gynecomastia is a premalignant state for carcinoma of the male breast is an attractive hypothesis which has earned little support. The degree of association varies with methods of establishing either the precedence or existence of gynecomastia. For example, Scheike and Visfeldt obtained a history of gynecomastia in only 10 of 265 men with breast cancer and saw only one example of coexisting clinical gynecomastia.[15] However, microscopic evidence of gynecomastia was found in 21 of 79 mastectomy specimens. A rare example of transition from gynecomastia to carcinoma may exist in Lyall's patient with gynecomastia associated with disseminated choriocarcinoma: there was ductal anaplasia which "at one point ... had advanced to the stage of definite malignancy."[16]

Genetic Influences

Little information is available on the family histories of men with breast cancer. In a survey of 2217 reported cases, breast cancer was described in 10 female blood relatives of 79 men with breast cancer.[5] Several examples of familial clustering among men have appeared. Marger et al. reported breast cancer in two brothers[6] and Everson et al. in two brothers and a son in one family and three brothers in another with no breast cancer among related women.[17] Mixed clustering with a male:female ratio of 1/9 in one family and 2/5 in another was reported by Haagensen.[18]

Geography

Some studies do suggest variations in risk by country of origin, such as a higher incidence of male breast cancer both in Jews residing in Israel and in Jews in the United States.[19,20] A slight excess of breast cancer among male immigrants to Israel of European contrasted to African or Asian origin has also been reported.[21] Two epidemiologic studies of breast cancer in men in the United States have produced conflicting conclusions. One showed morbidity to be higher in northern than in southern cities; mortality was found to be lowest in the southwest and lower for white than nonwhite men.[11] The other showed no association with geography, race, religion, or occupation.[22]

Ionizing Radiation

Exposure of women to ionizing radiation from atomic bombings, radiotherapy, or repeated fluoroscopy has been shown to lead to an increased incidence of breast cancer. Five examples in which men were exposed to significant radiation to the breast 20 to 25 years before appearance of breast cancer have been reported.[5] While this is insufficient evidence to establish cause and effect, history of radiation exposure calls for increased suspicion.

CLINICAL PICTURE

The presenting complaint in 90 percent of men with breast cancer is a painless mass beneath the areola.[5] Complaints of nipple or areolar abnormalities are part of the presenting symptom complex in nearly 20 percent of men; such symptoms are far more common occurrences than in women.[23] Nipple discharge occurs in 14 percent of men with malignant breast tumors and 2 percent in those with benign breast tumors, and is an early event in 80 percent of those with carcinoma.[24] Although serous discharge is most commonly associated with benign tumors, sanguine discharge is associated with carcinoma in 75 percent of carcinomas in men, three times the frequency found in women.[24]

Historically, men have delayed seeking treatment far longer than have women, but the discrepancy is disappearing. Delay averaged 18 months among 1228 male patients reported during the first half of this century, but was 10 months in those reported since 1951.[5] In their study of breast cancer in Philadelphia, Mausner et al. demonstrated significant delays in diagnosis in 77 percent of men compared to 60 percent of women, and delays of more than a year in one-third of men compared to one-fifth of women.[25] However, recent reports do not show significant differences in delay between men and women.[5,26]

PHYSICAL EXAMINATION

A mass beneath or adjacent to the nipple-areolar complex is the cardinal physical finding in men with cancer of the breast. Two instances of occult carcinoma of the breast presenting with palpable axillary lymph nodes have been reported in men,[5] and this rare phenomenon should be recalled in evaluation of men with histologically compatible regional node metastases.

Frequent and relatively early change in the nipple or areola is characteristic of breast cancer in men, and is a natural consequence of the close proximity of breast ducts to overlying skin. One-third of men with breast cancer present with inversion, fixation, encrustation, or edema, and one-fourth present with ulceration (Figs. 41-1 and 41-2).[5]

DIFFERENTIAL DIAGNOSIS

Benign true neoplasms are extremely rare in men, and include cystosarcoma phyllodes, florid papillomatosis, ductal papillomas, lipomas, and a number of other tumors not related to the breast as a specialized organ. Far and away the most common cause of a benign mass in the male breast is gynecomastia; this differential diagnosis can usually be made on the basis of age and physical examination. Characteristically, gynecomastia is a tender, symmetrical, discoid, and often bilateral enlargement beneath the nipple and areola. Carcinoma tends to be nontender, eccentric, and hard. Both

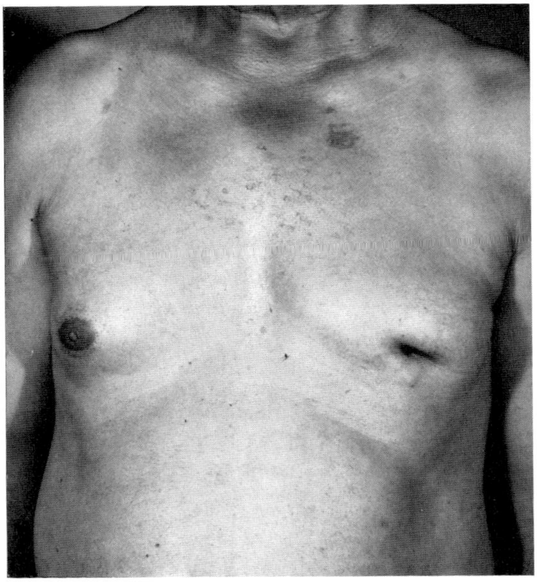

Figure 41-1 Nipple inversion from a carcinoma of the left breast which was not fixed to the pectoral fascia, but had metastasized to an axillary node and resulted in death 4 1/2 years later. (*From Crichlow RW, Kaplan EL, Kearney WH,*[90] *with permission.*)

may show some adherence to the overlying skin, but adherence to the pectoral fascia or nipple discharge, inversion, or ulceration indicate carcinoma. Aspiration biopsy is a simple method of identifying malignancy but cannot exclude it. Mammography has proven as useful in men as in women and the radiographic signs are similar in both sexes. While gynecomastia is characteristically seen in the midplane of the nipple radiographically, carcinomas are not.[27]

Although carcinoma of the breast has been reported in adolescent males,[5] the extraordinary rarity of carcinoma in the young makes a biopsy unnecessary to rule out carcinoma in a lesion showing all the characteristics of gynecomastia in this age group. The clinical differential diagnosis in older men is more difficult, and biopsy is certainly indicated if there is any suspicion of carcinoma.

PATHOLOGY

Virtually all pathologic types of carcinoma found in women have a counterpart in men (Fig. 41-3).[5] The relative frequency of each type is similar, except for lobular carcinoma. In its in situ form lobular carcinoma has not been reported in any men and in its invasive form is certainly less frequent than in women; a solitary report of invasive occurrence awaits confirmation.[28]

TREATMENT

There is no consensus for local regional management of carcinoma of the male breast. There are proponents of both conservative and radical surgery, with and without radiation therapy. Furthermore, treatment patterns which have evolved for women, especially modified radical mastectomy or primary radiotherapy, are not necessarily applicable to men, who present with tumors central and close to underlying pectoral muscle and overlying skin, an unusual presentation in women. If radical mastectomy is not chosen, excision of underlying pectoral muscle or postoperative radiation therapy to the chest wall should be strongly considered.

The initial operability of breast cancer in men does not appear to have changed significantly in the past three decades. In 1941 Sachs reported that 74 percent of 264 men had operable breast cancer,[29] and in 1974 Scheike found a prevalence of 78 percent in 253 men.[30] Of 495 male cases reported in the interval, 81 percent had operable breast cancer, with 68 percent undergoing radical mastectomy and 13 percent simple mastectomy.[1]

Axillary lymph node dissection for accurate staging is essential, as clinical assessment is inaccurate, and the presence of lymph node metastases has even greater impact on prognosis in men than in women. Lacour et al. from the European Cooperative Trial reported a 10-year survival rate of 25 percent in female patients

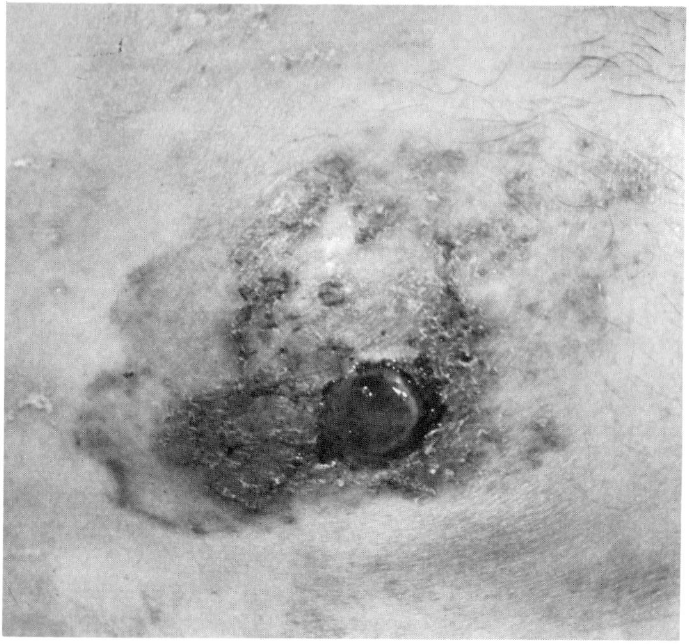

Figure 41-2 Nipple ulceration and adjacent infiltration resulting from an underlying carcinoma of the male breast. *(From Crichlow RW, Kaplan EL, Kearney WH,[90] with permission.)*

with both positive axillary and internal mammary nodes.[31] This is in contrast to the 10-year survival rate in men with positive axillary nodes of 14 percent (Table 41-1).

Postoperative radiotherapy to the internal mammary lymph nodes should be considered because of the central location of tumors in men. In the presence of tumor-positive axillary nodes, internal mammary nodes are positive in 25 to 50 percent of females with medial or central lesions.[31–34] When axillary nodes are tumor-free in similar lesions, the internal mammary nodes still contain tumors in 10 to 15 percent of patients.[32–34] Internal mammary nodes must reach at least 2 cm in greatest diameter to be seen on chest radiograph, and thus may first present as difficult management problems such as esophageal impingement, recurrent laryngeal nerve involvement, or parasternal mass. Therefore, postoperative radiation therapy should always be considered, and is indicated in the presence of positive axillary nodes unless supplanted by adjuvant chemotherapy.

There is no experience reported with adjuvant chemotherapy in men with axillary lymph node metastases. Comparable patterns of response to chemotherapy in women with metastatic disease, and some evidence for improved survival in women receiving postoperative chemotherapy, argue for use of adjuvant chemotherapy in men. Certainly, the dismal prognosis of men with lymph node involvement supports the use of any adjunct treatment which may improve outcome.

MANAGEMENT OF ADVANCED BREAST CANCER

Estrogen Receptors

In 1974, Wittliff provided the first report of the existence of cytoplasmic estrogen receptors in male breast carcinoma.[35] A total of 141 cases of male breast carcinoma for which estrogen receptors were assayed accumulated over the period 1975–1984 (Table 41-2). Of these, 127 (89 percent) contained cytoplasmic

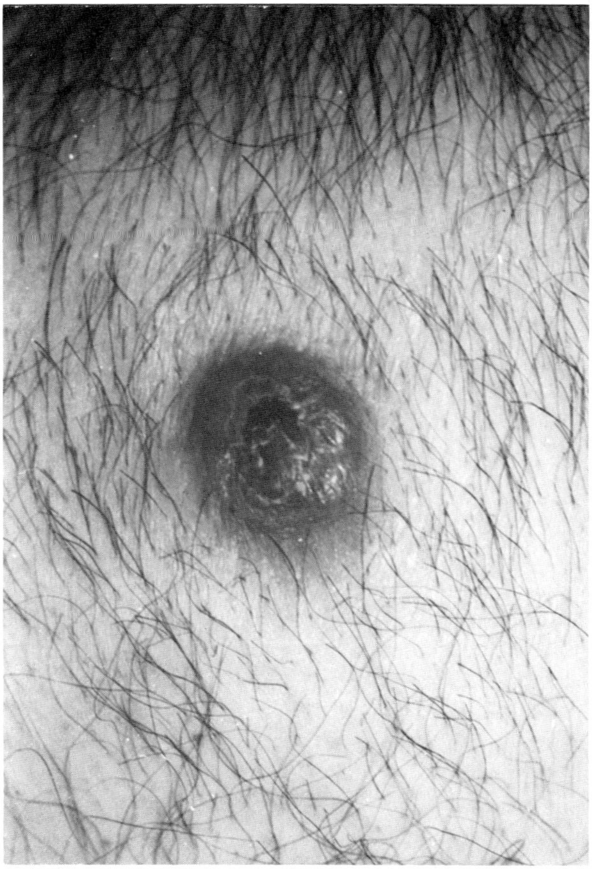

Figure 41-3 Excoriation and eschar of areola and nipple. (*From Crichlow RW, Czernobilsky B,*[91] *with permission.*)

estrogen receptors and 36 of 51 (71 percent) were positive for progesterone receptors. Nuclear estrogen receptors were studied by Pegoraro et al. and found to be present in eight of ten tumors.[36]

While data on estrogen receptor (ER) status and response to hormonal therapy are few, there appears to be a positive correlation between the two; 29/36 patients (81 percent) who were ER-positive responded to hormonal treatment (Table 41-2). Everson et al. found that patients with ER levels less than 30 fmol/mg protein failed to respond to hormonal therapy.[37] There was no significant correlation, however, between ER concentration and response duration.

Therapeutic Options

Patterns of metastases and recurrences of male breast cancer are similar to those in the female. Isolated metastases are best managed by excision or radiotherapy. For disseminated disease, the clinician faces a decision between ablative or additive hormonal therapy and chemotherapy.

Ablative Hormonal Therapy

Following the report in 1942 by Farrow and Adair,[38] orchiectomy became the accepted first-line treatment for disseminated male breast cancer. The procedure is technically simple,

Table 41-1 Relationship of Survival to Histopathology of Axillary Nodes

Reference	Node histology: Negative	Node histology: Positive
	Five-year survival	
1	$\frac{46}{58}$	$\frac{24}{85}$
65	$\frac{37}{41}$	$\frac{42}{40}$
64	$\frac{10}{13}$	$\frac{9}{24}$
89	$\frac{13}{23}$	$\frac{8}{26}$
60	$\frac{11}{17}$	$\frac{6}{11}$
Total	$\frac{117}{152}$ (77%)	$\frac{89}{186}$ (48%)
	Ten-year survival	
1	$\frac{16}{26}$	$\frac{1}{23}$
65	$\frac{13}{17}$	$\frac{2}{16}$
60	$\frac{10}{17}$	$\frac{4}{11}$
Total	$\frac{39}{60}$ (65%)	$\frac{7}{50}$ (14%)

associated with little morbidity, but limited by patient acceptance. Response rates have remained consistently high in reported series (Table 41-3). Treves found no relation between response and either age or histologic appearance of the testis,[39] so that unlike the female, the male's response to ablative therapy is not age-limited.

The role of adrenalectomy is less clear. Since the advent of hormonal and chemotherapeutic alternatives, adrenalectomy has become less popular. Limited experience with adrenalectomy, prior hormonal therapy, and lack of receptor correlation make the data difficult to review critically. Table 41-4 summarizes the results in 38 patients undergoing adrenalectomy. The response rate of 74 percent is noteworthy.

Hypophysectomy has been used less frequently than adrenalectomy, but with equal success. Meyskens et al. reviewed 17 cases;[40] of these there were ten responders with a median response duration of 20 months and a median survival from primary diagnosis of 90 months. Similar to adrenalectomy, seven of the ten responders to hypophysectomy had undergone prior orchiectomy. With the advent of the transsphenoidal approach, the morbidity and mortality of hypophysectomy are lessened; however, its use remains limited.

Additive Hormonal Therapy

Tamoxifen, similar to the other antiestrogens, clomiphene citrate and nafoxidine, is thought to act by binding to estrogen receptors, thereby blocking the uptake of estrogen by target tissues. Tamoxifen produces fewer side effects than the other two agents and has had more widespread use in women. To date, 61 men with metastatic breast carcinoma treated with tamoxifen have been reported, with a 46 percent response rate (Table 41-5).[41–53] Response to tamoxifen has been seen following both orchiectomy response and failure, suggesting that tamoxifen therapy and orchiectomy may be non-cross-resistant treatments.[49]

Limited experience with estrogen therapy has resulted in a poor overall response rate.[41,54] Ribeiro has reported the most encouraging results, with objectively assessed remissions occurring in 21 of 55 patients (38 percent).[55] Progestational agents, including medroxyprogesterone acetate[54,57] and megestrol acetate,[56] have produced more encouraging results in a small number of patients. Pannuti et al. reported a partial remission in five of six patients lasting a median of 7 months with high-dose medroxyprogesterone acetate.[56] Kantarjian et al. reported 6 responses in 14 patients (43 percent) with corticosteroids.[41] Of three patients who received them as the primary therapeutic modality, only one responded.

Chemotherapy

Yap et al. reviewed 29 chemotherapeutic trials in 18 men with breast carcinoma and found an overall response rate of 44 percent.[58] Both single- and multiagent regimens were used, and most of the patients had already undergone additive or ablative hormonal therapy. The median length of survival for those who demonstrated a chemotherapeutic response was 23 months.

Table 41-2 Presence of Cytoplasmic Hormone Receptors and Response to Hormonal Therapy

	Presence of receptors		Response* among individuals with receptors	
Reference	**Estrogen**	**Progesterone**	**Estrogen**	**Progesterone**
Contesso[67]	8/8	7/8		
Duffy[68]	3/4	2/4		
Ellison[69]	1/1	1/1	1/1	
Everson[37]	29/34	9/14	4/7	
Friedman[70]	12/12		2/2	
Gress[71]	0/1			
Grilli[72]	2/2			
Gupta[73]	5/6		4/5	
Hahnel[74]	0/2			
Hilliard[48]	1/1		1/1 †	
Korsten[75]	1/1		1/1	
Kraybill[54]	3/4		3/3	
Leclercq[76]	7/10			
Leung[77]	2/2		1/2	
Mitsuyasu[57]	1/1	1/1	1/1	
Mobbs[78]	1/1			
Moseley[79]	1/1		1/1	
Nomura[80]	2/2		1/2	
Ouriel[81]	8/10		2/4	
Pannuti[56]	1/1			
Patel[82]	3/3		3/3 (1†)	
Patterson[43]	5/8	2/3	4/5	2/3
Pegoraro[36]	12/13	6/9	3/3	
Raynaud[83]	8/8			
Ribeiro[50]	5/5	3/5	4/5	2/3
Rosen[84]	3/3			
Ruff[85]	14/14	8/12	2/2	
Saltzstein[86]	0/1			
Silvfersward[87]	5/5			
Thompson[88]	1/1	1/1	0/1	
Wittliff[35]	1/1			
Total	147/166 (89%)	36/51 (71%)	29/36 (81%)	4/6 (67%)

* Response = remission after hormonal therapy.
† No response to orchiectomy, subsequent response to tamoxifen.

Considering the therapeutic alternatives, variations in receptor status, and differing sites of metastatic spread, it is not surprising that a consensus for therapy of disseminated disease has yet to develop. If estrogen receptors are present, additive hormonal therapy with tamoxifen should proceed. Tamoxifen, well-tolerated and yielding a 46 percent response rate across the board (10/11 ER-positive), may well replace orchiectomy as the first-line therapy for systemic disease. With further progression, orchiectomy is indicated; adrenalectomy or hypophysectomy and chemotherapy should be reserved for subsequent treatment failures. The approach to receptor-negative patients with disseminated tumors remains less clear. While

Table 41-3 Remission of Breast Cancer Following Orchiectomy

	Response				Estrogen receptor status	
Reference	Fraction responding	%	Mean duration, months	Survival, months	Positive	Negative
Treves[39]	28/41	68	29			
Holleb[3]	17/38	45				
Crichlow[1]	17/29	59				
Meyskens[40]*	47/70	67	22†	56		
Everson[37]	5/13	38			5/13	
Kraybill[54]	11/23	49	27	58.4	3/3	0/1
Kantarjian[41]	8/25	32	17.5†	43.5		
Patel[82]	11/22	50	15		2/3	
Total	144/261	55				

* Collected series
† Median

none of five reported ER-negative patients responded to hormonal manipulation,[43,54,59] these scant data do not yet warrant exclusion of such patients. The high overall response to hormonal manipulation of advanced male breast cancer may be due to the preponderance of ER-positive tumors, and receptor-negative tumors may carry the same therapeutic implications as in the female.

PROGNOSIS

Prognosis in presumably localized male breast cancer is determined by a variety of factors, the most important of which is the presence or absence, by microscopic examination, of metastases in axillary nodes. Clinical staging by node palpation is useful for treatment planning but is not optimal for determining prognosis. Axillary dissection is needed to overcome the inaccuracies of clinical assessment of regional nodes.[60,61] The prognostic importance of the histopathology of axillary lymph nodes is illustrated in Table 41-1. The presence of metastases in axillary nodes affects survival substantially at 5 years and markedly at 10 years, to an extent far greater than in women.

Other factors also contribute to prognosis, probably by affecting the stage of initial presentation. The prediagnosis duration of symptoms is inversely correlated with survival.[60,62,63] Robinson found that patients with clinically

Table 41-4 Remission of Breast Cancer Following Adrenalectomy

	Response			
Reference	Fraction responding	%	Mean duration, months	Survival, months
Moseley[79]	1/1	100		
Meyskens[40]*	19/25	76	32†	42
Kraybill[54]	0/2	0		
Patel[82]	8/10	80	15	
Total	28/38	74		

* Collected series
† Median

Table 41-5 Remission of Breast Cancer Following Tamoxifen Therapy

	Fraction responding			Estrogen receptor status	
Reference	Overall	Before orchiectomy	After orchiectomy	Positive	Negative
Patterson[43]	12/22			3/3	
Becher[42]	2/2	2/2			
Tirelli[49]	2/4	0/2	2/2		
Kantarjian[41]	2/8	2/7	0/1		
Ribeiro[50]	9/24			6/7	0/3
Hilliard[48]	1/1		1/1	1/1	
Total	28/61 (46%)				

favorable stages of disease had an average delay in diagnosis of 10 months, whereas patients with locally or regionally advanced disease had an average delay of 18 months.[62] Appelqvist grouped patients according to duration of symptoms: up to 3 months, 4 to 11 months, and 12 months and greater; 10-year survival rates were 100, 50, and 25 percent, respectively.[60]

Differentiation of the carcinoma[60] and tumor size[64] are also related to patient survival. Yap noted that patients with primary breast lesions of > 5 cm diameter had a median time to first recurrence of only 5 months,[64] which is significantly different from the 41- and 25-month intervals reported for lesions ≤ 2 cm and 2 to 5 cm, respectively. Median survival time for lesions ≥ 5 cm in diameter was only 15 months.

The central location of breast cancer in men has been implicated in the decreased 10-year survival rate compared with females of the same pathologic stage.[65] One factor may be the greater risk of lymphatic spread by other than the axillary route. The sparseness of breast tissue in men places even a small tumor close to both overlying skin and underlying pectoral fascia without the separation afforded by the greater bulk of intervening breast tissue in women. Heller noted fewer men with T_2N_0 disease and more with T_1N_1 disease than in a similar group of women.[65] Since T_1N_1 disease has a poorer prognosis than T_2N_0 disease, this may contribute to the poor prognosis of men with stage II breast cancer.[65,66]

REFERENCES

1. Crichlow RW: Breast cancer in men. *Semin Oncol* 1:145, 1974.
2. Moss NH: Cancer of the male breast. *Ann NY Acad Sci* 114:937, 1964.
3. Holleb AI, Freeman HP, Farrow JH: Cancer of the male breast. Part II. *NY State J Med* 68:656, 1968.
4. De Waard F, Baanders-Van Helewijn EA, Huizinga J: The bimodal age distribution of patients with mammary carcinoma. *Cancer* 17:141, 1964.
5. Crichlow RW: Carcinoma of the male breast. *Surg Gynecol Obstet* 134:1011, 1972.
6. Marger D, Urdaneta N, Fischer JJ: Breast cancer in brothers: Case reports and a review of 30 cases of male breast cancer. *Cancer* 36:458, 1975.
7. Liechty RD, Davis J, Gleysteen J: Cancer of the male breast: Forty cases. *Cancer* 20:1617, 1967.
8. Symmers W ST C: Carcinoma of breast in transsexual individuals after surgical and hormonal interference with the primary and secondary sex characteristics. *Br Med J* 2:83, 1968.
9. Benson WR: Carcinoma of the prostate with metastases to breasts and testis: Critical review of the literature and report of a case. *Cancer* 10:1235, 1957.
10. Campbell JH, Cummins SD: Metastases simulating mammary cancer, in prostatic carcinoma under estrogenic therapy. *Cancer* 4:303, 1951.

11. Schottenfeld D, Lilienfeld AM, Diamond H: Some observations on the epidemiology of breast cancer among males. *Am J Publ Health* 58:890, 1963.
12. Jackson AW, Muldal S, Ockey CH, O'Connor PJ: Carcinoma of male breast in association with the Klinefelter syndrome. *Br Med J* 1:223, 1965.
13. Scheike O, Visfeldt J, Peterson B: Male breast cancer. 3. Breast carcinoma in association with the Klinefelter syndrome. *Acta Pathol Microbiol Scand* 81:3, 1973.
14. Davis JC, Wade AP: Discordant identical twins. III. Klinefelter's syndrome discordant for carcinoma of the breast. *Practitioner* 209:380, 1972.
15. Scheike O, Visfeldt J: Male breast cancer. 4. Gynecomastia in patients with breast cancer. *Acta Pathol Microbiol Scand* 81:359, 1973.
16. Lyall A: Choriocarcinoma of the testis with gynecomastia: Report of a case with early breast carcinoma. *Br J Surg* 34:278, 1947.
17. Everson RB, Li FP, Fraumeni JF, Fishman J, Wilson RE, Stout D, Norris HJ: Familial breast cancer. *Lancet* 1:9, 1976.
18. Haagensen CD: *Diseases of the Breast*, 2d ed. Philadelphia, W. B. Saunders, 1971, p. 780.
19. Lin RS, Kessler II: Epidemiologic findings in male breast cancer. *Proc Am Assoc Cancer Res* 21:72, 1980.
20. Steinitz R, Katz L, Ben-Hur M: Male breast cancer in Israel: Selected epidemiological aspects. *Isr J Med Sci* 17:816, 1981.
21. Modan B, Mintz U, Finkelman J: Male breast cancer in Israel: Selected epidemiological and clinical aspects. *J Chron Dis* 23:55, 1970.
22. Keller AZ: Demographic, clinical and survivorship characteristics of males with primary cancer of the breast. *Am J Epidemiol* 85:183, 1967.
23. Scheike O: Male breast cancer. V. Clinical manifestations in 257 cases in Denmark. *Br J Cancer* 28:552, 1973.
24. Treves N, Robbins GF, Amoroso WL: Serous and serosanguineous discharge from the male nipple. *Arch Surg* 73:319, 1956.
25. Mausner JS, Shimkin MB, Moss NH, Rosemond BP: Cancer of the breast in Philadelphia hospitals 1951–1964. *Cancer* 23:260, 1969.
26. Donegan WL, Perez-Mesa CM: Carcinoma of the male breast: A 30-year review of 28 cases. *Arch Surg* 106:273, 1973.
27. Kalisher L, Peyster RG: Xerographic manifestations of male breast disease. *Am J Roentgenol Radium Ther Nucl Med* 125:656, 1975.
28. Giffler FR, Kay S: Small-cell carcinoma of the male mammary gland, a tumor resembling infiltrating lobular carcinoma. *Am J Clin Pathol* 66:715, 1976.
29. Sachs MD: Carcinoma of the male breast. *Radiology* 37:458, 1941.
30. Scheike O: Male breast cancer. 6. Factors influencing prognosis. *Br J Cancer* 30:261, 1974.
31. Lacour J, Lê M, Caceres E, Koszarowski T, Veronesi U, Hill C: Radical mastectomy versus radical mastectomy plus internal mammary dissection: Ten year results of an international cooperative trial in breast cancer. *Cancer* 51:1941, 1983.
32. Handley RS: The early spread of breast carcinoma and its bearing on operative treatment. *Br J Surg* 51:206, 1964.
33. Caceres E: An evaluation of radical mastectomy and extended radical mastectomy for cancer of the breast. *Surg Gynecol Obstet* 125:337, 1967.
34. Lacour J, Bucalossi P, Caceres E, Jacobelli G, Koszarowski T, Lê M, Rumeau-Rouquette C, Veronesi U: Radical mastectomy versus radical mastectomy plus internal mammary dissection: Five-year results of an international cooperative study. *Cancer* 37:206, 1976.
35. Wittliff JL: Specific receptors of the steroid hormones in breast cancer. *Semin Oncol* 1:109, 1974.
36. Pegoraro RJ, Nirmul D, Joubert SM: Cytoplasmic and nuclear estrogen and progesterone receptors in male breast cancer. *Cancer Res* 42:4812, 1982.
37. Everson RB, Lippman ME, Thompson EB, et al: Clinical correlations of steroid receptors and male breast cancer. *Cancer Res* 40:991, 1980.
38. Farrow JH, Adair FE: Effect of orchiectomy on skeletal metastases from cancer of the male breast. *Science* 95:654, 1942.
39. Treves N: The treatment of cancer, especially inoperable cancer, of the male breast by ablative surgery (orchiectomy, adrenalectomy and hypophysectomy) and hormone therapy (estrogens and corticosteroids): An analysis of 42 patients. *Cancer* 12:820, 1959.
40. Meyskens FL, Tormey DC, Neifeld JP: Male breast cancer: A review. *Cancer Treat Rev* 3:83, 1976.
41. Kantarjian H, Yap H-Y, Hortobagyi GN, Buzdar A, Blumenschein G: Hormonal therapy for

metastatic male breast cancer. *Arch Intern Med* 143:237, 1983.

42. Becher R, Hoffken K, Pape H, Schmidt C-G: Tamoxifen treatment before orchiectomy in advanced breast cancer in men. *N Engl J Med* 305:169, 1981.
43. Patterson JS, Battersby LA, Bach BK: Use of tamoxifen in advanced male breast cancer. *Cancer Treat Rep* 64:801, 1980.
44. Aisner J, Ross DD, Wiernik PH: Tamoxifen in advanced male breast cancer. *Arch Intern Med* 139:480, 1979.
45. Jefferys DB, Epthimiou J: Carcinoma of the male breast and oestrogen metabolism. *Br Med J* 1:1697, 1978.
46. Morgan DAL: Carcinoma of the male breast and oestrogen metabolism. *Br Med J* 2:206, 1978.
47. Horrobagyi GN, Distefano A, Legha SS, Buzdar AU, Blumenschein GR: Hormonal therapy with tamoxifen in male breast cancer. *Cancer Treat Rep* 63:539, 1979.
48. Hilliard DA, Wilbur DW, Camacho ES: Tamoxifen response following no response to orchiectomy in metastatic male breast cancer: A case report. *J Surg Oncol* 25:42, 1984.
49. Tirelli U, Tumolo S, Talamini R, et al: Tamoxifen before and after orchiectomy in advanced male breast cancer. *Cancer Treat Rep* 66:1882, 1982.
50. Ribeiro GG: Tamoxifen in the treatment of male breast carcinoma. *Clin Radiol* 34:625, 1983.
51. Abel R, Alberto P, Megevand R: Carcinoma of the male breast and oestrogen metabolism. *Br Med J* 1:1697, 1978.
52. Cantwell BMJ, Tong D, Minton M, et al: Tamoxifen and male breast cancer. *Lancet* 2:582, 1978.
53. Sakai F, Cheix F, Clavel M, et al: Increases in steroid binding globulins induced by tamoxifen in patients with carcinoma of the breast. *J Endocrinol* 76:219, 1978.
54. Kraybill WG, Kaufman R, Kinne D: Treatment of advanced male breast cancer. *Cancer* 47:2185, 1981.
55. Ribeiro GG: The results of diethylstilboestrol therapy for recurrent and metastatic carcinoma of the male breast. *Br J Cancer* 33:465, 1976.
56. Pannuti F, Martoni A, Busitti L, Gramellini M, Piana E: High-dose medroxyprogesterone acetate in advanced male breast cancer. *Cancer Treat Rep* 66:1763, 1982.
57. Mitsuyasu R, Bonomi P, Anderson K, Fisher W: Response to megestrol in male breast cancer. *Arch Intern Med* 141:809, 1981.
58. Yap H-Y, Tashima CK, Blumenschein GR, Hortobagyi GN, Eckles N: Chemotherapy for advanced male breast cancer. *JAMA* 243:1739, 1980.
59. Gupta N, Cohen JL, Rosenbaum C, Raam S: Estrogen receptors in male breast cancer. *Cancer* 46:1781, 1980.
60. Appleqvist P, Salmo M: Prognosis in carcinoma of the male breast. *Acta Chir Scand* 148:499, 1982.
61. Cutler SJ, Connelly RR: Mammary cancer trends. *Cancer* 23:767, 1969.
62. Robinson FW, Farha GC: Carcinoma of the male breast. *Am J Surg* 113:394, 1967.
63. Roswell B, Edlis H: Carcinoma of the male breast: A thirty year experience and literature review. *Int J Rad Oncol Biol Phys* 4:711, 1978.
64. Yap H-Y, Tashima CK, Blumenschein GR, Eckles NE: Male breast cancer: A natural history study. *Cancer* 44:748, 1979.
65. Heller KS, Rosen PP, Schottenfeld D, Ashikari R, Kinne DW: Male breast cancer: A clinicopathologic study of 97 cases. *Ann Surg* 188:60, 1978.
66. Ribeiro GG: Carcinoma of the male breast: A review of 200 cases. *Br J Surg* 64:381, 1977.
67. Contesso G, Delarue J-C, Guerinot FM-L, Bohuon C: Recepteurs aux estrogenes et aux progestogenes en pathologie mammaire chez l'homme. *Nouv Presse Med* 6:1951, 1977.
68. Duffy MJ, Duffy GJ: Multiple steroid receptors in male breast carcinomas. *Clinica Chimica Acta* 85:211, 1978.
69. Ellison HS, Scheurer SA, Eichner ER: Metastatic breast carcinoma with positive estrogen and progesterone receptors in a man with Klinefelter's syndrome. *South Med J* 73:1393, 1980.
70. Friedman MA, Hoffman PG, Dandolas EM, Lagios MD, Johnston WH, Suteri PK: Estrogen receptors in male breast cancer: Clinical and pathologic correlations. *Cancer* 47:134, 1981.
71. Gress RE, Piantadosi CA, Skubitz KM, Hsu T-H: Breast carcinoma, thyroid carcinoma, and T_3 thyrotoxicosis in a male cretin. *Johns Hopkins Med J* 140:317, 1977.
72. Grilli S, De Giovanni C, Galli MC, et al: The simultaneous occurrence of cytoplasmic receptors for various steroid hormones in male breast carcinoma and gynaecomastia. *J Steroid Biochem* 13:813, 1980.

73. Gupta N, Cohen JL, Rosenbaum C, Raam S: Estrogen receptors in male breast cancer. *Cancer* 46:1781, 1980.
74. Hahnel R, Twaddle E: Estimation of the association constant of the estrogen-receptor complex in human breast cancer. *Cancer Res* 33:559, 1973.
75. Korsten CB, Englesman E, Persijn JP: Clinical value of estrogen receptors in advanced male breast cancer, in McGuire WL, Carbone PP, Vollmer EP (eds): *Estrogen Receptors in Human Breast Cancer.* New York, Raven, 1975, p. 93.
76. Leclercq G, Verhest A, Deboel MC, Van Schoubroeck F, Mattheiem WH, Heuson JC: Oestrogen receptors in male breast cancer. *Biomedicine* 25:327, 1976.
77. Leung BS, Moseley HS, Davenport CE, Krippaehne WW, Fletcher WS: Estrogen receptor in prediction of clinical responses to endocrine ablation, in McGuire WL, Carbone PP, Vollmer EP (eds): *Estrogen Receptors in Human Breast Cancer.* New York, Raven, 1975, p. 107.
78. Mobbs BG, Johnson IE: In vitro estrogen-binding by human breast carcinomas. *Can Med Assoc J* 114:216, 1976.
79. Moseley HS, Fletcher WS, Leung BS, Krippaehne WW: Predictive criteria for the selection of breast cancer patients for adrenalectomy. *Am J Surg* 128:143, 1974.
80. Nomura Y, Kondo H, Yamagata J, Takenaka K: Detection of the estrogen receptor and response to endocrine therapy in male breast cancer patients. *Gann* 68:333, 1977.
81. Ouriel K, Lotze MT, Hinshaw JR: Prognostic factors of carcinoma of the male breast. *Surg Gynecol Obstet* 159:373, 1984.
82. Patel JK, Nemoto T, Dao TL: Metastatic breast cancer in males: Assessment of endocrine therapy. *Cancer* 53:1344, 1984.
83. Raynaud JP, Ojasoo T, Delarue JC, Magdelenat H, Martin P, Philibert D: Estrogen and progestin receptors in human breast cancer, in McGuire WL (ed): *Progesterone Receptors in Normal and Neoplastic Tissues.* New York, Raven, 1977, p. 177.
84. Rosen PP, Monendez-Botet CJ, Nisselbaum JS, Schwartz MK, Urban JA: Estrogen receptor protein in lesions of the male breast: A preliminary report. *Cancer* 37:1866, 1976.
85. Ruff SJ, Bauer JE, Keenan EJ, Moseley HS, Fletcher WS: Hormone receptors in male breast carcinoma. *J Surg Oncol* 18:55, 1981.
86. Saltzstein EC, Tavaf AM, Latorraca R: Breast carcinoma in a young man. *Arch Surg* 113:880, 1978.
87. Silvfersward C, Gustafsson J-A, Gustafsson SA, et al: Estrogen receptor concentrations in 269 cases of histologically classified human breast cancer. *Cancer* 45:2001, 1980.
88. Thompson EB, Perlin E, Tormey D: Steroid-binding proteins in carcinoma of the human male breast. *Am J Clin Pathol* 65:360, 1976.
89. Ramantanis B, Besbeas S, Garas JG: Breast cancer in the male: A report of 138 cases. *World J Surg* 4:621, 1980.
90. Crichlow RW, Kaplan EL, Kearney WH: Male mammary cancer: An analysis of 32 cases. *Ann Surg* 175:489, 1972.
91. Crichlow RW, Czernobilsky B: Paget's disease of the male breast. *Cancer* 24:1033, 1969.

Part Nine

Support for the Breast Cancer Patient

42

The Psychological Aspects of Women with Breast Cancer

Adrienne E. Snyderman, M.S.W.
Reuven K. Snyderman, M.D.

INTRODUCTION

Breast cancer is a medical and a life crisis. Unfortunately, neither medical nor life issues are as yet thoroughly explored by those who are entrusted with the care of patients with breast cancer. The interaction between medical issues and life issues for the overwhelming proportion of breast cancer patients who are female is addressed here. Because of this interaction, the total care of the woman with breast cancer and her family must include consideration of psychosocial issues. The combination of psychosocial consideration and medical care is needed to help patients integrate, in a positive manner, their experiences with this disease. Furthermore, understanding that medical treatment is easier and perhaps more successful when the psychological needs of the patient are considered gives support to the interventions which include caring for the total needs of the patient.

A crisis is defined as a turning point where the future course may become either better or worse. Jacobson suggests that a crisis can lead to a time of adaptation, change, and growth. Whatever the outcome, this is a decisive time in the life of a breast cancer patient, both medically and psychologically. Therefore, the list of possible interventions for breast cancer must include all of those which can aid in promoting adaptation for the patient and her family.

Most people are closely involved with others whose influence, positive or negative, must be considered at all times, especially at times of stress. Thus total care for breast cancer may be defined as (1) considering the medical issues and options, (2) hearing the concerns of the patient, (3) understanding the issues for the breast cancer patient, (4) being aware of the impact of her whole situation on her social system, and (5) designing treatment with all of these considerations in mind.

THE ROLE OF THE PRIMARY PHYSICIAN

The first issue is that medical care be appropriate. Initially, a thorough evaluation and discussion with the patient of possible modes of treatment should take place. The issue of assessing and defining medical treatment often brings us face-to-face with the controversies about treatment. In some cases, the recommendation of a single treatment modality is obvious. In many cases, however, there are choices. When there are options or choices, they must be considered in both medical and psychological frames of reference.

A case of a recent patient demonstrates how medical and psychological considerations are combined. A woman in her late sixties who had had a mastectomy and adjuvant chemotherapy had been psychologically supported and encouraged by her husband during the extended period of diagnosis and treatment. A year or so later, an excisional biopsy of a mass in her neck confirmed a recurrence of the cancer. Her physician recommended a second course of chemotherapy, but the patient was emphatic that she felt unable to take chemotherapy a second time; even with the support of her husband, she had found it extremely difficult to sustain treatment in the first instance. Her husband had died in the interim. She felt alone and powerless because she had lost her vital support person. The agitated patient turned to her plastic surgeon. Because the surgeon felt unable to help the patient in her emotional state, he referred her to a counselor.

After fully reviewing the situation, the counselor proposed that the patient explore alternative treatment to the chemotherapy with her physician. The patient showed and expressed instant relief when she realized that the counselor had recognized her concerns. With the release of anxiety, the patient felt ready, comfortable, and able to participate in choosing appropriate treatment. The patient easily and comfortably tolerated radiation therapy because she felt that she had participated in an appropriate choice of treatment, one which was congruous with her real feelings.

This case study demonstrates that if a patient takes an active role in choosing her own treatment, she may be more comfortable, more compliant, and better able to withstand treatment. Therefore, physicians must continually be aware of the patient's feelings during the initial period of diagnosis and planning of treatment.

The research of the Simontons shows that patients who are actively involved in imagining their healthy cells engulfing their cancer cells survive longer and seem to control the course of their disease.[5] The patient who equates cancer with death dies. The patient who aggressively seeks to control the disease is able, in some way, to have an influence on the course of the disease. Thus, to have the patient emotionally involved in efforts to control her disease seems to promote the first goal of treatment, which is longevity. As for the goal of maintaining the quality of life, it is obvious that the patient whose emotions are considered as part of her total care is receiving treatment which is consistent with promoting a quality existence.

Another consideration is how the patient reacts, cognitively, to the positive diagnosis of breast cancer. As Schain notes, some patients have a cognitive style which makes it impossible to accept a recommended treatment without doing their own exhaustive investigation.[4] Their style of coping with anxiety makes monitoring every area of decision a requirement. In contrast, there are other patients who block out as many areas of decision making as possible. Their emotions are only kept under control by not dealing with issues. These patients want to be cared for without being too involved in making decisions. It is up to the primary care physician to judge where the patient lies cognitively. Thus, the physician has many important choices to make. These include assessing treatment choices and judging how this information should be presented to the patient. This kind of practice redefines the role of the physician as a *facilitator*, both in the process of choosing the best and most acceptable treatment and in curing the patient's cancer. When the physician begins to share responsibility for making decisions with the person whose life is in the balance, this redefinition can help the patient retrieve some control over her life. The physician is no longer the person who is totally responsible for both choosing treatment and curing the cancer. Instead, the patient and physician begin to form a team whose members also include the patient's family. The team's participants are available for mutual support during the whole period of involvement with the patient's disease.

THE ROLE OF THE PLASTIC SURGEON

It can only be presumed that women of the Halsted period had the same reaction to their mastectomies as do women today. At that time, however, most were unwilling to express their fear and anger to their physicians. Their surgeons probably gave little time or thought to their patients' emotions. There has been little or no information available about the psychological reactions of those women with breast cancer.

In the years when radical mastectomy was the only treatment for breast cancer, patients turned to plastic surgeons not only for breast reconstruction but also to help regain control of their lives. This was probably not a conscious choice for most women; but, because the consultation with the plastic surgeon was an option rather than a requirement of treatment for the disease, it served to promote a return of control to the patient and to make her feel restored both physically and psychologically. Though breast reconstruction at this time was anything but a cosmetic triumph, the return of some sort of breast represented a return of control to the patient who had been unable to make her own decision about the primary surgery.

The consultation with the plastic surgeon provided the patient with the opportunity to reconfirm that the mastectomy which she had undergone was, indeed, a necessary mode of treatment. The patient was also able to express her feelings to a member of the medical profession who would listen, understand, and empathize with her. The plastic surgeon had not been involved in her primary care and it was safe for the patient to express anger in his or her presence. Plastic surgeons became psychological support persons without even realizing that their functions in dealing with breast cancer patients were medical, physical, and psychological.

The modern era of breast reconstruction dawned in the 1960s following the development of the silicone implant. Though reconstruction had been carried out for many years, it had been a long, complicated procedure which required many hospital admissions. Because the silicone implant made breast reconstruction so much easier and faster, greater numbers of mastectomy patients began to choose this option as part of their treatment.

The sixties was also the time when the women's movement began to focus on the anger which women felt about lack of control of their own lives. Women began to question promotion of mastectomy as the treatment for breast cancer by the predominantly male medical establishment. Though some surgeons were reluctant to discuss breast reconstruction or advocate it, patients sought referrals to plastic surgeons. Plastic surgeons began to be aware that there were pressing physical and psychological issues for breast cancer patients that related to their diagnosis and treatment, and to the possibility of recurrence of their disease. Plastic surgeons began to notice that when patients received information about breast reconstruction they began to feel better, whether or not they opted for the reconstructive surgery. Some of what had been lost in the assault by the disease seemed to be returned to the patient who had a choice to make.

SOCIAL WORKERS

It soon became evident that the consultation with the plastic surgeon satisfied neither the patient's quest for information nor her eagerness to express her innermost feelings. At this juncture, specially trained counselors came to be seen as the appropriate people to help patients deal with their emotional aspects. The social worker or counselor could help both physicians and patients. By helping the patient and her loved ones express and share their feelings, the counselor provided service for the patient, her family, and the physician.

THE TEAM APPROACH

Women with breast cancer who are contemplating mastectomy with or without reconstruction, radiation treatment, or chemotherapy are in great need of adequate counseling. Most want to discuss their problems, not only with personnel of the medical field but also with other women who have undergone a similar experience. The Comprehensive Breast Center of the University of Medicine and Dentistry of New Jersey—Rutgers Medical School evolved for this purpose. General surgeons, plastic surgeons, chemotherapists, radiation therapists, diagnostic radiologists, social workers, psychiatrists, physical therapists, and a group of breast cancer patients join so that women with breast problems and their families have available a variety of services related to their diagnosis, treatment, and recovery from breast cancer.

THE CONSTANT FEAR OF CANCER

To recover or cope, the breast cancer patient must reorganize her feelings into a new reality which contains a revised view of how she sees her life and her body. The discovery of cancer means that the healthy body of the patient no longer exists. She must be concerned continually that there was or is cancer in her body. This fact confronts her for the rest of her life. Though treatment is aimed at curing cancer, she will always be concerned about recurrence and the possibility of eventual death from the cancer.

When not concerned about the possible ravages of the disease the patient is concerned about the physical changes which accompany breast cancer treatment. The integrity of her body is physically and psychologically shattered by this disease because treatment will effect at least some change in the patient's physical appearance. When the treatment is mastectomy, the loss of the breast in its entirety promotes a strong emotional reaction in the patient. The patient can still be overwhelmed emotionally, even when breast-sparing techniques are chosen as treatment. Thus, in the battle for emotional survival, interventions which will help patients and families find healthy adaptations to their situations and feelings are necessary.

In the context of relationships, both intimate and supportive, it is important not to overlook how valued breasts are both physically and sexually and, therefore, psychologically in western society. (See Chap. 1.) Changes in the physical person often necessitate a total readjustment for the patient in her feelings about her relationships. That there might be problems in adjustment in the area of intimate, sexual relationships is easily recognized, but how the world views a breast cancer patient also has tremendous impact. As the patient's need to reorganize her feelings about her relationships as well as other aspects of her life is added to her other pressing concerns, the breast cancer patient is often overwhelmed.

THE ROLE OF THE FAMILY

Patients who have not dealt physically with their mastectomies certainly have not been able to confront their own psychological issues. When these patients turn to breast reconstruction to take care of both physical and psychological problems, they are in need of counseling, for reconstruction of the body will not repair mental and emotional trauma. Because the patient has to deal with her own mortality, the physical insult, and the feelings about and results of physical treatment all at the same time, support seems not to be enough care. Thus, even without definitive research about the timing of intervention in the process of total care, a single counseling session with a trained, caring professional at the outset would provide an arena for the patient in which she could express her real feelings and could share her experience. Other members of the family or her husband could join the session so that all those who are concerned and involved could make use of the intervention.

Little is mentioned in the literature about helping the families of breast cancer patients. They too should have both supportive and helping services available. Understanding that their adjustment, like that of the primary patient, will take time means that services for the social system which surrounds the primary patient should be available in the same way and at the same time as for the patient. The counselor who is prepared to help families deal with their issues can help fill this void with both consideration and professional intervention.

"Significant others" most often feel that to choose breast reconstruction is a decision for the patient; they will support her whatever choice she makes. However, if support is not offered by those close to the patient, it can indicate that there is a relationship problem. Counselors and physicians should be aware that when families do not support the patient, a conflict exists which is an expression of problems which existed before the cancer was a concern for all.

Finally, adjustment for the patient and her social system does not mean being finished with the emotional overlay which is part of breast cancer. There is a definite, positive adjustment to the crisis of breast cancer. As Singer prescribes,[6] it is necessary to deal with reality and the feelings surrounding this reality in order to get relief from the volume of feelings evoked by cancer. Both families and patients benefit from the release of guilt, mourning, fear, anger, sadness, and loneliness that all those involved may be feeling. Though anxious feelings can be expected when medical checkups or treatments are to take place, dealing appropriately means that cancer is a part of life, but not the only part of life.

CONCLUSION

Raising the conciousness of patients and their families about the emotional issues which are part of dealing with breast cancer can provide the release of feelings. It is often the unexpressed feelings that cause tension and anxiety which are the emotional overlay of this group of patients. The simple intervention of asking what having breast cancer means can be a key to treatment and adjustment, which can limit fear rather than let fear overwhelm all who are concerned. By providing a mental health checkup as an intervention for breast cancer, the psychic component of illness and wellness receives appropriate attention. The value of understanding and sharing emotions to promote positive coping with the crisis of breast cancer cannot be overemphasized as a component of breast cancer treatment.

In time of crisis, it is necessary first to examine the whole picture and understand that those in crisis need help so that they can deal with the multiplicity of issues which are typical of crisis situations. Professional intervention is the way to help patients and families return to full, active lives as quickly as possible. This can change the focus of all who deal with breast cancer to the preciousness of life rather than the all-consuming fear of death. A positive adjustment to the life crisis of breast cancer can be promoted. Help with psychosocial issues is the key to promoting mental health as part of total care of breast cancer patients and their families.

REFERENCES

1. Jacobson EN: *Coping With The Crises In Your Life*. New York, Hawthorn, 1974.
2. Kubler-Ross E: *On Death And Dying*. New York, Macmillan, 1975.
3. National Cancer Institute, U.S. Department of Health and Human Services: *The Breast Cancer Digest*. 84:1691, 1984.
4. Schain WS: "Psychosocial Issues and Management of Breast Cancer." Belle Mead, N.J., Carrier Foundation, 1984.
5. Simonton OC, Mathews-Simonton S, Creighton JL: *Getting Well Again*. New York, Bantam, 1978.
6. Singer B: The psychological impact of cancer on patient and family. *J Med Soc NJ* 81:383, 1984.
7. Snyderman AE: Breast cancer management: How the social worker can participate, in *Cancer Update* vol. 4. American Cancer Society, 1984.

43

The Provision of Support to Patients and Their Husbands

Robert S. Weiss, Ph.D.

INTRODUCTION

For two decades this author's research group has been learning about the impact on people of life crises. Work has focused on the life crises of marital separation and conjugal bereavement and, to a much lesser extent, of other bereavements, of difficulties in work, and of geographical uprooting. We have developed principles that can help physicians and surgeons provide their patients with psychological and emotional help.

Physicians sometimes delegate responsibility for dealing with patients as people to psychiatrists, priests, and social workers. Often this practice can be justified: a physician's time is pressed; it would be poor resource management to spend it on a task others can do. Furthermore, providing emotional support may not be a skill the physician has developed. However, the physician sometimes is in a unique position to affect positively the emotional state of the woman with breast cancer and her husband and to facilitate their effective management of stress. Physicians should be able to recognize such occasions and should know how to deal with them.

In this chapter physicians are offered a few potentially useful principles for dealing with patients and their husbands. First, consider the situation of the patient with breast cancer who can be expected to be cured by treatment; and second, the unhappy event of the metastasizing of the cancer so that the patient has entered a terminal course.

THE PATIENT WITH SUSPECTED BREAST CANCER

Principle *In order to come to terms with a reversal, people have to have some understanding of how it happened.*

Explain to the patient the risk factors in cancer, as well as the probabilities that the patient will develop breast cancer given the risk factors. Describe the mechanisms by which breast cancer forms, so far as they are known. Ask the patient whether she is worried about the following as possible causes: nursing (or failure to nurse), sex play, an injury; each of these can be a reason for baseless blaming of the self or of others. In general, help the patient to establish an adequate account of the cause of the cancer.

Principle *Absence of anticipation of reversal leads individuals to generalized anxiety and sometimes to phobic or nearly phobic behavior.*

Being hit by a lightning bolt during a storm will make for caution and anxiety in subsequent storms. Being hit by a lightning bolt out of the blue will make for caution and anxiety always.

Inform the patients of anticipated events so that the events, when they occur, make sense to the patients.

1 Forewarn patients of surgical procedures. Detail is not necessary: some patients will want to know, others will not. (Those who want to know will express interest; those who do not want to know will not. If in doubt, it does not hurt to ask.) All patients should be told what will be the physical results of surgical procedures. If removal of a breast is indicated, patients should know this and have time to begin to come to terms with it.

2 Prepare patients for the postoperative experience. Tell them where they will be when they emerge from anesthesia, what will be attached to them, what they are likely to feel. Tell them who will be attending to them, how they can deal with discomfort, what will be the postoperative course, and how long they can expect each phase to be. Being given this information will not reduce their pain or discomfort, but it will reduce their anxiety and facilitate their emotional recovery.

Principle *Patients need support in dealing with the stress of a life-threatening illness and the further stress of its treatment.*

Here, patients who have a reasonably well-functioning marriage must be considered separately from patients who are unmarried or, if married, have marriages that are troubled or empty.

Among patients who have marriages that are of ordinary quality or better, the person the patient will most likely turn to for support is her husband. This should be acknowledged early. As soon as there is genuine reason to anticipate cancer, the husband should be informed or the patient asked to inform him. The point is to treat the husband as the patient's closest connection, the figure on whom will fall most responsibility for maintaining the patient's morale.

If surgery is anticipated, the husband should be informed. The husband, along with the patient, should be able to anticipate the patient's physical appearance after surgery. Pictures will be helpful. The patient should know that her husband is prepared.

Patients who do not have functioning marriages are encouraged to establish alternative sources of support. A close and trusted relative might do; so might a very good friend.

Principle *In addition to the help provided by discussion with her physician and by the reassurance of her husband's care and concern, a patient who must have surgical treatment can be helped by discussion with someone who has been through the experience (a "veteran") and also by contact with others currently going through the experience. The best source for such relationships is a self-help group.*

Every surgical patient should be told of the Reach-to-Recovery program of the American Cancer Society. (See Chap. 44.) Recommend to all but the best informed and best supported that they consult the program.

THE PATIENT WHO HAS ENTERED A TERMINAL COURSE

Principle *It is important to many patients to know their prognosis; it is also important to many patients to maintain hope in the future and to prevent others from treating them as* *dying. Patients will vary greatly in the extent to which they want a negative prognosis made explicit.*

In the provision of information, insofar as it is possible, follow the patient's lead. Where the patient asks directly, "What are my chances?" be candid (although note the next principle). Where the patient avoids asking directly about prognosis, but only asks, "What should I do now?" note the seriousness that the condition merits but do not insist on labeling it incurable.

Principle *Hope is an antidote to depression. To the extent it is possible, patients should be permitted to retain some hope.*

To a patient who has indicated a desire for "open awareness" (i.e., explicit acknowledgment of impending death), prognosis should be given in a way that permits hope; for example, "People with this condition may die within a year, but some live much longer than that." If spontaneous remission is a possibility, even an unlikely one, it is worth noting. To a patient who has clearly indicated a desire for "closed awareness" (i.e., avoidance of acknowledgment of impending death), a negative prognosis might be made by saying something like, "The disease has been progressing despite our efforts. What we now plan is . . . ."

Predictions of length of remaining life, even when made late in the course of a disease, have been shown to be inaccurate, frequently by many months.

Principle *Just as preparation facilitates recovery from surgery, so preparation facilitates recovery from loss.*

Husbands should be made aware that their wives may die. At the same time, patients' desires for closed awareness should be respected, insofar as this is possible.

If the patient accepts open awareness, give the husband and the wife the same information. If the patient so desires, talk to them together. If the patient wants closed awareness, the husband can be told something like, "Your wife's condition is very serious. This is what we have told her." His further questions can be answered candidly.

Principle *Husbands are likely to want to be protective of their wives to the end.* Husbands may feel they have failed their wives if they are not with their wives at the time their wives die.

With the patient's death imminent, let the husband be with her as much as the two want. Insofar as the husband indicates a desire to participate in the patient's nursing care, this should be permitted. Also, the husband should be permitted to remain with his wife when she dies.

Principle *Husbands will want to be able to reassure themselves that their wives were well cared-for and that as much was done for them as could have been done.*

If the husband was not present at the time of the patient's death, it should be the physician or another member of the medical staff who actually cared for the patient and whom the husband knows who tells the husband of the death. A reason for the death should be given, insofar as this is possible. The husband should be reassured that there was nothing more that could have been done.

The husband should also be reassured that the people who cared for his wife cared *about* her, that she mattered to them. If his wife had been respected, admired, or liked, this should now be said. If the physician or other members of the medical staff were personally desolated by his wife's death, this should also be said.

Principle *Death is always a shock, no matter how harrowing the illness. Loss is always unbearably painful, no matter how long it was anticipated.*

Even if the husband seems to be taking his wife's death well, it may be useful for him to sit and talk. Some men will not want this, but the man who is not averse to expressing his distress will be strengthened by talking with his wife's physician or someone else on the staff who had known his wife. A husband may be too stunned to cry, or may cry openly. In neither event is intervention indicated; all that is necessary is a sympathetic presence.

The physician might find it useful to keep in mind that grief is not a pathological condition, although it may produce symptoms that could also indicate pathology. Extreme agitation in someone who has just experienced loss does not require treatment (as by sedatives). It is properly responded to by sympathy and support.

44

Reach-to-Recovery Program of the American Cancer Society

Margery Wiesenthal

INTRODUCTION

The principle of the Reach-to-Recovery Program for women with breast cancer has always been simple: one woman reaching out to share with and support another in a time of need. The most important components of the program are the volunteers and their training.

TRAINING

The volunteer may be of any age. She must be well-groomed and well-spoken. She underwent a mastectomy at least one year before service, has adjusted to her surgery, and is emotionally stable. She has been approved for this program by at least one of her personal physicians. She must be warm, courteous, tactful and considerate. She should have a knowledge of professional ethics, understand the importance of confidentiality, and agree to participate in yearly training and update sessions. She has been interviewed extensively by American Cancer Society staff and her local unit and division Reach-to-Recovery coordinators. Though many women apply to be Reach-to-Recovery volunteers, not all can become *visitors*, due to the stringent selection criteria.

If she is accepted as one of the American Cancer Society's 12,000 Reach-to-Recovery visitors, the volunteer is prepared for her new role in a formal, eight-hour training session. After an introduction to the American Cancer Society, its structure, purposes, and goals, the volunteer receives her specialized training.

Much time is spent on what *not* to say when making a visit. The volunteer is taught and constantly reminded that a Reach-to-Recovery volunteer makes no personal comparisons and must refer all medical questions back to the proper medical personnel. She is taught never to anticipate patients' questions. Perhaps of most importance, she is taught to say, "I really don't know, but I will find out for you." As her primary expertise lies in issues relating to personal experience, she is taught to excel therein. She may meet questions such as: "What do I say to my friends?" "What will I wear?" "Will I ever look myself again?" "What will my boyfriend say?" "How do I act with my husband?" "What should I say to my children?" "Will I be able to swim, golf, play tennis, ski, and bowl?" "When I go back to work, what should I say to my coworkers?" "Will my arm ever work properly again?" "Am I going to live?" Through hours of instruction and role acting, supplemented by a thorough training manual, this new volunteer must become very comfortable with almost every conceivable question. Although the training is very professional, it is never forgotten that compassion, feeling, and "heart" play a most important part in the success of this program.

By the simple act of standing at the patient's bedside the Reach-to-Recovery volunteer answers many questions without words. The patient, seeing a woman like herself who is only a few years past surgery, who looks attractive, and can demonstrate exercises, often says to herself, "If she can do it, so can I!"

THE VISIT

The hospital visit, initiated only by the physician, takes place two or three days after surgery. This visit is carefully planned. A volunteer, matching the patient as closely as possible in age, interests, marital status, etc., is selected for the visit by an American Cancer Society Reach-to-Recovery coordinator who is contacted by the hospital. The selected volunteer makes the appointment with the patient for the visit. One of the most important subjects discussed at their meeting is the gift kit. This kit contains items of interest to the patient: a temporary prosthesis (and the volunteer demonstrates the use of this), a bra extender, and literature informing the patient where she can purchase personal effects and a permanent prosthetic form in her area. The volunteer offers to accompany the patient when purchasing the prosthetic form and explains the necessary exercises, if so requested by the physician. What these carefully trained women do to help can make such a difference in the rehabilitation of the patient.

LITERATURE

All Reach-to-Recovery literature has been updated. The patient guide is a general one, written for women of today. The book contains a pocket for any individualized information that is requested by the surgeon or that may be useful in particular situations. These pamphlets may be withdrawn, changed, or supplemented as needed. Available pamphlets cover a range of related topics: "What is Reach-to-Recovery?" "Helpful Hints and How To's," "Exercises After Mastectomy," "An Ounce of Prevention—Suggestions for Hand/Arm Care," "Breast Reconstruction—Some Questions and Answers." Another new pamphlet, "The Woman on Her Own," was developed to assist the thousands of women diagnosed yearly with breast cancer who are widowed, are no longer married, or have never married.

Three letters are available for the patient to use. At her request, letters to her son, daughter, and/or special love may be mailed. Patients often decide that these letters will be most helpful in explaining their recent surgery and feelings to those close to them.

Any postmastectomy patient who expresses an interest in breast reconstruction is offered the opportunity to visit with a trained, carefully selected Reach-to-Recovery volunteer who has undergone breast reconstruction. This new and much-needed addition to the Reach-to-Recovery visitation program has received many favorable comments from physicians and patients.

SUPPORT SESSIONS

Open forums or rap sessions where women gather to discuss various problems relating to mastectomy are very popular. Groups usually are led by Reach-to-Recovery volunteers, assisted by professionals. Meetings are well-publicized in local newspapers and are enthusiastically attended. The purpose of rap groups is to help women cope when mastectomy is new or when changes in lifestyle occur following breast surgery. They are not intended to serve as a substitute for professional psychiatric care.

MAN-TO-MAN PROGRAM

In 1976, Reach-to-Recovery's Man-to-Man program was developed and introduced. A trained husband of a Reach-to-Recovery volunteer speaks by telephone with a man needing answers to nonmedical questions. Little has been done to help emotionally the husband or lover of the woman who has just experienced breast cancer. Few think of his fears and suffering during this traumatic period. A telephone conversation with another man who has experienced the same problems can be most beneficial and rewarding. Common questions include, "How can I help my wife?" "What should I do and say to reassure her of my love?" "What do I do if she won't communicate with me?" "She is rejecting me sexually; how do I deal with this problem?" New emphasis will be placed on the Man-to-Man program in the coming years in order to use this valuable support program to its fullest potential.

PREOPERATIVE VISITS

Surgeons often request preoperative visits for their patients. Seeing a Reach-to-Recovery volunteer the night before surgery can mean much to a patient. These carefully trained "special volunteers" bring no kit and stay a short time. By their appearance, demeanor, and attitude alone, they try to alleviate many of the patient's fears. Recovery and rehabilitation can begin before surgery with the help of these preoperative visits. The visitor explains that she will return in a few days to talk at greater length about various subjects. This valuable program should expand significantly in the future.

HISTORY

The peer visitation program was the idea of Mrs. Terese Lasser. In 1952, after her own mastectomy, Mrs. Lasser had no one to emulate, no one to talk to about clothing and cosmetic problems, and no one with whom to discuss her concerns about body image and sexual feelings. Mrs. Lasser plowed her own road to physical and psychological recovery, gaining admiration from both lay and professional worlds. She soon was called upon to help other women after mastectomies. This "help" expanded into a program which grew and grew. The potential was obvious. In 1969 the Reach-to-Recovery Program became an integral part of the American Cancer Society. Since then it has been adopted throughout the world. The program has expanded greatly in recent years.

FUTURE PLANS

Reach-to-Recovery has extended its efforts to meet the needs of all women who have been treated for breast cancer. Visitation programs for those women who have had radiation therapy, chemotherapy, and/or lumpectomy in addition to or instead of mastectomy are now available. Volunteers for this program are selected and trained as rigorously as are other Reach-to-Recovery volunteers and are matched to appropriate patients.

45

The Law of Informed Consent and Mastectomy

Robert J. McKenna, M.D.
Nicholas J. Toghia, J.D.

INTRODUCTION

Breast cancer continues to be the most frequently encountered form of cancer in women and is a disease that women fear greatly. This fear is prevalent despite the fact that many women are now being cured of breast cancer. The combinations and permutations of treatment options available today for breast cancer number over 90. Treatment should be selected based on medical indicators (cancer size, stage, receptor status, multicentricity, etc.) and patient choice, rather than on emotion alone.[1] During the past decade, treatment of breast cancer has changed significantly[2] and therapy will continue to change. In the United States, breast cancer today is diagnosed at an earlier stage as a result of monthly breast self-examination and as a result of mammographic screening, especially of high-risk groups. Notwithstanding all of these improvements, biases concerning treatment continue to exist and may be expected to continue to exist for many decades. In addition, this field of medicine has been complicated by laws enacted by several states in an attempt to regulate the doctrine of informed consent.

HISTORICAL PERSPECTIVE

The paramount obligation of a physician, imposed by law and by oath, is the exercise of due care and skill in the treatment of patients. The physician's duty of due care includes, among other things, an obligation to inform fully the patient of her condition and to continue to provide for medical care once the doctor-patient relationship has been established.

The basic precepts of the doctor-patient relationship have undergone drastic changes during our lifetime. In part, this has been due to veritable quantum leaps in medical research and therapy; in part it is attributable to the proliferation of malpractice claims against physicians. The threat of medical malpractice suits against doctors was practically nonexistent before World War II. Only during the last thirty years have patients shown an increased willingness to take an adversarial position against their doctors in courts of law. This is partly due to the breakdown of the close, personal relationship between doctor and patient. The local family practitioner's office has been replaced by large and intimidating acute-care hospitals and research facilities. The personal touch, that relationship of trust and confidence, disappeared; the comforting persona of the family physician was replaced by unfamiliar faces dispensing treatment in an impersonal manner, and affection was supplanted by alienation. It is not hard to understand that, under these circumstances, some patients no longer felt restrained by personal loyalty and became more and more willing to attack the health care providers when the patients became dissatisfied with the care and treatment that they received, usually when the results were worse than what they expected.

THE GENESIS OF THE DOCTRINE OF INFORMED CONSENT

The legal premise of the theory of informed consent is that all adult persons of sound mind have a right to make major decisions on matters which involve their own bodies. One of the earliest judicial expressions of this legal principle came from the famous and respected jurist Benjamin Cardozo, then on the Court of Appeals of the State of New York, in the case of *Schloendorff v. Society of New York Hospitals.*[4] Cardozo wrote:

> Every human being of adult years and sound mind has a right to determine what shall be done with his own body; and a surgeon who performs an operation without his patient's consent commits an assault, for which he is liable in damages.

Although one could hardly expect a clearer and more precise statement, the doctrine of informed consent was relegated to obscurity and ignored in medical litigation until 1960, when the Kansas Supreme Court handed down its decision in *Natanson v. Kline.*[5] In that case, the patient had surgery for cancer. Following the operation, she received radiotherapy and was seriously burned. She had not been told anything about the risks of the treatment. The court held that the radiologist had a positive duty as a matter of law to disclose the risk. In this case the evidence indicated that if she had been properly informed, the patient would not have undergone treatment. The court stated:

> A man is master of his own body and he may expressly prohibit the performance of life-saving surgery or other medical treatment. A doctor may well believe that an operation or other form of treatment is desirable and necessary, but the law does not permit him to substitute his own judgment for that of the patient by any form of artifice or deception.

During the 20 years following the Kline decision, virtually every state has recognized in its decisional law the doctrine of informed consent, so that today it is permanently enshrined as an element of medical malpractice litigation.

THE INFORMED CONSENT STANDARD DEFINED

In most cases where the doctrine of informed consent arose, the patient was aware of the nature of the procedure to be performed and, in fact, signed a statement of consent to have it performed. The problem that the courts had to deal with was a claim by a patient that he or she did not understand that there was some risk of permanent damage. The California Supreme Court in the case of *Cobbs v. Grant*[6] recognized the problems inherent in the plaintiff's claim. The plaintiff held that he was not informed and did not understand the risks; therefore, he maintained, his was not an "informed consent." The court eloquently observed that

> The patient-plaintiff may testify on this subject, but the issue extends beyond his credibility. Since, at the time of trial, the uncommunicated hazard has materialized, it would be surprising if the patient-plaintiff did not claim that had he been informed of the dangers, he would have declined treatment. Subjectively, he may believe so, with the 20/20 vision of hindsight, but we doubt that justice will be served by placing the physician in jeopardy of the patient's bitterness and disillusionment. Thus, an objective test is preferable: i.e., what would a prudent person in the patient's position have decided if adequately informed of all significant perils.

In probing into the area of how much information needs to be communicated to the patient to achieve an informed consent and how much discretion should be left with the medical doctors to withhold information, the California Supreme Court in *Cobbs* set forth the following guidelines:[6]

> Preliminarily, we employ several postulates. The first is that patients are generally persons unlearned in the medical sciences and therefore, except in rare cases, courts may safely assume the knowledge of patient and physician are not in parity. The second is that a person of adult years and in sound mind has the right, in the exercise of control over his own body, to determine whether or not to submit to lawful medical treatment. The third is that the patient's consent to treatment, to be effective, must be an informed consent. The fourth is that the patient, being unlearned in medical sciences, has an abject dependence upon and trust in his physician for the information upon which he relies during the decisional process, thus raising an obligation in the physician that transcends arm's length transactions.
>
> From the foregoing. . . emerges a necessity, and a resultant requirement, for divulgence by the physician to his patient of all information relevant to a meaningful decisional process. To enable the patient to chart his course knowledgeably, reasonable familiarity with the therapeutic alternatives and their hazards becomes essential.
>
> Therefore, we hold, as an integral part of the physician's overall obligation to the patient, there is a duty of reasonable disclosure of the available choices with respect to proposed therapy and of the dangers inherently and potentially involved in each.

In *Cobbs*, the patient was not advised of the risks inherent in surgery for stomach ulcer. Because damage to the spleen resulted, a complication which may occur without surgical negligence in approximately 5 percent of cases, the court held that the physician had a duty to disclose to this patient "all information relevant to a meaningful decisional process." The same theory was adopted in *Wilkinson v. Vesey*,[7] in which a patient had a severe reaction in the course of radiation therapy. The court found that hers was not an informed consent because she had not been adequately advised of the risk of burns. Thus, the court stated, "the decision as to what is or is not material is a human judgment, in our opinion, which does not necessarily require the assistance of the medical profession. The patient's right to make up his or her mind should not be delegated to a local medical group—many of whom have no ideas about his informational needs."[7]

Thus, it appears that there is a growing trend suggesting that, in future informed consent cases, the physician will be less likely to be able to rely upon the community standard (i.e., the standard of care in the medical community as to what disclosure must be made by the reasonably prudent physician to secure an informed consent from the patient) when the physician determines what risks are material and therefore what should be disclosed to the patient.

LEGISLATIVE INVOLVEMENT WITH THE DOCTRINE OF INFORMED CONSENT

There is widespread agreement that informed consent is essential in current medical practice and demands good doctor-patient communication. At the same time it is self-evident that "cookbook medicine" should not be substituted for individualized, personalized therapy. Lawmakers have now trespassed into the province of the medical profession by enacting laws mandating informed consent relating to breast cancer.

In 1979 the Massachusetts State Legislature adopted a statute which affords patients the right to obtain full information about recognized alternative treatments for breast cancer. Since that time, several states have followed Massachusetts in adopting laws pertaining to disclosures with respect to alternatives to mastectomy. These include California, Hawaii, Kansas, Kentucky, Virginia, Georgia, and New York (Table 45-1). It is reasonable to assume that, within the next few years, other states will join the bandwagon.

The legislative enactments of these states differ in length, content, and consequence; they merit comparative analysis. Their purpose seems to be the same: to ensure that patients suffering from breast cancer receive information from their physicians, so that informed consent can be given to the proposed form of therapy or surgical treatment.

Initially, the reaction of the medical profession to breast cancer legislation was predictably negative. It was viewed by many as an unwarranted intrusion by government into the doctor-patient relationship and an undue interference with the practice of medicine.

The Massachusetts Law

The Massachusetts breast cancer law is part of the Patients' and Residents' Rights statute. It was adopted in 1979 and codified in the Massachusetts Public Health Code (Article III, Section 70E). It seems to follow generally the format and content of the "Patient's Bill of Rights" adopted by the American Hospital Association in 1972, which declares a patient's right to be informed of "medically significant risks" of a proposed procedure without any explicit limitation to customary disclosure practices.

The Massachusetts law is peculiar in that it provides the patient with a "right" to receive information without imposing a corresponding "duty" upon the doctor to provide such information. The plain language of the law affords these rights to inpatients and residents in a "facility," identified as any hospital, institution for the care of unwed mothers, clinic, infirmary maintained in a town, convalescent or nursing home, rest home, or charitable home for the aged that is licensed or subject to licensing by the Department; any state hospital; any private county or municipal facility, either departmental or ward, subject to licensing by the Department of Mental Health; as well as various soldiers' homes. The list conspicuously fails to include any private clinics or doctors' offices. Whether this omission was intentional or merely an oversight is a matter of conjecture since no reported court decisions construe this section of the law.

Further, the statute does not specify whether the information to be received by the patient should be in written or verbal form; nor does it prescribe its content. It does not state when the information shall be received by the patient, although the statute mandates that every patient or resident shall receive *written notice of the rights* "established herein" upon admittance into the facility (or, if the patient is a member of a health maintenance organization, at the time of enrollment in such organization). In addition, such rights are to be conspicuously posted in the facility.

The law states that violation of any provision thereof entitles the patient to bring a regular civil action as provided elsewhere in the code. However, the law does not seem to impose any administrative penalties against the doctor, nor does it indicate any licensure consequences.

Table 45-1 Comparison of State Breast Cancer Informed Consent Statutes

State	Year adopted	Content of information specified	Physician responsible to provide	Hospital responsible to provide	Consequences of non-compliance	Penalties against physician	State pre-emption of consent	Reduces risk of battery claim against doctor
Massachusetts	1979	No	No	Yes	Civil suit	No	No	Yes
California	1980	Yes	Yes	No	Administrative action	Revocation of license	Yes	Yes
Hawaii	1983	Not yet	Yes	Yes	Not specified	Not specified	Yes	Yes
Kansas	1984	Draft under way	Yes	No	Not specified	Not specified	No	Yes
Kentucky	1984	Board of Healing Arts to prepare	Yes	No	Administrative action	Revocation of license	Yes	Yes
Virginia	1984	No	Yes	No	Not specified	Not specified	No	Yes
Georgia	1984	No	No	No	None	No	No	Yes
Florida	Under study							
Maryland	Under study							
Michigan	Under study							
New York*	Under study							
Pennsylvania	Under study							

* Editor's Note: As of 1985, New York has adopted similar laws.

The relevant provisions state that

> every patient or resident of a facility shall be provided by the physician in the facility the right:
>
> (a) To informed consent to the extent provided by law...
>
> (h) In the case of a patient suffering from any form of breast cancer, to complete information on all alternative treatments which are medically viable.
>
> Any person whose rights under this section are violated may bring, in addition to any other action allowed by law or regulation, a civil action...

The California Law

The California breast cancer law was adopted by the legislature in 1980.[3] It has been codified as Section 1704.5 of the Health and Safety Code. In contrast to the Massachusetts law, it speaks not in terms of the patient's "right" to receive information but in terms of the adverse professional consequences to the doctor who fails to provide the information. Furthermore, it removes from the physician's prerogatives the determination of the substantive content or the form of the information to be given to the patient. Instead, the statute has designated the Board of Medical Quality Assurance of the California Department of Health and charged it with the responsibility to draft, print, and make available to physicians and surgeons a standardized written summary, in layman's language, of the alternative methods of treatment which may be medically feasible, including their advantages, disadvantages, and risks, as well as descriptions of procedures.

Thus, by a single stroke of the legislative pen, California not only regulated but, indeed, preempted the area of informed consent as it relates to the treatment of breast cancer. The long-range implications of this legislative intrusion into the medical profession can only be surmised. It should be noted, though, that the effect of this governmental regimentation of the private sector could be counterbalanced by the potential beneficial effects of the new law.

First, the law puts the burden upon a governmental agency to determine the content, form, length, vocabulary, level of sophistication, and other details of the information to be presented by the physician to the patient. Second, it lifts the responsibility from the doctor of making sure that the patient not only hears, but actually understands, the information being disseminated. Third, there is no prohibition against the doctor providing additional information, discussing the alternatives, or interpreting the content of this form for the benefit of the patient, although such activity is not required. Fourth, preserving in the charts maintained by the doctor a counterpart of the form dated and signed by the patient constitutes compliance with the requirements of the law and removes the potential for a claim against the physician based on lack of informed consent.

Thus, except for the imposition of another clerical function upon the physician, the operative effect of the law can be deemed beneficial to the practitioner. Most surgeons can recall trying to inform some patient of his or her condition and treatment options, and the process becoming so complex and lengthy that there was doubt in the mind of the doctor as to whether what was said was actually understood and retained by the patient. By following the requirements of the statute, this guesswork will be completely eliminated.

The text of the California breast cancer law is set forth, in part, below:

> The failure of a physician and surgeon to inform a patient by means of a standardized written summary, as developed by the department on the recommendation of the Cancer Advisory Council,... of alternative efficacious methods of treatment... when the patient is being treated for any form of breast cancer constitutes unprofessional conduct.... A standardized written summary in layman's language... informing the patient of the advantages, disadvantages, risks and descriptions of the procedures with

> regard to medically viable and efficacious alternative methods of treatment, which is given to the patient shall constitute compliance with the requirements of this section.

The Hawaii Statute

The state of Hawaii entered the arena of legislatively induced regulation of informed consent regarding breast cancer in 1983. A few years prior to that the legislature established criteria for informed consent and charged the Hawaii Board of Medical Examiners with the responsibility to establish standards for health care providers to follow in giving information to a patient and for obtaining the patient's consent.

The Hawaii statute contains an interesting feature. It provides that whatever standards the Board of Medical Examiners provides to reasonably inform the patient shall be admissible as evidence of the standard of care required of the health care providers in the state. In other words, the Board's criteria as to the condition being treated, the nature and character of the proposed treatment or surgical procedure, the anticipated results, the recognized possible alternative forms of treatment, and the recognized serious possible risks, complications, and anticipated benefits, including nontreatment, are to serve as the benchmark for malpractice because they establish the standard of care in the medical profession.

The specific provision with respect to breast cancer directs that the Board of Medical Examiners were to establish before January 1, 1984, standards to be followed by health care providers in giving information to a patient to ensure that the patient's consent to the performance of a mastectomy is informed. It provided that the standards must include the substantive content of the information, the manner in which it is to be presented, and the manner in which consent is to be given by the patient, and should include recognized alternative forms of treatment.

Thus, once the forms had been created by the Board of Medical Examiners, the clerical function of obtaining the signature of the patient would be left up to the doctor; by preserving an executed counterpart of the document the physician would establish compliance and have a defense against a claim of failure to obtain the informed consent of the breast cancer patient.

The Kansas Statute

In 1984, the state of Kansas promulgated a provision directed at informed consent in the treatment of breast cancer. The specific language was incorporated into the 1983 Supplement to Kansas Statutes Annotated, Section 65-2836. That statute generally deals with healing arts; grounds for revocation, suspension, or limitation of licenses; and standards of conduct in the medical profession. It provides that a medical practitioner's license may be revoked, suspended, or limited when the licensee has been found to have committed any of the enumerated acts or omissions. One of the grounds is the failure to inform a patient who is suffering from any form of abnormality of the breast tissue for which surgery is a recommended form of treatment of the alternative methods of treatment specified in the standardized summary supplied by the Board of Healing Arts.

The law provides that the information is to be given to the patient as soon as practicable and medically indicated following diagnosis. It also declares that giving the standardized summary constitutes compliance with the requirements of the law.

Curiously, the enactment contains a disclaimer intended to protect the Board of Healing Arts against being named a defendant in a lawsuit brought by a disgruntled patient. The legislature provided that the standardized summary should not be construed as a recommendation by the Board of any method of treatment. Ostensibly, this would provide the state a layer of immunity against tort actions arising out of some error or omission in the information to be disseminated to cancer victims. The wording of the Kansas statute states, in part, that

> Failure by persons licensed to practice medicine and surgery to inform a patient suffering from any form of abnormality of the breast tissue for which surgery is a recommended form of treatment, of alternative methods of treatment specified in the standardized summary supplied by the board. The standardized summary shall be given to each patient specified herein as soon as practicable and medically indicated following diagnosis, and this shall constitute compliance with the requirements of this subsection (o). The board shall develop and distribute to persons licensed to practice medicine and surgery a standardized summary of the alternative methods of treatment known to the board at the time of distribution of the standardized summary, including surgical, radiological or chemotherapeutic treatments or combinations of treatments and the risks associated with each of these methods. Nothing in this subsection (o) shall be construed or operate to empower or authorize the board to restrict in any manner the right of a person licensed to practice medicine and surgery to recommend a method of treatment or to restrict in any manner a patient's right to select a method of treatment. The standardized summary shall not be construed as a recommendation by the board of any method of treatment.

As of this writing, the Board of Healing Arts has not promulgated the standardized summary.

The Kentucky Statute

In 1984, the state of Kentucky also enacted a statute addressing informed consent relative to breast cancer. This statute, unlike all of the others examined, contains a preamble revealing the legislative intent behind the act. It is declared that much anxiety and fear about breast cancer is based on misinformation; that persons suffering from breast cancer have the right to receive all information available about the medical treatment of the disease; that standardized information about treatment alternatives assists the patient in thoroughly discussing with the physician treatment of the disease. Following this prologue, the Legislature ordained that, within one year after the effective date of the enactment, which was July 13, 1984, the McDowell Cancer Network, Inc., and the James Graham Brown Cancer Center were to jointly develop and submit to the Cabinet for Human Resources a standardized written summary, in nontechnical language understandable to the patient, of the advantages, disadvantages, risks, and descriptions of all medically efficacious and reasonable alternatives for the treatment of breast cancer.

It is noteworthy that the Commonwealth of Kentucky has delegated the responsibility of preparing the form and determining its content not to the Kentucky Board of Medical Licensure, but to two private cancer research organizations. As a consequence, it is reasonable to expect that the substance of the document will bear the stamp of medical practitioners most familiar with the problem as opposed to that of governmental officers or civil servants.

In the language of the law adopted by the Commonwealth of Kentucky,

> The cabinet for human resources, within ninety (90) days of receipt of the summary shall print and make available to all licensed physicians in the Commonwealth sufficient copies of the standardized written summary for distribution by such physicians to their patients.
>
> Upon receipt of the summary, any physician licensed under the laws of the Commonwealth who treats a patient for any form of breast cancer shall provide the patient with a standardized written summary, as provided under this section, informing the patient of medically efficacious and viable alternative methods of treatment for breast cancer which may include surgical, radiological or chemotherapeutic treatment or combinations thereof.

The Virginia Law

The Commonwealth of Virginia enacted its informed consent law regarding breast cancer in 1984. Of all statutes seen so far, it is by far the shortest and simplest. Its full text is as follows:

Informed consent for treatment of breast tumor; paragraphs required in form. Before a physician operates on a patient for a tumor of the breast, a consent form shall have been executed which includes the following:

"CONSENT FOR TREATMENT OF BREAST TUMOR

Sign option (a) or option (b), or option (a) and option (b).

(a) ______ breast biopsy (Side: right or left)

Patient's or other authorized persons's signature

(b) If it is determined that I have a malignant tumor in my breast or other breast abnormality requiring surgery, then I authorize Dr. ______ to perform such operations or procedures, including breast procedure:

____

____

Patient's or other authorized person's signature"

The Georgia Statute

In 1984, the Legislature of the State of Georgia enacted an amendment to Section 43-34-21 of the Official Code of Georgia Annotated; the amendment was sponsored by the Senate Committee on Human Resources. The sole purpose of the law was to authorize and direct the Composite State Board of Medical Examiners to develop and distribute an informational booklet on breast cancer and achievement thereof. The booklet

> shall contain a summary of the latest information on breast cancer and, in brief form, shall discuss the generally accepted and widely prevailing medical and surgical treatment for breast cancer. The booklet shall include a valid assessment of the relative risks and benefits of the accepted and widely prevailing methods of treatment. A copy of the booklet shall be made available by the Board [of Medical Examiners] to every appropriate physician in the State. A letter by the Board shall accompany this booklet stating that the Board urges the physician to distribute a copy of the booklet to each and every patient whose disease or course of treatment is covered by the material in the booklet. Copies shall also be made available to any person upon request at a fee prescribed by the joint-secretary sufficient to cover the cost of printing and distribution. The booklet shall be updated and redistributed at such times as the Board shall deem necessary.

The booklet could not be compiled until funds were specifically appropriated for such purpose. Thus, if the legislature were not to allocate any money for the project, the booklet would not come into existence. The statute imposes no mandatory duties upon any physician or the medical profession. It provides that the booklet be made "available... to every appropriate physician," but does not define or describe who is "an appropriate" doctor (it could mean that those practioners not connected with oncology would have to pay some fee, designed to cover the cost of printing and distribution, in order to obtain the booklet).

Neither the content, the format, nor even the time for publication of the booklet is specified. No guidelines are established for its use; no enforcement procedure is established and no penalties are prescribed for noncompliance. The statute is at the most lenient end of the spectrum when compared with the specific provisions enacted by the other states that have legislated on this subject.

CONSEQUENCES OF A CLAIM BASED ON LACK OF INFORMED CONSENT TO THE PRACTITIONER

Because of the recent origin of the statutes on informed consent, it is necessary to look at prestatutory judicial interpretations of this doctrine to put into proper perspective its relevance for the medical practitioner. The law books are replete with lawsuits wherein the plaintiff's claim against the doctor for malpractice was coupled with a claim for assault and battery based on lack of informed consent. Close scrutiny of these judicial decisions reveals that some courts have treated lack of informed consent in the matrix of traditional negligence;

others have dealt with it in the context of assault and battery. The consequences of judicial attitudes treating lack of informed consent as an act of negligence on the one hand or assault and battery on the other can be enormous for the physician-defendant.

The negligence standard is failure to comply with the applicable standard of due care, since a medical doctor is not an insurer of results. Assault and battery is "unauthorized touching that is offensive or harmful"; it is not related to any community standards, but is an absolute: the degree of inviolability of the patient's body does not depend on the intent of the physician. A review of some of the trendsetting court decisions on these divergent tort concepts reveals lack of consistency or clear direction. It naturally follows that the defense strategy of the suit from the standpoint of the doctor will be dramatically different depending on whether the plaintiff is suing the doctor for negligence or for assault and battery.

First, punitive damages are almost never awarded in cases of medical negligence, but are not infrequently given in substantial amounts in cases of ordinary assault. Punitive damages cannot be awarded against a demonstrably negligent physician unless there is conduct indicating a reckless disregard for, and complete indifference to, the patient's welfare. There are only a handful of cases where jury verdicts of punitive damages against health care providers were upheld on appeal. The majority of these were against pharmaceutical companies, hospitals, or clinics, rather than physicians.

Second, the statutes of limitations are usually different for battery cases and those applicable to negligence actions, and the time elapsed before the suit was filed may be the controlling factor in a given situation. Thus, there may be a technical defense available to the doctor in a negligence action, which would not apply to a battery claim.

Third, most malpractice insurance policies specifically exclude coverage for battery cases; therefore, if a patient recovers damages for assault and battery, the doctor's insurance carrier will undoubtedly refuse to pay any judgment.

Fourth, proof of battery does not require expert medical testimony on behalf of the plaintiff. Lay witnesses alone, usually the plaintiff him- or herself, are sufficient to prove the facts. However, with the demise of the community standard of disclosure in informed consent cases and the increase in the number of decisions which hold that no expert testimony is necessary to prove what "the prudent patient would have found to be a material risk," this distinction between assault (intentional act) and negligence (unintentional act) is rapidly disappearing. On the other hand, in jurisdictions where the community standard of disclosure still prevails, prosecuting a claim on an assault-and-battery theory is one way to vitiate this requirement if no expert witness can be located to testify on behalf of the plaintiff.

One of the most favorable things that can be said about the statutes dealing with informed consent for the breast cancer patient is that if the doctor complies with the letter of the law applicable in the jurisdiction where he or she maintains a practice, the probability of a claim against the doctor for assault and battery is, for all practical purposes, nonexistent. The obvious relief to both doctor and malpractice insurance carrier should be enormous if the charts maintained by the careful practitioner contained written proof that the doctor observed all of the clerical requirements of the law and that the patient signed the form describing the alternative treatment options mandated by the informed consent statute.

REFLECTIONS AND OBSERVATIONS

The legislative enactments by the states of Massachusetts, California, Hawaii, Kansas, Kentucky, Virginia, and Georgia mandating patient education regarding breast cancer treatment evidence a growing trend of governmental regulation of the medical profession.

Compliance with the law varies, accompanied by considerable misunderstanding by physicians, hospitals, and other health care providers. The California statute resulted in what so far appears to be the best document dealing with breast cancer treatment alternatives; but even it fails to distinguish between primary therapy and ancillary therapy, nor does it interpret choices in relation to prognostic factors (size, stage, receptors, etc.).

A two-step procedure, first, a diagnostic biopsy, and second, treatment, should eliminate most patient apprehension and decision making until treatment options are discussed and evaluated. This protocol satisfies the legitimate objectives of the informed consent laws for breast cancer.

We believe physicians can better inform breast cancer patients through education than through legislative fiat; selected patient education materials are listed in Table 45-2. There remain many individuals who are not informed about breast cancer, but the requirements posed by the various state statutes do little or nothing for patient education. Further, only the Virginia and Georgia laws contain an explicit provision for keeping up with the state of the art, by requiring regular updating or reevaluation of the informed consent documents which they mandate. Legislators are not likely to have current knowledge of cancer treatment and therapy; the same can be said about the clerical and administrative staffs of those states where these laws have become effective. The ultimate question to be addressed is whether state government should mandate for the patient with breast disease some general disclosure pamphlet which could educate the patient.

Public health education may be achieved by nonlegislative means (Table 45-3). These laws set a dangerous precedent. A single pamphlet is impractical for all forms of cancer and the choice of treatment available; further, it can be safely asserted that state governments will prove to be too slow to keep up and respond with current information about medical advances. These laws, unless carefully consolidated by updating and reevaluation, therefore stand to victimize the very class of the population they intend to protect by the enactment of informed consent statutes.

Table 45-4 enumerates some of the advantages and disadvantages of breast cancer informed consent laws. No pamphlet can substitute for dialogue between patient and physician. At best, its value is restricted to providing a limited reference source. The personal experience of most practicing physicians is that there is no substitute for frank discussion between doctor and patient, which is sometimes enlarged to include members of the family, the primary care physician, and even friends of the patient. No pamphlet can truly place into perspective the exact prognosis, and the multitude of options available for treatment of breast cancer of varying stages. Thus, some pamphlets may do more harm than good by creating confusion and alarm.

It may be argued that regulation of medical practice in the area of breast cancer is discriminatory. All of the statutes examined are directed against the specialist practicing oncological surgery; against a single disease, breast cancer; against a single modality of treatment, mastectomy. All protect a single anatomical part of the human body, the female breast. Some commentators involved in the issue claim that there are no broad public policy values to justify the discriminatory treatment of the surgical oncologist. As has been observed by one commentator, "it is worth noting that debate about radical prostatectomy versus irradiation for the local control of primary prostate cancer is not tinged with anything like the emotionalism that similar options evoke for primary breast cancer."[1] Further, the breast cancer laws have been held to carry the serious potential to adversely impinge on communication between

Table 45-2 Educational Materials for Patients with Breast Problems

Source	Title
American Cancer Society	"If You Find a Lump in Your Breast" by Martha McLean "How to Examine Your Breasts" "Breast Reconstruction Information"
National Cancer Institute	"Questions and Answers about Breast Lumps" "If You've Had Breast Cancer . . ." "Breast Cancer: We're Making Progress Every Day" "What You Need to Know about Cancer of the Breast" "Progress Against Breast Cancer"
Women's Breast Cancer Advisory Center, Inc.	"If You've Thought about Breast Cancer"

doctor and patient and can never be an adequate substitute for good dialogue between the two.

It has been noted that the protocol for treatment options for breast cancer have been viewed by some women's groups in terms of feminist issues. There have been comments that the geneses of the Massachusetts and the California statutes are attributable to two seperate campaigns waged by two women who disagreed with their physicians that they needed a mastectomy. What might be described as two women's separate experiences with, perhaps, insensitive physicians have led to some strident rhetoric and emotional reaction. The result, for good or ill, has been governmental direction of the doctor-patient relationship.

Breast cancer law would appear to be unnecessary in cases of benign breast problems, although the breast cancer brochure would be given to such patients. It is unclear whether physicians are in violation of the law when a biopsy alone is done and the state pamphlet is not given to the patient until after the diagnosis is established.

Table 45-3 Breast Cancer Informed Consent Law

Purposes of the law	Alternatives to the law
Patient education	Physician's explanation to patient supplemented by pamphlets from American Cancer Society and National Cancer Institute
Physician education	Medical society and association educational programs
Maintenance of uniform content	Health education by American Cancer Society and National Cancer Institute
Vindication of women's rights	Monitoring of abuses through professional societies and licensing agencies

Table 45-4 Advantages and Disadvantages of the Breast Cancer Informed Consent Laws

Advantages
State-mandated brochure possibly sole source of patient education
Minimized legal risk to doctor for failure to give sufficient information to patient to obtain valid consent
Response to women's concerns about potentially unnecessary mastectomies
Potential to stimulate patient awareness and public concern about breast problems
Disadvantages
Incomplete breast cancer information in brochure
Failure of brochure to differentiate various breast cancer modes and individualized treatment
Interference with doctor-patient relationship
Potentially reduced level of communication between doctor and patient; encouragement of complacency
Validity or constitutionality not yet scrutinized by the courts
Usefulness not yet evaluated by the medical profession
Lack of mechanism to update brochures in order to reflect advances in breast cancer therapy
Potential discouragement of use of alternative patient educational materials available from American Cancer Society, National Cancer Institute

Notwithstanding the criticisms presented, the breast cancer informed consent statutes have been incorporated into the legal fabric of at least seven states. So far, no one has challenged their validity or constitutionality. Indeed, it has been reported that several other states, including Florida, Maryland, Michigan, New York, and Pennsylvania, are also considering breast cancer legislation. Thus, the medical profession may be in for further regulation as government attempts to safeguard public health.

REFERENCES

1. Carter S: The California breast cancer law and government-mandated patient education. *CA* 32:173, 1982.
2. Patterns of care of carcinoma of the breast. *Bull Am Coll Surg* Publ 159, No 4, 1984.
3. Breast cancer treatment. Summary of alternative effective methods: Risks, advantages, disadvantages. Report of the California State Department of Health Services, 1983.
4. *Schloendorff v. Society of New York Hospital*, 211 N.Y. 125 (1914).
5. *Natanson v. Kline*, 186 Kan. 393 (1960) *clarified* 187 Kan. 186.
6. *Cobbs v. Grant*, 8 Cal 3rd 229 (1972).
7. *Wilkinson v. Vesey*, 110 R.I. 606 (1972).

Index